The U.S. Health System: Origins and Functions

The U.S. Health System: Origins and Functions

Marshall W. Raffel, Ph.D.
Professor of Health Planning
and Administration
College of Human Development
The Pennsylvania State University
University Park, Pennsylvania

A WILEY MEDICAL PUBLICATION
JOHN WILEY & SONS
New York • Chichester • Brisbane • Toronto

Library of Congress Cataloging in Publication Data:

Raffel, Marshall W.
  The U.S. health system.

  (A Wiley medical publication)
  Includes index.
  1. Medical care—United States. 2. Public health
—United States. I. Title.
RA395.A3R33   362.1'0973   80-86
ISBN 0-471-04512-8

Printed in the United States of America

10 9 8 7 6 5 4 3 2 1

To Norma
and
Robert, Dorothy, and Timothy

Preface

... [I]n reality, complete freedom from disease and from struggle is almost incompatible with the process of living.

Life is an adventure in a world where nothing is static; where unpredictable and ill-understood events constitute dangers that must be overcome, often blindly and at great cost; where man himself, like the sorcerer's apprentice, has set in motion forces that are potentially destructive and may some day escape his control. Every manifestation of existence is a response to stimuli and challenges, each of which constitutes a threat if not adequately dealt with. The very process of living is a continual interplay between the individual and his environment, often taking the form of a struggle resulting in injury or disease. The more creative the individual the less he can hope to avoid danger, for the stuff of creation is made up of responses to the forces that impinge on his body and soul. Complete and lasting freedom from disease is but a dream remembered from imaginings of a Garden of Eden designed for the welfare of man.

René Dubos
Mirage of Health

This process of living, with its inevitable spin-offs of injury and disease, has led to the establishment of one of society's largest industries: health. To prevent, to cure, to maintain to the greatest extent possible, have led the American people in 1978 to allocate $192,400,000,000 to the health sector of the economy. This represents 9.1% of the Gross National Product—9.1% of the value of all goods and services produced in the United States that year. Quite a sum! Quite an industry!

It is an industry that is labor intensive at all levels, from the most highly trained professional to the unskilled, with an estimated 1 out of every 14 employed persons in the United States in a health related occupation. It is an industry forever changing in response to new health problems, to new knowledge, which permits the treatment of old problems in new or more effective ways, and to new technology. It is an industry constantly striving to improve the quality of professional education and the quality of professional care. It is an industry pressured by more and more people needing care or demanding care, and it responds as positively as it can, although its responses are limited by the knowledge at its disposal and by the resources available to utilize the knowledge it has.

It is an industry beset by growth, increasing complexity, limited resources, and rising costs, which result, inevitably, in problems of citizen access to services, in problems of raising money to pay for services, and in the need for increased coordination of a complex system in terms of ongoing operations and development. These are essentially administrative and planning problems, and the industry is turning more and more to people trained in these areas.

As part of the effort to train health administrators and health planners, an increasing number of colleges and universities are offering introductory courses on the health system in order to provide students in health administration and health planning, as well as students in other allied health programs, with an opportunity to learn more about this enormous industry and to understand its development, its operations, its problems, and its trends. This text is designed to be a resource for those students.

Major portions of the text were critically reviewed by my colleague at Penn State, Stanley P. Mayers, Jr., and by Harold J. Cohen of Ithaca College. Their critiques were both thoughtful and helpful, and their efforts are much appreciated. Also at Penn State my colleagues Joel Lee and Andreas Muller were helpful, at various stages, as I sought to check interpretations and to verify facts. They are not responsible, however, for the interpretations or for any remaining errors; for these, I alone am responsible.

A special debt is owed to the baccalaureate students of HPA 101, from Cindy and Cheryl to the hundreds who followed. They may not know or fully appreciate it, but they were all the inspiration.

Marshall W. Raffel, Ph.D.
University Park, Pennsylvania

Contents

1

History of Medical Practice and Medical Education in America

MEDICAL PRACTICE AND TRAINING IN COLONIAL AMERICA

The physician today is a person vastly different from the practitioner in seventeenth- and eighteenth-century America. Today's medical practitioner has pursued a vigorous course of study and clinical practice under the close supervision of faculty who are typically at the forefront of the health professions. Not only must today's medical practitioner pass courses in a premedical curriculum at a college or university and those offered by the medical school, but he or she must also pass the state licensing exam. Nearly all practitioners, moreover, now undertake at least three years of additional supervised specialty training in a nationally accredited residency training program on completion of medical school. The end result is a person licensed by the state government to practice medicine, a physician who, it can safely be assumed by the patient, is competent to diagnose and treat most illnesses and to know when to refer the patient for specialist care.

This is not to suggest that every physician is excellent, that all are competent, that all provide the best possible medical care, or that diagnostic and treatment errors are not made. It is to say, rather, that the physician who is consulted is probably a competent physician and that the patient has reasonable grounds for believing this.

Not so in colonial America. In that period, most "physicians" were trained under an apprenticeship system, and there was no organized method for testing the competence of those practitioners or their students, nor were there effective licensing bodies that could attest, by the granting of a license, to the physician's

1

competence. Packard quotes from William Smith's 1758 *History of New York* (1, p.284):

A few physicians among us are eminent for their skill. Quacks abound like locusts in Egypt, and too many have been recommended to a full practice and profitable subsistence; this is less to be wondered at, as the profession is under no kind of regulation. Loud as the call is, to our shame be it remembered, we have no law to protect the lives of the King's subjects from the malpractice of pretenders. Any man, at his pleasure, sets up for physician, apothecary, and chirurgeon. No candidates are either examined, licensed or sworn to fair practice.

Smith's reference to "physician, apothecary, and chirurgeon" reflects the then British categorization of practitioners. The physicians typically held university medical degrees and practiced what we would now call internal medicine. The apothecary was not a physician or university trained. He was trained as an apprentice and was concerned with the dispensing of drugs. Like today's pharmacist, people frequently sought medical advice from the apothecary, and the apothecary became, in Britain, the equivalent of a general practitioner. The chirurgeon, or surgeon, was also apprentice trained.

These distinctions became blurred in colonial America, for very few physicians came to the New World, and there were, at Smith's time, no medical schools in America to train them. Furthermore, at Smith's writing, there was only one hospital in all the colonies, the Philadelphia Hospital, and it had been open for only a few years.* The first medical school was established in 1756 at the College of Philadelphia (later, University of Pennsylvania). The second school was King's College (later, Columbia University), founded in 1768. By the time of the Revolutionary War, neither school had made significant medical manpower contributions to the total number of medical practitioners in the colonies; accurate figures are hard to obtain, but it would appear that the Philadelphia school graduated fewer than ten students a year from 1768 to 1773; the first class at King's College in 1769 consisted of two.

Shryock notes that on the eve of the Revolutionary War, "it has been

---

* Today, the physician and surgeon are both graduates of accredited medical schools and hold either the degree of Doctor of Medicine (M.D.) or Doctor of Osteopathy (D.O.). In American terms today, the physician is any M.D. or D.O., whereas in Britain the physician is still the equivalent of our specialist in internal medicine. The surgeon in America is thus a physician, with the added specialty qualifications in surgery. The apothecary has, in America, become the pharmacist and is the graduate of a university pharmacy program.

estimated that . . .there were about 3,500 established practitioners in the colonies and that not more than 400 of these had received any formal training. Of the latter, only about half—or barely more than 5 per cent of the total— held degrees" (2, p.9). Most of the 200 degree holders in medicine were from European, and mainly British, medical schools.

Some of the early nonmedical degree practitioners were simply learned men* — ministers, planters, lawyers, teachers—who could gather a smattering of knowledge from books they read and apply that knowledge because there were no alternatives. As Shryock puts it

A man who had graduated from an arts college, read in medicine, and acquired some experience was the nearest thing to a formally trained practitioner that the colonial environment produced before the 1760s. As late as about 1830, it may be added, the University of Virginia still provided instruction in medicine for all its undergraduate students (2, p.16)

Others who aspired to medical practice apprenticed themselves for a number of years to established physicians. Upon completion of the training period, during which time the apprentice would watch and assist his preceptor and read his books, the physician would give the apprentice a signed testimonial that would constitute the certificate of proficiency. The real competence of the "graduate" from apprentice training would be as good or as bad as the preceptor, as the books available, and as the conscientiousness of the apprentice.

Samuel Treat, for example, apprenticed to Dr. John Redman in Philadelphia and received his medical certificate in 1765 after nearly four years' service. Treat was fortunate in being able to learn from more than just one teacher: the Pennsylvania Hospital opened in 1752, and Treat was afforded the opportunity to attend there during his apprentice period. He was also fortunate in being in Philadelphia where some learned physicians began to offer lectures in various subjects. Treat attended the anatomical lectures offered by Dr. William Shippen, Jr. Treat's medical certificate was thus signed by many, as quoted in Packard(1, p.278):

---

*At this point, the use of the word *men* is appropriate, for medicine was a male domain. Female involvement in "medical" matters was confined to midwifery, and to the extent that some of them received formal training, it was frequently provided by medical practitioners. The first female medical-school graduate was from the Geneva Medical College around 1850. See Shryock, R.H.: "Women in American medicine," *Journal of the American Medical Women's Association* Vol. 5; No. 9 September 1950: (reprinted in Shryock, R.H.: *Medicine in America*. Baltimore, Johns Hopkins Press, 1966).

MEDICAL CERTIFICATE TO MR. SAMUEL TREAT, 1765. PHILADELPHIA.

This is to certify to all whom it may concern that Mr. Samuel Treat hath served as an Apprentice to me for nearly four years, during which he was constantly employed in the practice of Physic and Surgery under my care, not only in my private business, but in the Pennsylvania Hospital, in which character he always behaved with great Fidelity and Industry. In Testimony of which, I have thereunto set my hand this first day of September, One Thousand Seven hundred and Sixty-five.

(Signed)   John Redman.

We whose names are under written do Certify that Mr. Samuel Treat hath diligently attended the practice of Physic and Surgery in the Pennsylvania Hospital for several years.

(Signed)   Thos. Cadwalader,
Phineas Bond,
Th. Bond,
Wm. Shippen,
C. Evans.

This is to certify that Samuel Treat hath attended a course of Anatomical Lectures with the greatest diligence and assiduity.

(Signed)   William Shippen, Jr

More commonly in the colonial period, the medical certificate was signed by only one physician. Still others, as Corner notes (3, p.3) "probably had no other qualifications beyond an interest in the sick and assurance enough to hang out a shingle."

Apprenticeship to a single physician was the more common approach to training for a long period of time because there was, until 1752, in Philadelphia and 1791 in New York, no institution that could rightly be called a hospital.* With the opening of the Pennsylvania Hospital, however, a significant new pattern of training began to develop. Physicians not only began to take their apprentices with them to the hospital to assist (as Dr. John Redman did with

---

*The New York Hospital apparently served briefly during the Revolutionary War as an American Military hospital until the British occupied New York, at which time it became for seven years a barracks, and possibly also a military hospital, for British and Hessian soldiers. It was not until 1791 that the hospital admitted its first civilian patient. See *Hospital Care in the United States*, Commission on Hospital Care. New York, The Commonwealth Fund, 1947, p.439.

Samuel Treat) but also they began to allow other students to follow them as they examined and treated their hospital patients. So many students sought this privilege that the hospital resolved in 1763: It is the unanimous opinion of the Board that such of them at least who are not apprentices to the Physicians of the House, should pay a proper Gratuity for the Benefit of the Hospital for their privilege (1, p.323).

By 1773, the hospital decided to regularize this system so that an aspiring physician could pay a fee to the hospital and be formally apprenticed to the insitution for five years, upon completion of which the institution would grant a certificate. With the establishment in 1765 of the medical department at the University of Pennsylvania, the hospital apprentices attended lectures there. Packard states that this practice continued until 1824, when the hospital required that future residents had to be regular graduates from the medical college before taking up their hospital appointment. (1, p.327). Packard also provides us with a sample Pennsylvania Hospital certificate (1, p.281):

This is to Certify that . . . , son of . . . , West Jersey, entered regularly as a pupil of the Pennsylvania Hospital, . . . , 1763, and continued his attendance with Diligence and Application, to . . . , 1764, during which time we hope and have reason to believe he has made considerable Progress in the Knowledge of Anatomy and the Practice of Physick and Surgery, therefore wishing Happiness and success we give from under our hands and the seal of the Corporation, this Testimonial of our Esteem and Approbation.

Lecture series on various medical subjects were sometimes provided by the better-trained physicians in the larger cities long before the founding of medical schools. The lecturers were mostly physicians trained abroad, some of whom were products of colonial apprentice training who went overseas subsequently for the additional training, chiefly to Scotland and England. Typically, fees were collected for their lectures, and even after the founding of medical schools, professors were paid by the students for the privilege of attending their lectures.

Many of these early practices continue today in a somewhat modified form. Aspiring physicians are now apprenticed not to individual physicians or to hospitals, but to an entire faculty, and the assisting process in the treatment of patients continues as an important part of clinical training in all medical schools. Students also pay today fees for lectures and for apprenticing, but instead of paying individuals, the preceptor, the lecturer, or the hospital, the fee is now given as tuition to the medical school.

NINETEENTH-CENTURY DEVELOPMENTS

The development of medical schools during the eighteenth century was slow. We have noted already the schools in Pennsylvania and New York. The only other schools to be developed were at Harvard (1783) and at Dartmouth (1797). We should not think of these schools as being like those today. Three or four faculty members were sometimes all that were available. But not always, for Corner tells us that Dartmouth "appointed the formidable Harvard graduate Nathan Smith to be a one-man medical faculty. For ten or twelve years he alone ably taught all the courses" (3, p.57). The science and art of medicine were extremely limited in what they could offer by way of cure, and one can appreciate, therefore, the great appeal in the nineteenth century of cultists and quacks. However weak as the first schools were, they marked an important forward step. Stevens notes that "the foundation of the medical school in Philadelphia . . . was a part of the movement by university-trained physicians to organize and rationalize medicine on a European model and to institute recognizable educational standards" (4, p.17). The early medical faculties at Pennsylvania, Harvard, and Columbia and even at Dartmouth were dominated by men with European medical training. Indeed, as the number of medical schools grew, and as more and more American medical graduates went abroad—to Edinburgh, London, Paris, and other cities of Europe—many returned and gravitated to the medical-school faculties, and they championed reform.

It is typical of most endeavors that those who are most expert seek to raise standards, to elevate the level of practice. So it was in medicine. It was evident in the founding of university medical schools, the early establishment of medical societies, and the initiation of medical journals—all designed to share knowledge, to communicate, to improve quality.

Medical licensure was rarely effective in the colonial and postcolonial periods in large measure because there was an insufficient number of well-trained practitioners. Early attempts at licensure included the establishment of state licensing boards, granting authority to the medical society, and recognition of the university M.D. degree both as entitlement to a license and as an alternative to licensure by the medical society or state licensing board. Georgia was the first state to restrict medical licenses to graduates of medical schools (1821). However, opposition to licensure was strong from the apprentice-trained physicians, to whom licensure loomed as a threat, from other kinds of quasi-health practitioners, whose practices were threatened, as well as from many segments of the lay population that resented medical elitism. Resentment against the profession is illustrated on the matter of vital-statistics registration: "In Georgia . . . the legislature 'fairly hooted' when a registration bill was introduced in 1849, and the whole matter was viewed as just another 'trick of the doctors'." (5). By the middle of the nineteenth century, many licensure acts either had been repealed or so drastically altered that they were rendered ineffective. (4, pp. 26-28)

But the trend toward formalized medical education was firmly established. As the decades advanced in the nineteenth century, more and more medical practitioners came from medical schools; a decreasing percentage came from the apprenticeship system. In the absence of a strong licensing mechanism, the measure of a physician's competence came to rest on the standard of whether or not the physician had graduated from a medical school with an M.D. degree.

This encouraged development of a large number of new medical schools, some at universities that were ill-equipped to support and nourish them and a great many free-standing schools with no university ties.

The notion of university-based medical education, it should be remembered, came to this country primarily from Scotland; University of Edinburgh-trained physicians strongly influenced the structuring of the schools at Pennsylvania and Columbia. University-based medical education was also dictated by the absence of strong hospitals in colonial America that could provide the milieu for excellence. In England, however, there developed a number of medical schools around such long-established hospitals as St. Thomas' and Guy's, from which came the acceptable model of free-standing and hospital-based schools in nineteenth-century America. By then, hospitals were more common in the states than they were in the latter part of the eighteenth century, though not all of the new medical schools could claim meaningful hospital affiliation.

Some of the new non-university schools were good and had reputable faculties. Some of the schools were weak and were alledgedly set up to make money since the professors in most all of the schools (good and bad) were mostly paid directly by each student for attendance at lectures. Stevens cites the first of the proprietary schools as one established by three local physicians in Castleton, Vermont, in 1818 (4, p.25). Whether it was an improvement over apprenticeship to a single physician we can only guess, but the school did survive until 1862. Norwood, moreover, tells us that for some time the school was, in form, the medical department of Middlebury College and that some of its faculty were people of considerable ability (6, pp.204-208). In Boston, among the better private schools, Packard cites the Tremont Street School, established in 1838 by four physicians, including Oliver Wendell Holmes, and the Boylston Medical School (1, pp.446-447).

The Tremont Street School flourished and offered, over time, lectures in embryology and anatomy, surgical pathology, chemistry, auscultation and percussion, and microscopic anatomy. The faculty was mostly moonlighting Harvard faculty, something we should not be surprised at, since rarely did a faculty member in those days rely solely on medical-school income. The school thus had a close relationship with Harvard and eventually became Harvard's summer program.

The Boylston Street School opened in 1849. Despite opposition from Harvard, it got degree-granting authority in 1854. It had a good faculty, illustrated by the fact that soon after receiving degree-granting authority, Harvard recruited the best of them, and the school "faded out of existence" (1, p.447).

But even the quality of education at the "better" schools left much to be desired. Burrow tells us (7, p.9):

When Charles Eliot became president of Harvard in 1869 (the year that the institution provided its first microscope for medical students), his early effort to institute written examinations for medical degrees met opposition from the director of the medical school who asserted with little exaggeration that a majority of the students could hardly write.

Under such conditions, one can sympathize with those in the population who relied on quacks of various sorts or who cherished their apprentice-trained doctors as being as good as any coming out of a university medical school. Medical science was rather primitive or, at best, only beginning to emerge into the mainstream of medical education.

During the next decade, Harvard increased its length of training from two to three years, instituted written exams, and then required for admission a college degree or the passing of a qualifying exam. In 1892, the length of training was lengthened again, to four years.

It was noted previously that a great many of the early leaders in American medical education received training in Britain and France. In the latter part of the nineteenth century, the development of scientific medicine reached its height in Germany and Austria. Bonner has estimated that some 15,000 Americans undertook serious medical studies in German-speaking universities, 10,000 of these drawn to Vienna. Many others (over 10,000 more in Vienna), he estimates, familiarized themselves with the medical scene from short visits and vacation tours, and the medical faculties at Johns Hopkins, Harvard, Yale, and Michigan were dominated by professors who had spent time at German-speaking universities (8, pp.39,60-64,69). How many others received training during this period in France, Britain, and other centers of European excellence is not known. But the German influence at this stage was critical. Shryock states (9, p.30)

German-trained leaders in the better schools (Hopkins, Harvard, Michigan) found the continued mediocrity of medical education intolerable. Medical professors in this country still retained private practice, although incomes from apprentices vanished when this practice declined, after 1870, with the lengthening of the curriculum. Hence, professors were able to infiltrate the medical societies as practitioners, and appealed to the AMA (American Medical Association) to reform the schools. The latter [schools], because of their power to license, were primarily responsible for the low state of both training and practice; and the reformers—consciously or unconsciously—returned to an earlier program in appealing for control by medical societies. The latter, in turn, succeeding in persuading most states to re-establish the examining and licensing boards which had earlier been abandoned; and such bodies (1875 to 1900) were able to exert some pressure for better educational standards. By 1900, moreover, liberals in the AMA secured its reorganization, and in 1904 set up a Council on [Medical] Education which began to rate the various schools.

Although the AMA at its founding in 1847 had as a primary goal the reform of medical education, its efforts were diluted for many years because so many of its members had an interest of one sort or another in the continuance of the weaker schools. One can surmise that this vested interest was not only financial investment and return but also included a desire to buy time so that the improvements could be made, an emotional tie by some practitioners who did not want to see their schools put out of business, and a certain skepticism about what reform would accomplish, for the discoveries of Lister on antiseptic surgery and Pasteur on germs were not to come until the 1860s, and anesthetic was introduced into surgery only in 1846. One can also speculate a sometime resistance resulting from impolitic expressions from medical-school faculty whose words seemed arrogant and condescending to the more traditionally trained physician.

A similar problem arose in 1876 when 22 medical schools organized the Association of American Medical Colleges (AAMC) as part of the effort to improve the quality of medical education. Coggeshall notes that "the embryo organization soon foundered over an issue involving its principal concern for higher standards. The question was whether graduation requirements should be extended to three years rather than two" (9, p.49).

Both the AMA and the AAMC thus encountered the problem that besets all representative bodies: to continue to exist, the organization, like the elected politician, must retain the support of its constituency: get too far ahead and the

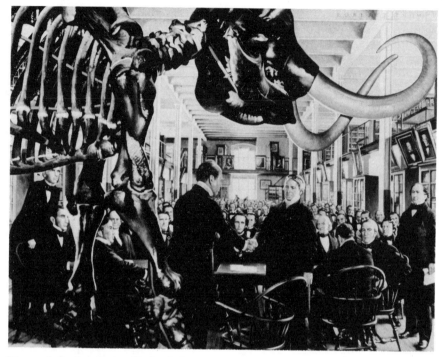

Figure 1–1. American Medical Association. First meeting, Philadelphia, 1847. (Reprinted with permission from the American Medical Association.)

effort will founder because it will not enjoy support from the majority of the membership. Standards thus tend to be minimal, such that most of the present members can meet. Progress is still made, as it was by the AMA and the AAMC, in incremental steps by which the constituency is persuaded that it is to its interests to support whatever it is that is being proposed.

Sometimes an organization can make little progress on an issue. Individual members may charge ahead, but there may simply not be enough support for the entire group to do so. The reluctance of the entire group to move may be based on any number of reasons, such as not being convinced that the proposed course of action is merited or wise, fear that the course of action may produce undesirable outcomes, fear that the action will harm or destroy the efforts of individual members, as well as satisfaction with the way things are at present. In such instances, an organization may simply have to tread water until some other body is able to make the necessary breakthrough, on the assumption that a breakthrough is appropriate. Reform of medical education is a good illustration of this.

Despite the fact that Harvard lengthened its curriculum to three years in the early 1870s, it and others could not move the AAMC on this matter in 1876. Not until 1891 did the AAMC support a three-year training period, only to have Harvard a year later again go its own way and lengthen its curriculum to four years. In 1893, Johns Hopkins University launched its pioneering effort in medical education with a four-year curriculum, one which became, as we shall see, the model used to reform all medical education. The AAMC was persuaded in 1894 also to support a four-year curriculum. The organization played an important role, increasingly so from the 1890s on, but clearly it did not have enough clout to bring about the necessary reform by itself. It was at this point that the AMA played a significant role. As we have seen, it, too, was restrained by its rank and file, but some leadership was evident, since it was able to establish the Council on Medical Education, which became a semi-independent body with strong leadership.

The beginnings of AMA leadership are described by Johnson in Fishbein's history of the AMA. (10, pp.887-899)

THE AMA AND MEDICAL EDUCATION

At the organizational meeting of the AMA in Philadelphia in 1847 (Fig. 1-1), a Committee on Medical Education was established. The first pronouncement of the committee was to decry "medical instruction which does not rest on the basis of practical demonstration and clinical teaching; . . .it is . . .the duty of the medical schools to resort to every honorable means to obtain access for their students to the wards of a well regulated hospital" (10, p.888).

In its 1872 report, the Committee on Medical Education observed that "it seems much easier to show the defects in our present system than to advise a suitable and practical remedy" (10, p.890). The influence of the medical-school professors "has always been so great in the Association as to prevent its doing what it should have done long ago, viz, establishing a national standard for medical teaching and demanding that colleges shall accept it or not be recognized" (10, p.890).

In 1901, the association was restructured to become a more representative body, with business transactions conducted by a House of Delegates consisting largely of elected representatives from the states but also including a representative from each of the scientific sections of the association and from each of the federal government health services (Army, Navy, and Public Health). This reorganization made the association a more representative national body, lessening the domination by those close to the city in which the annual meeting was being held; the reorganization also lessened the influence of medical educators in the governing House of Delegates. In 1904, the House of

Delegates acted on a report of the Committee on Medical Education and created a new Council on Medical Education whose functions were, as quoted by Johnson (10, p.892):

---

1. To make an annual report to the House of Delegates on the existing conditions of medical education in the United States.
2. To make suggestions as to the means and methods by which the American Medical Association may best influence favorably medical education.
3. To act as the agent of the American Medical Association (under instructions from the House of Delegates) in its efforts to elevate medical education

---

The first council consisted of four medical-school professors and one dean, from what might fairly be cited as the more reputable schools, that is Rush, Harvard, Pennsylvania, Michigan, and Vanderbilt. The council still exists, and its annual report, published toward the end of each year in the *Journal of the American Medical Association (JAMA)*, offers, without question, the most definitive account of the current state of medical education.

But even before the council's work began, leadership in the AMA was making progress. Beginning in 1902, JAMA published medical-school failure statistics on state board licensing examinations, a form of exposure that could not help but embarrass and lead to institutional reform. In 1907, the assessment of schools was made even easier by grouping the schools into four classes. Class 1 had fewer than 10% failure; class 2 has 10-20% failure; class 3 had more than 20% failure; class 4 consisted of a miscellaneous grouping of smaller schools (fewer than 10 graduates) and not otherwise classifiable institutions (11, p.895).

The council subsequently decided to rate each school based not only on the state board exam performances but also on such factors as entrance requirements, medical curriculum, laboratory facilities, hospital facilities, faculty quality, library, research. The resulting scores would place each school in one of three categories: class A (acceptable, with a point score above 70); class B (doubtful, with a score of 50-70); and class C (unacceptable, with a score of less than 50). Each school was visited; in 1907, the findings were reported.

The council chairman noted that "the Council was very lenient in its markings," and of the 160 schools, Fishbein reports that 82 were in class A, 46 in class B, and 32 in class C. The classifications were not published, though each school was notified of its standing. The council chairman, some years later, stated:

As a result of the report of this first inspection a great wave of improvement in medical education swept over the country. Fifty schools agreed to require by 1910, or before, at least one year of university physics, chemistry and biology and one modern language as a preliminary education before matriculating in medicine. Immediately a number of consolidations were arranged in many cities having several schools. A number of schools, as a result of state boards refusing examinations to their graduates, went out of business and it became evident that the 160 schools would be reduced within a short time to probably less than a hundred (10, p.897).

The improved situation was evident. The AMA's work was clearly facilitated by effective leadership in the organization as well as by medical educators from some of the better schools who were also working within the AAMC. The AAMC began to inspect the schools and put pressure on the poorer schools to improve or else get out of the association. There was, however, a clear political constraint on the AMA classification of schools. The ratings were made leniently perhaps in recognition of the fact that it had to take one step at a time if it was to be effective and that to be successful in this, a clear majority of schools had to be acceptable, and so it was: 51% of the schools (82) fell in the acceptable class; only 20% (32) were unacceptable; the remainder, while doubtful, could pass muster if they improved. This, then, was perhaps as far as the AMA could go by itself. Johnson notes that there was considerable resentment over these reports by many of the colleges, and as a result of this, he quotes the council chairman, who said years later (10, p.897): "It occurred to some of the members of the Council that, if we could obtain the publication and approval of our work by the Carnegie Foundation for the Advancement of Teaching, it would assist materially in securing the results we were attempting to bring about."

Johnson then quotes from the minutes of the council meeting held in New York in December 1905 (10, p.897):

At one o'clock an informal conference was held with President Pritchett and Mr. Abraham Flexner of the Carnegie Foundation. Mr. Pritchett had already expressed, by correspondence, the willingness of the Foundation to cooperate with the Council in investigating the medical schools. He now explained that the Foundation was to investigate all the professions, law, medicine and theology. He had found no efforts being made by law to better the conditions in legal education and had met with some slight opposition in the efforts he was making. He had then received the letters from the Council on Medical Education and expressed himself as most agreeably surprised not only at the efforts being made to correct conditions surrounding medical education but at the enormous amount of important data collected.

He agreed with the opinion previously expressed by the members of the Council that while the Foundation would be guided very largely by the Council's investigation, to avoid the usual claims of partiality no more mention should be made in the report of the Council than any other source of information. The report would therefore be, and have the weight of an independent report of a disinterested body, which would then be published far and wide. It would do much to develop public opinion.

It was considered wise to withhold publication of the list of satisfactory colleges until the Carnegie report comes out . . . (so that) . . . that report would make the Council's report at a later date more effective.

THE FLEXNER REPORT AND REFORM

The study was begun almost immediately. In January 1909, Flexner—not a physician but an educator, the holder of a baccalaureate degree from The Johns Hopkins University and a master's degree from Harvard—began the first of his medical school visits. On most, if not all, of his visits, he was accompanied by Dr. N.P. Colwell, who was the secretary of the AMA's Council on Medical Education. In his autobiography, Flexner tells us how he carried out his survey (11, pp.120-122). He notes that it was essentially an educational survey, not a medical one. He identified five factors that would provide him with conclusive data as to the quality of a school:

First, the entrance requirements. What were they? Were they enforced?

Second, the size and training of the faculty.

Third, the sum available from endowment and fees for the support of the institution, and what became of it.

Fourth, the quality and adequacy of the laboratories provided for the instruction of the first two years and the qualifications and training of the teachers of the so-called preclinical branches.

Fifth and finally, the relations between medical school and hospitals, including particularly freedom of access to beds and freedom in the appointment by the school of the hospital physicians and surgeons who automatically should become clinical teachers.

Much of the data he sought was secured through interviews with the dean and a few of the faculty. A "stroll through the laboratories" revealed to him much about the availability of equipment and specimens, and a "whiff" revealed something about the teaching of anatomy. He goes on to say:

In the course of a few hours a reliable estimate could be made respecting the possibilities of teaching modern medicine in almost any one of the 155 schools I visited in the United States and Canada. Having visited perhaps half a dozen schools, sometimes more, I would return to New York and set my facts in order—never the same facts respecting any two of them. These brief summaries I returned to the dean of the school by mail with the request that he correct any misstatements. I had the feeling during the whole time that the faculties were more than candid with me, because though I endeavored to disabuse them of the idea, they were convinced that Mr. Carnegie, having once made a gift to a medical school in Atlanta, contemplated further activities of the same kind.

His autobiography describes in vivid terms the conduct of his study and is rewarding to read. Flexner's formal reports, *Medical Education in the United States and Canada,* was published by the Carnegie Foundation in 1910. Though more controlled in language than the accounts given in his autobiography, it nonetheless provided a candid, searing critique of medical education in both the United States and Canada. It named schools, their assets and their liabilities, and it offered a prescription for each school, for each state and region, and for the country as a whole. Where the schools were no more than business ventures (such as the Jenner Medical College in Illinois and Still College of Osteopathy in Iowa), he said so. Regarding the California Medical College, he stated that "the school is a disgrace to the state whose laws permit its existence." The Los Angeles College of Osteopathy had all the aspects of a "thriving business." Chicago was described as "the plague spot of the country" in terms of medical education, and the provisions of the Illinois state law "are, and have long been, flagrantly violated" with the "indubitable connivance of the state board."

Small wonder Flexner's life was threatened and a libel suit filed and other suits promised. But not all was so negative. With regard to Dartmouth, he noted the difficulties that the institution had of attracting a sufficient number of medical cases for teaching purposes because of its remoteness and expressed doubt about a compulsory fifth-year internship in a large hospital. The college's preclinical training in the basic sciences was excellent. He concluded (12, pp.264-265):

That the school cannot much longer continue in its present stage is clear; for with the requirement of two years of college work for entrance in 1910, it asks a student to spend six years to get a degree in medicine, in attaining which he can enjoy only a very limited opportunity to learn internal medicine. It is safe to predict that on that basis the present facilities will not hold the student body together during the third and fourth years.

Subsequently, Dartmouth took Flexner's observations to heart and abandoned clinical instruction, retaining only the two years of preclinical instruction in what is known as a school of basic medical sciences, with the students transferring to some other schools for the third and fourth years of clinical instruction. Many other schools could expand their clinical classes on two accounts: the big blockages in medical education are the very expensive preclinical labs and clinical training is easily expandable in the larger centers because of the availability of a larger population base with a plentiful range of medical and surgical cases and of hospital beds. Because of population growth and improved transportation, Dartmouth went back to a four-year curriculum in the 1960s.

Other schools, which showed weaknesses but also promises, received constructive criticism. At Yale, for example, the teaching staff was cited for being "overworked and without a proper force of assistants." At New Haven Hospital, there was a good use of the available beds, but criticism was registered, "the obstetrical and gynecological wards . . . are not used for teaching; nor is there a contagious disease pavillion. Post-mortems are scarce" (12, p.200). At Columbia, the criticism was also constructive: there was no real medical library, endowments were insufficient (but, he felt, readily correctable); but more serious was a problem regarding "rights" in the hospitals in which the teaching was carried out.

Some institutions received high praise, particularly Harvard, Western Reserve, McGill, Toronto, and Johns Hopkins. It was Johns Hopkins School of Medicine, launched only 17 years earlier (1893), that was singled out and became his preferred model for medical education. In addition to requiring a bachelor's degree for admission, Flexner states (12, p.12):

This was the first medical school in America of genuine university type, with something approaching adequate endowment, well equipped laboratories conducted by modern teachers, devoting themselves unreservedly to medical investigation and instruction, and with its own hospital, in which the training of physicians and the healing of the sick harmoniously combine to the infinite advantage of both. The influence of this new foundation can hardly be overstated. It has finally cleared up the problem of standards and ideals; and its graduates have gone forth in small bands to found new establishments or to reconstruct old ones.

Following publication of the Flexner report, schools began to close and to consolidate. Some allegedly closed before the report's publication in order to escape the criticism. In his autobiography, Flexner notes many schools quietly went out of existence; others merged. In Chicago, where there had been 15 schools, he tells us that the number was reduced to 3 (11, p.31). In all, Flexner recommended that the number of schools be reduced from 155 to 31. By 1920, the number of schools was down to 85. By that time, however, the need for more than 31 was apparent due to population increases and new knowledge, which permitted more to be done for patients.

The report, coming from an independent body, strengthened the hand of medical reformers in the AMA, and AAMC, state medical societies, and importantly, state licensing boards. Licensing legislation in the states mandated more rigor. The council, moreover, leaned on people in the state societies, even before the Flexner study, to see to it that reform-minded people got appointed to state licensing boards. Stevens notes (4, p.68):

In 1905 only five schools had required any college preparation for admission. Ten years later eighty-five schools prescribed a minimum of one or two years' college preparation; by 1932, every recognized medical school and most of the state licensing boards required at least two years' college work, many required three, and several a college degree ... by 1925, forty-nine boards required candidates for their examinations to be graduates of a medical college, and forty-six states refused to recognize low-grade schools as a preparation for the license. Since the only national rating of colleges continued to be that of the AMA Council on Medical Education, the profession by then held effective monopoly control of educational regulation.

The increased leverage provided the work of the AMA and the AAMC was evident in their increased coordinative efforts, leading, in 1942, to the establishment of a Liaison Committee on Medical Education, which developed educational program guidelines, inspected schools, and became the official accrediting body for medical schools. Their efforts were supported by the growing number of medical graduates from the better schools who in their own ways were persuasive within their state societies, before legislative bodies, and to the public.

But the final lever for reform came from the foundations and from individuals whom the foundations could persuade. Flexner's influence here was a critical factor—his report and his person. Shortly after his report, he joined the General Education Board, a Rockefeller charity, which poured enormous sums into medical education. Flexner estimated that the General Education Board's 50 million dollars for medical education had been successful in getting other contributors to come up with half a billion dollars or more from 1919 to 1928, a period when the dollar bought much more than it does today. His role in the allocation of these funds and in persuading others to complement the board's contributions are described in his autobiography *I Remember*. The monies, of course, went to the better schools and to those that showed promise of moving in the direction laid out in his report. The monies were also strategically allocated where they would do the most good in terms of influencing reform at nearby institutions: the grant to the University of Rochester, for example, was designed to stimulate the reform of all New York schools; the grant to the University of Iowa was meant to do the same in the Middle West (11, p.296).

Our story of medical schools might appropriately end here while we backtrack to look at the development of medical specialties. We'll return to medical schools in a later chapter.

THE DEVELOPMENT OF MEDICAL SPECIALTIES

Most physicians in the colonial and postcolonial periods were general practitioners. This was the great need at the time; moreover, it was made necessary because the state of medical science was rather primitive, hardly justifying a specialist, and because surgical practice was limited until 1846 by the absence of anesthesia. Where physicians did develop special skills or interests and became known for them, they remained, first of all, general physicians and practiced their specialties (such as obstetrics or surgery) only on occasion. As to the state of medical science, Shryock reminds us that this was the age of bleeding and purging (the former carried on as late as the 1870s), when illness was attributed to some generalized problem such as "impurities of the blood or the existence of excessive tension or laxity in the nervous and vascular systems (13). Under such a philosophy, there was little need for specialists. Surgery inside body cavities would be pointless as well as painful, and surgery was thus limited largely to trauma. Benjamin Rush, besides being a signer of the Declaration of Independence and a prominent Philadelphia physician, was a great advocate of both bleeding and purging. A contemporary critic of Rush (William Cobbett) described his mode of practice as "one of those great discoveries which are made from time to time for the depopulation of the earth" (2, p.70). The unpleasantries of such treatment and the risks they entailed made the milder treatments offered by quacks and cultists seem appealing.

During the first half of the nineteenth century, a growing number of American physicians went to France for advanced study. It was during this period that French investigators were effectively proving the errors of bleeding and purging as well as the ineffectiveness of many drugs then in common use. Their investigations pointed to specific pathology in different locations and in systems of the body, there being no single, let alone simple, explanation for disease. These findings, of course, made the whole notion of specialization appealing to those physicians whose interest was excited by special health problems.

But old ideas die hard, and it was not until the 1860s that specialties began to make headway on the medical scene. Resistance to specialties was, at times, vigorous, and the issues were complex. Fishbein, in his history of the AMA, summarizes the issues as contained in a report at the association's 1866 meeting in Baltimore (13a, pp.74-75):

This year was notable for the majority and minority reports of the Committee on Medical Ethics dealing with specialization. The majority report listed the advantages of specialization as including minuteness in observation, acuteness in study, wideness of observation, skill in diagnosis, multiplicity of invention and superior skill in manipulation. The disadvantages were a narrowness of view, a tendency to magnify unduly the diseases which the specialty covers, a tendency to undervalue the treatment of special diseases by general practitioners, some temptation to the employment of undue measures for gaining a popular reputation and a tendency to increased fees. The advantages far outweighed the disadvantages from the point of view of the patient and of the advancement of the specialty. The committee felt that these disadvantages could be overcome if the specialist would begin as a general practitioner and gradually grow into his specialty.

The committee was especially concerned with the means by which the specialist made himself known to the community. They felt that there should be no advertising either in newspapers or medical journals.

The minority report was signed by Dr.Henry I. Bowditch. He considered that the whole tendency of modern science was toward specialism but he felt also that the Association had no business passing on the question of the advertisements unless they were evidently of a mountebank character. It was his opinion that "any Association would be better occupied in the hearing of able papers and in discussions on all subjects connected with medicine than in any movements for the mere discipline of erring members."

To some of these issues and related ones there are no easy or hard and fast answers, and many persist to this day. Should a patient go first to the general practitioner or directly to the specialist? Will the specialist treat the whole patient? Should a specialist be permitted to advertise, and how? Will the surgeon cut because that is what a surgeon is taught to do? Does specialty practice lead to unnecessary procedures? Will the higher fees accorded specialists lead people into medicine and the specialty for the sake of money? But don't we want the best medical care, and isn't the specialist the best?

It was only six years earlier (1859) that the scientific sections of the AMA began to be set up. Initially, they focused on what were then well-defined areas of scientific interest as the AMA delegates saw them: anatomy and physiology, chemistry and materia medica, practical medicine and obstetrics, and surgery. Obstetrics became part of the new section of Obstetrics and Diseases of Women and Children in 1873. *Children* were broken out to become a section on Diseases of Children in 1879. Ophthalmology, laryngology, and otology sections were formed in 1878, and so on. The AMA's responses to specialty interests were often slow because of the sometime reluctance of AMA membership to recognize the validity of the specialty. Is there such uniqueness in diseases of children, for example, to justify the problems being spun off from general practice to be treated as a specialty? Will the specialist become so narrowly focused that he or she might miss the critical contributions that can be made by those more generally oriented? While it is true that the specialist may tend to draw paying patients away from the general practitioner, it is also true that there is considerable evidence to suggest that a specialist practicing in too isolated an environment runs grave risks of practicing bad medical care due to the tendency to magnify concerns of the specialty and to be insensitive to the contributions and skills of other specialties. The resistance to some specialty development was thus genuinely concerned with quality of patient care as well as being rooted in the economics of medical practice.

Concern by general practitioners on the economic score was also well founded, for by the mid-twentieth century, general practitioners were squeezed out of hospitals by the specialists in some of our larger cities. The argument advanced by the specialists was: If you're sick enough to be in the hospital, you're sick enough to need a specialist. This led the general practitioners to fight back, organizing in 1947, the American Academy of General Practice (AAGP), with state and local chapters, and applying pressure for hospitals to add departments of general practice. To prove their worth, members of the academy were required to have 150 hours of approved continuing education credits every three years. In 1969, general practice—now family practice—

became a recognized specialty. The AAGP is now the American Academy of Family Physicians (AAFP).

Because of the slow response by the AMA to specialty interests, the specialists began to form their own societies and associations. These groups, by and large, did not fight the AMA but simply went their own way. Not infrequently, some held leadership positions both in the AMA and their specialty group. The specialty organization could focus more quickly than the more generally oriented AMA on the problems and concerns of the specialty. Some of the early specialty groups were the American Ophthalmological Society (1864), the American Otological Society (1868), the American Gynecological Society (1876), the American Association of Obstetricians and Gynecologists (1888), and the American Pediatric Society (1888). There were also state and local specialty societies, some established before the national body, some later. Specialty journals followed; in many cities, the specialty was advanced by the presence of specialty hospitals and clinics. Indeed, in most large cities today, one can find specialty hospitals still thriving or only recently merged with other hospitals. Eye and ear hospitals are the most common example.

These special hospitals and clinics became, in the late nineteenth and twentieth centuries, the foci for training in those specialties, for at those institutions, generally speaking, were the most outstanding practitioners. This is not to suggest, however, that some outstanding specialists did not practice and train others in the more generally oriented hospital; they did.

There was, of course, no standard at the turn of the century for what constituted adequate training in a specialty. Courses were offered by medical societies, hospitals, specially founded schools, and by universities. The programs of study lasted anywhere from a few weeks to three years. Flexner described some of these in his report (12, pp.174-177):

THE POSTGRADUATE SCHOOL

The postgraduate school as developed in the United States may be char-acterized as a "compensatory adjustment." It is an effort to mend a machine that was predestined to break down. Inevitably, the more conscientious and intelligent men trained in most of the medical schools herein described must become aware of their unfitness for the responsibilities of medical practice; the postgraduate school was established to do what the medical school had failed to accomplish.

"When I graduated in the spring of 1869," says Dr. John A. Wyeth,* "I can

---

* Proceedings of the Nineteenth Annual Meeting of the Association of American Medical Colleges, pp.25,26 (abridged).

never forget the sinking feeling that came over me when I realized how incompetent I was to undertake the care of those in the distress of sickness or accident. A week later, after arriving in my native village in Alabama, I rented a small office and attached my sign to the front door. Within two months, the tacks were withdrawn by the hand which had placed them there and the sign was stowed away in the bottom of my trunk. Two months of hopeless struggle with a Presbyterian conscience had convinced me that I was not fit to practise medicine, and that nothing was left for me but to go out into the world of business to earn money enough to complete my education. I felt the absolute need of clinical experience, and a conviction, which then forced itself upon my mind, that no graduate in medicine was competent to practise until he had had, in addition to his theoretical, a clinical and laboratory training, was the controlling idea in my mind when, in later years the opportunity offered, it fell to my good fortune to establish in this city the New York Polyclinic Medical School and Hospital."

The postgraduate school was thus originally an undergraduate repair shop. Its instruction was necessarily at once elementary and practical. There was no time to go back to fundamentals; it was too late to raise the question of preliminary educational competency. Urgency required that in the shortest possible time the young physician already involved in responsibility should acquire the practical technique which the medical school had failed to impart. The courses were made short, frequently covering less than a month; and they aimed preëminently to teach the young doctor what to "do" in the various emergencies of general practice.

As the general level of medical education has risen, the function of these institutions has been somewhat modified. The general course, aiming to make good deficiencies at large, has tended to give way to special courses adapted to the needs of those inclined to devote themselves more or less exclusively to some particular line of work. Simultaneously, as the facilities of the schools have enlarged, they have become centers to which at intervals men practising in isolated places may return for brief periods in order to catch up with the times. Once more the training offered is of a practical, not of a fundamental or intensive, kind. It is calculated to "teach the trick"—or, perhaps better, to exhibit an instructor in the act of doing it. For, as nothing is known of individuals in the stream of students who course through the schools, it is impossible to give them an active share in the work that goes on at the bedside or in the operating-room. Their part is mainly passive; they look on at expert diagnosticians or operators. The danger of permitting an unknown student, tarrying for a brief stay, to participate at close range is prohibitive. In surgery the so-called practical courses are not usually worked out in such fashion that cadaver work, animal work, and service as dresser might prepare for actual participation: the school lacks means and facilities; the students lack the time. In medicine the absence of sufficient material, the lack of proper hospital organization and equipment, the scrappiness of professional service, combine to prevent a systematic, thorough, and intimate discipline.

Of the thirteen postgraduate schools,* the best of them reflect the conditions and purposes above described. The Postgraduate and Polyclinic of New York and the Polyclinic of Philadelphia command large dispensary services and considerable hospital clinics, partly in their own hospitals, and partly in public and private hospitals in the city. No unkind criticism is intended when the teaching is characterized as too immediately practical to be scientifically stimulating: it has the air of handicraft, rather than science. Comparatively little is done in internal medicine: surgery and the specialties predominate. The courses, being practical and definite, are disconnected; the faculties are huge and unorganized. In the main, demonstrative instruction is offered to small bodies of physicians, who come and go uninterruptedly through the year. Only one of the three—the Philadelphia school—has a laboratory building, and in that no advanced work is in progress; the two New York schools have laboratory space or equipment adequate only to routine clinical examinations. The teaching is in the main more elementary than the upper class instruction of a good undergraduate school of medicine. It is, of course, also at times more special in character. With the exception of the New York Postgraduate, these schools are without endowment: they live on fees, donations, and hospital receipts.

Two departmental postgraduate schools are conducted by the government at Washington for those accepted for service in the army or navy medical corps. Eligible for these appointments are graduated physicians who have had a year of hospital experience or three years of practice. Excellent practical instruction is furnished by way of supplementing the usual undergraduate course. The needs of the services can be very definitely formulated; the course worked out aims to meet them. The accepted surgeons get in this way a concentrated practical drill in bacteriology, hygiene, and military surgery. The laboratories are excellently equipped, though cramped for space. The army school enjoys the advantage of contact with the great library and museum of the surgeon-general's office. The schools, as yet in their infancy, may not improbably develop into research laboratories dealing with the specific

---

* Four are situated in Greater New York; (1)The New York Polyclinic Medical School, (2)New York Postgraduate Medical School, (3)Brooklyn Postgraduate Medical School, (4)Manhattan Eye, Ear, and Throat Postgraduate School: four in Chicago: (5) Postgraduate Medical School, (6)The Chicago Polyclinic, (7)Illinois Postgraduate Medical School, (8)Chicago Ear, Eye, Nose and Throat College; one each in Philadelphia, (9)The Philadelphia Polyclinic; Kansas City, (10)Postgraduate Medical School; New Orleans, (11)New Orleans Polyclinic (affiliated with Tulane University); and two in Washington, (12)Army Medical School, (13)Navy Medical School. A number of schools offer special courses to graduates, in special summer and regular winter sessions.

problems that crop up in naval and military service in various quarters of the globe.

Postgraduate, like other schools, vary in character. We have spoken of the best. The others are weak concerns wearing a commercial hue. The Brooklyn Postgraduate School, for instance, entertains less than half a dozen students on the average at a time, in a wretched hospital, really a death-trap, heavily laden with debt, and without laboratory equipment enough to make an ordinary clinical examination; the Kansas City affair had, when visited, no students in its improvised hospital containing 25 ward beds, only 13 of them occupied; it ekes out its opportunities with clinics at the public hospital. Chicago, varied and picturesque in this as in all else pertaining to medical education, supports four postgraduate institutions. None of them has a satisfactory plant. All are stock companies. Only unmistakable scientific activity could dislodge the unpleasant suspicion of commercial motive thus suggested. No such activity is in any of them observable. A cynical candor admits in one place that "it pays the teachers through referred cases;" in another, "it establishes the reputation of a man to teach in a postgraduate school;" in a third, "it pays through advertising teachers." In one a youth was observed working with a microscope. Inquiry elicited the fact that he was the teacher of clinical laboratory technique, lecturing in the absence of the "professor." The following dialogue took place:

"Are you a doctor?"

"No."

"A student of medicine?"

"Yes."

"Where?"

"At the Jenner Night School."

"In what year?"

"The first."

A first-year student of medicine in a night school was thus laboratory instructor and pro tempore lecturing professor in clinical microscopy in the Chicago Polyclinic.

Improved medical education will undoubtedly cut the ground from under the independent postgraduate school as we know it. This is not to say that the undergraduate medical curriculum will exhaust the field. On the contrary, the undergraduate school will do only the elementary work; but that it will do, not needing subsequent and more elementary instruction to patch it up. Graduate instruction will be advanced and intensive,—the natural prolongation of the elective courses now coming into vogue. For productive investigation and intensive instruction, the medical school will use its own teaching hospital and laboratories; for the elaboration of really thorough training in specialties resting on a solid undergraduate education, it may use the great municipal hospitals of the larger cities. But advanced instruction along these lines will not thrive in isolation. It will be but the upper story of a university department of medicine. The postgraduate schools of the better type can hasten this evolution by incorporating themselves in accessible universities, taking up university ideals, and submitting to reorganization on university lines.

The "repair shop" to which Flexner referred was also the rationale in the latter part of the nineteenth century for the internship, which over time became standard practice—the requirement of an additional year of supervised training to give the medical graduate (still, in a sense, a student) that extra bit of on-the-job training. The need for some practical on-the-job training was necessitated by the adoption of medical schools of the Harvard practice of not requiring an apprenticeship before medical school. This need for additional training was also, in part, what motivated many other physicians to go abroad. As Stevens notes (4, p.117), the internship tended to emphasize either medicine or surgery and thus became an introductory phase of specialization. (If we might jump ahead in time, we might note this in terms of internships in the second half of the twentieth century. They are of three types: the straight internship, which until very recently was in one of four areas—surgery, pediatrics, internal medicine, pathology—and which led the way into most all of the approved specialties; the rotating internship, in which the intern rotated through a number of hospital clinical departments; the mixed internship which reduced the number of clinical rotations permitting more concentrated training. In recent years, the rotating internship has lost its appeal since most all physicians now train for one specialty or another.)

Note might also be taken of Flexner's view of postgraduate university medical education, an ideal that has not yet been achieved but that medical schools today are vigorously pursuing. More will be said of this later.

Early specialty training was thus erratic, and in the absence of accepted standards, the quality of specialty care ran from excellent to complete incompetence. Perhaps the best assessment was made by the United States Army in 1917. Stevens cites army sources and tells us (4, pp.127-128):

The army acted as a filtering system for quality. No one reached the medical training camps unless they were initially felt to be desirable (thus eliminating the obviously incompetent, the sick, those of bad character, alcoholics, drug addicts, and so on), were from reputable medical colleges, were licensed to practice in the state in which they lived, were already in active practice, and had passed an examination before a local board. At the camps many more were rejected; physical unfitness rather than professional incompetence was used as the reason for rejection wherever possible, to avoid embarrassment.

Specialist qualifications received searching examination. The surgeon general's office card-indexed men whose reputation seemed to warrant their acceptance as specialists, but so many were found to be overrated that the specialists' divisions agreed to make specialist appointments conditional on examination. The results were appalling. Some of the "specialists" examined were found to be unfit to practice any branch of medicine in the service. A study of the examination results at Camp Greenleaf in 1918 revealed only one medical officer in three qualified to do independent surgery, and only about 6 percent were rated as high-class surgeons; there was a similarly small proportion of really high-grade men in internal medicine. Seventy percent of the otolaryngologists, 51 percent of the ophthalmologists, and 38 percent of those who said they were plastic and oral surgeons were rejected. Thus the extent of educational deficiency was glaringly acknowledged—and at the same time directly linked with the potential danger to the public if such practices were to continue.

All these factors were to deepen concern over the preparation and role of the specialist in postwar prosperity, not only in relation to the kinds of intraprofessional questions which had stimulated the surgeons and ophthalmologists to develop separate organizations but also in relation to the provision of high-quality medical care to the public.

But the army's findings described sets of circumstances that were well known by the leaders in many specialty areas. Anyone who wanted to become a specialist did so. There was no mandated course of study or training, nor was a license granted for specialty practice. State licensure acts focused on the basic qualifications for medical practice. A physician, once licensed, had no legal constraints placed on him or her but could legally do all that fell within the definition of medicine and surgery.

To be sure, many, perhaps even most (we have no way of really knowing), of the specialists were conscientious. They sought to learn through special courses, by going abroad, and by reading books and journals. They sought further information and fostered research through local, state, and national specialty societies. When one of their members secured a reputation for special skills, others went to work with that person. Bond, for example, writes of "an enthusiastic pioneer in gynecological surgery, and one of the founders of the Woman's Hospital" who, in the latter half of the nineteenth century, would journey to New York from Baltimore "every year . . .for several weeks to familiarize himself with any new advances in his specialty, in that birthplace of American Gynecology, where Marion Sims labored and suffered in his earlier years" (14, p.73). With the advent of anesthesia, antiseptic techniques, new instrumentation, and new technology learned from the Civil War battle casualties as well as from European research, a new era began to open up. Hospitals grew in number because now people could go to them for general and special surgery with less fear of pain and more assurance that from the encounter the patient would likely survive and improve.

But this new era posed new problems. The new opportunities unlocked the specialties, but the advances in most of the specialties entailed surgery. Surgery used to be the domain of the general practitioner—sewing a laceration, setting a bone, or amputating. Now, however, surgery became more complicated, and the better surgeons wanted to restrain not only the general practitioners (GPs) but the less qualified surgeons as well.

As noted earlier, this could only mean cutting the volume of paying patients for the GP. It meant that the GP's image to the public might be lowered, that the GP might come to be viewed as a less than complete physician. (By 1947, the Council on Medical Education had to issue a special report on the prestige of general practitioners [4, p.307]). The better surgeons, on the other hand, argued that GPs had no business inside the belly, and this led, as noted earlier, to the attempt to keep the GP out of the urban hospitals and, in many areas of the country, to restrict the practice of the GP in the hospital to nonsurgical cases. There are still, however, today small community hospitals in which the GP does general surgery because the GP has always done it, because there are no specialists, because some procedures are relatively simple even though in the abdominal cavity, for example, appendectomy, and because some patients want their doctor to do the cutting.

A number of practices developed, however, around the turn of the century that were considered unethical. One practice was ghost surgery. Another was fee splitting, and still another was unnecessary surgery.

Ghost surgery is surgery performed by a surgeon other than the person the patient thinks did the operation. If, for example, a patient needed abdominal surgery, and the GP was uncomfortable undertaking it, the GP might take it on "to save face" or to satisfy the patient, and when the patient was under anesthesia, the hired surgeon would come in to do the job. The patient would never see the ghost surgeon. This practice is probably non existent today.*

---

*A television documentary in 1977 described ghost surgery as surgery performed in a teaching hospital in which the actual work is done by the surgical resident and not the surgeon. The essential difference between this practice and what I have defined as ghost surgery is that in the teaching hospital instance the surgical resident is under the guided direction of a qualified surgeon and in all probability sees the patient preoperatively and postoperatively. The resident, moreover, is paid these days by the hospital on a salary basis. At issue in the television documentary was that the patient had not clearly been informed that the resident would be a key person on the case. There is an ethical issue here as well as a possible legal issue relating to civil liability under modern doctrines of informed consent.

Fee splitting is a practice in which the surgeon's fee is divided with other physicians without the knowledge and consent of the patient. In its most pernicious form, it was a kickback from the surgeon to the referring physician as payment for the referral. One might describe it as a bounty system. But one might also describe it as a mechanism for discouraging surgery by GPs, saying to the GP, in effect, Don't do surgery because you are not really trained to do it, but to stabilize your income and to encourage you to refer patients, we'll give you a payment for every case referred. Fee splitting has long been a violation of the AMA's code of ethics, but it was believed to be widespread at least until the Second World War.

Fee splitting has also been carried out above board. In this instance, the family doctor refers the patient to a surgeon. The surgeon tells the patient that a medically qualified operative assistant would be desirable and that the surgeon would like the family doctor to be that assistant. In such a case, the division of the fee would be with the knowledge and, presumably, consent of the patient and would, therefore, not be a violation of the AMA's code of ethics. The surgeon's wish in this case might well be in the patient's interest. Then again, it could also be a splitting of the fee as payment for the referral. The latter practice is probably not significant today because most referring physicians have all they can do and make enough without having to seek this form of fee splitting. Whether it was ever widely practiced, I doubt anyone can tell.

Unnecessary surgery is an issue that still troubles the nation. We shall deal with it later in the text. Suffice it to note here that specialists do what they are trained to do, and a surgeon is trained to treat medical problems surgically. There have undoubtedly been some unscrupulous surgeons who operated knowing that there were no medical indications for surgery, but probably more of the unnecessary surgery (that is truly unnecessary) is due to inadequate diagnosis. I have used the phrase "that is truly unnecessary" because, as shall be noted in the later discussion, much of the unnecessary surgery today is not factually based; rather, it is based on different judgments.

Some of the surgical leaders moved vigorously to address the above evil practices. It was done through the American College of Surgeons (ACS), which was established in 1912. It moved vigorously against fee splitting and unnecessary surgery. It also established standards for surgical training and developed a mechanism (fellowship) for recognizing those who were judged by the college to be acceptable surgeons. The AMA did not lag on the issue of fee splitting; it condemned it officially in 1913, stating that "any member of the American Medical Association found guilty of secret fee splitting or of giving or receiving commissions shall cease to be a member of the American Medical Association" (13a, p.953). But it had, in fact, acted even earlier, supporting, in 1902 the expulsion of fee splitters from local medical societies and, in 1912, making fee splitting a violation of its ethical code. In working toward this position, the association's Judicial Council conducted a survey of prominent members of the profession. The results were reported by the Judicial Council: "It is interesting to note that in the replies given stating whether or not secret fee splitting was justifiable, there was 77.3 percent who answered in the negative, 13.4 percent who ansered in the affirmative, and 9.3 percent who were doubtful" (13a, p.952).

Why did the AMA act so late? Simply because it was a relatively new practice and problem.

The AMA's principles of ethics had always condemned unnecessary surgery, as had the profession from at least the times of Hippocrates. While the AMA and the ACS condemned it, however, it was difficult to get a handle on the problem until the specialty of pathology was well developed and used and until the mandated recording of pathology reports on all hospital surgical cases in the 1950s by the hospital accrediting body (the Joint Commission on Accreditation of Hospitals [JCAH]). The JCAH not only forced hospitals to monitor surgical practices but also sent inspection teams in as part of the accrediting process. Hospitals more or less had to go along if they wanted to be accredited, and this they wanted in order to get paid by Blue Cross and other health-insurance companies. But even then the problem persisted in large measure because of disagreements on the indications for surgical intervention. As one specialist in internal medicine told the author, "everyone has hemorrhoids, but that doesn't mean that everyone should have a hemorrhoidectomy." The issue of unnecessary surgery will be discussed more extensively in a later chapter.

Ghost surgery apparently was not recognized as a problem until the 1930s. The practice died out with the widespread acceptance of hospital accreditation and acceptance by the GPs of their newly defined role.

Perhaps the most significant contributions of the ACS were the requirements it established for fellowship in the college. Stevens notes that "prerequisites included a one year internship, three years as an assistant, fifty case abstracts, visits to surgical clinics, and for graduates of 1920 and after, two years of college before medical school" (4, p.92). This suggested a pattern for the certifying specialists, the first specialty-certifying board being established in 1917. Clearly, the ACS requirements were devices for the employment of peer pressure to improve. While the college could not license surgeons, it could pass professional judgment and approve of accomplishments and of behavior. As a voluntary group, however, it could only judge those who appeared voluntarily before it. Once accepted into fellowship, there was little that could be done in the beginning to monitor continued excellence; this came much later. All these developments by the ACS were important but not enough. The next step was to inspect the places in which internships were provided, that is, in the general and special hospitals around the nation. Both the AMA and the ACS moved on this front.

The AMA began to pay attention to the internship at the time it established its Council on Medical Education. The council surveyed hospitals that were offering internships and in 1914 published its first list of approved internship hospitals. At about the same time, the ACS began to think about establishing hospital standards for surgical practice; in 1916, it received a Carnegie grant for this purpose. Stevens tells us that at one point the ACS asked the AMA to provide leadership with regard to hospital standardization but that the cost appeared too much for AMA resources and the ACS was forced to go it alone (4, p.119). The first list of hospitals that the ACS felt met its standards was ready in 1919, but the conditions reported were so bad that the college suppressed the list. In 1924, the Council on Medical Education began to approve hospitals for residency (specialty) training programs. A key requirement at that time was that the hospital must first have approval for internship programs.

These advances did not, of course, take place in a vacuum. Other forces were at work among the ophthalmologists, National Board of Medical Examiners, Federation of State Medical Boards, and others.

THE DEVELOPMENT OF SPECIALTY BOARDS

Treatment of eye conditions was the domain of many. Optometrists, who were not medically qualified, were active in the field, as were general practitioners. The specialty within medicine only began to emerge during the latter part of the nineteenth century, aided greatly by the developments of the ophthalmoscope and anesthesia.

Over the years, those physicians who developed a special interest in problems of the eye organized specialist organizations. There were three principle organizations. The AMA had within its scientific groups a Section on Ophthalmology. Then there were the American Ophthalmological Society and the American Academy of Ophthalmology and Otolaryngology. There were, in addition, a number of regional and state groups. Concern within each of these groups over the quality of ophthalmologic training and practice and the appropriate role for the nonmedically qualified optometrists led the three national bodies to get together and to recommend, in 1915, to each of their organizations that a single specialty board be sponsored, the board to consist of three representatives from each of the societies, and that "the board would appoint examiners, hold examinations, and determine requirements; that it would grant a certificate or diploma; and that the specialty societies should limit their membership to diplomates" (4, p.113). The two societies and the AMA Section on Ophthalmology approved, and, in 1917, the first specialty board was incorporated, the American Board for Ophthalmic Examinations, which was renamed, in 1933 the American Board of Ophthalmology.

Societies of a closely related group of physicians incorporated the second specialty board in 1924, the American Board of Otolaryngology. They were closely related because many specialists in this area also include ophthalmology in their practices. Younger specialists in these areas today are either ophthalmologists or otolaryngologists, the latter known as ENT (ear, nose, throat) specialists. It is not uncommon, however, to find some older physicians who consider themselves EENT (eye, ear, nose, throat) specialists. But they are a dying breed. It was not until the 1930s that other specialty boards were established.

The American Board of Ophthalmology set the pattern for specialty recognition in the nation, that is, a national body sponsored by the generally recognized (i.e.,recognized by widespread peer reputation) specialty groups. These groups consisted in each case of the one or more specialty societies and the appropriate specialty section of the AMA. The logic for legitimacy was simple: any specialist worthy of recognition belonged to one or more of the sponsoring groups. This did not mean that a physician could not be a competent specialist without belonging, but it did say that if that self-styled specialist wanted outside professional recognition of competence, he or she had to belong to one of the societies or to the AMA scientific section. If the specialist belonged, then the society or AMA section, as a representative body, could legitimately sponsor a specialty board.

Over a span of time, each of the specialty societies modified their requirements for membership. One common element, however, became that of certification by the appropriate specialty board.

The number of specialty boards in 1978 stands at 22; 20 of these boards are *primary* boards. Two of the boards are *conjoint* boards. These two are the American Board of Allergy and Immunology (a conjoint board of the American Board of Pediatrics and of the American Board of Internal Medicine), and the American Board of Nuclear Medicine (a conjoint board of the American Board of Internal Medicine, the American Board of Pathology, and the American Board of Radiology). The latter is also sponsored by the Society of Nuclear Medicine.

A new specialty is in the advanced stages of development; the American Board of Emergency Medicine, which was initially sponsored by three groups: the AMA's Section on Emergency Medicine, the American College of Emergency Physicians, and the University Association of Emergency Medical Services. The application by this developing board was submitted to the Liaison Committee for Specialty Boards (LCSB), which body is the joint creation of the AMA's Council on Medical Education and of the American Board of Medical Specialties (ABMS). The latter (ABMS) is a coordinative body representing the 22 existing approved specialty boards, with five cooperating or associate members who are there for liaison purposes: the American Hospital Association, the Association of American Medical Colleges, Council of Medical Specialty Societies, the Federation of State Medical Boards of the USA, and the National Board of Medical Examiners. The application of the American Board of Emergency Medicine is somewhat controversial in that some of the existing specialties believe that, at most, it should be a subspecialty of one or more of the existing boards. In 1977 Emergency Medicine was disapproved as a primary specialty, but its sponsors persisted, and in early 1979 it received tentative approval as a *conjoint* board. Final approval is scheduled for September 1979. In addition to the three sponsoring societies the new board will consist of representatives from seven primary specialties boards, including the specialties of family practice, pediatrics, and surgery, which had earlier opposed elevation of Emergency Medicine to specialty status.

Table 2-4 lists the approved boards in the medical specialties and subspecialties as of late 1978. Table 2-5 lists the specialties and subspecialties for osteopathic medicine.

When the ABMS was established (as the Advisory Board for Medical Specialties) in 1933, there were only four existing certifying boards: Obstetrics and Gynecology, Ophthalmology, Otololaryngology, and Dermatology and Syphilology, (later renamed Dermatology). But the trend toward establishment of specialty certifying boards was clearly established, and to keep some sense of order, the existing boards met in 1933 with representatives from other organizations. The Advisory Board of Medical Specialties resulted, with the then four specialty groups as founding members plus the American Hospital Association, the Association of American Medical Colleges, the the Federation of State Medical Boards, and the National Board of Medical Examiners. In 1970, the board was reorganized and became the American Board of Medical Specialities with the AHA, AAMC, FSMB, and the NBME as associate members. A fifth associate member joined in 1973, the Council of Medical Specialty Societies. The regular members consist of representatives from each of the approved primary and conjoint medical specialty boards. It will be noted that the AMA is neither a regular nor an associate member. Hence, the need for the LCSB, which was formally established in 1948, although both groups collaborated from the beginning.

The *Annual Report* of the ABMS states the organization's purpose (15).

The Statement of Purpose included in the Articles of Incorporation is:

- To improve the standards of medical care.
- To act as spokesman for all approved specialty boards, as a group.

- To resolve problems encountered among and between specialty boards.
- To deal with the applications for approval of proposed new specialty boards, subsidiary boards, new types of certification, modification of existing types of certification and related matters.
- To endeavor to avoid duplication of effort by specialty boards.
- To establish and maintain minimal standards of organization and operation of specialty boards.

The *Annual Report* also describes the nature and function of specialty boards:

The primary objective of specialty boards is improvement in the quality of medical education and medical care.

The primary function of each of the specialty boards is to evaluate candidates in its field who appear voluntarily for examination, and to certify as diplomates those who are qualified. To accomplish this function, specialty boards determine if candidates have received adequate preparation in accordance with established educational standards; they provide comprehensive examinations to evaluate such candidates; and they certify physicians who have satisfied the requirements.

In collaboration with other organizations and agencies concerned, the approved specialty boards assist in improving the quality of medical education by elevating the standards of graduate medical education and approving facilities for specialty training.

The actual accreditation review for approval of residency programs in each specialty is carried out by a Residency Review Committee on which each Specialty Board has equal representation with the Council on Medical Education and in some cases, with a related specialty society as well.

Each individual specialty board is composed of specialists qualified in the particular field represented by that board. Their members are derived from the several national specialty organizations in related fields and related sections of the AMA. They endeavor to maintain on the board appropriate representation of specialists according to their:

- geographic distribution,
- type of practice and academic relationships,
- qualification in the appropriate subspecialties,
- demonstrated motivation and ability in assisting in the evaluation procedures leading toward certification.

In addition to approval by and membership in the American Board of Medical Specialties, all such boards are also approved by the American Medical Association.

Finally, the ABMS *Annual Report* prints an official policy statement on the significance of certification in medical specialties:

A. GENERAL PRINCIPLES

Medical specialty certification in the United States, from its inception has been a voluntary precedure. Since the establishment of the first nationally recognized medical specialty board in 1917, some physicians have elected to seek formal recognition of their qualifications in their chosen specialty fields by presenting themselves for examination before specialty boards comprised of their professional peers. The definitions of each of the specialties and of the educational and other requirements leading to eligibility for board certification have been developed by consensus within the medical profession and, to date, the certification of a medical specialist has remained separate and distinct from licensure by civil authorities of professionals qualified to practice medicine within their jurisdictions.

The voluntary nature of specialty certification is attested to further by the fact that as of December 31, 1973, only 46 percent of the 308,127 physicians not in training included in the national registry of physicians maintained by the American Medical Association are diplomates of one or more of the 22 member Boards of the American Board of Medical Specialties. Yet, as Levit, et al., have recently demonstrated, the trend toward specialty board recognition is accelerating and during the current decade "virtually all United State graduates will undertake residency training and seek specialty certification."

The growth in medical specialty certification must be differentiated from the parallel increasing trend of physicians voluntarily to designate special areas of interest or areas of special practice to which they devote the largest segment of their professional time, whether or not they are diplomates of the 22 member boards of the American Board of Medical Specialties. For such purposes the American Medical Association has expanded its list of specialty designations to 67 categories to assist the individual physician in describing his primary field of medicine for listing in the American Medical Directory. There are no professional or legal requirements for a licensed physician to seek specialty board certification in order to offer his professional services in his specialty.

Many thoughtful observers, both within and outside of the profession, caution that the progressive fragmentation of medicine into more and more medical specialties and subspecialties is contrary to the best interests of the public. Nevertheless, the established specialty boards—as well as the American Board of Medical Specialties itself—increasingly are facing concerted pressures to offer certification in additional specialty or subspecialty categories. This is occurring despite the fact that accreited educational programs and the evaluative examinations on which general certifications are based assign appropriate emphasis to each of the subspecialties—or areas of special competence—identified with the corresponding primary field. Accordingly, diplomates holding general certification normally acquire, to a greater or lesser degree, all of such special competencies in their educational and specialty practice experience.

There is no requirement or necessity for a diplomate in a recognized specialty to hold special certification in a subspecialty of that field in order to be considered qualified to include aspects of that subspecialty within a specialty practice. Under no circumstances should a diplomate be considered unqualified to practice within an area of a subspecialty *solely* because of lack of subspecialty certification.

Specialty certification in a subspecialty field is of significance for physicians preparing for careers in teaching, research, or practice restricted to that field. Such special certification is a recognition of exceptional expertise and experience and has not been created to justify a differential fee schedule nor to confer other professional advantages over other diplomates not so certified.

Concentration of practice in a field acceptable for the award of a certificate of special competence may connote expertise in the use of special devices, techniques, or methodologies associated with that field. However, recognition of a subspecialty by the American Board of Medical Specialties must be based on broader principles than such expertise alone. The essential nature of an accepted discipline relates to the body of knowledge or philosophy of action which it encompasses.

Physicians wishing voluntarily to limit their practices to the use of special devices and techniques or methodologies are free to do so, but if they wish to have specialty board certification, it should be within one of the specialties which includes the use of the related device, technique, or methodology, along with the more basic body of knowledge that is applied through their use.

Approval of a new area for special certification, sometimes identified as subspecialty certification or as certification of special competence, signifies that there has been a thorough and critical review of the proposals by Committee on Certification, Subcertification, and Recertification, by the Executive Committee, and by the full Membership. This critical review includes recognition of the fact that such approval is accompanied by related decisions by educational institutions to provide training in such areas.

Chart 1-1.

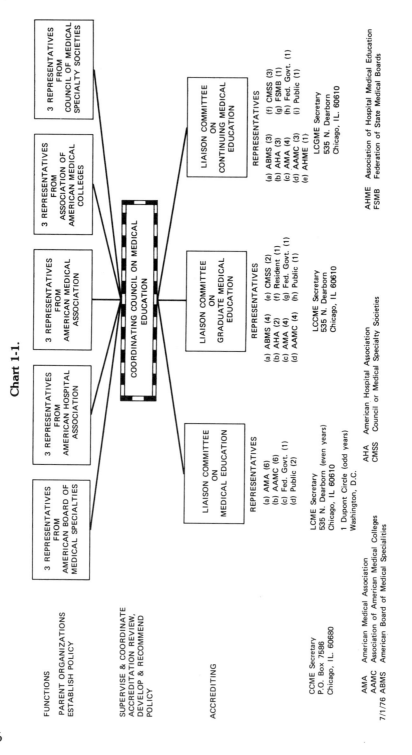

FUNCTIONS

PARENT ORGANIZATIONS
ESTABLISH POLICY

3 REPRESENTATIVES FROM AMERICAN BOARD OF MEDICAL SPECIALTIES

3 REPRESENTATIVES FROM AMERICAN HOSPITAL ASSOCIATION

3 REPRESENTATIVES FROM AMERICAN MEDICAL ASSOCIATION

3 REPRESENTATIVES FROM ASSOCIATION OF AMERICAN MEDICAL COLLEGES

3 REPRESENTATIVES FROM COUNCIL OF MEDICAL SPECIALTY SOCIETIES

SUPERVISE & COORDINATE ACCREDITATION REVIEW, DEVELOP & RECOMMEND POLICY

COORDINATING COUNCIL ON MEDICAL EDUCATION

ACCREDITING

LIAISON COMMITTEE ON MEDICAL EDUCATION

REPRESENTATIVES

(a) AMA (6)
(b) AAMC (6)
(c) Fed. Govt. (1)
(d) Public (2)

LCME Secretary
535 N. Dearborn (even years)
Chicago, IL 60610

1 Dupont Circle (odd years)
Washington, D.C.

LIAISON COMMITTEE ON GRADUATE MEDICAL EDUCATION

REPRESENTATIVES

(a) ABMS (4)   (e) CMSS (2)
(b) AHA (2)   (f) Resident (1)
(c) AMA (4)   (g) Fed. Govt. (1)
(d) AAMC (4)   (h) Public (1)

LCCME Secretary
535 N. Dearborn
Chicago, IL 60610

LIAISON COMMITTEE ON CONTINUING MEDICAL EDUCATION

REPRESENTATIVES

(a) ABMS (3)   (f) CMSS (3)
(b) AHA (3)   (g) FSMB (1)
(c) AMA (4)   (h) Fed. Govt. (1)
(d) AAMC (3)   (i) Public (1)
(e) AHME (1)

LCGME Secretary
535 N. Dearborn
Chicago, IL 60610

CCME Secretary
P.O. Box 7586
Chicago, IL 60680

AMA	American Medical Association
AAMC	Association of American Medical Colleges
ABMS	American Board of Medical Specialties

7/1/76

AHA	American Hospital Association
CMSS	Council or Medical Specialty Societies

AHME	Association of Hospital Medical Education
FSMB	Federation of State Medical Boards

B. THE RESPONSIBILITY FOR SELF-REGULATION OF SPECIALIZATION IN MEDICINE

Various specialty boards, with approval of the American Board of Medical Specialties, have been developing and offering increasing numbers of special certifications in the past several years. The reaction to requests for such recognition and special competence has varied in different boards from quite free acceptance to considerable resistance.

It is only realistic to recognize that subspecialization in many of the areas covered by the various American Boards is already established. The realities and complexities of evolving medical knowledge and practice may well justify the creation of more areas of certification; however, the cost of disciplinary integrity, ready accessibility to definitive medical care by the public, and the expense of the delivery of health care should be carefully considered in the recognition of any further subspecialties.

A practical approach would undoubtedly demand that the American Board of Medical Specialties should exercise control in this area by critical evaluation of all future proposals rather than by attempts to develop too rigid a policy on the establishment of new certifications or by withdrawing recognition of presently established subspecialties. Initiation of an action by a Member Board to withdraw existing certification in the presently established subspecialty should be encouraged if appropriate.

It is the policy of the ABMS that recognition of special certification should be primarily for individuals who are devoting a major proportion of their time and efforts to that restricted special field. Special Certification should be granted only after education and training or experience in addition to that required for general certification in the discipline.

Adopted September 18, 1975

Some additional issues surfaced in the development of specialties. First, establishment of many specialty boards inevitably led to conflicts over definition of the specialty. So long as the specialty, however defined, did not pursue a formal legitimizing process, the need for precise definitions was not imperative, but once the boards were established, definitional or domain or turf problems arose. Many groups experienced these difficulties. Stevens ably recounts the controversy as it developed between the optometrists and ophthalmologists, noting, also, that the controversy there still persists. Controversy developed as well among other medical specialists. Stevens notes, for example, that in the area of surgery, a great many of the medical specialties have surgery as an integral part of the specialty. Most of these specialties were incorporated before the American Board of Surgery (1937). Each carved out for itself a piece of the action, leaving little that can be considered unique to general surgery. With the renaming of the Advisory Board of Medical Specialties to the American Board of Medical Specialties in 1970, the umbrella agency's role was strengthened by receiving authority to coordinate the boards.

A second item to note is that there were a great many organizational conflicts. One can view these conflicts in a negative or positive way. Negatively, they appear as power plays by a body that wishes to dominate. Positively, and I believe more appropriately, they can be viewed as the result of disagreements on how best to do the job. The AMA, for example, at many points, sought to bring things under its umbrella, believing that the stronger the AMA was, in terms of being *the* voice of American medicine, the more persuasive it could be in bringing about lasting improvements. Others, on the other hand, saw movement outside the AMA, but not in opposition to the AMA, as a more effective mechanism. Sometimes the disagreement over strategies were in part conflicts of longterm versus shortterm objectives. Clearly, the AMA was not altogether happy that the specialties developed outside its structure, for it wanted a unified medical profession. On the other hand, during the period the specialties were developing, the AMA's principal support came from its rank-and-file general practitioners, whose anxieties may not have been as great as were those physicians who saw themselves as specialists. One notes in this regard that the AMA's view of its scientific sections was that the sections should primarily be focal points for the dissemination of knowledge to all physicians and not just serve the needs of the highly trained specialists (13a, p.288). Hence, specialty societies and, in time, specialty boards. A major step was taken by the AMA in late 1977 to bring the specialty societies into its policymaking framework. As reported in the AMA's newspaper to its members (16, p.1):

After nearly three hours of heated debate, the AMA's House of Delegates totally revamped the section council system and set specific criteria for giving specialty societies direct representation in the AMA.

The actions, approved by the house at its interim meeting in Chicago, eliminate delegates to the house from the 28 section councils and instead will enable any specialty society that meets the criteria to request the seating of its own delegate.

The move is a major policy change that can greatly expand specialty society representation in the AMA, and in doing so can provide a stronger, more united voice for American medicine, proponents said.

Urging delegates to accept the plan that was drafted by the Council on Long Range Planning and Development and which was hammered out in numerous discussion sessions among many concerned groups, Trustee Joseph F. Boyle, MD, said:

"No other organization is capable of providing the strength of leadership as the AMA. Specialty societies do want to become active participants.

"But they are quite ready to turn elsewhere and in some instances are (if their interest is not encouraged)," he said.

"You have a real chance, that may be fading if you don't seize it now, to accomplish the long-time objective of a strong federation for American medicine in this house," Dr. Boyle warned.

As one looks at the sweep of history, despite some competitiveness and disagreements, the AMA and most all of the organizations sought ways to work together for both the good of their profession and of the public as they saw it. This is evident in the representatives on various committees, set up from time to time by the various organizations. These organizations saw themselves as part of a community in which, to survive, they had to get along with those of standing. The fringe areas, of course, where there may not even be medical qualifications—chiropractors and the like—the AMA and others felt could be attacked, for these peripheral groups were not perceived as legitimate parts of the medical community.

The third item to note relates to specialty terminology. A physician who has completed all specialty requirements except the final board examination is said to be *board eligible* in that specialty. Some specialties, such as orthopedic surgery, require the person to be a board-eligible practitioner in the specialty area before being permitted to take the exam. In other cases, the board-eligible person practices in the specialty area until the exam is scheduled and results reported. In some cases, the board-eligible person never bothers to take the exams. The author of a major textbook on pediatrics who was also professor and head of a university medical school department of pediatrics was, for example, only board eligible. This type of case is, however, relatively rare today. Since *board eligible* can cover a multitude of competencies as well as sins (including those who fail the board exams), there is a move by specialty boards to drop use of this phrase. When the physician passes the specialty exam and is awarded a diploma, he or she is then said to be a *diplomate* (holder of a diploma) or *board certified*.

The fourth item to note is that the time required for training in a specialty varies with the specialty. The training program is known as the *residency* in a particular clinical area. The person being trained is a graduate of a medical school and while in the residency is known as a *resident*. Normally, an appropriate internship is accepted as the equivalent of the final year of residency training. The requirements for each specialty are spelled out in the *Directory of Medical Specialists,* which is published every other year for the ABMS, and they are also published each year by the AMA in its *Directory of Approved Residencies.*

Fifth and finally, we should note that since 1975, the AMA would not approve internships unless they were part of, or led to, specialty training. Before the rapid rise and expansion of the specialties, the graduating physician typically undertook a year of postgraduate supervised training in an approved hospital. This was the internship. Now, however, practically all physicians go on for specialty training. The internship has thus become somewhat redundant for these people, and no specialty board today requires an internship before entering residency.

FEDERATION OF STATE MEDICAL BOARDS AND NATIONAL BOARD OF MEDICAL EXAMINERS

In the last half of the nineteenth century, licensing boards were established and/or reestablished in many of the states. But not all states at the turn of the century required passing a state board licensing exam as illustrated by the following letter to the editor and answer in *JAMA* in 1901 (17, p.817):

Please let me know where a graduate in medicine could practice without the State Board examination.

Answer. The laws of the following states admit graduates to practice medicine without examination, under varying conditions: Arkansas, Colorado, Kentucky, Michigan, Nevada, Nebraska, Oklahoma, Rhode Island, South Dakota, and Wyoming. In some of the states only diplomas from certain schools are recognized: thus in Michigan the diplomas of some forty or fifty schools only are accepted and in Rhode Island similar scrutiny is exercised. In nearly all, more or less discrimination is made in regard to certain schools, but in these states more particularly than others.

Womack notes that Texas was the first of the state boards of medical examiners in this renascence period, beginning in 1873. He goes on to say that (17, p.819)

---

by 1901, 23 states required more than a diploma for licensure, and there were 37 states requiring certain credentials for licensure. By the turn of the century, already a few states had formed groups that could exchange the recognition of credentials, an action that became known as "reciprocity."

Such a cooperative venture was at that time not too successful, for the legislation governing the qualification for medical practice differed widely in the various states, as did the effectiveness of the examination. Some examining boards scrutinized a candidate with unusual care. Others did not. Some did not require an examination. Others did. Some examining boards quickly became the pawn of political influence and, too often, could not maintain the type of respect from other boards that would be needed to make reciprocity universal. By 1900, in many areas, the situation was not a happy one.

The need for some kind of national standard was apparent to many. But to bring this about was not easy. As with so many change efforts in all fields, resistance is often encountered. The National Confederation of Medical Examining and Licensing Boards, for example, had considered the question of a national examining board but had disapproved the idea. Some states still wanted something done in this regard, and Derbyshire states that the Wisconsin board worked out an exchange plan with the Michigan board in 1901 (18, p.50). The following year, these states met with representatives from Illinois and Indiana, and they established the Confederation of Reciprocating State Medical Examining Boards. Derbyshire states that soon afterward "its membership was increased and its aim broadened to include efforts to improve educational standards and to promote uniform legislation for medical licensure." Merger of the two organizations was achieved in 1912 with the formation of the Federation of State Medical Boards. By 1914, 26 boards were members. Despite many developmental problems over disagreements as to the aims of the federation, by 1978, all medical (MD) boards were members; there are, as well, eight member osteopathic examining boards.

During the early part of this century, there was interest on the part of some in the AMA in national licensure, but this never became a strong movement because of constitutional concerns over the question of state rights. This is a nice way of stating two related points of view: concern over federal bureaucratic control of the right to practice and concern by state boards not only over their rights (self-preservation) but also the belief held by many that the state boards were better able to assess the competence to practice medicine. One should not snicker at the defensiveness of some state boards on this issue. If, after all, standards were generally low nationally, any national system would have to have standards low enough so that most states could qualify. Otherwise, a national system would not be acceptable. Why, then, should a state board with very high standards opt for a system that would lower that state's standards? This is in part why the federation's early successes were limited.

Reformers wanted to see a raising of standards throughout the nation, however, and, with that, increased reciprocity. In addition, they wanted some mechanism to assure high-quality physicians in the federal services. The idea, then, of some kind of national examining system as a means for comparing medical graduates from the different schools had a lot going for it, and this led, by 1915, to the formation of the National Board of Medical Examiners (NBME). The initial board included, among others, representatives of the navy, army, Public Health Service, the Federation of State Medical Boards, the AAMC, the ACS, and the AMA. The critically important position of secretary was filled by Dr. William L. Rodman, who announced the formation of the NBME (a month after its establishment) during his presidential address at the AMA meeting in San Francisco in June 1915. Rodman labored hard to develop this new organization. He served as professor of surgery at a number of medical schools, was president of the AAMC in 1903 and 1904, active in AMA clinical affairs and politics, serving in the House of Delegates from 1900 to 1903 and for many years as chairman of its Committee on Reciprocity, and was a founding fellow of the ACS. In 1915 he became the sixty-seventh president of the AMA.

Rodman's career is interesting because it illustrates the kind of pathways through which many medical leaders worked and still work. They wear many hats, some of them at the same time. One person is thus able to exert influence in a number of organizations. One can hypothesize, also, that the whole idea of federal representation on the NBME stemmed from a 1902 editorial in JAMA, which has been attributed to Rodman, that called for a national board to examine the qualifications of physicians who serve in the federal services, and this was, in part, prompted by Rodman's experiences previously as an army surgeon. While early federal-government representation later caused some concern in the ranks of medicine, Womack notes that in some of the developmental stages of the NBME, these representatives provided needed consistent support (17, p.821).

The AMA's endorsement of the NBME came in 1916, and with that endorsement, the NBME was fully legitimized. The AMA noted in its resolution of endorsement that two legal forces—government medical services and state licensing boards—were represented on the NBME and that "finances have been generously provided for its maintenance for a number of years (17, p.820). Who provided that generous financial support? None other than the Carnegie Foundation for the Advancement of Teaching.

The NBME quickly began work administering the first exam in late 1916. Thirty-two applicants asked to take the exam, but only 16 were considered sufficiently qualified. Womack reports that only 10 took it, and only five passed. "Between 1916 and 1921, 11 examinations were held. There were, in all, 498 applicants, 427 qualified to take the examination; 325 appeared and 269 passed (17, p.820). Initially, eight states indicated that they would accept NBME test results for licensure. Over the years, as testing procedures improved, as state boards were reassured that the NBME would not usurp their prerogatives and become the licensing agency, more and more states accepted the results. By 1965, all but six states licensed physicians who passed the NBME exams. But there were many variations, and some states insisted on setting their own exams, constructed from the NBME pool of questions, graded by NBME, but administered by the states under their names. Some states, moreover, insisted on special basic-science examinations, a barrier to licensure, which is, Derbyshire states, a matter of increasing exasperation to medical educators and physicians. "In these days of rapid growth of medical knowledge, the burgeoning of medical education, and the increasing mobility of the population, basic science requirements are considered by many to be anachronistic stumbling blocks to medical licensure (18,p.118). The original intent of these laws was to deal not so much with physician deficiencies but with chiropracters, cultists, and the like. In states that have these laws, a certificate of proficiency is given by the examining board and must be presented when applying for a license to practice one of the healing arts.

Despite the significant advances brought about through the NBME exams, state structuring of some exams (from NBME questions) by boards whose personnel were always changing and who generally had no expertise in testing procedures, coupled with state determination of pass levels, prompted concern. Derbyshire notes, for example, that some states rarely failed applicants. Other states had high failure rates, and one state apparently gave special treatment (favorable) to its native sons. These variations posed very real problems in terms of facilitating reciprocity (endorsement). In addition, the NBME exams were not given to graduates of foreign medical schools—during the late 1940s, there began a pattern of foreign medical-graduate movement to the United States.

We should note at this juncture that we do not usually refer to graduates of Canadian schools as foreign medical graduates (FMGs). Because of the similarities between the educational systems and the medical-school accreditation process (which was until recently the same accreditation body), graduates of approved Canadian schools are considered eligible to be examined by all state boards on the same basis as U.S. graduates, and about half of the states will grant reciprocity. In recent years, this receptivity by the United States of Canadian graduates has not been viewed sympathetically by the Canadian government because of the talent drain to the south.

The problems that arose, from variations between the states that adapted the NBME tests to their uses, concerned enough of the state boards so that a move began to improve on the situation by creating one national test. The vehicle for this effort was the Federation of State Medical Boards of the United States, which developed the Federation Licensing Examination (FLEX), and FLEX is now accepted by all state boards for medical licensure. The exam is developed nationally by the federation from NBME questions. It is administered by each state and graded by the NBME; scores are recorded by the federation for reference purposes and are reported to the appropriate state boards, which determine their own pass levels. Thus, a state does not have to endorse another state's license (since the latter's pass score may not be acceptable to the former) but can simply refer to the federation records to ascertain the candidate's performance on FLEX and thereby determine whether or not the candidate meets its pass standard. Graduates of foreign medical schools are now able to take a standardized national exam.

FLEX is described by the federation as "an objective, multiple choice comprehensive examination designed to test knowledge and ability in the basic medical sciences, the clinical sciences and competence in patient management" (19, p.5). It is a three-day examination. The first day covers basic science material relating to anatomy, physiology, biochemistry, microbiology, pathology, and pharmacology. The questions, moreover, may cut across disciplinary lines. The second day covers the traditional clinical subjects of medicine, obstetrics and gynecology, pediatrics, preventive medicine and public health, psychiatry, and surgery. The third day tests clinical competence (19, p.5):

Day III uses techniques designed specially to test clinical competence and ability to manage patients. The first section consists of objective questions related to graphic and pictorial materials such as roentgenograms, gross lesions, gross and microscopic pathological specimens, blood smears, graphs, etc. The other two sections use a form of programmed testing by erasure technique whereby the examinee is presented with a description of a clinical situation and then given the opportunity to choose or reject procedures or modes of management from a list of offered choices, in such a manner that the results of his selections are reported to him.

The NBME exams are also still administered. They are in three parts: part I, taken toward the end of second-year medical school; part II, toward the end of the last year; and part III, during or on completion of the internship or first year of residency training. There is an obvious advantage to the National Boards in that the candidate takes part I, the basic science portion, when the material is freshest. As is noted in the next chapter, however, taking part I may not be practical, given changes in some medical curricula, and a single exam, given at the end of the undergraduate medical education process is now being considered. As this happens, the need for both National Boards and FLEX will undoubtedly come into question.

It should be noted, finally, that both exams are under regular revision and that changes are made on the basis of new knowledge, new views as to what a physician should know, and as new testing techniques become available or recognized. The change process, however, is a slow one because the federation is a representative body of autonomous state licensing boards, and each of these boards has to deal with their own state licensing laws, change of which is not always easily accomplished because of differing views, usually honestly held, as to what should be required for licensing of a physician.

Is the time now at hand for a national licensing system? The idea of national licensure of physicians has been bandied about for nearly a century. While some of the objections that were previously noted may no longer be valid, a move for national licensure would require, in all probability, an amendment to the U.S. Constitution. A proposed amendment, moreover, would inevitably raise the question of national licensure for all other practitioners—in health, law, engineering, and so on. In view of the deep-seated tradition of states' rights, a national licensing system is a remote notion.

CONCLUSION

At any point in time, the health system seems riddled with weaknesses, but when it is studied over a long period of time, enormous changes for the better can be seen, changes brought about by health professionals working through a variety of professional bodies. Leadership within the medical profession, and particularly within the AMA, has had an enormous positive impact. The changes that have been brought about were, by and large, not sweeping. Each change was, rather, an incremental, negotiated step that most who might be affected could accept and support. The role of government, except for the army and navy chiefs, is significant by its absence. The prevailing view of the times was that health matters were the domain of the physicians, that what they decided or wanted was appropriate. It is for this reason that state licensing, like state boards of health, fell under the early control of the medical profession.

Shortcomings in our health system still exist, and change is occurring. As in the past, the change is usually a negotiated settlement, negotiated not because some don't want to act but because there are disagreements over how best to act.

REFERENCES

1. Packard, F.R.: *History of Medicine in the United States*. New York, Hafner Publishing Co., 1963.
2. Shryock, R.H.: *Medicine and Society in America, 1660-1860*. New York, New York University Press, 1960.

3. Corner, G.W.: *Two Centuries of Medicine, A History of the School of Medicine—University of Pennsylvania*. Philaelphia, J.B.Lippincott Co., 1965.

4. Stevens, R.: *American Medicine and the Public Interest*. New Haven, Yale University Press, 1971.

5. Shryock, R.H.: The Early American Public Health Movement. Am J Public Health, October 1937 (reprinted in Shryock, R.H.: *Medicine in America* Baltimore, Johns Hopkins Press, 1966. p. 131).

6. Norwood, W.F.: *Medical Education in the United States Before the Civil War*. Philadelphia, University of Pennsylvania Press, 1944.

7. Burrow, J.G.: *American Medical Association—Voice of American Medicine*. Baltimore, Johns Hopkins Press, 1963.

8. Bonner, T.N.: *American Doctors and German Universities*. Lincoln, University of Nebraska Press, 1963.

8a. Shoyock, R.H.: *Medicine in America*. Baltimore, Johns Hopkins Press, 1966

9. Coggeshall, L.T.: *Planning for Medical Progress Through Education*. Evanston, Association of American Medical Colleges, 1965.

10. Johnson, V.: The Council On Medical Education and Hospitals, Fishbein, Morris (ed.): *A History of the American Medical Association, 1847-1947*. Philadelphia, W.B. Saunders Co., 1947.

11. Flexner, A.: *I Remember*.New York, Simon and Schuster, 1940.

12. Flexner, A.: *Medical Education in the United States and Canada,* bulletin 4. New York, The Carnegie Foundation for the Advancement of Teaching, 1910.

13. Shryock, R.H.: The American physician. *JAMA* 134: May 31, 1947; (reprinted in Shryock, H.R. *Medicine in America*. Baltimore, Johns Hopkins Press, 1966, p. 168.)

13a. Fishbein, Morris (ed): *A History of the American Medical Association, 1847-1947*. Philadelphia, W.B. Saunders, Co. 1947.

14. Bond, A.K.: *When the Hopkins Came to Baltimore*. Baltimore, Pegasus Press, 1927.

15. American Board of Medical Specialties, *Annual Report,* 1976_1977, Evanston, Ill.

16. *American Medical News,* December 12, 1977.

17. Quoted by Womack, N.A.: The evolution of the National Board of Medical Examiners. *JAMA,* 192: June 7, 1965

18. Derbyshire, R.C.: *Medical Licensure and Discipline in the United States*. Baltimore, Johns Hopkins Press, 1969.

19. *FLEX,* 4 ed. Description of Examination, The Federation of State Medical Boards of the United States,

2
Medical Education

The medical-education continuum consists of four segments: premedical education, undergraduate medical education, graduate medical education, and postgraduate or continuing medical education.

PREMEDICAL EDUCATION

The first segment in the medical-education process is the premedical school or premedical period of study. This is undertaken in colleges and universities and leads to a baccalaureate degree. At this stage, there is no commitment to the student that he or she will be able to go on to become a physician. While most premedical students tend to major in the sciences, they can, in fact, major in most any academic program so long as they take the needed science and other courses that medical schools require for admission. About 7% of the entering medical students do not hold a baccalaureate degree. These are generally students in a number of integrated medical-premedical programs typically covering six calendar years of study instead of eight.*

Because medicine is a high-prestige and well-paying profession and because, for the foreseeable future, most all physicians will be able to make a good living, the supply of physicians never really exceeding the demand, becoming a physician is attractive to many students. Because of this, the competition for entrance to medical school is very intense, and it is becoming more intense as the opportunities that medicine offers increase and as the appeal of other fields lessen due to oversupply of people and lack of work in those other fields. The AMA's Council of Medical Education reports some interesting data (from which

---

*The data, unless otherwise specified, refer to the medical schools that grant or will grant the M.D. degree. The osteopathic schools do not always have comparable data.

I have structured Table 2-1), which reflects on the competitive situation vis-à-vis medical-school application and admissions (1).*

Applications peaked in 1974-1975 and dropped slightly over the next three years. However, the number of applications per individual rose, reflecting a recognition on the part of applicants as to the difficulty in getting admitted. Also, the premedical grade-point averages of those matriculating clearly rose.

Medical-school admission is based, however, on a number of factors in addition to grade-point average. These other factors include performance on the Medical College Admission Test (MCAT), which nearly all accepted applicants take, recommendations, and interviews. The MCAT is an objective test of verbal ability, quantitative ability, general information, and science. Table 2-2 shows a rise in the mean test score of accepted applicants for all categories except general information, which peaked in 1968-1969. One might hypothesize that the decline of the test scores for general information and the rise in other categories reflects the intense pressure under which most premedical students operate.

Another weighted factor is the report to the medical school from the students' premedical advisers. In many schools, this confidential report is a committee report, which serves to minimize risks of bias. Interviews by the medical schools of applicants are also considered important by many as a mechanism for assessing personality factors on which tests and recommendations may not shed adequate light. Not all schools or medical educators are satisfied with the interview mechanism because it is fraught with the risk of interviewer bias, and the search continues, therefore, for other methods of assessment of these factors.

For many years, medical schools were dominated by white, middle-class men. The cost of going to medical school contributed to the middle-class element; race and sex discrimination contributed to the other elements.

Deliberate discrimination against racial minorities has virtually been eliminated. Whether there is unconscious discrimination because of the grade and testing factors long accepted for selection of applicants is a matter of some debate. To the extent that medical schools rely on grades and MCAT scores, they are relying on fairly objective factors, although some argue that objective tests are frequently culturally biased—particularly the general-information sections—and are therefore not truly objective.† As many families will attest, it is

---

*Most of the data in this chapter are drawn from this report. The data were generated by AMA and AAMC staffs. This report is updated and printed annually in *JAMA*.

†Course grading is more objective than most students would grant. There are, to be sure, errors and variations between instructors. Over the long haul, however, a student's college record with some 40 + courses tend to show a pattern. In a sense, the student is judged by 40 + jurors over a four-year period. The individual course grade, while sometimes painful and sometimes flattering, is simply one event in a game of 40 + events.

Table 2-1. Medical School Admissions

First-year Class	Applicants	Applications per Individual	Number Accepted	Number Matriculating	Premed Grade-Point Average of Class (Percentage)			
					A	B	C	Unknown
1956-1957	15,917	3.8	8,263	8,014	—	—	—	—
1965-1966	18,703	4.7	9,012	8,769	12.7	76.7	10.6	—
1968-1969	21,118	5.3	10,092	9,863	16.8	75.9	7.3	—
1974-1975	42,624	8.5	15,066	14,963	39.3	50.8	3.0	6.8
1976-1977	42,155	8.8	15,774	15,667	46.0	47.3	2.7	4.0
1977-1978	40,569	9.2	15,977	16,134	50.4	43.0	1.6	5.0

"A": 3.6-4.0 on a four-point scale.
"B": 2.6-3.5.
"C": less than 2.6.

Source: Medical education in the United States, 1977-1978: 78th Annual Report on Medical Education. JAMA, 240: 1978.

Table 2-2. Mean MCAT Scores of Accepted Applicants for Selected Years

Year	Verbal	Quantitative	General Information	Science	Number Taking MCAT	Number Accepted
1956-1957	525	525	526	519	8,012	8,263
1965-1966	541	583	565	549	8,983	9,012
1968-1969	556	600	570	577	10,010	10,092
1974-1975	563	611	559	603	14,943	15,066
1976-1977	573	633	549	618	15,584	15,774
1977-1978	580	633	559	639	15,524	15,977

Source: Medical education in the United States, 1977-1978 78th Annual Report on Medical Education. *JAMA*, 240: 1978.

far better to rely on objective factors than on religion, complexion, or the sound of the name, all of which were once used to exclude a number of religious groups and a great many Americans of Asiatic and European origins. The dilemma facing medical schools, as well as others, is how to increase the opportunities for racial minorities through the identification and elimination of nondeliberate, racially discriminatory practices without, at the same time, opening the door for reintroduction of some of the evil practices that once prevailed. Virtue, when once attained, is not a constant. In the attempt to increase opportunities for racial minorities, the medical schools have made significant progress to the extent that 12.6% of the 1977-1978 first-year class could be classified as being from racial minorities. Problems, however, have existed relating to academic performance in that 8.5% of the minorities in the first-year class were repeating the first year studies due to previous unsatisfactory performance. This compares to 1.6% report for other first-year students(1, p. 2824). The earlier discriminatory practices of medical schools contributed to the development of a number of Afro-American medical schools, two of which still exist: Meharry and Howard. A third predominantly black school is being developed in Georgia at Morehouse College. Also under development is the American Indian Medical School in Arizona.

Discrimination against women has been pronounced, more so in the United States than in many of the European countries. A number of factors undoubtedly entered into the exclusion of women, and the literature quoting some of the reasons is quite humorous, provided one can find humor in the widely held male notions about the intellectual inferiority of women and their need to maintain modesty and to preserve their delicate nature. The exclusion of women led to the development of a number of women's medical colleges, the last of which, the Medical College of Pennsylvania, still survives. It is, however, no longer exclusively a female institution; the 1976-1977 entering class is only 67% female(1, p. 2893). In most recent times, exclusion of women from medical schools was dictated, at least in part, by the belief that if women completed their training, they would probably get married, have children, and be a loss to the active medical profession. Firm data to support such a position were hard to come by; in the 1970s, under increasing pressure from women, medical-school barriers began to crumble. In 1959-1960, the entering medical-school class was 6% female; in 1976-1977, the percentage rose to 25.7%(1, p. 2823).

The attrition or dropout rate from medical school for all students is of some interest. In the early 1960s, it ran between 10 and 12% nationally. It is currently 2%, and most of these students are in the first year(1, p. 2825). Some withdrew because of their poor academic record, others to pursue advanced study in other areas; relatively few withdrew for financial reasons. Why the drop in attrition rate? Competition and improved selection processes account for some of the drop, as well as a more lenient, more understanding, and more tolerant approach to those whose first-year level of performance is not as satisfactory as would be desired. The latter is reflected in the practice of allowing students to repeat the class.

Many critics assert that the current methods for selection place too much emphasis on grades and test scores, excluding from the field of medicine many who would make excellent physicians. They are saying, in other words, that the selection measures are not valid indicators as to which students will make good physicians. While there may be merit in this assertion, changes in the selection processes are not easily accomplished. The facts are that the current methods have served to reduce the attrition rate and have facilitated elimination of many of the irrational, subjective, and discriminatory measures once employed. While medical schools would generally be amenable to use of alternative selection methods, no satisfactory ones have yet been identified.

The premedical student is an undergraduate, working toward graduation with some kind of baccalaureate degree. Baccalaureate graduates who then go on not to medical school but to a graduate school in, say, nutrition or philosophy and who study for a master's degree or doctor of philosophy degree are during this period of study called graduate students. Not so medical students. Although they typically hold a baccalaureate degree, in medical school they are considered undergraduates; hence, undergraduate medical education refers to medical schools and their training of physicians who will, on graduation, be awarded a doctor of medicine (M.D.) or doctor of osteopathy (D.O.) degree.

Graduate medical education refers to formalized training post MD or DO in an approved internship or residency. Postgraduate or continuing medical education refers to formalized training on a short course or short-term basis for physicians who have completed a period of graduate medical education and are generally viewed as refresher courses or as intensive courses to develop new skills.

UNDERGRADUATE MEDICAL EDUCATION

For the 1977-1978 academic year, there were 120 fully accredited medical schools in the United States and 16 additional fully accredited schools in Canada (Figs. 2-1 and 2-2). 112 of the accredited U.S. schools and the 16 Canadian schools were accredited to award the M.D. degree. Eight of the fully accredited U.S. schools were accredited to award the degree of Doctor of Osteopathy (D.O.). There are, in addition, 11 U.S. medical (M.D.) schools and six osteopathic (D.O.) schools with provisional accreditation; that is, they have admitted students, will probably become accredited, but can't be until they have graduated their first class. There are also in the developmental stages at least three M.D. schools.

Accreditation of the M.D. schools is by the Liaison Committee on Medical Education (LCME), which is a joint committee established in 1942 by the AMA Council on Medical Education and the AAMC. Each organization has six representatives, and there are, in addition, two public representatives and one from the federal government. The legitimacy of accreditation by the LCME stems from its recognition for this purpose by the United States Commissioner of Education and the Council on Post-secondary Education. Before 1942, the AMA was the only body to inspect medical schools. It wasn't until 1969 that the U.S. Office of Education began to recognize accrediting agencies. In 1976, the Federal Trade Commission (FTC) challenged the appropriateness of the LCME as the official accrediting body, contending that AMA participation might represent a conflict of interest. The FTC conceded that although it didn't have any evidence of misconduct on the part of AMA, the potential for misconduct nevertheless existed. The Office of Education, however, granted continued recognition of the LCME. Instead of the usual four-year recognition, however, it was granted for only two years, and the LCME was asked to correct certain deficiencies relating to its autonomy. Whether the FTC is paranoid or not is yet to be determined, though the author suggests later on in this chapter that alleged AMA restriction of physician supply is not a crucial matter of concern at this time.

Accreditation of the D.O. schools is granted by the American Osteopathic Association (AOA), and its legitimacy in this role has also been acknowledged by the U.S. Commissioner of Education. It might be appropriate at this point to digress a bit and to explain a few things about osteopathic medicine.

Osteopathic Medicine

Osteopathic medicine represents an approach to medical practice employing all the methods traditionally associated with physicians—drugs, laboratory tests, x-ray studies, surgery, and so forth—but advocates also the value of manipulative procedures in the diagnosis and management of disease and injury. The osteopath is a physician, licensed in all of the states to practice medicine and surgery. The osteopath is trained in essentially the same way as the allopathic physician (the osteopathic word for the physician trained in the M.D. schools) and in most of the same specialties.

As a school of medicine, osteopathy developed following the Civil War under the leadership of a former army physician, Andrew Taylor Still. Because his theories received little support from the established schools, Still branched off and opened the first osteopathic school in 1892. Others followed. The osteopathic schools took the same kind of drubbing from Flexner as did the allopathic schools, and osteopathic reform began also to take place.

Osteopathy was strong in the Midwest, where most of the schools were, and still are, located. Because it was a competing approach to medical practice, and because the AMA long sought a unified voice for medicine, there developed over the years considerable antagonism between the two groups. For many years, osteopaths were unable to secure licenses in some states and were given limited licenses in some other states. Today, however, the licensing barrier is down, and they are licensed in all states with the same rights and responsibilities as the M.D.s. In eight states, they are licensed by an M.D. medical board, probably because there are not enough D.O.s in those states to justify a separate or a joint board. In 25 states, there is a joint M.D.-D.O. board. In the remaining states, the osteopaths have their own licensing boards.

The fight between the M.D.s and D.O.s has in recent years subsided. Each group has now inspected each other's schools and satisfied themselves that each is worth associating with the other and that each could serve on each other's faculties and in the same hospitals. Before that, osteopaths had to develop their own hospital system. Occasionally, we hear of an allopathic hospital that won't give privileges to the osteopathic physician, but this is increasingly rare. The wounds were opened for a while in California where the osteopaths could trade in their degrees and be given an allopathic degree in return; the D.O. school became an M.D. school; the state law then provided that new D.O.s could not practice in California. Since 85% of the 3,000 D.O.s had converted to M.D.s, that left only 450 D.O.s who held firm and who could continue to practice with assurance that their numbers in California would not increase and that they were a dying breed. The California law was declared unconstitutional in 1974 by the California Supreme Court.

While the AMA apparently wanted to absorb the osteopathic movement, the latter felt it better to stay apart, believing that it could work for objectives it valued if it stayed outside the AMA framework. D.O.s were thus prohibited by the AOA from joining M.D. medical societies, but enforcement of this prohibition was apparently ignored in states where there were relatively few osteopaths perhaps because it was believed that it is important for physicians to associate professionally with other physicians, and if there aren't many D.O.s, then M.D.s will do! The AOA prohibition against D.O. membership in the AMA and other allopathic societies was dropped in the summer of 1979.

Is there any real difference between what an osteopath does and what an allopath does? Osteopathic philosophy speaks of understanding the whole person and treating the patient as a total unit. But the allopaths believe this, also, so there is nothing unique on this score. Manipulative therapy is considered unique, but some of this seems to be part of physical medicine and rehabilitation (a specialty within allopathic medicine) and is used to some extent when the

M.D. calls on the physiotherapist. It seems that the average M.D. is not trained to use manipulative therapy at this time, but some osteopaths assert that they really don't use it, anyway.

What is clear, however, is that the osteopathic school, while encompassing all of the traditional medical specialties, does seem to stress family practice more than does the allopathic approach. Approximately 75% of the osteopaths are in primary-care fields, while the percentage of allopaths in primary-care fields is only around 44%. This difference, however, may be a passing one because Bowers notes that "new graduates in osteopathy are showing a greater preference for the nonprimary care specialties" (2, p. 88). In addition, there is growing pressure for and interest in the primary-care specialties within allopathy.

The osteopathic movement is an important one. Osteopaths represent only about 5% of the medical practitioners today, and the percentage may rise slightly as the osteopathic schools expand, but it is not likely to exceed 6% for quite some time.

Most of the data that will appear with regard to medical education will relate to allopathy since the published data by the AMA are more complete than the data available through the AOA.

It should be noted that the osteopath is very different from the chiropractor. The osteopath is a licensed physician; the chiropractor is not. The chiropractor uses manipulative procedures; some use physiotherapy, and some are permitted to take x-ray films for diagnostic purposes.

Medical-School Curriculum

The typical undergraduate medical-education program lasts four years, covering 36 months in all. Some schools permit students to attend during the summer, thus enabling a person to graduate in three calendar years; at seven schools, the three-year curriculum is mandated. Bowers notes, however, that "the 3-year curriculum is losing popularity in some of the schools that adopted it, primarily because of the unduly heavy demands on faculty and students," as well as because "the Federal financial inducement was suddenly withdrawn" (2, p. 74).

Until the 1960s, most medical-school programs followed a basic pattern: Two years were devoted to preclinical studies, mostly in the basic medical sciences (anatomy, physiology, biochemistry, histology, pharmacology, etc.), and two years in the clinical sciences (pediatrics, internal medicine, obstetrics, gynecology, surgery, etc.). Although a lock-step approach, it had one advantage in that it proved easy for students to transfer from a two-year school of basic medical sciences to the third-year class of a four-year school. The basic medical-science area was the big block to expansion of class size in medical school because of the dependence on costly laboratories. If a university could handle that portion of training through a school of basic medical sciences, a medical school in an urban center could easily expand its clinical teaching commitment since large centers have ample hospital patients available for teaching purposes and also have a reservoir of able clinicians who could assist in the teaching process.

While many schools still adhere to some extent to this pattern because full appreciation of clinical medicine requires a grasp of the basic science underpinnings, most schools have broken the traditional lock-step approach through the introduction of students to patients in the first year and through the wide use of electives. As put by Bowers (2, pp. 69-70):

The traditional rigid departmentalization has also largely vanished. Correlation, integration, and interdisciplinary instruction have become the currency of medical education, with interdisciplinary courses in cell biology, growth and development, and neural sciences established in most schools. Further, it has been nationally accepted that there should be a core curriculum which includes the information in the basic sciences that should be required of all students.

The second year of medical school is usually an introduction to clinical medicine through the study of the physiological basis of disease. There is a basic clerkship in medicine, surgery, pediatrics, psychiatry, and obstetrics-gynecology, with the latter an elective in some schools. The subspecialties have largely disappeared from the required curriculum but are offered as electives.

The basic clerkship is a major strength of American medical education. Students are assigned patients on whom they conduct histories, physical examinations, and essential laboratory procedures. The students are active participants in the diagnostic and therapeutic programs, working under the supervision of residents and faculty members. Formal lectures are held to the minimum and diseases are discussed in small seminars . . .

Bowers goes on to state that in nearly all schools medical students have at least one year of elective study, but he also notes that this is an expensive system in terms of faculty time and that it poses frequent logistic problems in terms of when an elective is available.

The innovations have apparently created some problems with regard to national testing of student performance. Most medical schools had been using parts I and II of the NBME tests to evaluate students and to compare performances with other schools. Part I covered the basic medical sciences and was typically taken toward the end of the second year. Part II covered the clinical sciences and was typically taken toward the end of the fourth year. Part

III was a clinical test taken during or after the completion of the internship. As curricula were reshuffled and electives introduced, taking parts I and II—as was traditional—proved to be somewhat dysfunctional. Bowers states that consideration is now being given to a single test, replacing part I and part II, to be given on completion of medical school. Most states, it will be recalled, accepted these test results for licensure if the tests were passed by the candidate with a state-acceptable score. An alternative state licensing exam is FLEX, which was discussed in the previous chapter.

Cost of Medical Education

In early 1974, the Institute of Medicine of the National Academy of Sciences made public the results of a study of the costs of medical education. It found that the average annual cost of undergraduate medical education was $12,650. Depending on the school in its 14-school sample, the costs ranged from $6,900 to $18,650. The study also found that the average annual cost of osteopathic training came to $8,950. The $12,650 average cost per student dropped to $9,700 when the income from research and patient care was taken into account. The AAMC, a few months earlier, released its own study based on a sample of 12 schools. It found that the annual cost per student ran from $16,000 to $26,000.*

Since that time, costs have, of course, soared considerably. But even those figures indicate that the cost of medical training is high. Tuition costs in 1977 ranged from $267 a year at Texas Tech to $12,500 a year at Georgetown University. The AMA, citing an AAMC study, reports (3, p. 8):

The median tuition among public medical schools for in-state residents is now $1,319, which is about 10% higher than last year's median tuition of $1,200.

For out-of-state residents at public medical schools, median tuition this year is $2,840, 17% higher than last year's median of $2,426.

At private medical schools, median tuition this year is $5,000, up 11% from last year's median of $4,500. . . .

AAMC officials say the big tuition increases are a result of rising costs combined with declining federal capitation support, which provides flat grants per student enrolled. Two years ago, medical schools received $2,000 per student per year; last year the capitation dropped to $1,050.

*Both studies were reported in the *Bulletin of the Association of American Medical Colleges*, Vol. IX, Number 3, March 1974.

Without some kind of subsidy, becoming a doctor would be the privilege of the wealthy. Because this is not a socially acceptable policy, and because the well-to-do probably can't supply our physician needs in any event, subsidies of medical education have been commonplace. They are most prominent at public universities where the tuition is pegged well below cost, with the legislature appropriating tax monies to help keep the school going and tuition costs down. The subsidies also exist in the form of scholarships and loans, enabling the tuition level to stay higher than it could otherwise be. Subsidies also come from patient income, from the monies received by the salaried faculty for patient care, and from federal appropriations. But the federal subsidy is somewhat elusive, as noted above, where the capitation grants were cut almost in half, at the very time overall costs were rising. Further subsidies came from writing off education costs on the hospital charges for patient care. Perhaps one of the largest subsidies comes from research grants and contracts from the National Institutes of Health (NIH) and other federal agencies. These grants pay the salaries of researchers, who also do teaching. While a comprehensive picture of the costs of medical education is not really possible, the Division of Operational Studies of the AAMC has provided some insightful data, which is abstracted and shown in Table 2-3 (1, p. 2779).

The figures in Table 2-3 relate to medical school activities. How much is vital to the training of a competent physician cannot be ascertained. Any figure is bound to be largely judgmental in any event. But it should be clear that when costs go up, and federal or state appropriations go down, a medical school heads for financial difficulty.

For a great many years after World War II, expansion in medical education was heavily fueled by federal monies coming in via research contracts and grants. These monies came from a variety of federal agencies, including the Defense Department. But the principal vehicle was the NIH. Freymann observes (4, pp. 86-87):

The seed of university-based medical research, originally imported from Germany, had been sown across the land by Flexner and the General Education Board between 1910 and 1940 and had been germinating all those years. NIH money only fertilized a field already sown. Furthermore, in any consideration of the deleterious effects federal research support had on education, one must never forget that NIH support almost single-handedly brought about the upgrading of the nation's medical schools which occurred between 1945 and 1965. Although research undoubtedly deflected the interest of many faculty members away from teaching, I agree with Chapman that "as a direct consequence of federal support of research and researchers, the medical student has, since the war, been actively exposed to and in direct contact with an infinitely broader galaxy of teachers than was the case before 1946."

The monies paid the salaries of faculty (who were also permitted to teach), secretaries, and equipment and even built buildings. Without these monies, the expansion could not have taken place. These monies came not to the deans of the medical schools but to the individual researchers, which, of course, created a number of little kingdoms within each school. These centers of power carried enormous influence in shaping the course of medical education. The most adept could get the grants, and thereby hire more faculty, travel to meetings, and attract more residents, who were also paid out of grants. It certainly made attractive the highly specialized areas. Reinforcing this was the reward system. Medical schools were reflecting the universities of which they were a part; the rewards of promotion and salary increases went to those who pulled in the money and who published.

Freymann points out that before 1951 there were relatively few full-time salaried faculty in American medical schools despite what Flexner recommended 40 years earlier. In 1954, out of 80 schools, 15 had no full-time faculty; by 1968, 48% of the faculty had all or part of their salaries paid from federal funds (4, p. 87). "The proportion of each school's total salary budget derived from federal assistance ranged from 7% to 69%" (4, p. 91). Relatively small amounts of this federal money went directly for support of medical education; most of it was for research, which was indirectly used to subsidize the costs of medical education.

During the early 1960s, change was beginning to occur. Legislation in 1963 provided for direct federal assistance to medical schools in terms of construction grants, student loans, and financial distress grants. Some voices were raised at about this time as to whether all the research was doing much good as far as improving the health of people. By 1966, this came to be a dominant theme in federal circles, with the surgeon general of the Public Health Service moving his office to the grounds of NIH in an attempt to gain control of the NIH genie and by the development of new programs designed to emphasize the application of research findings in the delivery of health services. There was also growing concern over the availability of primary-care physicians. At the same time, the costs of the Vietnam War and, a few years later, the costs of Medicare and Medicaid, proved to be so great as to necessitate cost controls in other areas. But the control of NIH was not easily accomplished; with the retirement of its powerful director, James Shannon, directors turned over several times before the president felt he had enough control of the agency or at least had

Table 2-3. Summary of Medical School Sources of Revenue, 1967-1968 to 1976-1977*

Source	1967-1968		1975-1976		1976-1977	
	Amount	(%)	Amount	(%)	Amount	(%)
Total Revenue, $	1,175	(100.0)	3,353	(100.0)	3,901	(100.0)
Federal contracts and grants	619	52.7	1,244	37.1	1,262	32.4
For research	390	33.2	656	19.6	746	19.1
For teaching and training	154	13.1	290	8.6	206	5.3
For public service	...†		94	2.8	88	2.2
Recovery of indirect costs	75	6.4	204	6.1	222	5.7
Nonfederal contracts and grants for restricted programs	108	9.2	561	16.7	502	12.9
Nonfederal contracts and grants for public service	...†		293	8.7	230	5.9
Nongovernment contracts and grants for research	70	6.0	151	4.5	151	3.9
Nonfederal contracts and grants for teaching and training	17	1.4	82	2.4	79	2.0
State, city, and county contracts and grants for research	13	1.1	16	0.5	23	0.6
Recovery of indirect costs on nonfederal contracts and grants	8	0.7	19	0.6	18	0.5

Medical school/university activities	236	20.1	811	24.2	1,263	32.4
Tuition and fees	48	4.1	155	4.6	192	4.9
Professional fee (medical service plan)						
Income	48	4.1	399	11.9	541	13.9
For general operations	48	4.1	399	11.9	440	11.3
For restricted programs	...	...	...	...	101	2.6
Income from college services	21	1.8	62	1.8	37	0.9
Income from endowments	30	2.6	53	1.6	48	1.2
Hospitals and clinics	...	...	...	...	249	6.4
For general operations	...	...	...	...	196	5.0
For restricted programs	...	...	...	...	53	1.4
Other income	89	7.6	142	4.2	196	5.0
For general operations	89	7.6	142	4.2	170	4.4
For restricted programs	...	...	...	...	27	0.7
Other sources of funds	173	14.7	738	22.0	872	22.4
State appropriations to public schools	143	12.2	628	18.7	724	18.6
State, city, and county grants-in-aid, or subsidies to private schools, or payments via interstate compacts	16	1.4	81	2.4	92	2.4
State funds for restricted programs	...	...	...	...	20	0.5
Unrestricted gifts	14	1.2	29	0.9	36	0.9

*Dollars are given in millions. Totals may not equal the sum of the parts because of rounding.

†Data not available in this detail; therefore, total revenue is not equal to the sum of the subtotals.

Source: Medical education in the United States, 1977-1978: 78th Annual Report on Medical Education. JAMA, 240: 1978.

gone as far as he thought he could politically go. In 1971, Congress moved more directly to aid medical schools by appropriating capitation grant monies by which each school received a certain amount for each student. As Table 2-3 indicates, however, federal grants for teaching and training have declined considerably and represent today a less significant part of the medical-education subsidy.

Capitation grants occasioned a shift of some power from departmental faculty to the deans, facilitating administrative direction of the medical-education process. Frequently, this direction was prompted by the strings attached to the federal capitation grants monies. Put another way, by shifting from indirect support (still substantial) via research grants to direct capitation support, Congress was able to specify the activities it expected schools to engage in in return for the federal monies. As we shall see, grants of money may not be an unmixed blessing.

The AMA's report, *Medical Education in the United States 1971-1972*, summarizes some of the provisions of the 1971 Comprehensive Health Manpower Act (5, p.963).

The legislation also marked the first time that federal support had been tied specifically to requirements that certain activities be carried out by the instituions receiving the funds. Accordingly, it marked the first time that there has been intervention by federal agencies in the internal program decisions of the educational institutions.

According to the provisions of the capitation grants, the grants may not be received unless an institution presents a plan to carry out projects in at least three of nine categories described in the law. These include such things as shortening the length of training; establishing interidsciplinary training and the use of the team approach to the provision of health services; training new types of health personnel including physician's assistants; offering innovative educational programs including those in the organization, provision, financing, or evaluation of health care; increasing the enrollment; increasing the enrollment of disadvantaged students; training primary-care health professionals; and establishing programs in clinical pharmacology, drug use and abuse, and in the science of nutrition.

Specific provisions are contained in the legislation for incentives to increase the enrollment of students and to increase the number of graduating students. Expansion of enrollment is required for every school that receives a capitation grant, but special bonuses are provided for enrollment increases over the required minimum. Special project grants and health manpower education initiative awards are available for many of the categorical purposes listed above as well as certain others. A special section is provided for grants to initiate, expand, or improve professional training programs in family medicine. Student loan and scholarship provisions are expanded and extended under the new legislation.

When fully implemented, the new Comprehensive Health Manpower Training Act will provide a substantial portion of the operating support of virtually all educational institutions in the health professions field. Initial appropriation and expenditure of funds has been at a level substantially below that authorized by the legislation, but these amounts may be expected to be greater in subsequent years.

With the Health Professions Education Assistance Act of 1976, Congress assumed an even more vigorous role. It mandated that medical schools give greater emphasis to primary care by allocating 35% of their first-year residency slots to primary-care specialists (family practice, internal medicine, pediatrics), the percentage rising to 50 by 1980. This may have been a locking of the barn door after the horse had bolted in that many perceived movement in this direction long before the legislation. The legislation also provided that as a condition for receipt of capitation grant monies, medical schools would have to agree to accept into their third-year class American students who had taken two years of medical studies abroad and that the Department of Health, Education, and Welfare (HEW) would make the assignments. The number of Americans going abroad to study had been growing considerably due to the limited number of places in American schools. Italy, the Dominican Republic, and Mexico have been the major training outlets for Americans. This provision of the act (the "Guadalajara Clause" after the Universidad Autonoma de Guadalajara in Mexico where a large contingent of Americans—an estimated 2,600— were studying) was so onerous that a significant number of schools announced that they would forego capitation grants rather than allow HEW to become the admissions director for their schools. These schools also suggested that it was unfair to admit such students simply because they had enough money to go abroad to study. In late 1977, the uproar had become so great that implementation was deferred. The episode does illustrate rather well the risks involved when one welcomes such bearers of gifts.

Dr. John Cooper, president of the AAMC put the issue pointedly in an editorial in the association's *Journal of Medical Education* (6, pp. 69-70):

The long-awaited health manpower law, in many respects infinitely better than earlier bills considered by the House and Senate, was seriously flawed by the now infamous "USFMS provision." While the schools were unanimous in their opposition to its infringement on the fundamental academic decision-making process, it was not clear how many institutions would or could refuse to comply. Even less clear was how the program would operate, if it could be administered at all. The confusion over this section was best summarized by Federal District Court Judge Edward Becker, who, in ruling against Guadalajara students seeking enforcement of the provision in 1977, called the law "far from a model of lucidity."

The officers and Executive Council of the Association of American Medical Colleges wrestled uncomfortably with the political dilemma of seeking amendment of the law at the risk of gaining little or nothing while sacrificing other provisions. While working to obtain legislative relief, we also labored hard to get regulations which would make this program manageable and maximize its acceptability to the schools. The Congress was finally convinced to reexamine this section of the manpower law and to approve constructive amending legislation. But the medical schools may yet pay a price for this activity. With the law now reopened for amendment, Congressional reconsideration of other capitation conditions has been promised for 1978. It appears that we will have rolling legislation, subject to review and change each year, providing little of the stability for which we had hoped.

Congressional leverage vis-à-vis the medical schools is weakened, however, by the decreasing importance of capitation grants in overall school finance. These grants are reflected in Table 2-3 under "for teaching and training."

In the 1977-1978 academic year, there were 401 American students who transferred from foreign to U.S. medical schools; 201 were sponsored by COTRANS, a program initiated by the AAMC that permits transfer to a U.S. medical school with advanced standing. Required is a passing grade on part I of the National Board Examinations and acceptance by a medical school. The remaining 200 transferred without COTRANS sponsorship. (In 1976-1977, of the students permitted to sit for part I of the National Board Examinations by COTRANS, only 52% passed. By contrast, of students in American schools, 85% passed.) The number of students transferring from foreign medical schools fluctuates; during the late 1960s, fewer than 100 transferred each year. During the 1970s, it varied from 139 to 297 a year, with a major jump in 1976-1977 to 494. In 1977-1978, however, the number of transfers dropped to 401. Whether there is any significance to this due to medical-school resistance or to new restrictions by the Italian schools cannot be determined at this time. Many of the Americans in foreign medical schools may be opting for the Fifth Pathway program, offered by about one-third of the schools in the United States.

The Fifth Pathway program provides a one-year clinical clerkship to Americans who have graduated from foreign medical schools but who completed their premedical training in the United States. They must pass either the ECFMG exam or part I of the National Board Examinations, whichever the U.S. school specifies. The number of Fifth Pathway applicants in 1976-1977 nearly doubled from the preceding year, rising to 1,339. In 1977-1978, the number jumped to 2,400. These 2,400 applicants competed for 628 slots.

Development of New Schools

It was noted at the beginning of this section that there were at least three M.D. schools in the planning or developmental stages (Figs. 2-1 and 2-2). There is, in addition, one accredited school of basic medical sciences offering the preclinical course work so that its students might transfer to the third-year class of a four-year school. This school might, if history is any guide, become, in time, a four year school. How many other schools are being planned but have not emerged to public view is not known. There are a number of Caribbean or offshore medical schools that regularly advertise for students. Most of these are business operations. In Puerto Rico, there are two unaccredited schools (as well as one school that is accredited at the University of Puerto Rico).

Control in the number of schools is not by the AMA. Despite its role in the accreditation process, neither it nor the AAMC can prevent a school from developing. Neither may be happy about a new school, particularly if it means sharing available revenues, but both bodies are constrained by the accreditation

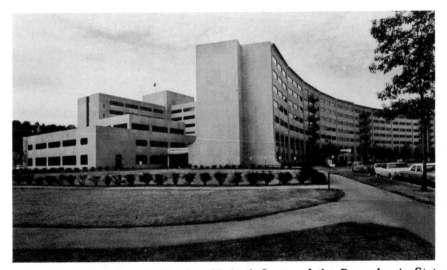

Figure 2–1. The Milton S. Hershey Medical Center of the Pennsylvania State University is one of the newer medical schools. The medical school hospital is in the foreground. (Courtesy of The Milton S. Hershey Medical Center.)

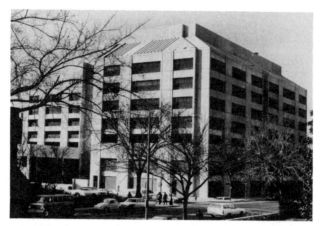

Figure 2–2. The Walter G. Ross Hall; the new George Washington University School of Medicine building in Washington, D.C. (Courtesy, George Washington University School of Medicine.)

criteria, which must be fairly applied. If not fairly applied, litigation can follow or complaints filed with the Office of Education, which could lead to the loss of LCME accrediting legitimacy. In addition, the ability of the population to use doctors suggests that physician incomes are not likely to be affected should new schools develop and more physicians be graduated.

The real control today on the development of new schools, as well as the number of physicians new and old schools turn out, is money. One cannot enter the medical-education game lightly. Apart from the cost of building medical-school buildings, the average U.S. medical school in 1976-1977 had average operating expenses of $19.2 million.

GRADUATE MEDICAL EDUCATION

Graduate medical education consists of a period of supervised training in an approved clinical setting following graduation from medical school. While the laws on licensure vary from state to state and thus present a rather complicated picture, it should be noted that while nearly all medical graduates complete some form of graduate medical education, it is required by 36 states for licensure of American medical school graduates and by nearly all states for graduates of foreign medical schools. There are two types of graduate training: the *internship* and the *residency*.

The internship is the old standby of American medicine, an experience that most physicians went through until very recently. In its early form, the internship was a *rotating* one in which the intern rotated through the various clinical departments of the hospital, securing that extra bit of on-the-job supervised experience before going out on his or her own into general practice. In some respects, the rotating internship was less than satisfactory because the intern would be spending so little time in each department that the value of the experience was open to some question. This was increasingly a concern as clinical departments expanded and as specialties increased in number. The rotating internship, as a consequence, began to evolve to an experience wherein the intern limited himself or herself to some two or three clinical services. This became known as a *mixed* internship. As specialties further developed, so, too, did another type of internship, the *straight* internship, in which the intern specialized in one of four clinical areas: internal medicine, surgery, pediatrics, or pathology.

But the number of internship slots around the country were more than the number of U.S. medical graduates. Doctors and hospitals frequently wanted a supply of interns for night and weekend coverage as well as for the routine work-up on patients. As important, perhaps, was that, via the internship program, communities felt they would be in a stronger position to persuade a physician to establish his or her practice in that community upon completion of the internship. The AMA describes the internship evolution and resulting problems in these words (7, p. 123):

The internship, since the turn of the century an integral feature in the education of a physician, has been the subject of much critical discussion and study, particularly in the last few years. The improvement of clinical clerkships on the one hand and the marked expansion of residency training programs on the other have altered the intern's position as a member of the hospital staff.

When the internship became a generally recognized part of the education of a physician some 40 years ago, it was designed to provide the graduate's initial contact with patients, including responsibility for their care. It no longer constitutes such initial contact nor is it any longer the final step in the formal education of most physicians. Rather it is now only one of several graded steps toward the assumption of total responsibility for patient care. As such, it remains an essential part of the education of a physician but should be redesigned to fulfill its present purpose. With this concept in mind, it is evident that the internship can be conducted only in those hospitals in which the educational benefits to the intern are considered of paramount importance, with the service benefits to the hospital of secondary importance.

One aspect of intern education which warrants consideration is the growing discrepancy between the number of internships offered in hospitals approved for intern training and the number of applicants available to fill them. While this disparity, *per se*, is of no great import, its effect on the stability of internship programs throughout the country is of serious consequence. It is obvious that a sound educational program cannot be maintained if the number of interns the hospital is able to appoint varies from none at all one year to a full complement the next. Further, it is unlikely that a hospital can conduct a satisfactory program with substantially less than its normal complement of interns. To attract a full intern staff, many hospitals have begun to offer excessive stipends, bonuses, or other rewards of a non-educational nature. Such practices all too often result in an undue emphasis being placed on the intern's services to the hospital, while the educational aspects of the program are neglected.

The larger general hospitals, particularly those affiliated with medical schools or those that had also approved residency training programs, attracted the American and Canadian medical graduates. The other internship slots were filled, if at all, largely by foreign medical graduates. In the former, there was usually a salaried full-time director of medical education who saw to it that the educational experiences of both interns and residents were appropriate In the latter hospitals, the director of medical education typically filled that role on a voluntary or part-time basis.

The need for reform was evident to many medical educators and leaders of the AMA. The movement for reform proceeded along two paths: The AMA commissioned a Citizens Commission on Graduate Medical Education, chaired by John S. Millis, who was then president of Western Reserve University. The commission consisted of eleven members, only three of whom were physicians. In the preface to the commission's report *The Graduate Education of Physicians,* Millis stated (8, pp. v-vii):

A principal motive for the founding of the American Medical Association was a concern for the character and standards of medical education and thus for the qualifications of the future members of the profession. Twice in the twentieth century the Association has requested an external examination of the state of medical education and has sought recommendations for changes to ensure an increasing excellence. In the first decade of the century the Association took advantage of the interest in education for the learned professions of Mr. Henry Pritchett, President of the Carnegie Foundation for the Advancement of Teaching, to obtain a study of the medical schools of the nation. The report of this study, known universally as the Flexner Report, was wholeheartedly supported in its implementation by the American Medical

Association. It had profound effect upon the development of American medical education and, therefore, upon the medical care of our citizens.

In the seventh decade the Association has again expressed its continuing concern by requesting an external examination of the internship and the residency, the constituent parts of graduate medical education. In the five and a half decades which have passed since the Flexner Report, the sytem of graduate medical education has become established and now constitutes the larger half of the formal education of the physician. In this development a process of specialization and consequent fragmentation has occurred so that responsibility is diffuse and authority divided. Once again, the American Medical Association sought external examination and asked for the formation of the Citizens Commission on Graduate Medical Education to make recommendations for the improvement of this phase of medical education. In requesting this study, as in supporting the Flexner study, the American Medical Association has demonstrated its deep concern not only for the profession which it represents, but also for the public good.

For any learned profession there are but two alternatives for establishing standards of practice and education. Responsibility can be assumed by society as a whole, operating through government, or can be assumed by the organized profession through a voluntarily accepted self discipline. There are no other alternatives, for, if the profession does not take responsibility, society will surely demand that the vacuum be filled and the government assume the responsibility. It is the conviction of the Commission that the profession of medicine should assume the responsibility for its standards of education and should have a mechanism adequate to the full discharge of these responsibilities. The recommendations of the Commission set forth in the following pages are designed to provide such a mechanism. The mechanism, we believe, is capable of assuming clearly and effectively the necessary responsibilities, and is of such independence that it can be free of special interests and serve both the interests of the profession and the public welfare.

The Citizens Commission on Graduate Medical Education has operated as a committee of the whole and has not employed a staff. Data, opinions, and relevant evidence have been presented to the entire Commission. Thus, the ensuing report represents the conclusions formed by the members. It is not a staff report in which a committee has concurred. In its attempt to understand the changes which have occurred in medical education, the Commission has endeavored to delineate the forces which are operating at present and to take account of those which may operate in the foreseeable future. The recommendations, we believe, will make it possible for graduate medical education to enjoy an orderly adaptation to the changes required by a burgeoning science and an evolving society.

Special thanks must be given to Dr. Dael Wolfle, the Commission member who served as draftsman of the report. Credit for the lucid presentation of the report belongs to him. The Commission is grateful for the constant interest and helpful counsel of Dr. Walter S. Wiggins, who served as consultant. Further, the Commission is grateful to the many people representing all parts of medical education and practice who shared their knowledge and experience with us.

With regard to internships, the commission observed (8, pp.11-14):

From the comparative uniformity of medical schools to the great diversity of internship programs is a huge jump, both for the young physician and in terms of organization and control. Where undergraduate medical education is concentrated in fewer than 100 schools of medicine, internships are offered in almost 800 approved teaching hospitals. Where medical school curricula are the corporate responsibilities of faculties, internship programs are often devised by single services or single individuals.

When the internship first became an established part of medical education, its purpose was straightforward and uniform: a year of hospital training, with nearly equal portions devoted to medicine, surgery, and obstetrics-gynecology, provided the first extended clinical experience and the first supervised responsibility for the welfare of living patients. These experiences were deemed necessary, and usually sufficient, to complete the preparation of a young physician for independent practice.

The purpose of an internship is no longer clear and it is far from uniform. The internship no longer provides the student's first practical experience with problems of diagnosis and treatment; that function is now served by under-graduate clinical clerkships. Nor is it sufficient to provide the final educational experience preceding independent practice; the additional training of a residency is generally considered necessary to fulfill that purpose.

Because nearly all students now go on from an internship to a residency, the nature of the internship has changed. The original, or rotating, form provides from 12 to 24 months of experience in medicine, surgery, pediatrics, and obstetrics-gynecology. More recently, two other forms have come into use: mixed internships—which resemble rotating internships in providing training in two or three fields, but differ by requiring that from six to eight months be spent in one field; and straight internships—which are devoted entirely to single areas, such as medicine, surgery, or pediatrics.

When a student progresses from medical school to an internship, he leaves an institution devoted primarily to education and enters one devoted primarily to medical care. Hospital experience is essential, but unless the internship is truly educational, it fails of its principal purpose. Within the context of the *Essentials of an Approved Internship* (published annually in the *Directory of Approved Internships and Residencies*), the responsible staff members of a teaching hospital determine their own educational processes and standards, and decide how an intern's time and responsibility are divided between education and service. The responsibility for reviewing internship programs in an attempt to make certain that they meet minimum acceptable standards has been assumed by the Council on Medical Education of the American Medical Association. In deciding whether to approve of disapprove a particular internship program, the Council relies heavily on the advice of the Internship Review Committee, which consists of representatives of the Council on Medical Education, the Association of American Medical Colleges, the American Hospital Association, the Federation of State Medical Boards, and the field of general practice.

The hospitals in which internships are offered are also subject to review and approval by several other bodies. The American Hospital Association accredits hospitals on the basis of such criteria as the number of beds and the types of services offered, but does not examine the efficiency or efficacy of these services. The state health departments approve hospitals on the basis of sanitation, safety, and similar criteria. The Joint Commission on Accreditation of Hospitals accredits in terms of the quality of medical service rendered, but not in terms of educational criteria. Thus, a hospital that offers internship training is subject to periodic examination by several different reviewing bodies. But only one of these bodies, the Internship Review Committee, bases its decisions on the quality of education being offered.

To complicate the system further, the educational quality of a straight internship is usually not the responsibility of the hospital as a whole, but of an individual service—surgery, medicine, pathology, or another—or of the head of that service. Rotating and mixed internships are usually the successive and unrelated responsibility of several independent services. Unlike a school of medicine in which the faculty takes corporate responsibility for the educational program, a hospital is more likely to consist of a federation of separate services in which each is responsible for its own standards and policies, with relatively little help, counsel, or criticism from other services.

An inevitable result of such highly individualistic and fragmented responsibility is that internship programs vary widely in the extent to which they duplicate the experience already gained in the clinical clerkship, in the amount of routine and sometimes menial service required, and in their educational quality.

The commission has this to say about residencies (8, pp. 14-17).

After the internship comes the residency. The typical medical school graduate now follows his internship with three or more years of residency training. In 1965, residencies were offered by more than 1300 American hospitals, of which approximately half offered residencies but not internships, and half offered both.

The function of residency training has changed greatly since its start half a century ago. At that time the internship normally marked the completion of preparation for medical practice; a residency was something extra, a special period of added clinical education for a few particularly promising and scholarly young physicians who wished to become the teachers or leaders in advancing the science and art of medicine. Even as late as 1927, when a list of approved residencies was first published, the number was only a third as great as the number of internships. Now the ratio is exactly reversed; there are three times as many residents as interns. Residency training has become standard for the rank and file of physicians, and is no longer exclusively for a few selected individuals.

The expansion of residency training has largely resulted from the growing desirability and importance of specialization and certification by a specialty board. Most young physicians aspire to certification and most of them succeed, if not on the first attempt, on the second or third. In 1945, the specialty boards certified 1308 candidates as specialists. In the year 1955, the number was 3843. And in 1965 it was 5386, a number equivalent to approximately 80 percent of the medical school graduates six years earlier.

The rise in specialization has been accompanied by an alarming decline in the number of physicians who devote themselves to continuing and comprehensive care of the whole individual.

Although in theory teaching hospitals are free to determine the nature and duration of their residency programs, in actual practice their freedom is limited by the powerful influence of the specialty boards, for completion of an approved residency is one of the requirements for certification.

As previously observed, internship programs are usually treated as the independent responsibilities of individual services rather than as the corporate responsibility of the hospital. This division of responsibility is even more common in residency programs, for residency training is always specialized— in one or another of the 25 recognized specialties and subspecialties. Accordingly, responsibility for reviewing and approving residency programs is divided among 19 independent residency review committees. Each residency review committee includes some members appointed by the Council on Medical Education and some appointed by the appropriate specialty board. Some of the committees also include members appointed by the association or society of the particular specialty. In general, however, each review committee owes its fealty to the corresponding specialty board, and these specialty boards are autonomous.

The review and approval of residency training programs is, therefore, quite unlike the review and approval of schools of medicine or internship programs. All schools of medicine are reviewed by one body and all internship programs by another. In contrast, responsibility for the approval of residency programs is greatly fragmented, and neither the Council on Medical Education nor any other organization has insisted upon agreement and consistency among the several residency review committees.

Emphasis in this description has been on the great diffusion of responsibility for offering, directing, appraising, and approving programs of graduate medical education and on the fact that the two stages of graduate medical education, the internship and the residency, are separate from each other in planning and control, and separate also from undergraduate medical education.

Lawyers, ministers, engineers, physicists, historians, and other professionals are educated in a system under which the whole course of education, undergraduate and graduate, is a continuing responsibility of educational institutions, in which each department functions not only as a unit but also as an integral part of the whole university whose institutional standards and policies must be satisfied, and which, in turn, must meet external standards of review and accreditation.

Medical education differs from other professional education in the extent to which the young physician must have many opportunities to observe and work upon living patients who are suffering from a variety of afflictions. So great is this difference that it may not be possible or even desirable to organize and structure graduate education in medicine in the same pattern as in other fields. However that may be, it must be emphasized that graduate medical education is unique among the fields of graduate and professional education in being a responsibility of institutions which have service rather tha education as their primary function. It is unusual, in that responsibility is divided among more than a thousand hospitals instead of among a few score universities or medical schools. It is in a class by itself in the extent to which responsibility reposes in individuals rather than in faculties.

These characteristics of graduate medical education have given rise to a number of problems that will be examined in later chapters.

After reviewing the major trends in medical education and practice, evolving goals, and related matters, the commission focused on steps to improve residency and internship training (8, pp.57-72):

The basic soundness of the residency system deserves a strong vote of confidence. Responsible, supervised, and varied hospital experience gives a resident progressively increasing responsibility, opportunity to observe and work with accomplished senior men, experience in solving problems, and practice in using the facilities of a hospital and the special competence of other physicians. A good residency offers opportunities for gaining in technical skill, for acquiring the kind of vocational training that is a necessary and proper part of medical education, and for combining that training with the more abstract aspects of a scientific-medical education. At its best, a residency program permits of much flexibility to adjust to the different interests and skills of different residents and the different facilities and problems of different hospitals and types of practice.

Any basically sound system may, however, have troubles, and this one has its share. The hospitals that offer residencies differ widely in quality, size, opportunity for diverse and progressive responsibility, and in commitment to educational objectives. In some teaching hospitals too few of the attending physicians are interested in teaching. In some there is little if any full-time staff. In some the resident's educational experiences and practice are poorly supervised and coordinated. In others the senior staff members are too involved in research to have adequate time for treating patients or for teaching residents. Many hospitals have difficulty in finding patients adequate in number and variety who can be assigned to the residents as their responsibilities.

A basic problem is the confusion, and sometimes the direct conflict, between the hospital's goal of education and its goal of service to patients. A hospital—any hospital—exists for the primary purpose of housing and providing for people who need medical care. It is organized, equipped, and staffed for these purposes, and must always be judged on the quality of its medical services.

Some hospitals have assumed the additional function of training young physicians. One reason for the spread of residency training to more and more hospitals seems clearly to have been the desire to secure junior staff members to help carry the patient load. A conflict between service and educational goals has inevitably resulted, and this conflict cannot be resolved by contending that service and education are identical, for they are not. The service a house officer renders may be useful to the hospital and its patients, but it will not be maximally useful to him unless it is truly educational, and this it cannot be unless it is consistently planned and thought of as part of his graduate medical education. The governing board and staff of any hospital that assumes responsibility for interns or residents therby become obligated to offer graduate education of high quality.

House officers may not always be impartial judges of how effectively their time has been spent, but it is pertinent to consider their comparisons of what they have learned with the amount of service they have rendered. In a study conducted by the Bureau of Applied Social Research of Columbia University, only a small minority of the interns and residents felt they were being exploited, yet only about a quarter of them considered what they were learning to be very much worth the time spent providing services for the hospital.

There will always be qualitative differences among hospitals and the training programs they offer. Individual shortcomings may never be eliminated. But there are more general faults to consider. One concerns the way in which the residency program is considered by the staff members responsible for its planning and direction. Typically it is planned, monitored, and appraised only by members of one individual medical service; it is treated as the responsibility of an individual service rather than of the hospital as a whole. And sometimes responsibility seems to be centered almost entirely in the single individual who serves as chief of service.

There may have been a time, when the body of medical knowledge was smaller, when a young apprentice could learn all he needed to know from one older master. Now, no master knows enough; the intellectual content is too great; apprenticeship is no longer satisfactory. The house officer learns from several seasoned physicians, from his fellows, from patients, from the library, the laboratory, the journal club, visiting lecturers, and other sources.

Half a century ago it came to be generally recognized that the proprietary, apprenticeship system of training physicians in the vocational skills that were then recognized as necessary could no longer be tolerated. Rather quickly, the requirements for admission to medical schools were elevated, substantial courses in the biomedical sciences were developed, and responsibility for planning and conducting medical education was assumed by medical school faculties instead of by practicing physicians acting individually or in small groups.

It is now time for comparable changes in graduate medical education. After a young physician graduates from medical school, he still has much to learn— much theory, principle, scientific knowledge, as well as much art and skill. No one physician can teach him all he needs to learn. No amount of practice will suffice. Even the best imaginable apprenticeship would be insufficient. He needs a planned, progressive, integrated educational program that benefits from the contributions of a variety of able and imaginative medical scientists and practitioners. This need leads directly to the changes that are recommended in the remainder of this chapter.

CORPORATE RESPONSIBILITY

A first principle to insist upon is that every teaching hospital demonstrate, through its plans and actions, that it understands and has accepted the obligations and responsibilities of an institution giving graduate medical education. The board of trustees, the administrator and the senior professional staff must recognize that they are assuming a serious and costly obligation above the costs of patient care itself. They must be prepared to devote a reasonable portion of the hospital's resources to the proper discharge of this obligation. Unless a hospital offers a truly educational program, it is not a good place for interns or residents.

> We recommend that each teaching hospital organize its staff, through an educational council, a committee on graduate education, or some similar means, so as to make its programs of graduate medical education a corporate responsibility rather than the individual responsibilities of particular medical or surgical services or heads of services.

CONTINUITY OF GRADUATE MEDICAL EDUCATION

A second principle to establish is that any program of graduate medical education should be planned as a unified, progressive sequence. It is not so today. Instead it is two separate stages—an internship and a residency—and the connection between the stages is too loose.

Specialty boards require an applicant for certification to have served an approved internship and an approved residency. With one or two exceptions, however, the nature of the internship is not specified. Any internship that continues for a sufficient number of months meets the requirement. The Board of Neurological Surgery requires a surgical internship. A few boards prefer a straight or rotating internship. But with these exceptions, any internship—straight, mixed or rotating—meets the requirement. The specialty boards seem to have agreed that the internship provides a useful year of hospital experience, but that the particular nature of that experience is not important. The residency, in contrast, must meet the specific requirements of a particular specialty board.

The internship was originally devised to give the medical school graduate supervised opportunity to practice applying the knowledge and theories he learned in school. It gave him some, though limited, progressive personal responsibility for real patients with real medical problems. This experience was expected to transform him from a student into a physician. In older, simpler years it was accepted as enough, but it no longer is. Initiation into hospital work now begins in the clinical clerkship, which is an integral part of the medical school program. After the internship, in order to obtain the progressive experience in patient care now considered necessary to develop mature competency, residency training is required. The internship, therefore, has come to occupy an intermediate position, overlapping in some respects the clinical clerkship and in others the first year of a residency.

As a consequence, there has been much change in the way the internship year is used. The classical rotating internship is losing ground to mixed and straight internships, especially the latter, which are, in effect, the first year of a specialized residency.

The question therefore arises: is it necessary or desirable to continue the internship as a separate, freestanding part of medical education?

> We recommend that the internship, as a separate and distinct portion of medical education, be abandoned, and that the internship and residency years be combined into a single period of graduate medical education called a residency and planned as a unified whole.

Because state licensure acts usually require service of an internship and in some cases specify its nature, and because certification requirements also include service of an internship, there will be a period of transition during which the name "internship" will have to be retained. Even during this period of transition, however, there can be rapid progress toward unifying graduate medical education into the new kinds of residencies that will span the entire period of graduate medical education.

> We recommend that state licensure acts and statements of certification requirements be amended to eliminate the requirement of a separate internship and to substitute therefore an appropriately described period of graduate medical education.

GENERAL AND SPECIALIZED STAGES OF MEDICAL EDUCATION

Abandonment of the separate internship will help to clarify the allocation of responsibility for the general and the specialized stages of medical education.

Medical schools operate on the assumption that a graduate will be qualified to enter any internship, rotating, mixed, or straight, and that his medical school experience has been sufficiently broad, basic, and nonspecialized to prepare him to enter whatever graduate program he considers most attractive.

Some medical educators have advocated the prolongation of undifferentiated education into the graduate period. For example, some would require a rotating internship or an internship in internal medicine for all young physicians, regardless of their later specialties.

As a countertrend, some differentiation is found among schools of medicine and among students in the same school. Large amounts of money for research have led some medical schools to place heavy emphasis upon research and specialization, and this emphasis has become a major reason for the lack of interest among students in preparing themselves for general or family practice and the increasing tendency to prepare for specialized practice. Thus, so to speak, specialization has already been started during the medical school years. Some students already know the directions they will want to follow later. By the selection of elective courses, clerkships, and topics for individual study, they begin early to prepare for later specialization.

Thus, there is no point that uniformly marks the transition from general to specialized medical education. Many medical school graduates start specialized training immediately after graduation with a straight or mixed internship, and some have begun even earlier to prepare for specialty training. Others, who take rotating internships, defer specialized training for a year or more after graduation.

Intimately involved in this general problem is the length of the whole process. Lengthening of the period of education for physicians has gone as far as it should go. From kindergarten to completion of residency spans 25 years of education. This is long enough, or too long. Future accommodations to advances in knowledge and future efforts to establish higher standards must not require a still longer period of formal education. Two other means should be used. One is to improve continuing education for men in practice so that it will become more systematic, more prevalent, and more effective. If better and more widespread opportunities for further learning are provided to mature practitioners, there will be less pressure for lengthening the period of formal education.

The other improvement is to achieve greater knowledge and higher competence by the time of completion of medical school. There is a strong trend in education to teach topics earlier than formerly. This trend, supported by intensive efforts to improve the education offered at elementary, secondary, and collegiate levels will mean that students entering schools of medicine can be expected to be better educated than were students of earlier years. By building upon this better preparation, taking advantage of improved methods of instruction, and giving students greater opportunities and encouragement to learn on their own, schools of medicine should continue to complete in not more than four years the general medical education that precedes specialization. The general period should include not only education in basic medical knowledge but also, largely through the clinical clerkship, a supervised introduction to the application of this knowledge to the practice of medicine.

> We therefore recommend that graduation from medical school be recognized as the end of general medical education, and that specialized training begin with the start of graduate medical education.

Agreement upon this division of responsibility will make it easier to plan for the future of both undergraduate and graduate medical education.

The statement above that schools of medicine should continue to complete general medical education in not more than four years and the recommendation that graduation from medical school be recognized as the end of the general or undifferentiated period do not mean that we attribute any magical qualities to the number "four" or that we think that the continuous processes of education can or should be completely separated into two utterly distinct stages. Several schools of medicine are experimenting with programs that allow some students to complete their collegiate and medical school work in less than the traditional eight years. Some medical educators have proposed a shortening of the medical school curriculum and the introduction of a greater amount of flexibility to meet the needs of students who have different interests and plans. Our use of the terms "four years" and "general or undifferentiated period" is in no way a criticism of efforts to develop more effective and more efficient programs of undergraduate medical education. We are certainly not trying to freeze any medical school into its present mold. We applaud experimentation.

BASIC RESIDENCY TRAINING

Abolishing the internship as a separate and free-standing year of training and incorporating that year into a progressively planned residency will open the way to a greater amount of flexibility and coordination in the planning of residency programs.

The stated requirements for most types of residencies testify to the importance of knowledge in related specialties. Candidates for certification in pediatric allergy and pediatric cardiology must be previously certified by the American Board of Internal Medicine or the American Board of Pediatrics; residents in child psychiatry must already be certified by the American Board of Psychiatry; and those in thoracic surgery must meet the certification requirements of the American Board of Surgery. Each of these specialties is thereby recognized as constituting an extension or a subspecialty of a broader specialty.

Even in cases which do not involve a sequential relationship, the statements of residency requirements indicate the importance of study in related fields.

A resident in general surgery is expected to gain experience in several of the specialized fields of surgery. Residents in internal medicine spend part of their time in psychiatry, neurology, dermatology, or pediatrics. Those in psychiatry are expected to be "competent in and responsible for the medical examination and treatment of their patients." Residents in orthopedic surgery are advised, and those in otolaryngology are required, to have a year of residency in general surgery. In short, no specialty is an island unto itself, complete and independent of other specialties.

It is possible for each medical service to teach its own residents the selected portions of neighboring specialties considered most essential. It is also possible for residents in one specialty to spend a portion of their time in a related service. Both methods of teaching are widely used, and both have shortcomings. The danger of the first procedure is superficiality and of the second, disjointedness and repetition.

Both dangers may be reduced by organizing those elements of residency training that must be mastered by residents in several related specialties into a basic program common to those specialties.

Residents in obstetrics and gynecology "must understand and be trained in the care of emergencies, shock, hemorrhage, blood replacement, electrolyte and fluid balance, protein and nitrogen balance, choice of anesthetics, chemotherapy, acidosis and alkalosis, wound healing, etc." Residents in other surgical specialties must also understand and be trained in these matters. Part of the necessary understanding and training can be acquired in the undergraduate years. Part probably must be reserved for the training and experience that are unique to a particular specialty. In between lies a substantial area that could be planned as part of the education of residents in several related specialties. For example, a period of fundamental training in general surgery (two to four years) before branching into the specialized surgical areas is advisable, and a basic period of perhaps two years in medicine would advantageously precede branching into the medical specialties. It is not necessary that only two basic residency programs be considered. Perhaps some other number, some other way of grouping specialties, would offer greater educational advantages.

This recommendation has been made many times. As long ago as 1945, representatives of five of the surgical specialty boards agreed that basic surgical training was an essential prerequisite to sound training in all of the surgical specialties. Despite this agreement in principle, the boards could not agree upon the details of a plan to put the principle into effect.

Most residency requirements permit great flexibility with respect to specific content, methods of teaching, variety of experience, and organization of the program. From this standpoint there is little to inhibit a hospital from exploring the possibility of a basic residency training with subsequent branching into more specialized training. In another respect, however, the stated requirements impose some limitations. Generally speaking, a residency program is not approved unless it is directed by a senior physician who is certified or recognized as highly qualified in the particular specialty. Modification of this requirement would be necessary to permit residents who plan later to enter several different specialties all to take the first portion of their residency training in a program common to those specialties.

The details of this proposal must be determined by the staffs of individual hospitals, and it is desirable that the details be neither rigid nor uniform from hospital to hospital. Neither is it essential that all specialties within a group branch off the common stem at the same time. A hospital might find it profitable to organize a basic program for residents in four specialties, to have residents in two of these specialties leave the basic program at the end of two years to begin concentrated training in their specialties, while residents in the other two specialties continued together for another year before separating.

Three advantages should accrue from such basic residency programs. One is combined planning. For example, gynecologists, orthopedists, and other specialized surgeons as well as general surgeons would jointly plan the basic surgical residency. In general, teaching physicians in related groups of specialties would be forced to give concerted thought to what they wished to include in their residency programs and how the agreed upon content could best be organized and taught. This is always a healthy exercise.

The second advantage is that gaps and redundancies would become evident. Sending residents around from one service to another is likely to result in several repetitions of the same material at about the same level of detail. Better organization might save time and enable the student to reach a greater depth of understanding.

The third advantage would lie in the better utilization of the patient population for teaching purposes. There would be less compartmentalization of patients of particular types, greater flexibility in their use, and thus opportunities for broader and more varied experience on the part of each beginning resident. As an example of present difficulties, one consultant informed the Commission that "Because of the divisions of training programs and surgical staffs, the general surgery resident is not allowed to gain experience in pelvic surgery. Each service jealously guards its domain and sees to it that there is no crossing of lines." There should be some crossing of lines. A basic surgical residency prior to later specialization would make that possible.

We recommend that hospitals experiment with several forms of basic residency training, and that the specialty boards and residency review committees encourage experimentation by interpreting liberally those statements in the residency requirements that now inhibit this form of educational organization.

The desirability of basic residency programs seems clear. In fact, it almost seems axiomatic that with proper basic training in medicine or in general surgery the trainee will learn his subspecialty more rapidly and more efficiently. But no one can foretell with assurance the ideal duration or number or organization of basic residency programs. Experimentation is therefore in order, and we encourage teaching hospitals to undertake a variety of experiments.

THE DURATION OF RESIDENCY TRAINING

Most young physicians now spend four or more years in internship and residency training. The time has been lengthening in response to three factors: the growing amount to be learned; hospital needs for house staff; and the attitude that "my field is more difficult than yours, so the residency should be longer, and anyway a long residency looks good and adds to prestige."

Only the first of these reasons has any legitimacy. Hospital service is an important problem, but a separate one. A certain amount of rivalry among specialties is commendable, but residents should not have to pay the bill. Only the educational values should be considered in determining the length of residency training.

If the internship, as a separate part of graduate medical education, is abolished and if the residency period begins immediately following graduation from medical school, there should be opportunities to shorten the length of graduate medical education. It is not clear that a full year would be saved in all specialties, but is quite possible that abolition of the internship, together with the development of the basic residency period recommended above, would allow that much saving.

It is too soon to state with assurance just what changes in normal or average duration would be possible or desirable. Decision can be postponed for a time, for there is an alternative procedure that has merit in its own right.

> We recommend that the specialty boards, in amending their regulations concerning eligibility for examination for certification, not increase the required length of residency training to compensate for dropping the requirement of a separate internship. This can be done by retaining present wording concerning length of residency training and deleting statements concerning internship training.

This recommendation does not propose that every resident finish a year sooner. It merely proposes that the formal requirement of internship plus residency be shortened by a year. Residents vary in ability, in the speed with which they learn, and in the amount of time they wish to devote to research or to more extended opportunities to study particular areas of their specialties. The resident and the physicians under whom he is working can exercise judgment concerning the length of time he should spend in residency. Reducing the formal requirement would not suddenly shorten the training period of all residents. It would permit shortening for those who could successfully complete the program in less time. Now, with rare exceptions, the best and the poorest all serve the same time.

The American Board of Neurosurgery has been experimenting with a technique that merits broader trial. With the help of the National Board of Medical Examiners, a written examination for prospective neurosurgeons is given during the course of their residency. These examinations have no weight in later applications for certification; they are progress examinations, the results of which are communicated only to the individual and to the head of his training program. To both they offer guidance on how the remainder of the residency period can most profitably be spent, or whether it should be extended.

Through the more widespread use of such examinations, through elimination of the internship, through the wise use of opportunities for basic residency training, and—most fundamental of all—through consistent and clearheaded emphasis on the educational values involved, the time required for graduate medical education can be shortened for many physicians. It should even become possible to use accomplishment instead of time as the criterion for completion of graduate medical education.

Turning to the teaching hospital, the Millis Commission recommended that "programs of graduate medical education be approved by the residency review committees only if they cover the entire span from the first year of graduate medical education through completion of the residency"(8, p. 73).

Then, noting that good programs depend on more than just the resources in the specialty under review, the commission went on to recommend that "programs of graduate medical education not be approved unless the teaching staff, the related services, and the other facilities are judged adequate in size and quality, and that, if these tests are met, approval be given to the institution rather than to the particular medical or surgical service most directly involved"(8, p. 74).

The Millis Report is an excellent example of a health plan, and it proved to be one that was successfully implemented. The report was persuasive as a plan should be, and in late 1970 the AMA's House of Delegates endorsed the concept that the first year of graduate medical education be in a program approved by the appropriate residency review committee rather than by the Council on Medical Education. As Bowers notes, "Its acceptance by the House of Delegates permitted both the integration of internships and residencies and the elimination of the internship in hospitals that did not have residency programs." As a result, a number of the specialty boards reduced the span of their training and "by 1975 most of the specialty boards had redefined their requirements to include one year of broad clinical experience" (2, pp. 90-91).

This was one arm of the reform movement in graduate medical education. The other arm came from the AAMC. It appointed a committee of medical educators under the chairmanship of Lowell T. Coggeshall. As an education body, it addressed the role of the university medical school vis-à-vis graduate medical education (9, pp. 41-43):

Perhaps the clearest implication of emerging trends is the need for medical education in all its aspects to center in the university. As just noted, only the university can integrate instruction and research. The university alone comprises all the fields of knowledge and disciplines related to health. The university alone can encompass the education required for all health fields. Only through the university—the locus of research—can the full benefits of scientific advance be brought to the future physician and the practitioner.

The modern university represents the most and probably the only effective organization for coordinating all of the intellectual resources in the total spectrum of health services. Furthermore, the university is the best setting for the maintenance and evaluation of professional education. In the words of Barry Wood, "If medical education is to continue to flourish, the educational policies of medical schools must remain in the hands of faculties. Only teachers devoting their lives to the core of learning are close enough to the problems to plan wisely."

The atmosphere of the university provides important stimulation to scholarship, to research, and to teaching. The function of the university as an external arbiter of standards for all the disciplines serves as a useful antidote to the tendency of medical schools to become parochial. Through it, the medical school faculty have membership in an institution which recognizes as scholarly peers, persons both within and outside the medical profession. The university ideal of a community of scholars dedicated to truth should be increasingly important to medical schools as their responsibilities and their horizons enlarge.

There are many advantages to offering multiple health programs in a single setting. Specifically:

- The scope of the educational program can be better for each discipline, because of the ready availability of qualified teachers on a wide variety of health topics.
- The scope and quality of research programs is enhanced by the presence of this assembly of faculty.
- The scope and quality of patient care are benefited, and a referral center for patients for diagnostic and treatment problems results.
- Students in the several health disciplines can learn to understand and respect the contributions which other health disciplines can give, and the health team which is so important at the community level can be started in the educational setting.
- There are economies in the use of common facilities and services—for example, the library, extension department, and computer center.
- In some ways, the various disciplines stimulate each other to higher accomplishments.
- Demonstrations of excellence or "models" can be provided to lead others to improve the ways in which medicine is practiced and comprehensive health care provided.

However, the universities cannot extend their facilities to produce all the large numbers of health service personnel required by society. The universities should educate the teachers, research workers, and administrators for the allied health professions and occupations, and should develop and accredit educational programs in these disciplines for colleges and junior colleges to train the majority of practitioners. The recent expansion of junior college nursing schools has demonstrated the excellent potential of these institutions for training certain types of health personnel. Community hospitals in affiliation with medical schools should also be regarded as part of the training base for practicing allied health personnel.

To make the relationship meaningful, the medical school, and with it the hospitals and other units that make up the medical center, should become increasingly established within the framework of the university. Human biology and the emerging concept of total community health as a preventive-therapeutic continuum should receive contributions from economics, sociology, anthropology, psychology, regional planning, and many other disciplines, in addition to the traditional biomedical fields. The distinction between the "professional schools" of health sciences (e.g., medicine, public health, nursing, dentistry, and pharmacy) and other elements of the university should become diffused and the preparation of these specialists should be the combined responsibility of many departments, colleges, and schools.

Curricula should be interwoven to provide a community of mutual under-standing among all health-oriented disciplines, and the programs of each specialty should include direct experience in how to function as a member of a cooperative team.

Through operation of university hospitals for teaching and research—the essential classrooms for education in all health disciplines—and through maintenance of highest professional standards in affiliated institutions, the university exemplifies the best in health care. By making available its expert service to the community as a model, the university gains access to the social laboratories in which students and faculty can study the natural history of health as well as of disease.

It is clear that establishing the university as the effective center of medical education is the greatest need and the most important challenge to the field of medical education today. Now, and in the years ahead, the effort must be made to carry this development beyond the developments envisioned even by Flexner.

Bowers notes that the Coggeshall Report met with some initial resistance from department heads in medical schools who feared loss of control to the school administrations, from some hospital administrators who feared loss of some of their independence, from some medical-school deans who worried about the financial stress these measures might bring about, from nonuniversity-affiliated hospitals which were reluctant to defer to the medical schools, and from some specialty boards that also feared loss of autonomy. But Bowers concludes that "these tensions are easing . . . and control of graduate education by academic medical centers is approaching reality" (2, p. 91).

Although the words "intern" and "internship" will undoubtedly persist for some years, the AMA has ceased to refer to them in its directory of graduate medical education programs since "the first year of graduate medical education is part of a continuing period of graduate medical education, or residency rather than a separate and independently approved year" (7, pp. 35-36). The AMA goes on to say:

The first graduate year will be reviewed by residency review committees as part of the review of the residency programs which sponsor and supervise that first year.

Three types of first graduate medical education years will be listed in the Directory and will form the basis for the National Intern and Resident Matching Plan. They are as follows:

1. *Categorical First Year*—These are first-year programs planned, sponsored, and conducted by a single approved residency program as part of that residency. The content of such a first year will be limited to the specialty field of the sponsoring residency program.

2. *Categorical First Year*—The asterisk designates a first-year program that will be planned, sponsored, and supervised by a single, approved residency program as part of that residency's program of graduate medical education, the content of which will not be limited to the single specialty of the sponsoring residency program but may include experience in two or more specialty fields as determined by the sponsoring program.

3. *Flexible First Year*—The first year will be sponsored by two or more approved residencies and will be jointly planned and supervised by the residencies that sponsor it. Such a first year is designed to give a broad clinical experience for: (1) Students who feel the need for this type of first year: (2) Program directors who feel that such an experience will best serve the purpose of subsequent graduate education in their field; and (3) Students who have not yet decided on their specialty but may wish to choose among several fields during their first graduate year. The content of a flexible first year must include four months of internal medicine, but the remainder of the year may be designed in accordance with the purposes of the two or more sponsoring residency programs, and the interests and needs of the student.

It should be understood that the standards for approval of residency programs are separate from the requirements established by the various specialty boards for the certification of individuals in a particular specialty.

The National Intern and Residency Matching Plan referred to by the AMA is a computerized matching of resident applicants and approved hospital training programs. The aim is to meet the desires of the hospitals and the would-be residents to the greatest extent possible. The aims also are to eliminate, if possible, pressures and special inducements that tended to skew the distribution of interns and residents, leaving some hospitals with many unfilled slots and other hospitals oversubscribed. (With the movement away from the free standing internship, the NIRMP has been renamed the National Residency Matching Plan.)

Both intern and resident have historically been required to work a demanding time schedule. Work weeks to 80 and 100 hours were not uncommon, and uninterrupted sleep was not designed for either. In 1975, a group of interns and residents (commonly referred to as *housestaff* because they are staff employees of the house, i.e., the hospital) persuaded the Physicians' National Housestaff Association to vote support of a union to represent their interests, that is, improved patient care, better hours, and more money. What the long-term impact of this unionization movement will be, only the future will tell. At the time of this writing (September 1979), the position of the National Labor Relations Board (NLRB) is that housestaff are students and not employees and therefore not protected under National Labor Relations Act.

As a final note on graduate medical education, it should be noted with respect to residencies that not all training programs are in general or special hospitals. The American Board of Preventive Medicine is not a clinical specialty, and its residents are typically trained in nonhospital settings.

The process for reviewing and approving a residency training program requires, as with so many activities, coordination with a number of independent organizations and interest groups. The residency review committees cited in the Millis Commission Report lost some of their autonomy in 1975 when the approval of each program shifted from the residency review committee to the Liaison Committee on Graduate Medical Education (LCGME), which is a representative body of the AMA, AAMC, ABMS, CMSS (Council of Medical Specialty Societies), and the American Hospital Association (AHA). There is, in addition, a representative of the federal government and one of "the public." The LCGME is to graduate medical education what the Liaison Committee on Medical Education (LCME) is to undergraduate medical education.

Established at the same time (1972) as the LCGME was the Coordinating Council on Medical Education (CCME), which has the same body of representatives as the LCGME, though not necessarily the same people. The CCME was designed to be a coordinating and supervising agency "concerned with policy matters and accreditation of all levels of medical education" (10, p. 3). Shortly after its establishment, the CCME moved to establish a Liaison Committee on Continuing Medical Education (LCCME) consisting of representatives from the AMA, ABMS, AHA, AAMC, CMSS, Federation of State Medical Boards, and the Association for Hospital Medical Education, as well as the public and federal representatives. In August 1979 the AMA pulled out of the LCCME and proceeded to establish its own accrediting body—the Committee on Accreditation of Continuing Medical Education. The pull-out was controversial, apparently stemming in part from the AMA belief that the LCCME was not sufficiently sensitive to the views of the AMA which was, after all, the representative body for the practitioners who would be taking continuing education programs and the organization which provided the bulk of the financial support for the liaison committee's work. There were a number of issues that bothered the AMA, one being the AMA wish to have the accrediting authority delegated to state medical societies rather than to new regional groups representing all of the constituent members of the LCCME. This was not just a desire for AMA domination, but rather a concern over how the continuing education courses would be organized. *Medical World News* (August 20, 1979) reported AMA concern that the liaison committee's approach would "change the nature and structure of CME [continuing medical education] to resemble didactic medical school courses . . ." Whether there will be a rapprochement between the AMA and LCCME, whether the LCCME will fold, or whether the two bodies will continue to accredit programs independently with confusion reigning—is not known as of September 1979 (Chart 1-1).

Table 2-4 is a listing of approved examining boards in the various M.D. specialties and the subspecialties in which certification is currently possible. Table 2-5 lists the specialties and subspecialties in osteopathy. It should be noted that many osteopathic physicians are completing their graduate training in allopathic residency programs. Most of the M.D. specialties will examine D.O.s for certification upon meeting their respective requirements. Comparison of the two tables indicates remarkable similarities. Osteopathic subspecialties do not seem as well developed. There is no osteopathic general surgical specialty, and most of the surgical specialties are coordinated through the American Board of Osteopathic Surgery. This kind of grouping also exists for EENT. Allergy and immunology have not developed as an osteopathic specialty nor has preventive medicine.

POSTGRADUATE OR CONTINUING MEDICAL EDUCATION

Keeping up to date has always been an important responsibility for all professional people. Physicians have sought to do this in a variety of ways. We saw in the last chapter how the establishment of medical societies and of journals were important steps for the dissemination of knowledge, enabling a physician to acquire new knowledge and to refresh one's memory about many clinical matters.

With the legitimate focus of the profession on improving the quality of undergraduate medical education, development of rigorous specialty training requirements, and the improvement of the sites of specialty training programs that has just been described, the matter of continuing education received relatively little organized attention.

Hospitals, of course, usually mandate that physicians on the staff attend the periodic medical staff meetings where, among other things, there would be some continuing education activity, such as the presentation by the pathologist of some interesting case(s) or the showing of a film on some medical topic by the representative of one of the pharmaceutical manufacturers. Like the exhibits (Fig. 2-3) and lectures at the annual meeting of the state medical society or other society, attendance was spotty, and the programs themselves often left

Table 2-4. Approved Examining Boards in Medical Specialties and Subspecialties for Which the Boards Certify

American Board of Allergy and Immunology*
American Board of Anesthesiology
American Board of Colon and Rectal Surgery
American Board of Dermatology
American Board of Family Practice
American Board of Internal Medicine
   Allergy and Immunology
   Cardiovascular Disease
   Endocrinology & Metabolism
   Gastroenterology
   Hematology
   Infectious Disease
   Medical Oncology
   Nephrology
   Pulmonary Disease
   Rheumatology
American Board of Neurological Surgery
American Board of Nuclear Medicine**
American Board of Obstetrics and Gynecology
   Gynecology
   Obstetrics
American Board of Ophthalmology
American Board of Orthopedic Surgery
American Board of Otolaryngology
   Endoscopy
American Board of Pathology
   Anatomic Pathology
   Anatomic Pathology and Medical Microbiology
   Anatomic Pathology and Clinical Pathology
   Anatomic Pathology and Forensic Pathology
   Anatomic Pathology and Neuropathology
   Chemical Pathology
   Medical Microbiology
   Medical Microbiology and Medical Chemistry
   Clinical Pathology
   Dermatopathology
   Forensic Pathology
   Radioisotopic Pathology
   Hematology

Table 2-4. (continued)

American Board of Pathology (*cont.*)
  Anatomic Pathology/Hematology
  Clinical Pathology/Hematology
  Neuropathology
  Anatomical, Clinical, and Forensic Pathology
  Blood Banking
  Clinical Pathology/Blood Banking
American Board of Pediatrics
  Pediatric Allergy
  Pediatric Cardiology
  Pediatric Hematology/Oncology
  Neonatal/Perinatal Medicine
  Pediatric Nephrology
American Board of Physical Medicine and Rehabilitation
American Board of Plastic Surgery
American Board of Preventive Medicine
  Aerospace Medicine
  Occupational Medicine
  Public Health
  General Preventive Medicine
American Board of Psychiatry and Neurology
  Psychiatry
  Neurology
  Child Neurology
  Psychiatry & Neurology
  Child Psychiatry
American Board of Radiology
  Diagnostic Roentgenology
  Diagnostic Radiology
  Medical Nuclear Physics
  Radiological Physics
  Radiology
  Radium Therapy
  Diagnostic Radiological Physics
  Roentgen Ray and Gamma Ray Physics
  X-Ray and Radium Physics
  Roentgenology
  Therapeutic Radiology
  Therapeutic Roentgenology
  Therapeutic Radiological Physics

Table 2-4. (continued)

American Board of Radiology (cont.)
  Therapeutic & Diag. Radiological Physics
  Diagnostic Radiology with Special Competence in Nuclear Radiology
American Board of Surgery
  Pediatric Surgery
American Board of Thoracic Surgery
American Board of Urology

*A conjoint board of the American Board of Internal Medicine and the American Board of Pediatrics.

**A conjoint board of the American Board of Internal Medicine, the American Board of Pathology, and the American Board of Radiology.

Source: Directory of Accredited Residencies 1977-78. Chicago American Medical Association, p. 368. 1978.

something to be desired. During the 1950s, beginning with the American Academy of General Practice (later, American Academy of Family Physicians), an increasing number of organizations began to require their members to take a specified number of approved continuing education courses. Over the years, the trend accelerated. At least 17 state medical societies now require continuing medical education for maintenance of membership. At least 18 states require it for renewing one's medical license. Some specialty boards now also require this of their members as part of the developing trend for specialty recertification. The American Board of Family Practice, interestingly enough, having as one of its sponsoring societies the pioneering American Academy of Family Physicians, was the first board to set a recertification exam. It might be noted that in 1970 the AMA House of Delegates urged all medical specialty boards to consider the desirability of periodic recertification.

When this movement first began, many of the continuing education programs were of questionable value. The AMA began to move directly on this matter in 1961 by accrediting continuing medical education programs. In 1975, the LCCME was established. In 1979 as we noted above, the AMA withdrew from the LCCME and reestablished its own accrediting mechanism.

Similar developments have occurred within the osteopathic movement.

FOREIGN MEDICAL GRADUATES

The United States has always attracted graduates of foreign medical schools, and they came for a variety of reasons: to escape wars, religious persecutions, and other repressions, as well as to seek new opportunities that frontiers

Table 2-5. Approved Examining Boards in Osteopathic Specialties, and Subspecialties

American Osteopathic Board of Fellowship of the American Academy of Osteopathy
American Osteopathic Board of Anesthesiology
American Osteopathic Board of Dermatology
American Osteopathic Board of General Practice
American Osteopathic Board of Internal Medicine
American Osteopathic Board of Neurology and Psychiatry
   Neurology
   Psychiatry
   Neurology and Psychiatry
   Child Psychiatry
American Osteopathic Board of Nuclear Medicine (conjoint board)
American Osteopathic Board of Obstetrics and Gynecology
   Obstetrics and Gynecology
   Obstetrical-Gynecological Surgery
American Osteopathic Board of Ophthalmology and Otorhinolaryngology
   Ophthalmology
   Otorhinolaryngology
   Orofacial Plastic Surgery
American Osteopathic Board of Orthopedic Surgery
American Osteopathic Board of Pathology
   Anatomic Pathology
   Clinical Pathology
   Forensic Pathology
American Osteopathic Board of Pediatrics
American Osteopathic Board of Proctology
American Osteopathic Board of Radiology
   Diagnostic Roentgenology
   Roentgenology
   Radiation Therapy
   Radiology
American Osteopathic Board of Rehabilitation Medicine
American Osteopathic Board of Surgery
   Neurological Surgery
   Orthopedic Surgery
   Plastic and Reconstructive surgery
   Thoracic Surgery
   Urological Surgery

Source: J Osteopath. Assoc. 77, (Suppl. to No. 8): 1978.

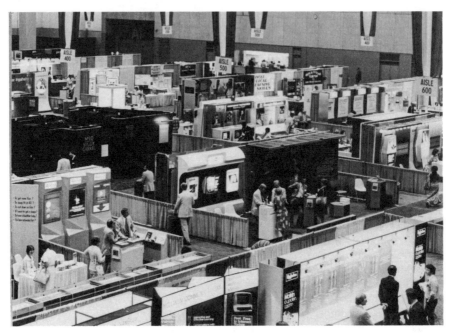

Figure 2–3. Commercial exhibits at a meeting of the AMA at which physicians can learn about new drugs, new instruments, new equipment, and new therapeutic approaches. (Reprinted with permission from the AMA.)

frequently offer in terms of adventure, economic well-being, etc. In the eighteenth and nineteenth centuries, these physicians often provided a level of expertise very needed in this land. Following the Second World War we began to experience a new wave of physician immigration, graduates of European schools who sought to establish a new life in America in large measure as a result of the dislocations resulting from the war or of the economic chaos that reigned in the postwar period. As Europe was reconstructed, the flow of physicians waned. Bowers notes that the flow of physicians from both Latin America and Canada also tapered off from the mid-1960s through 1972 (2, p.92). The Latin influx probably reflects the surge of Cuban refugee physicians before our break with Cuba.

But a new group of physicians began to come to the United States to establish new lives and to get advanced training; some, under the guise of advanced training, hoped to stay. They came from Asia. During the 1950s and 1960s, the flow from Asia did not contribute much to the permanent physician supply in the United States because our immigration laws were weighted heavily against Asians and Africans. Changes in 1968 and 1970, however, opened the gates to immigration from all countries. Physicians came heavily from a former American colony (the Philippines), from newfound military allies (South Korea, Thailand, Iran, Taiwan), and from India. We welcomed them, for they helped fill the physician shortage that we were beginning to experience as a result of a rapidly growing population, hospital expansions to meet its needs, and added expansions due to research and technological advances that enabled physicians to help people in ways that were not previously feasible. Many, if not most, of these physicians came from medical schools that were relatively unknown to us, and many—again, if not most—of the physicians, also had language difficulties (though not the Indians, who, thanks to British imperialism, had received excellent English-language training). The unknown quality of the foreign schools raised legitimate questions about the adequacy of their student training and of their graduates' competence. The language barriers caused communication problems between doctor and patient, as well as between the foreign medical graduate and his or her American colleagues.

To deal with the uncertainties of foreign training and with the language problems (12, pp. 16-17):

In 1956, a Cooperating Committee on Graduates of Foreign Medical Schools (including members of the American Medical Association, the Association of American Medical Colleges, the American Hospital Association, and the Federation of State Medical Boards) endorsed the concept of an examination program to identify those FMGs (both U.S. and foreign-born) who are most likely to benefit from graduate medical training in the United States. The Educational Council for Foreign Medical Graduates (ECFMG) was set up to organize and administer a certification program which included a medical and English examination and a reivew of credentials; it began operation in October 1957. . . .

The medical examination questions are drawn from the pool of questions used in the tests given by the National Board of Medical Examiners. The standard for passing is set such that an expected 2 percent of U.S. medical students would not achieve the cut-off score of 75. FMGs have the option of retaking the examination until they achieve this passing score; more than 40 percent of the foreign physicians sitting for each examination are repeaters.

The ECFMG has become a major professional organization, giving examinations twice a year (usually February and September) in 42 centers in the United States, 7 in Canada, and over 125 in other countries. By the end of 1973, about 178,325 foreign-trained physicians had sat for the examination, and over 119,800 (or 67 percent) ultimately passed. In 1972 alone, 37,000 foreign-trained medical graduates took the examination, slightly more than one-half for the first time. Over the years, the percentage of candidates passing has varied from a low of 31 (in 1971) to a high of 46 (in 1967). The overall pass rate indicates that the examination does serve as a screening device, although there have been recommendations that it be made even more stringent . . .

Once the candidate passes the test, produces the required professional credentials, and clears his financial account, he is eligible to receive the ECFMG standard certificate. He can be awarded an interim certificate pending clearance of his financial account.

The ECFMG certification process is necessary in two different (although related) areas, namely, State licensure and appointment to hospital training programs. With regard to the former, ECFMG certification is listed by almost all of the 55 State and Territory licensure boards as part of the requirements for permanent licensure for physicians trained outside the United States or Canada . . ., although it can be waived in individual cases by all but 13 boards. . . . With regard to the latter, hospitals wishing to retain approved internship or residency programs and to appoint foreign-trained physicians to those programs must appoint only those with ECFMG certification or those with full and unrestricted State license to practice . . . (The latter requirement is relaxed somewhat for U.S. citizens.) Similarly, accreditation of hospitals by the Joint Commission on Accreditation of Hospitals is dependent to some degree on hospitals employing only those foreign medical graduates with valid State licenses or ECFMG certification.

An "agreement of combination" was signed in November 1973 mandating the merger of the ECFMG and the Commission on Foreign Medical Graduates; the latter had been formed originally as an outgrowth of one recommendation of the 1967 National Advisory Commission on Health Manpower. The functions of the two organizations will continue, and the name will become the Educational Commission on Foreign Medical Graduates. The merger is expected to become effective by summer of 1974.

The ECFMG exam has been criticized by many on a number of accounts. Some, for example, feel that many foreign physicians are not accustomed to the objective-question-type exam. Others cite language barriers as creating difficulty in understanding the questions. Still others feel that it is not fair to ask foreign physicians, who may have been out of school for many years, questions that we give not to practicing physicians but to medical students who are at the time on top of the subject matter. To some of these objections, there is merit, but they do not by themselves justify abandonment of the exam unless an alternative screening device is developed. We can be comfortable, for example, with the 86 physicians from Malaysia who took and passed the 1972 ECFMG exam (12, pp.73-81). No Malaysian failed that year. And we can be comfortable with the 89 (out of 101) University of Singapore graduates who passed and of the four out of four from Kenya. But we don't know how representative their performances are compared with all the graduates of those schools. We might hypothesize that it is probably fairly representative because the schools are in former British colonies, and we do know that British schools are very similar to ours and that of 700 United Kingdom graduates who took the exam, 646 (over 92%) passed. But then again, the British influenced India, and of 4,078 Indians who took the exam in 1972, only 1,667 passed. We don't inspect those schools, and we probably couldn't if we wanted to either because the pride of nations may not allow foreign (U.S.) inspection or because the nations aren't interested in training physicians for the United States. The simplest solution for the United States, then, is to screen would-be residents and immigrants.

The development of FLEX has introduced a new element that affects FMGs (11, p. 17):

One problem facing FMGs, in particular those FMGs desiring to remain as permanent residents and practice medicine in the U.S., has been the wide variation among States in licensing requirements. A desire to bring some degree of standardization into State requirements led to the development in 1968 of a new examination, the Federation Licensure Examination (FLEX). Like the ECFMG examination, it is based on the current pool of questions from the National Board of Medical Examiners; the FLEX questions are chosen to be of middle range in difficulty with emphasis on their practical value and clinical applicability ... FLEX is given in June and December of each year, over a three-day period. It is open to graduates of U.S. medical schools and to FMGs and is designed for physicians who are in house staff positions or already in practice. By December 1973, all States (except Florida and Texas), the District of Columbia, Puerto Rico, and the Province of Saskatchewan, will use FLEX as their official board examination, and thus it will become the standard test for licensing for physicians who do not or cannot take the National Board examination. Legislation is required in the other two States and then FLEX will become universal. The total number of State licensure examinations administered in 1972 was over 18,500, the great majority being FLEX. Because of other requirements for licensure heretofore incumbent upon FMGs but not USMGs, however, it is not clear whether States will accept FMGs taking FLEX on the same terms as USMGs taking FLEX.

Some coordination between the ECFMG and FLEX is beginning to take hold. For example, the ECFMG will now accept for certification, any FMG who has passed FLEX with a grade of 75 or better and does not require him to take the ECFMG's own examination.

But the problem or issue of FMGs does not end here. The states are the licensing authorities, and the shortage of physicians in some areas has prompted the licensing authorities to issue temporary licenses. Very often, these licenses are issued to physicians who seek to take positions in state-run mental hospitals, positions that carry low salaries (by American standards), and an inadequate environment for an effective therapeutic program (by American standards). American physicians shy away from such positions, but FMGs are attracted to them, for the pay is good by their standards, the facilities and support services better than anything they have known, and the position represents an entrée to the United States. In some states, nearly all the medical staffs of state mental hospitals are from foreign medical schools. Since the therapeutic processes in psychiatry depend so much on verbal communication and an understanding of the patient's social milieu, alarm over the quality of care by FMGs is well founded. The situation in Illinois and the questions raised regarding professional competence were described by the *American Medical News* (13):

All 127 unlicensed physicians working for state mental hospitals in Illinois failed their licensure test, and another 63 did not even take it.

The physicians, mostly foreign-born and all foreign trained, should be fired from their positions, according to a 1972 Illinois law concerning special-permit physicians. Such a mass firing, however, could jeopardize the state's entire psychiatric program, said Robert DeVito, MD, director of the state Dept. of Mental Health.

The 190 physicians were required by the 1972 law to replace their special permits for state hospital work with an Illinois license by 1976. The National Board of Medical Examiners devised a test for them in 1974 and administered it last year. The examination drew questions from the psychiatric/neurology and general medical sections of the clinical competency portion of the FLEX.

All the physicians failed the clinical portion, "and not just by a couple of points, but with appallingly low scores," said a spokesman for the director of the Dept. of Registration and Education, the licensing arm of the state.

Scores reportedly were as low as eight points out of a possible 800, with an average score of 227 on the medical and 245 on the psychiatric sections. Six physicians passed the psychiatric portion.

Dr. DeVito said that the physicians did so poorly because "they responded to the notification of the test with an intense degree of anxiety. They didn't read the questions as clearly as they should have. They said they only had an average of 45 seconds for each question.

"In terms of their competency . . . every three months they are examined by licensed physicians," Dr. DeVito said. "They are then repermitted every year based on the four evaluations."

The Illinois State Medical Society (ISMS) asked that the Dept. of Mental Health initiate steps to replace unqualified permit doctors rather than rely solely on efforts to upgrade those now practicing in state mental hospitals.

"Efforts to upgrade permit doctors previously have failed," said ISMS President Joseph Skom, MD. "While the ISMS supports the department's efforts to obtain a temporary extension of full licensure requirements and avert a crisis, we believe this deplorable situation must be permanently resolved."

Dr. Skom also said that "the major problem is lack of funding. We believe that the state can attract qualified physicians if it is willing to pay the going rates."

Dr. DeVito met with Gov. James Thompson March 2 to ask his help in sponsoring emergency legislation that would enable the unlicensed physicians to continue working in the state institutions.

"The governor and I have agreed that the goal of the new legislation is full licensure and to replace the permit system," Dr. DeVito told AMN.

The governor's office said legislation has been drafted "that would allow these people to continue in service until June 1. And there's the possibility that they could be fired, that they be retained, that the test was invalid, that they be retested, or that they be kept on until 1980," the spokesman said.

"Our main concern is the patient," Thompson's spokesman said. "The governor has stressed that he wants the best care available given the resources."

Until the issue of new legislation is resolved, all 190 physicians will continue practicing in the state hospitals.

The issue of FMGs is hotly debated in medical circles. A recent exchange in the "Letters" section of *JAMA* is worth quoting (14, p.106):

To the Editor.—In his commentary "A Prescription for the Rising Cost of Medical Care" (237:2383-2384, 1977), Vernon H. Mark, MD, states that "all too often, when they finish their educational program, they enter the American medical system in areas where they are least needed." This quote is in reference to the ever increasing number of foreign-born medical graduates (FBMGs) who are swelling the physicians' ranks in this country. Even if this allegation is correct, in part or whole, Dr. Mark's proposed solution to this problem is wrong both in principle and practice. He proposes to limit the FBMG to two years postgraduate training in this country: "This would prevent them from becoming Board-certified" and theoretically discourage their entry into the "American medical system."

In his aside concerning the surgical and medical specialties as well as elsewhere in his commentary, he favors simple solutions for complex problems. The problems he addresses are not so easily remedied; otherwise they would have been already. I find it regretable that Dr Mark chooses to single out the FBMG in his discussion of the problems of specialization. It is not my experience that the FBMG seeks to contribute to the maldistribution of medical care in this country. I find, rather, that the FBMG is exploited and scapegoated both in educational and service settings. The American medical system accepts the FBMG ambivalently and then often showers on him or her condescension and derision. Dr Mark should know that large numbers of FBMGs who continue to remain in this country do so either as a result of the personal choice to become a citizen or as a result of our exploitation of them in educational and service settings.

In my opinion exploitation of and the second-class professional status accorded the FBMG is undeserved and not in accord with the moral and ethical responsibilities of the medical community. We as physicians have responsibilities to patients, colleagues, and our communities. We have not consistently been ethical or honorable in the discharge of these responsibilities as they relate to our foreign-born medical colleagues. It is time that the FBMG be seen as a colleague and that our exploitation of the FBMG stop.

I would suggest in the future whether or not an FBMG returns to his country of origin is not a question to which the medical community may ethically address itself. How the FBMGs are welcomed into and treated by the medical community of this nation is the question that we ought to continuously address. If we find that an FBMG does not fulfill the standards we set for a physician, then before we permit him or her to enter into the American medical system, it is incumbent on us to assist him or her to the degree needed as we would any native-born physician.

My thanks to Dr Mark for sharing his provocative and stimulating formulations.

BRUCE R. HOLZMAN, MD
Columbia, SC

In Reply.—Dr Holzman's statement that I singled out the foreign-born medical graduates in my comment on specialization is inaccurate. I mentioned them only as one facet of the problem. Dr Holzman's sympathy for these physicians is commendable, and his assertion that they are exploited is true, at least in some cases, but the exploitation is not one-sided. Many FBMGs are also exploiting their own countries by leaving them with the ostensible purpose of getting more education but with the actual intention of immigrating to the United States.

At first glance there may seem to be nothing wrong with this kind of exploitation. After all, our country was built by immigrants; furthermore, educated immigrants would appear to make desirable citizens. However, there are two aspects that Dr Holzman overlooks in his defense of the FBMG. Many of them come from underdeveloped and economically poor countries that have expended their meager resources to educate their citizens so that their physician population could be maintained or increased in undeserved areas. The immigration of these physicians is especially unfortunate because it deprives their own countrymen of needed services. Also, these immigrants have taken places in their country's medical schools that could have been held by others who would be more faithful to national medical needs.

Equally important is the fact that FBMGs fill positions in this country that should be held by American physicians. Every year thousands of well-qualified applicants to American medical schools are turned away, and at the same time many foreign-born physicians are imported to fill positions in private and public hospitals. Our system should be altered to correct this inequity.

There should be some exceptions to the immigration ban on FBMGs. Those who are escaping from political tyranny and cannot return to their native countries could be welcomed like any other refugees. However, the other foreign physicians should be encouraged to come to this country only to study in a temporary resident status. In this capacity they will be giving service as well as gaining education; then they should return to their countries of origin. A two-year limit on their training and stay would ensure this.

VERNON H. MARK, MD
Boston City Hospital
Boston

The FMG situation is exacerbated by the FMG underground. Speaking to this in 1973 before the U.S. Senate Committee on Labor and Public Welfare, Dr. Robert Weiss, from Harvard University's Center for Community Health and Medical Care, said (15, pp. 126-129):

The problem of the quality of health care delivered is not only fundamental but is complex. Control of the quality of health care is being approached by various methods, and the enactment of PSRO legislation is proof of the Congressional concern about this subject.

It is obvious that the effect of measures such as peer review hold promise of being able to contribute to quality control of health services in the future, but most experts in the field agree that the methodology that is necessary to accomplish this is not fully developed and will require a great deal of research before fulfilling its potential.

In the meantime, the controls which have been responsible for the development of high quality medical care in the United States have been seriously eroded by the application of a double standard in the control of the process of education of physicians entering the United States health care system.

I am referring to the dilution effect on quality of physician manpower by the large increase in the importation of Foreign Medical Graduates from widely varying educational systems. Since the Flexner Report in 1910, American medical education has been subjected to a whole series of controls on the process of education. Requirements include selection for admission to an undergraduate college which has been subjected to outside accreditation; certification of the student by the faculty of that institution; selective admission to an approved United States medical school whose instructional content and methods are subject to a continuous review by an outside accrediting body; and certification by the faculty of that approved medical school before graduation. Only then is a United States graduate eligible to sit for our licensing examinations. It is clear that control of a minimal level of educational process and certification does assure that United States medical graduates have been observed and certified on their professional competence before being tested on just their level of medical knowledge.

There are increasing numbers of Foreign Medical Graduates (FMGs) immigrating to the United States educated in medical schools in developing countries. Most of these countries do not exercise any control over student selection or the educational process. This has resulted in a serious dilution in the quality of physician manpower in the United States. Last year approximately 80 percent of the FMGs entering the United States had been educated in the Asian countries. The substitution of the Educational Council for Foreign Medical Graduate (ECFMG) examination for the complex system of controls developed for United Stated medical graduates as the sole measure of the FMG's competence to enter the United States health care system has resulted in a double standard for the minimal control of physician manpower.

In addition, even those FMGs who pass the ECFMG and go through approved United States postgraduate training programs perform much worse on licensure and specialty board examinations than United States medical graduates. FMG's have a six-fold greater failure rate on State Medical Licensure examinations than United States medical graduates, and the experience of the specialty boards reveals that the overall failure rate of FMGs is 63 percent while the failure rate for United States medical graduates is 27 percent.

The above figures relate to the best of the FMGs. In addition, there were, in 1971, 69,188 FMGs in the United States of which 15 percent (10,360) were not fully licensed and were not in approved training programs. Of these, 51 percent reported their primary activity as direct patient care. The number of FMG's known to the American Medical Association (AMA) who are not fully licensed and are not in approved training programs has risen to over 14,000.

In a study published in the June 20, 1974, issue of the New England Journal of Medicine, my colleagues and I report on a study which indicates that there is an ever increasing group of non-ECFMG certified physicians working in the United States health care field with direct patient care responsibilities and with unsupervised physician responsibility. They are employed with non-physician titles and work as physicians in a "medical underground."

A written questionnaire was distributed by the ECFMG to 4,035 Foreign Medical Graduates taking the January 1973 examination in United States centers. Fifty-eight percent of the 2,500 permanent residents taking that examination were working in the health field. Those working in the health field had a lower pass rate on the examination than those not working (15 percent versus 26 percent).

The questionnaire was followed by telephone interviews of a sample of 850 respondents designed to obtain more detailed information about job duties. Seventy-three percent of the 513 FMGs who reported working in the health field were involved in direct patient care and 64 percent of these were employed in hospitals. Analysis of specific job duties revealed large numbers functioning independently and in unsupervised settings.

The results suggest that serious problems exist in the control of the quality of care delivered in the United States health care system . . .

Senator Kennedy: There are FMGs that are practicing medicine today that have not completed their examinations, State licensing examinations?

Dr. Weiss: There are 14,000 that are listed by the AMA who are not fully licensed. They probably have temporary licenses, but they are not in approved training programs, which means that they are practicing medicine in an unsupervised setting.

Senator Kennedy: Where?

What sort of places?

Dr. Weiss: They are in all sorts of settings.

They tend obviously—you will hear, I am sure, about some of them in the mental hospitals, it was of some concern to me that it is just not in mental hospitals but they are in general hospitals, city hospitals, county hospitals, State hospitals.

Senator Kennedy: What are they doing there?

Dr. Weiss: Their jobs include, as they are usually employed under titles which are non-physician titles, but we interviewed those physicians, a sample of those physicians, and used interviewers who are proficient in the foreign languages of the foreign medical graduate and those physicians are taking night calls, covering emergency rooms, sewing lacerations, doing general practice, in charge of emergency rooms, delivering babies, prescribing pre-anesthetic medication, giving anesthesia, writing xray reports.

They are doing history and physical examination. Some of those known as pathology assistants are reading frozen sections on which a surgeon bases a determination to do a radical procedure or not.

Some of them are doing flouroscopy. These are those that are totally unknown to the AMA. These are the ones who are [not] even ECFMG certified, which is the examination that only permits the Foreign Medical Graduate to enter an approved training program on the supposition that they will benefit from postgraduate medical education in the United States and deliver care in a supervised setting, so that in addition to these who are non-ECFMG certified, we also have that large number of 14,000 who are ECGMG, probably many of them ECFMG certified, known to the AMA, who are not fully licensed, meaning that they probably hold temporary licenses in their States, temporary, partial or limited licenses.

Senator Kennedy: What other kinds of people they are practicing medicine on?

Are these upper income people, in the suburbs? Scarsdale?

Dr. Weiss: It is a leading question, Senator, obviously.

It is obvious that we do not have exact data and specifically because we maintain confidentiality on exactly the hospitals that these physicians are practicing in by name.

But it is certainly true that the new flux of Foreign Medical Graduates has resulted in primarily because of the demands made in urban settings in inner city hospitals for service, and in many cases, because the physicians are overloaded, and I would suggest that in the State mental hospitals, which will be referred to, I am sure, by another member of this panel, they are taking care of the sickest and the poorest of the patients in the United States.

The comment was made in a statement of the relation to those in psychiatry, that they were second class physicians taking care of second class citizens.

I do not believe these are second class citizens. I think these are poor people who unfortunately are not able to get decent care.

Senator Kennedy: Why are the States not doing something?

Dr. Weiss: Well, sir, I think it is both the State and Federal governments' responsibility and it is obvious from the previous testimony that the Administration has not taken a policy which would do something about the problem. It is perfectly obvious since most of them are working in hospitals, that they could not work there without other physicians and hospital administrators knowing about it.

I think what happens is that they get in and are given assignments and they do the jobs that American physicians would rather not do; and as a result I think it has already been true that many of our municipal, State and Federal authorities—these people are paid lower salaries. They are exploited in the sense that they do not come up to standard and they cannot demand the same wage that they would get, although they are paid higher wages than they would be paid in their own countries, which is one of the reasons why indeed they continue to come . . .

Mr. Goldman, *Subcommittee Staff Director:* Dr. Weiss, would you think there is variation in the quality of medical services offered by FMGs State to State depending on whether they happen to be not licensed, partially licensed or fully licensed?

Dr. Weiss: I do not think there is any question about it. Of those people who have not even passed the ECFMG—well, they have not in any way satisfied any requirement, and are employed with non-physician titles, and that is a totally unknown number in terms of this one examination, and we found of 3,935 that 1,905 were in the health care field delivering patient care.

Mr. Goldman, *Subcommittee Staff Director:* Is the lack of uniformity from one State to another fairly marked or not marked with respect to licensing of FMGs?

Dr. Weiss: The lack of uniformity is marked. It bears on the question of national licensing. There is no question that what happens is that many State licensing boards, medical boards, act as States happen to see its priorities for staffing in public institutions, and very often look the other way, and bend the requirements, so one has considerable variation in terms of how licenses are given . . .

In 1910 when the Flexner Report was published, we were inundated with poorly trained physicians from proprietary medical schools, as you know.

In 1947 I believe there were still 3,000 physicians practicing in the United States who had been graduates of unapproved and unaccredited medical schools, and any delay would mean that it would take 40 years before these people are out of the system.

In other words, if the average of coming in is 25, and they practiced to age 65, it is 40 years more that they are in the system. So that I think that despite the fact that there will be severe dislocations, and in a paper to appear this coming Thursday, we pose some of the many implications and problems which will be inherent in applying for rigorous standards and getting unqualified people out of the system.

On the other hand, I think the time has long since passed for us to begin to act. I am happy to see that this legislation addresses itself to the question.

In regard to our production of physicians, in the 1950's there were about 128 physicians for 100,000 in the United States. In 1970 there were 150 physicians per 100,000 in the United States.

However, there were only 126 U.S. medical graduates per 100,000, so that the production of U.S. physicians in the United States medical schools has not kept pace with the growth of the population, so that I think that we have avoided the issue consistently by allowing ourselves to take an expedient route and expedient solution.

I feel that while there are qualified FMG's in the system, unquestionably, there are so many that are unqualified, and so little way of controlling at the present time that it is terribly important to impose the kind of restriction that is contained in the current bill that Senator Kennedy and Senator Javits are jointly sponsoring.

Congress took steps to deal with the problem of FMGs in the Health Professions Educational Assistance Act of 1976 (P.L. 94-484). The law provided that FMGs who wished to enter the United States as immigrants on the basis of their skills must pass parts I and II of the National Board exams or an equivalent acceptable to the secretary of HEW and be competent in written and oral English. In addition, the law set a similar requirement for those coming for residency training except that the alien may no longer apply for permanent residence status while here but must, rather—after two or in some cases three years—return to his or her country of origin for at least two years and then apply for an immigration visa. There were, of course, a number of special qualifying provisions, including a number of waivers, that could be employed until 1980, but the essence of the law was clear.

A Visa Qualifying Examination (VQE) was subsequently developed and certified as the equivalent of parts I and II of the National Boards. It was administered in 27 centers around the world in September 1977; 4,611 FMGs took the exam, 75% failed. The overall failure rate jumped to approximately 80% for the 1977 and 1978 combined test results. Those who failed will not be able to enter the United States as exchange visitors or as physician immigrants. Whether all, who were already in the United States and who were supposed to take the test, did, in fact, take it is not known. It did not, of course, deal at all with the medical underground. The president of the NBME noted, after the 1977 test results were in, that the results showed that FMGs performed better on the clinical portion than on the part testing basic medical-science knowledge.

More reassuring, however, was a study reported in the January 1979 issue of the *American Journal of Public Health* in which investigators found "no consistent and generalized pattern of differences" between U.S. and foreign-trained physicians (16, pp. 57-62).

It is safe to say that we have not heard the end of the FMG issue. The legislation was controversial because it sought to curb a flow of physicians who were sought by state mental hospitals and by many teaching hospitals that had only nominal, if any, university medical-school ties.

The waivers and grandfather clauses did not, moreover, deal with the competence of those who have already been licensed under weaker conditions, and as the testimony cited earlier indicates, it is likely to take 40 years before these physicians are out of the system.

As in other areas in the evolution of medical practice in the United States, however, we may find leadership in further reform shifting to other, but related, areas, for example, change dictated by almost universal specialty certification, increasing control of specialty training by medical schools, the movement for continuing education required by more and more specialties and medical societies and some states, and a developing movement for periodic reexamination of physicians.

CONCLUSION

Reform in medical education continues. Leaders are constantly seeking new ways to deal with the problems that they perceive to exist, problems that interfere or prevent the training of the best possible physician, and problems that interfere with the practice of high-quality medicine. By and large, the problems of the pre-Flexner era are gone, and those of graduate medical education are infinitesimally small compared with what they were in the early part of this century. The principal focus now is postgraduate medical education and a related issue of FMGs.

REFERENCES

1. Medical education in the United States, 1977-1978: 78th Annual Report of Medical Education. *JAMA* 240: 1978.
2. Bowers, J. Z.: *An Introduction to American Medicine, 1975,* DHEW Publication No. (NIH) 77-1283, U.S. Department of Health, Education and Welfare, 1977.
3. *American Medical News,* October 17, 1977.
4. Freymann, J. G.: *The American Health Care System: Its Genesis and Trajectory.* Baltimore, Williams and Wilkens, 1974.
5. *JAMA* 222: 1972.
6. *JME* 53: 1978.
7. *Directory of Approved Residencies, 1974-1975.*
8. *The Graduate Education of Physicians.* Citizens Commission on Graduate Medical Education. Chicago, American Medical Association, 1966.
9. Coggeshall, L. T.: *Planning for Medical Progress Through Education,* Evanston, Association of American Medical Colleges, 1965.

10. Medical education in the United States, 1973-1974: 74th Annual Report on Medical Education, *JAMA* 231: 1975.

11. *Foreign Medical Graduates and Physician Manpower in the United States,* DHEW Publication No. (HRA) 74-30, U.S. Department of Health, Education and Welfare, 1974.

12. *Medical Licensure Statistics for 1972,* Council on Medical Education of the American Medical Association, 1973.

13. *American Medical News,* March 7, 1977.

14. *JAMA* 239: 1978.

15. *Report No. 93-133, Health Professions Educational Assistance Act of 1974,* U.S. Senate Committee on Labor and Public Welfare.

16. Saywell, R. M., Studnicki, J., Bean, J. A., and Ludke, R. L., A performance comparison: USMG-FMG attending physicians. *A. J. Public Health* 69:1979.

3

Medical Practice

There are somewhere between 400,000 and 425,000 physicians in the United States. As one looks at published data on the number of physicians, however, one has to be extremely careful because of how the data are aggregated. The figures just given include D.O.s and M.D.s, federal and nonfederal physicians, active and inactive physicians, as well as those whose addresses are not known, and they include physicians in Puerto Rico and U.S. outlying areas. The federal physicians include those in the United States and on overseas assignment. The figures do not, however, include physicians with "temporary" foreign addresses. Depending on the purposes for which a table or report is prepared, the data may consist of any combination of the above elements.

The gross number of physicians is typically used as a basis for projecting future physician needs. In 1950, for example, there were about 233,000 physicians, which represented a physician-to-population ratio of 149 physicians per 100,000 people. This was a marked change from 1940 when the ratio was 133 per 100,000 population. Since 1940, the ratio has risen steadily to 197 per 100,000 persons at the end of 1976. Projections for 1985 indicate that the physician/population ratio will reach somewhere between 207 and 218 per 100,000 population. The 1985 projections all assume there will be a net decline in the flow of foreign medical graduates to the United States.

What is the meaning of the physician/population ratio? It is a gross, an unrefined figure enabling planners to compare physician availability from one year to the next. Its value is very limited, and particularly so when applied to state populations; when applied to subunits of states, it is of slight, if any, value.

There is no optimal ratio. One needs a supply of physicians adequate for a population so that it has easy access to care and so that the full state of medical science can be applied. The number of physicians needed will be affected by the level of our knowledge and technology: new knowledge and new technology permit physicians to do what was previously not possible, and the need for more physicians becomes necessary. But determination of need is complex and, one might say, elusive. It is affected not only by the limits of our knowledge and our technology but also by the health problems that exist and that the population recognizes as problems. It is affected by the extent to which physicians are willing to use other health workers, by the population's willingness to accept other kinds of practitioners, and by the expectations of the population.

To illustrate the difficulty in relying on physician/population projections, we might note that the AMA reports a total of 348,443 physicians as of December 31, 1976 (1, p.12). Not included in the AMA count, however, are osteopaths, inactive physicians (22,117), unclassified physicians (30,129), and those with unknown addresses (8,757). The General Accounting Office, in its report to Congress, *Are Enough Physicians of the Right Types Trained in the United States?* totals those categories (409,446) and adds the number of osteopaths (15,436) to develop the physician population ratio of 197. But how appropriate is it to count the inactive physicians, the nonclassifiables, and the address unknowns? As our population, including physician population, ages, we may be misleading ourselves. But even the AMA figure of 348,443 poses some problems, for only 318,412 are in patient care: 6,935 are in teaching; 11,689 are in administration; 8,514 are in research; and 2,893 fall into a miscellaneous "other" category.

Need projections derived from manipulation of physician/population ratios also fail to take account of need in light of the potential contribution from other health practitioners, in particular, nurses and physician assistants. In 1974, for example, there were approximately 22,000 pediatricians in the country; studies have shown that a pediatric-nurse practitioner can do 82% of what a pediatrician does: 71% on the nurse's initiative, an additional 11% after telephone consultation with the pediatrician. What does this say about the need for pediatricians? Could the same kinds of results be found if appropriately trained nurse practitioners worked in obstetrics and gynecology (over 21,000 obstetrics-gynecology specialists) and family or general practice (approximately 80,000 M.D.s and D.O.s)? These questions are simply introduced to indicate that determining the need for physicians is exceedingly complex, the variables are many, and reliance on physician/population ratios is much too simplistic for an industrial society.

In recent years, health planners have tended to shy away from physician/population ratios, to focus instead on the availability of primary-care physicians. In part, this was in recognition of the limitations of the ratios; more importantly, it was in recognition of the facts that rural areas and inner cities were having difficulty recruiting and retaining physicians who were in primary care, because general or family practice lacked appeal, as evidenced by the increasing number of physicians who sought specialty training, and because rising costs seemed to bear a direct relationship to the growth of the medical specialties.

HOW PHYSICIANS PRACTICE

Most physicians are in the *solo practice of medicine,* that is, they practice alone, by themselves. Most are, moreover, paid a *fee for service.* These are the time-honored methods of practice and payment. They are not without their critics.

The chief criticism of solo practice is that the physician practices in an unchallenged setting wherein he or she is not accountable to peers for either comprehensiveness or quality of care. The physician, instead, has only to satisfy the patient; as a lay person, the patient is not in a position to judge either. In such settings, critics will note, sloppy and inappropriate care can too easily develop. This is a widely held belief by those who are not in solo practice. Critics of solo practice typically go on to say that the quality of care in group or hospital-based practices is superior to that provided in solo practice. This, too, is a widely held belief by those not in solo practice, but data to support this conclusion are hard to come by. Mechanic correctly points out, however, that "the major foundations of solo practice are ... undermined by technical developments and the growing complexity of treatment and rehabilitation, and new incentives encouraging more organized practice" (3, p.286), but he also notes (3, p.36):

There is reason to believe that salaried group practitioners are somewhat less responsive to their patients than private fee-for-service physicians, and that the efficient organization of such practices can stimulate bureaucratic barriers that undermine a sympathetic approach to the patient. Such problems are in no sense insurmountable but require organizational mechanisms that insure the quality of responsive care. These mechanisms become costly and begin to consume some of the savings that result from more efficient organization. In short, although organized group practice appears to offer possible advantages for high quality care which surpass those available under existing conditions, it is not at all evident that such care, if it is to be effective and conform to high expectations of preventive and responsive care, can be provided at significantly reduced cost.

"Reduced cost," and, as also suggested, although the potential for improved quality of care exists, the data to support this are sparse at best. Silver reminds us that "the advantages and disadvantages of this system have been argued for generations. It is not likely that they will be settled in this generation. There are strong partisans on both sides" (4, p.98).

So, too, on *fee for service.* Critics assert that it encourages a physician to overservice because the physician is paid for each service. This may mean added units of service during each visit, or it may mean follow-up visits, and there are no controls except the conscientiousness of the physician and the limits of patient tolerance. Abuses of Medicare and Medicaid and of some health insurance policies lend support to these criticisms. But how widespread the abuses are, no one really knows. These abuses, however, can exist in group-practice settings just as easily, particularly the ordering of extra services for which charges can be made. But whether extra visits or services are ordered because they are judged to be clinically necessary or as a safeguard against possible malpractice suits (the physician practicing in this instance what is known as *defensive medicine*) or to earn the extra payments is not easily determined except in the most glaring cases of abuse.

It is fairly well agreed within professional circles that physicians are not as sensitive to cost implications as they might be: Their training never focused on what services cost; they just ordered tests and services to explore all avenues as part of the learning process. Recognition of this weakness in physician education has prompted some to argue for introducing this issue into the educational process.

Fee for service can be viewed, positively, as a symbolic contract, binding the physician to the patient in terms of attention, care, and confidentiality. As Mechanic suggested, there is reason to believe that fee-for-service physicians are more responsive to their patients. If the patient doesn't like the physician's attention, the patient can go elsewhere. So, too, if the patient doesn't like the care or the way the care is delivered. While patient choice is built into most large group-practice arrangements, there are bureaucratic constraints that may govern regardless of who the physician is.

Fee for service is also a vehicle for strengthening the confidentiality of patient records: If the patient contracts with a physician for certain services, the contract being consummated by payment of the fee, the patient has a right to confidentiality. No one has a right to that information without the patient's consent. Typically, patients authorize release of information in order to have the fee covered by insurance, but if the patient asks no one to pay the fee, then the patient is assured by contract that no one will have access to that information. This is not a matter of theoretical concern. Many patients will not submit claims to the insurance company because of the possibility that their employers might gain access to that information. Similarly, many workers will not consult company physicians for some ailments for the same reason: Can one be absolutely certain that the boss won't be able to pressure the company physician into releasing the medical information on an employee?

Finally, on fee for service, we might note that, historically, physicians charged on a *sliding-fee scale,* the poor paying less (if at all) than the more affluent. With the widespread growth of health insurance, and now Medicare and Medicaid, sliding-fee scales are much less common. Sliding-fee scales are different from *relative-value scales,* which have been employed to express a value relationship between various medical and surgical procedures. Under relative-value scales, a number is assigned to each task or procedure that expresses its value in relation to other tasks. Thus, a simple task may have a unit value of two, whereas a more complex procedure might have a unit value of four, and one, still more complex, a value of eight or nine. The fee a physician chooses to charge is arrived at by the physician setting a dollar value to the unit service. Relative-value scales have been challenged by the U.S. Justice Department as constituting price fixing, and their legality is in doubt: while a number of medical organizations capitulated to government pressures and abandoned their scales, the American Society of Anesthesiologists went to court on the issue and won in July 1979.

An increasing number of physicians are functioning in *group-practice,* which is generally viewed as consisting of three or more physicians of the same speciality or of different specialties who choose to practice together. They choose to do this for a variety of reasons, including ease of consultation with colleagues, coverage on nights and days off, sharing of equipment and support personnel, and intellectual stimulation. Physicians in group-practice typically charge a fee for service (or the group makes the charge), but how they divide the income varies from fee for service to straight salary to salary plus a percentage of the group's incomes. In a growing number of group-practices, however, the group contracts with a population to provide complete medical services (including preventive and family-medicine services) in return for regular payments whether the enrolled person uses the service or not; hence, no fee for service. These kinds of groups are called *health maintenance organizations* (HMOs) because of their emphasis on prevention. Physicians working in HMO settings are usually salaried. Some of the physician-run HMOs are also known as *foundations for medical care.* Some foundations for medical care do all that HMOs do but do not underwrite the risk for the population, and not all are comprehensive. An increasing number of physicians are entering *hospital-based practice.* Some of these are in hospital-based HMOs but where they are not in HMO practice, the patient typically pays a fee for service, but how the physician is paid varies.

There were approximately 8,483 groups identified by the AMA in 1975 with some 66,842 physicians (5, p.31). Not all of these physicians, however, were in full-time group practice. About 8% of these groups with about 20% of the group-practice physicians (13,534) were formally associated with prepayment health-insurance plans and clearly represent larger group practices. About 54% of the groups surveyed in 1975 were single specialty groups, and about 10% were limited to general practice (6, p.49). Nearly 40% of the groups consisted of only three physicians; 75% consisted of from three to five physicians. Goodman (5, p.43) concludes his analysis by stating,

Prepaid groups tend to be much larger than other organized forms of group medical practice, are more likely to reimburse their member physicians on the basis of a straight salary, and are more likely to have a legal affiliation for the provision of medical services with either a hospital, university, labor union, or industry. In addition, prepaid groups tend to provide a broader range of social and counseling services and to utilize a more formal management structure. Thus, it is evident that prepaid groups are distinct from other forms of group practice in terms of these attributes.

MEDICAL SOCIETY MEMBERSHIPS

Most physicians find it essential to belong to the county or city medical society in the area in which they practice and to their state medical society. Only slightly more than half elect to join the AMA. A variety of factors influence the latter choice: Many disagree with the AMA's policies (although the association probably truly represents the views of its members), others are more interested in their specialty society, while others are concerned over the rising costs of membership, particularly in view of the many other memberships a physician feels he or she must maintain. The AOA claims that approximately 80% of all osteopaths belong to the AOA. AOA is, of course, a much smaller body with a smaller constituency; it is less active in the political arena, and it does not engage in the breadth of activities that engages the AMA.

Membership in the local and state societies is more vital for the practicing physician. These organizations serve a number of purposes. First, and perhaps most important, these organizations enable the physician to meet his or her colleagues, to learn about the skills and abilities of other physicians, and vice versa. This is a vital element in building the practice of a specialist, enabling other physicians to size one up to permit them to decide whether or not they have confidence for purposes of referring their patients. A second element in society membership is that it facilitates an intellectual interchange between physicians that has always been a key element in the continued learning process of physicians. Indeed, this has been formalized in most societies, whereby the society sponsors regular continuing medical education programs, an increasingly important and necessary activity for professional practice. Many local medical societies and all state societies also issue medical journals for dissemination of knowledge and of other matters of concern to the profession. Third, medical societies provide an organizational focus for representation of medical view-points on matters affecting the health of the population as well as on the viewpoints of the physicians on other matters of interest or concern to them. Related to this is that if any body—government, industry, or others—wishes to communicate something to the medical community, the medical society is perhaps the most effective vehicle. Fourth, membership often enables the physician to receive such financial benefits as group life, health, and malpractice insurance. A fifth function of the medical society is social.

Laws and society rules governing memberships vary from state to state. Some states allow membership in the local society only. Other states have a unified local/state membership. Some have a unified local/state/AMA membership. Generally, membership in the state society or AMA requires membership in the lower units. One AMA exception is direct AMA membership for federally employed physicians.

Physicians often belong to other medical societies, depending on their interests and on their specialties. Among the many other societies is the National Medical Association (NMA), an association representing the special interests of black physicians.

It was suggested above that the policies of the AMA probably truly reflect the views of its members, suggesting that it is a very democratic organization. It is. We can perhaps begin to understand this if we begin to look at the lowest level of medical society organization, the county or city medical society.

When a physician first enters practice, he or she tends to join the local and state medical societies for reasons that have been cited. The local society carries out a variety of society activities, and these activities will vary from society to society. But they might include working with the local health department to assist it in carrying out its functions, for example, assisting the health officer with an immunization program, helping with athletic physicals, and so on, making representations to the local government on behalf of some voluntary agency that is seeking government help, assigning representatives to serve on the boards of directors of various community agencies, investigating complaints against physicians involving medical ethics or malpractice, organizing continuing education programs for members to help them keep up to date, participating in public and school health-education programs, or editing the local medical journal or newsletter. The local society will have its officers and will be entitled to send a certain number of delegates to the state medical society's legislative body, often called the House of Delegates. Each of these activities—some to serve the public's interest, some the medical profession's interest—requires time on the part of the local members. If the physician participates, accepting her or his share of the society's work load, the physician can be influential and help shape the policies that are formulated by the local body and the positions taken by the local delegates to the state society. To the extent the physician ducks local assignments, that physician's influence is reduced accordingly. I recall the story told about one group of physicians who could never activate their local society around a particular set of issues that concerned them; one society member observed about that group of physicians: "They never assumed a role in society affairs, they never came to meetings except when they wanted the society to do something for them, so it should have been no surprise to them that the membership was lackluster in its responses."

As in most voluntary groups, leadership falls to those who take the time, who make the effort to help the organization. All too often, the critics of organizations, including medical societies, remove themselves from meaningful participation and are, therefore, unable to exercise influence.

State medical associations or societies are similarly structured except that their legislative bodies are not the total membership present and voting as at the local levels but the House of Delegates from the constituent local medical societies. State society delegates meet usually once or twice a year to conduct the legislative business of the association and at other times when necessary. The state associations tend to have a broader range of activities and larger paid staffs. (Large local medical societies have well-paid executives, usually nonmedical; state societies have larger nonmedical staffs to execute the directives of the House of Delegates and officers. Some state societies may have employed physician executives.) The state associations concern themselves mainly with state issues: advising and negotiating with state agencies, testifying and lobbying at the state legislative sessions, proposing new policies and new legislation, negotiating as appropriate with the state hospital association, helping to devise solutions to problems that impact on society members, organizing the annual meeting of the association for the conduct of association business, and continuing medical education activities. Increasingly, the state associations are involved with health planning issues and, in particular, with the state health planning and development agencies. State medical journals also represent an important medium of communication to association members, with scientific articles, book reviews, editorials, communications from the state health agencies (which may consist of reporting on new health problems, new state services, as well as rules and regulations regarding diseases that must be reported to the state, etc.). Some of these journals are of exceptional quality, the *New England Journal of Medicine* (the journal of the Massachusetts Medical Society) being one of the world's leading medical journals.

Much of the work of state medical societies is carried out by committees drawn from the general membership. The committees are assisted by the paid staff, and the committees serve generally in an advisory capacity to the House of Delegates or to carry out the mandates of the House. Here again, the ability to influence the state society or association depends on the willingness of the membership to get involved.

Each state society elects a certain number of delegates to serve as its representatives in the AMA's House of Delegates (Fig. 3-1). The AMA functions

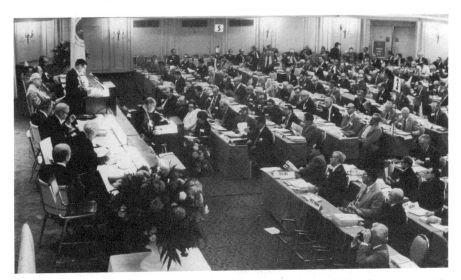

Figure 3–1. A meeting of the House of Delegates of the AMA. (Reprinted with permission from the AMA.)

as does the state societies except that, as a national body, it deals mostly with national issues, and it has a larger paid staff with many more functions to perform.

The extent of AMA activities were described by the AMA's executive vice president for the period of July 1971 through November 1972 as follows:

The AMA is a large and complex organization whose wide-ranging, diversified activities are probably unmatched by any voluntary agency in the world. Here is a kaleidoscope of AMA:

1. In one day at the AMA there are 700 long distance telephone calls received. Membership Services gets 137,000 per year. That's 545 per working day.
2. 8,000 to 10,000 pieces of first class mail come in to the AMA every day. Membership Services gets 855 per day or 212,000 per year. This is 6,000,000 pieces of incoming mail every year for the AMA total.
3. Each year we receive 50,000 requests from the general public for help and information, and many thousands more requests for information are received from physicians.
4. In the AMA master listing of physicians, 8,000 changes are made every week to update home and office addresses.

5. Your AMA Library, with quiet efficiency, each month processes and responds to: 3,000 research requests, 700 requests for books, photocopy requests for approximately 25,000 pages of material, and a steady stream of requests for use of the 4,500 available films.
6. The AMA is one of the world's largest publishers and about one third of our budget goes into the paper, printing, and mailing of what is published.

- American Medical News has a circulation of 20,000,000 newspapers per year.
- We produce approximately 1,300 different pamphlets on child care, health education, health tips, sex education, first aid, and many other subjects.
- We have mailed 5,000,000 pamphlets on "The Pill" alone.
- The magazine Today's Health reaches several million readers per month.
- "Horizon's Unlimited," a brochure on health careers, has been sent in the amount of two million to schools, colleges, and medical societies.
- The Journal of the AMA distributes 12,000,000 copies per year.

7. Throughout the course of the year the AMA sponsors 400 scientific lectures, 400 scientific exhibits and 300 exhibits on drugs.
8. The AMA-ERF Student Loan Program has arranged over $54,000,000 in loans to over 23,000 medical students, interns, and residents . . . 47,000 loans. We have received and distributed over $35,000,000 to medical schools in this country.

In addition to these on-going services, some of the special activities during 1972 were:

The "Quality of Life"

The AMA's Congress on the Quality of Life conducted in Chicago in March 1972 was structured to provide national impetus to a better quality—and therefore improved health—at the beginning of life. Some 50 national organizations co-sponsored this meeting under AMA leadership. It was an extraordinary success, with over 1,000 participants, and extensive national coverage.

A seminar on the Quality of Life was also held in San Francisco in June. The second Quality of Life Congress, emphasizing the middle years of life, will be held in the Spring of 1973.

Maternal and Child Health

AMA's Committee played an important role in promoting the above-mentioned Quality of Life Congress. During the last year it also stimulated the establishment of centralized community or regionalized intensive care centers for infants born at risk, a program which will have a dramatic effect on the USA infant mortality rate once it has been implemented in all key areas.

Blood Banking

Our Committee on Transfusion and Transplantation is conducting a survey of 6,000 blood banks to provide up-to-date information. A current directory of such facilities will be published by the end of 1972.

Human Sexuality

An AMA committee has completed a text on this subject to aid physicians dealing with human sexuality and family counseling. We predict that this text will be a best-seller to the medical profession, other professions, and the public.

Scientific Assembly and Postgraduate Education

For the first time, postgraduate courses were offered at the 1972 Annual Convention. All seven courses were sold out a month before the meeting. This is one of many changes in our Scientific Assembly that the Board of Trustees and Council on Scientific Assembly are considering as efforts are made to improve programs and increase attendance.

Nomenclature

The effort to bring order into the nomenclature morass in which our profession finds itself was more frustrating than ever during the last year.

The AMA publication of Current Procedural Terminology, now moving toward its 3rd edition, was the focal point of intense controversy as varied interests maneuvered for control of the basic input. A systematic nomenclature for processing of claims, for peer review, and for effective accumulation, evaluation, and communication of medical information was impeded by the impasse. Accurate identification of the services provided by physicians was suffering delay because of the clash of differing objectives. The AMA, with the support of most of the medical specialty societies, at times found itself embroiled in a conflict of divergent interests, with the National Assn. of Blue Shield Plans, the American College of Surgeons, the Commission of Professional and Hospital Activities, and the federal government.

Prescription Drugs

The first edition of AMA-Drug Evaluations was distributed to 230,000 physicians, the most widely circulated single edition of a medical text ever published. A revised, updated 2nd edition will be published in 1973. The

Council on Drugs and staff have made a major contribution to the quality of medical care and therapy by this effort.

Medical Education

The Council, its Committees, and staff are an integral part of America's medical educational effort. Without the daily application of these enormous resources, the production of new physicians, and their subsequent graduate and continuing education would experience a sharp setback. No aspect of the education and credentialling of physicians is untouched by the diverse activities of AMA's medical education arm.

The establishment of two new committees called the Coordinating Council on Medical Education and the Liaison Committee on Graduate Medical Education, which include representation from the AMA, American Hospital Association, the Council of Medical Specialty Societies, the Association of American Medical Colleges, and the American Board of Medical Specialties, was an historic change.

Education of Allied Health Professions and Services

Nineteen medical specialty and allied health associations cooperated with AMA in setting standards and approving educational programs for 18 allied health occupations.

International Medicine

(1) The first meeting of the new National Council for International Health, comprising the major national agencies active in this area, was held at AMA Headquarters this year. AMA provided the initial impetus to develop this coordinating activity, and is furnishing staff for the Council.

(2) The recent USA-Russian accord will open up bilateral opportunities for both countries. The President of the AMA and the Chairman of our Committee on Community Emergency Services left for Russia on July 8 to conduct an in-depth survey of the Russian program which has received praise from American observers.

(3) Chinese medicine, including acupuncture for anaesthesia, is the subject of discussions between representatives of China, the USA, and the AMA. You will be hearing much more about that in the near future. In October 1972, a delegation of Chinese physicians visited AMA Headquarters as a part of their tour of U.S. health and medical facilities.

(4) In Vietnam, AMA continues to provide volunteer practicing physicians for provincial hospitals, and, with academia, shares American medical edu-

cation expertise to help operate the medical school in Saigon. These are two positive programs that all observers have applauded.

Interns and Residents

The unique problems and interests of house officers have resulted in recent House of Delegates' actions and intensified AMA staff activity to respond to their needs.

Three mailings have been made to 51,000 interns and residents urging AMA membership and active participation in organized medicine locally. This staff activity is just beginning and will receive continued emphasis.

Membership Recruitment

Another subject of intense preoccupation is our level of dues paying members. In 1971, following the dues increase and the unique situation in New York, where the existing unified membership was declared illegal because of a local statute, AMA lost 12,000 dues paying members. As of June 16, 1972, we were 4,821 members ahead of the comparable figure at this time last year and we are confident that this upward trend will continue through 1973.

AMA conducted its first membership recruitment campaign this year. 50,000 non-members of AMA who are members locally are being urged to join. This program was carried out in cooperation with 850 medical societies who bill physicians on behalf of AMA. We expect some innovations in billing procedures that should have a salutary effect on membership totals.

Public Affairs—Washington, D.C.

The Washington Office staff operation is an integral arm of the public affairs program. During the last year national health insurance legislation, HMOs, PSRO, chiropractic in Medicare, catastrophic expense coverage, medical manpower proposals, cancer and heart research support, and many other controversial issues have kept our Washington staff constantly busy. Due in no small measure to their dedicated efforts, no significant legislation opposed by AMA has passed Congress in this session. Conversely, many bills have become law, due in part to our support and related staff activity.

Legislation

2,300 bills with medical interest have been reviewed by our Council on Legislation and staff. An increasing responsibility of the Legislative Department is the critical review of government regulations which often subtly create new law.

Fiscal Control

The Office of Finance came of age in 1972. Internal auditing procedures and budget control were established throughout the Association. Assembling of expenditures by program, in addition to accountability, facilitated priority planning.

Center for Health Services Research and Development

This AMA Center has become one of the leading medical socioeconomic research and development activities in the U.S. Here are a few selected items from an extensive program: (1) Staff support is provided our representatives on the Committee on the Health Services Industry; (2) the recent poll of AMA members was developed and processed by the Center; (3) over 25 medical societies have received assistance in the design of surveys and the collection of data, and twenty have prepared grant requests with the aid of the Center; (4) eight volumes have been published on the socioeconomics of medical practice; (5) the important research project being conducted with the University of Southern California on the "economies" of different types of medical practice is still in process, and no final conclusions are available yet.

Foundations for Medical Care

This challenging new development in medical society guidance of delivery systems, medical care financing, peer review, and a variety of other programs is receiving close attention from the Council on Medical Service and staff.

Rural Health

The Council on Rural Health is the focal point of activities to promote the best possible medical care and health in rural America. It is now developing "models" of effective rural medical care delivery systems in Adams and Lincoln Counties in the State of Washington.

Communications

This year has brought new and improved communications contact with the public and the profession: (1) The informational program to the public through paid messages has covered overeating, exercise, the environment, quality of life, Anatomy of a Doctor, and other subjects. 160,000 people have asked for materials from AMA based on these messages. It has been a successful effort but the cost is high.

AMA Update

This new monthly publication reaches 14,500 public opinion leaders in and out of government. It is being widely quoted by the press.

Radio News Telephone Service

Any radio station in the country can call AMA over a toll-free telephone hook-up and receive a taped interview on health subjects designed to be integrated into a station's local newscasts. An average of 250 calls is received a week. During the Annual Convention well over 500 calls were received.

Every segment of American life that involves health is touched by some AMA program. Is Dr. Welby accurate scientifically in his medical comments? AMA's Physicians Advisory Committee on Television, Radio and Motion Pictures in Hollywood reviews every word of the script and advises the producer. Does a dermatologic residency program need review? AMA staffs and finances the review committee, and all the other specialty review committees at an annual cost of almost $500,000. What kind of medical care is given to prisoners in our federal and local prisons? AMA and the American Bar Association have joined forces to study the problem and report to the nation. When the Epilepsy Foundation of America wonders what the other national voluntary health agencies are doing and planning, it attends a meeting sponsored by the AMA's Council on Voluntary Health Agencies, composed of the medical directors of 30 voluntary agencies, and reports on that AMA meeting in its national newsletter. Whether it is the accreditation of hospitals, the prevention of automobile injuries, the protection of athletes, the promotion of environmental and occupational health, or whatever, AMA is involved and is productive. It is a record of continuing accomplishment of which the House, the Board, all the Committees, Councils, Commissions, ad hoc groups and every member physician can be proud.

We often hear critics of organized medicine attack the AMA as a control center, pulling strings that fan out to all corners of the nation and dictating policies to the state and local levels. More often than not, the facts indicate that the AMA has taken up the cudgels on issues raised by local medical societies, issues that have implications extending beyond the local or state area, and the chief legitimization for AMA action was the AMA's *Principles of Medical Ethics.* MacColl notes that "the AMA code is a guide for the state and local societies which must include in their own codes all the principles in the AMA standards, but may expand provisions to meet local needs. Quackery, advertising, fee-splitting, patient stealing, promoting fraudulent remedies and devices and developing undue personal publicity have all been pretty well curbed through the application of these codes" (7, p.136). The AMA became directly involved in a local issue during the 1930s, and was found guilty of restraint of trade in 1941. The case involved the AMA and the District of Columbia Medical Society in their actions relating to the Group Health Association of Washington (GHA).

THE AMA, GHA, AND THE D.C. MEDICAL SOCIETY

MacColl notes that opposition to the GHA by the D.C. Medical Society arose almost immediately after the GHA was organized. The society notified "all the physicians in the area that the plan was unethical. GHA's physicians were expelled from the Society, and a list of 'reputable physicians' was circulated to all the hospitals for their guidance" (7, p.140). The D.C. Medical Society and the AMA were subsequently indicted, found guilty, and fined for having conspired to monopolize medical practice. MacColl goes on to note that the GHA physicians were later admitted to the society and had no subsequent difficulty over hospital privileges. In other parts of the country, specifically Seattle and San Diego, the local medical societies and not the AMA were the defendants, and in each case the medical societies lost in their efforts to block development of group health plans.

THE COMMITTEE ON THE COSTS OF MEDICAL CARE AND CONTINUED OPPOSITION TO GROUP PRACTICE

Behind these medical society actions was the specter of the 1932 report of the Committee on the Costs of Medical Care (8). That report recommended that medical care should be provided by organized groups of physicians, dentists, nurses, pharmacists, and others. These groups, moreover, should be organized so that they can provide comprehensive care in the home, physician's office, and hospital; preferably, these groups should be organized around a hospital. The report also recommended that the cost of care should be financed through some form of prepayment mechanism. In all, the report provided the first comprehensive review of the health needs of the American people. I have summarized only those recommendations that are germane to the discussion that follows.

The committee (omitting those who died during the study and those who resigned) consisted of 48 members, representing private medical practice, dental practice, public health, institutions and special interests, nursing, economics and sociology, and the public. One of the designated public representatives was Ray Lyman Wilbur, a physician who was President Hoover's secretary of the interior. Secretary Wilbur was chairman. Of 48 members, 25 held an M.D. degree, but institutional and professional loyalties were divided among these 25; One of the M.D.s was also a dentist and was dean of a dental school; three M.D.s were in public health and not in the clinical practice of medicine; one was a hospital administrator; one was secretary of the AMA. Only 15 were listed as in the private practice of medicine. Nine members of the committee, including eight physicians (seven of the 15 in private practice, the eighth being the AMA secretary), filed a dissent.

In their dissent, the minority noted its support for many of the conclusions and recommendations. They objected, however, to what they perceived as the tone or trend of the report as well as to some of the recommendations.

We call attention to the fact that neither scientific medicine nor the organized profession have been unprogressive. They have assumed initiative and have maintained leadership in the advancement of scientific knowledge and in improving the methods of its application to human welfare. In the opinion of the minority the general trend of the majority report makes it appear that the medical profession has been static and unprogressive. This implication we believe to be unjustified by the history of medical progress (8, pp.152-153).

Two of the private practicing dentists supported the nine dissenters in this point, noting in their dissent "that the attitude of the majority is unduly critical of the professions, and that this attitude has developed a bias in some of the statements in their report (8, p.185).

To what extent the report's *perceived* abusive language in respect to the professions colored or distorted the views of the dissenters to the main recommendations is not known. So often when things have gone wrong or problems develop we look for the villains on whom to place the blame when in fact there may be no villains because the evils just grew and developed as a result of one-time limitations of our knowledge, absence of technology, or changes in society at large. In eagerness to place blame, we sometimes alienate those who could have been supportive, and this may have been a factor with this report, for the dissenters went on to argue against the committee's recommendation for organized group practice and against "the corporate practice of medicine, financed through intermediary agencies . . .as being economically wasteful, inimical to a continued and sustained high quality of medical care, or unfair exploitation of the medical profession" (8, p.150). The dissenting group accused the majority, among other things, of being visionary, impractical, biased, and failing to understand some of the real lessons to be learned from European experiences. The dissent was vigorously stated and also offered some positive alternatives, but the medical profession by and large felt challenged and on the defensive.

In 1933, the AMA declared that groups of physicians in salaried practice were considered unethical. It was unethical, as the dissenters had noted.

---

when there is solicitation of patients either directly or indirectly . . .when there is competition and under-bidding to secure the contract . . .when compensation is inadequate to secure good medical practice . . .when there is interference with reasonable competition in a community . . .when free choice of physicians is prevented . . .when the contract because of any of its provisions or practical results is contrary to sound public policy (8, p.156-157).

This change on the part of the AMA reflected widespread concern within the profession, which hit the boiling point in Washington D.C., Seattle, and San Diego. The concern was professional as well as economic, although critics all too frequently focus on the economic component, ignoring the professional objections. MacColl notes that after the AMA fine in the GHA case the AMA disengaged from "further legal entanglement." He goes on to note that it fell to the local societies to interpret or misinterpret the code of ethics and that at times the interpretations were to serve the ends, and the fears and pressures, at the local level.

The objections to group practice at times took on rather nasty aspects. In metropolitan New York, for example, the Health Insurance Plan (HIP) was established in the mid-1940s as a demonstration project for national health insurance. HIP, the fiscal agent, contracted with medical groups, paying each group so much for each person on its list. How the group divided the money was up to the group. In return for the capitation payment, the group was responsible for providing comprehensive physician services, preventive and treatment. For hospital care, most HIP subscribers were covered by Blue Cross. While the local medical societies might not have been able to keep HIP physicians from joining, they could ostracize them socially. I recall the medical society meeting in the 1950s in Garden City, New York, where, at lunch, the HIP physician sat alone while his "colleagues" enjoyed fraternal relations with each other. As late as the 1960s, HIP physicians were denied hospital privileges. The intensity of local medical feeling did not need AMA fuel, for HIP, at its inception, had proclaimed itself a demonstration project for a national system, and there were many physicians in New York who were accustomed to government systems before coming to the United States. In addition, the economic pressures on physicians in New York City were considerable, for many believed in the 1950s that New York City had an oversupply of medical practitioners. At every turn, HIP was challenged by non-HIP physicians. While Blue Shield, which was sponsored by the medical profession, used paid salesmen and advertising, when HIP did this, "the charge of unethical conduct was raised. Ben E. Landis, one of the HIP physicians, took the matter to the Judicial Council of the AMA, which ruled in his favor, finding that HIP was a legally organized plan and had as much right to advertise as did Blue Shield so long as the personal qualifications of the physicians were not promoted" (7, p.139). By the 1970s, in New York, except on Staten Island, all wounds were healed, and HIP physicians were fully accepted by medical societies and hospitals.

The AMA's Judicial Council, in addition to the Landis case, also reversed, on appeal, the earlier expulsions from the Los Angeles County Medical Society of the developers of the Ross-Loos Medical Group.

In Baltimore, by way of contrast with New York, the state of Maryland, in consultation with the state and city medical societies, established a medical-care program to pay physicians for care of the poor. Physician payments were on a capitation basis—so much a year for the complete care of each person on the physician's list. Outside Baltimore, a different program existed, paying physicians on a fee-for-service basis. Some years after the program became operational, some physicians, in what had evolved into a more conservatively oriented state society, raised objections to the system of capitation payments, but the city physicians were satisfied with the program at the time, and there was not much the state society could do about it.

To return to the concept of group practice medical service plans, in 1948, the Massachusetts Medical Society accepted free choice of medical group as the equivalent of free choice of physician; in 1959, the AMA ended its opposition by adopting the report of its Committee for the Study of Medical Care Plans, commonly referred to as the Larson Report. MacColl notes that the Larson Report advised medical societies "to exercise great caution in blanket condemnation and the use of the term 'unethical'" (7, p.137).

CONDITIONS OF WORK FOR OFFICE-BASED PRACTITIONERS

Most physicians, it was noted, are in solo practice. Most see patients on an appointment basis. House calls by family physicians are pretty much things of the past: The physicians can be more efficiently engaged if the patient rather than the doctor travels for the consultation, and the physician can be more effective in whatever he or she does if the full armamentarium is available, as in the office, rather than the limited resources in the little black bag. Generally, solo-practice physicians have developed relationships with other physicians for coverage when away. Such coverage is considered a legal obligation, although the need for such arrangements has lessened as general hospitals establish full-time, medically staffed emergency rooms. Group-practice physicians have a built-in system of professional coverage, and the patient may benefit from the covering physician's access to the patient's medical record, which would typically not occur in solo practice. Many physicians are locating their offices in medical-office buildings, which frequently facilitate patient access to radiology, laboratory, and consulting services.

The AMA periodically surveys a sample of physicians (AMA members as well as nonmembers) on how they practice, and the results are very informative. The eleventh survey results and other data were published by the AMA under the title of *Profile of Medical Practice, 1978,* and the data that follows in this section are drawn from that volume and reprinted with permission from the AMA.

The AMA projections found that the 216,533 active, office-based, federal and nonfederal physicians in 1976 were distributed among the specialities as follows:

Specialty	N
Total	216,533
General practice	46,628
General surgery	19,864
Internal medicine	28,170
Obstetrics-gynecology	15,995
Radiology	7,028
Psychiatry	12,432
Anesthesiology	9,074
Pediatrics	12,981
Other	64,361

It should be noted that the above breakdown is a projection from the responding sample. It does not include some 130,000 active physicians who are in hospital-based practice (including 63,000 residents), administration, research, and other professional activities.

The average physician worked 47.2 weeks per year in 1975. (Data for 1976 were not reported.) The weeks per year varied from specialty to specialty from a low of 46.2 and 46.9 weeks for anesthesiologists and surgeons to a high of 47.4 weeks for general practitioners, radiologists, and psychiatrists. If looked at from the point of view of solo versus group practice, physicians in groups of five or more averaged a little less work—about a week—than those in smaller groups and solo practitioners.

The average physician worked 52.2 hours per week in 1976. The average varied considerably from specialty to specialty as the following indicates:

Specialty	Hours
General Practice	51.4
Internal Medicine	55.7
Surgery	54.4
Pediatrics	49.8
Obstetrics-gynecology	54.3
Radiology	48.4
Psychiatry	48.1
Anesthesiology	51.1

The data on hours worked per week in 1976 by size of group and solo practice are not terribly meaningful: according to the AMA's survey, groups averaged from 51.2 to 54.3 hours per week; solo practitioners averaged 51.2 hours per week.

In 1976, approximately 89% of the average physician's working hours (46.5 out of 52.2 hours) was devoted to direct patient care. Of the 52.2 hours averaged per week, 55.8% (29.1 hours) was spent in the office, 23.9% (12.5 hours) in the hospital seeing patients and 9.6% (5 hours) on the business-administration aspects of medical practice. House calls and other activities consumed the remainder of the time.

The average physician in 1976 made 128.5 patient consultations or visits per week, about 69% (88) of them office visits. But the average number here varied considerably by specialty from a high of 167.8 visits per week for family or general practitioners (177.2 in 1975) to 146.1 for pediatricians, 207.1 for radiologists (138.8 in 1975), 133.2 for specialists in obstetrics-gynecology, to 124.3 for internists, 122.2 for surgeons, and then a big drop to 50.6 and 33.8 for psychiatrists and anesthesiologists. (The 1975 figures are shown in the preceding sentence in which a significant change occured.) Many factors can, of course, account for yearly variations.

Average fees for an initial office visit in 1976 were up over those of 1975:

1975 (dollars)	1976 (dollars)	Specialty
13.10	14.80	General or family practice
26.11	31.27	Internal medicine
20.81	23.29	Surgery
16.18	17.45	Pediatrics
23.57	27.41	Obstetrics-gynecology

Follow-up-visit fees were considerably less than fees charged for the initial visit by from 28% to 50%, depending on the specialty. The average initial fee for all practitioners ($24.90) did not vary by more than $1 from solo to group practice except in the very large groups (26 physicians or more) in which the average was $29.10.

It costs money for a physician to maintain a practice: office rent, utilities, drugs and supplies, laundry, secretarial and nursing services, and sometimes the services of other health professionals, for example lab technician or physician's assistant. In 1975, the average physician had professional expenses of $38,481. For 1976, the projected average was $42,443, and projections by specialty were:

Dollar Amount	Specialty
42,407	General or family practice
45,567	Internal medicine
54,779	Surgery
36,624	Pediatrics
54,377	Obstetrics-gynecology
19,842	Psychiatry
22,207	Anesthesiology

Of the average professional expense reported in 1974 in *Profile of Medical Practice, 1977* ($33,985), the largest office expense was for nonphysician payroll, including employee fringe benefits; this averaged over $13,445. Drugs and medical supplies accounted for $3,813; malpractice insurance, $2,523; office equipment and supplies, $6,033; legal and other nonmedical professional services, $1,337; lab and x-ray services, $1,946; office insurance, $920. The AMA notes that the sum of these items is less than the total average expense due to nonreported expenses and incomplete information from some physicians. However, the figures are useful in getting some idea of practice expenses. Expenses vary, of course, among the specialties, malpractice insurance (professional liability) being very low for internal medicine ($1,256), pediatrics ($1,050), and psychiatry ($638) but comparatively high for higher-risk specialities such as anesthesiology ($5,791), obstetrics-gynecology ($4,985), and surgery ($4,090). Except for overall professional expenses ($42,443 for 1976) and for malpractice rates, figures in this paragraph are not available for 1976. For 1976, malpractice insurance expenses for internal medicine averaged $2,537; for pediatrics, $2,323; psychiatry, $1,140; anesthesiology, $10,596; obstetrics-gynecology, $8,198; surgery, $7,774.

The average net income for physicians for 1974 and as projected for 1976 was reported by the AMA as $51,997 and $59,554 and by specialty as:

1974 Income (dollars)	Estimated 1976 Income (dollars)	Specialty
44,727	47,438	General or family practice
51,390	60,459	Internal medicine
60,510	73,245	Surgery
42,112	46,962	Pediatrics
61,693	65,800	Obstetrics-gynecology
41,258	47,565	Psychiatry
54,365	60,059	Anesthesiology

The 1974 income figures are given to facilitate analysis with the earlier breakdown on professional expenses. For detailed analysis, however, the original AMA documents should be used.

Income figures are terribly deceptive and, like figures on weeks and hours worked, need to be taken with caution. There is, for example, a difference between urban and rural practitioner incomes, but the differences may not be significant because of lower living costs in nonmetropolitan areas—lower taxes, auto insurance rates, and so forth. The AMA's projected 1976 mean average net income for nonmetropolitan physicians is $54,571; for metropolitan physicians, it is $58,819 and $63,158, the larger figure for those practicing in metropolitan areas of less than one million people. For all physicians, the projected average is $59,544. (Note: the AMA 1976 figures on income are projected because its survey was conducted in November 1976).

Another reason for cautionary treatment of these income figures is that they do not reveal the nontaxable income that may accrue to the physician. Depending on the structure of the practice, the physician may or may not be the recipient of such nontaxable benefits as retirement contributions, life insurance, health insurance, car, and so on. In the very large group practices (26 or more physicians) and in salaried, hospital-based practice, these benefits are probably greatest. In business and industry, it is not uncommon to have such fringe benefits valued at 20%-25% of the taxable income paid to an employee.

The figures given by the various surveys are reported averages. Many within each speciality earn at a very high end of the spectrum, and their earnings are balanced by those at the low-income end. Typically, the highest earners in primary care at least have a very high patient volume; put another way, they really hustle.

As one might expect, there are geographical or regional variations in income and variations by physician age. On the latter, while the mean average income for 1976 was $59,544, the averages by age group were projected as follows:

Age Group	Income (dollars)
35 and under	53,480
36-40	66,526
41-45	67,653
46-50	67,432
51-60	61,209
61 and over	42,556

The younger physician's income begins low and rises as his or her practice is built up, and the older physician's income tends to taper off. The oldest physicians may, in addition, not be getting as many referrals since there may be a tendency for the bulk of physicians (who are younger) to relate more to their age peers than to the "old-timers." This is, of course, speculation.

The magazine *Medical Economics* conducts annual surveys of physician incomes, but its response rate is only 15%, whereas the AMA's response rate is 33%. *Medical Economics* reports the median income; the AMA reports the mean. The difference for 1974 was $2,143, the mean average income being $51,997, and the median, $54,140.

The AMA average income for 1976 was $59,554; *Medical Economics* found for 1976 an average income of $62,800. The AMA, however, includes salaried physicians whose reportable incomes tend to be lower, while *Medical Economics* excludes this group. With such a low response rate in both surveys, the question of reliability exists. Some believe that among the nonreporting physicians may be those whose incomes are the highest. In addition, both surveys depend on the information voluntarily supplied by physicians. There is no check on accuracy of reporting. However, the figures are about the best available. The Council on Wage and Price Stability in March 1978 cited "a study of physician's income in 1965 in which income data from a sample of physician's income tax returns, the *Medical Economics* median income estimate for each of the nine specialties was found to be within 10% and for all physicians within 3% of the IRS based estimate" (9, pp.141-143).

There was, however, another survey of physician incomes, a sample of 1,000 fee-for-service-based physicians. This survey was conducted by a consulting firm under contract with HEW (10). It found an average net income of $53,600, with distribution among the specialties as follows:

Specialty	Average Net Income
General and family practice	44,800
Internal medicine	53,900
Surgery (general)	61,300
Pediatrics	50,100
Obstetrics-gynecology	64,600

At least there seems to be some agreement that among these specialties, obstetrics-gynecology secures the highest net income; comparatively speaking, neither pediatricians nor family practitioners do very well. This survey, unlike the other two, finds the pediatricians doing better financially than the family practitioners.

Neither the AMA nor the *Medical Economics* and HEW surveys report on two of the most highly remunerated specialties: pathology and radiology. The Council on Wage and Price Stability, however, does report some previously unpublished data for those who are hospital based and whose earnings are on other than a fee-for-service basis. Their incomes appear in Table 3-1. Whether those pathologists and radiologists who do their own billing have higher average incomes or not is unknown. This table is worth examining, also, because of what it tells us about general hospitals.

The lowest earnings are for *salaried* pathologists and radiologists, those in

Table 3-1. Earnings and Reimbursement Arrangements of Hospital-Based Pathologists and Radiologists, Fiscal Year 1975

Physician Group	Mean Earnings[a] of Hospital-Based	
	Pathologists	Radiologists
All physicians	$98,400	$102,300
Compensation arrangement		
Salaried M.D.s	49,200	52,600
Percentage arrangement M.D.s	138,200	122,400
Teaching vs. nonteaching		
Teaching hospital	67,200	81,200
Nonteaching hospital	133,300	118,900
Hospital size		
Less than 100 bed hospital	107,500	125,300
100-299 bed hospital	143,300	110,600
300 or more bed hospital	66,600	90,200
Reimbursement arrangement (%)		
All reimbursement arrangements	100	100
Salary	27	16
Percentage of gross or net revenue	37	37
Fee for service	14	28
Salary + percentage of gross or net	22	19

[a]Excluding fee-for-service physicians, who bill patients directly.

*Source:*Unpublished data provided by the Health Care Financing Administration of the U.S. Department of Health, Education and Welfare.

teaching hospitals, and those in the largest hospitals. The largest hospitals tend to be teaching hospitals because they generally have the range of clinical cases that permit well-rounded teaching programs, and they have the patient load sufficient to justify development of strong supporting services and departments for the clinical services and the teaching programs. These hospitals are also the ones that tend to have a higher proportion of full-time salaried physicians. They are able to attract physicians on a lower income basis because they have other inducements: advanced technology, stimulating intellectual environment, research opportunities, fringe benefits, paid vacations, and time off for professional meetings.

The Dyckman Report on physician fees, which was issued by the Council on Wage and Price Stability, was controversial. A sensitive nerve was touched within medical circles at its suggestion that in terms of surgical-fee inflation, a possible explanation may be that "physicians have a target level of income. And when demand for their services is insufficient to achieve that income level, they raise their fees in order to achieve it" (9, p.ii). Another controversial point was the seeming acceptance of the alleged anticompetitive forces in organized medicine as exemplified by the codes of medical ethics and the efforts opposing federal subsidies for medical education and opposing expansions of medical schools. The controversy on these points stem from the medical profession's view that many of its anticompetitive actions could also be viewed as mechanisms to control the quality of medical care in the absence of anyone else doing anything to control quality. Concern by the AMA for the economic welfare of its members is, of course, a legitimate function for an association, but whether the opposition of the AMA to medical-school expansions and federal subsidies was economically motivated or motivated by professional concerns is debatable. In any event, in reading this report and others, one can't help but feel that to some extent the positions of the AMA 20, 30, and 40 and more years ago are not clearly indicated as being different from the positions of the AMA today, that the positions today may have been as reasoned as they were in years past. One senses that critics want to find the devil in the figure of the AMA.

Despite the controversies surrounding the Dyckman Report, the introduction and summary which follow, are worth studying.

ARE ENOUGH PHYSICIANS OF THE RIGHT TYPES TRAINED IN THE UNITED STATES?*

The cost of physcian care is increasing at a distrubing rate. Last year alone, physician fees rose 9.3 percent—50 percent more than other consumer prices. The 1977 increase followed a pattern that spans nearly three decades. In fact,

---

*This section is the full introduction and summary to the Dyckman report.

ever since 1950, physician fees have consistently outpaced overall inflation except during the 1971–74 period of wage and price controls. Over the entire 1950-77 period, physicians' fees increased 43 percent faster per year than non-medical care prices.

All medical care services have long been a major source of inflationary pressure in our economy. Sharply rising medical care prices have contributed to a steady increase in the share of GNP represented by health care outlays, going from 4.5 percent of GNP in 1950 to 9.3 percent today.

Previous Council reports dealt with hospital cost inflation and private sector efforts to contain health care costs.[1] This report deals primarily with physician fee inflation and its principal causes.

Consumer outlays for physician services have risen even faster than fees, increasing from $2.7 billion in 1950 to about $35 billion in FY 1978. Sixty percent of the increase in consumer dollars paid to physicians is the result of higher fees, with the remainder accounted for by population growth and an increase in the quantity of physician services, such as diagnostic tests and more frequent visits.

Physicians' incomes have grown rapidly as the result of fee inflation. The median income of self-employed physicians—$63,000 in 1976—is higher and has risen faster than that of any other major occupational or professional group for which historical income data are available. This trend has been developing for many years. In 1939, physicians' earnings were less than twice as great as those of a broad group of professional and technical workers. But by 1975, physicians' earnings were four times as great.

Moreover, there is substantial income variation among specialties within the profession and the variations do not appear to be related to supply conditions. Supply, in fact, seems to have little bearing on fee structures and incomes. While surgeons are in greater relative supply than primary care physicians, income levels of surgeons are considerably higher than those of internists, general practitioners and pediatricians.

Pathologists and radiologists have the highest earnings among broad specialty groups; one study estimates their mean earnings at about $100,000 annually in 1975. Hospital-based pathologists and radiologists whose incomes are derived from percentages of department revenue contracts with hospitals earned $138,000 and $122,00, respectively, in 1975.

One explanation for high physician income is that it is necessary to attract an adequate supply of applicants into the profession. This notion is disputed, however, by several studies. Rates of return on investment in medical training are far in excess of rates of return for educational training in other fields.

This report also examines geographic variation in surgical fee levels.[2]

---

[1]See *Complex Puzzle of Rising Health Care Costs* and the *Rapid Rise of Hospital Costs.*

[2]Comparable data on hospital and office visit fees are not available.

Average surgical fees are more than twice as great in some large cities, such as New York, than in some smaller communities. After accounting for both metropolitan area size and cost-of-living differences, fees are still more than 50 percent greater in some locations than in others. There is no statistical evidence that fees are lower where relative surgeon supply is greatest. In fact, when variations in cost-of-living for different areas are not taken into account, fees are found to be higher where the relative physician supply is greater. This is consistent with the view that normal market forces are weak or almost non-existent as constraints on surgical fee inflation. One possible explanation for this is that physicians have a target level of income. And when demand for their services is insufficient to achieve that income level, they raise their fees in order to achieve it.

The report also concludes that after adjusting for differences in cost-of-living and other factors, surgical fees are found to be highest in the West, in very large cities, and in areas experiencing the most rapid recent population growth. Area-wide income levels show no consistent relationship with fee levels.

The principal causes of rapid physician fee inflation and growth in consumer outlays for physicians' services have changed dramatically since 1965. During the 1950s and early 1960s, the relatively high rates of physician fee inflation could be traced in large part to the anticompetitive practices of organized medicine, designed in some measure to increase both fee and income levels of practicing physicians. Through control of medical school accreditation, the American Medical Association reduced the number of medical students during the 1930s and restricted medical school growth during the 1940s and 1950s. Partly because of these restrictions, the physician-population ratio was lower in 1960 than in 1950. With per capita demand for medical services increasing because of substantial growth in disposable income and health insurance coverage, a declining supply of physicians per capita resulted in both higher fees and incomes. Physicians' fees rose 60 percent between 1950 and 1965, compared to 30 percent for non-medical care prices. And physicians' incomes increased 230 percent between 1947 and 1965, compared to 120 percent for average earnings of all U.S. workers.

At the same time, state and local medical societies put additional upward pressure on doctor bills by discouraging both price competition among physicians and the establishment of prepaid medical group practice, the forerunner of the health maintenance organization.

Since 1965, the number of medical students and the per capita supply of physicians have increased substantially, and anticompetitive practices of organized medicine have ceased to be an important source of physician fee inflation. These past practices, however, are partially responsible for the high *levels* of prevailing physicians' fees that contribute to the current $185 billion nationwide medical care bill.

A primary cause of rapidly increasing physicians' fees and growth in expenditures for physicians' services since the mid-60s has been the growth in private and public health insurance ocverage and changes in methods of insurer payment for physicians' services. While increased insurance coverage enabled many people to receive required medical care, it also, to a large extent, exempted physicians' fees from the usually restraining effects of market forces that exist for most other consumer products and services.

Between 1950 and 1960, the number of persons covered by surgical insurance doubled (54 million to 112 million), while the number with insurance for non-surgical services almost quadrupled (22 million to 83 million). Currently 160 to 170 million persons, about 80 percent of the population, have private health insurance covering physicians' services. While the number of persons insured for physician expenses grew most rapidly during the 1950s, the comprehensiveness of insurance coverage improved most sharply after 1965. Along with greater comprehensiveness of coverage came a change in the method of paying for physicians' services, and this significantly reduced consumer incentives to resist higher costs of physician services.

During the 1960s and early 1970s, the principal method used by health insurers in paying for physicians' services changed. Instead of paying fixed dollar amounts under a fee schedule—amounts that were usually substantially below the physicians' customary or "list price" fee—many insurers adopted a "usual, customary and reasonable" (UCR) fee. Insurers using the UCR method typically reimburse 80 to 100 percent of the fee charged by the physician, as long as this fee is not among the highest 10 percent of fees for that service in the area. In a market where about 60 percent of the cost of services is reimbursed by either private insurance or public health benefit programs, a payment mechanism based on a physician determining his own fee can be expected to result in high rates of fee inflation. This is especially true in those specialties for which the proportion of total revenue from third party payors is greatest— in some cases 80 percent or more—such as surgery, radiology, anesthesiology and obstetrics-gynecology. It is less pertinent to general practice, pediatrics and psychiatry, where direct consumer payments typically comprise a greater share of the total doctor bill. Earnings of physicians in specialties for which third party payments are the primary source of revenue are substantially greater than earnings of physicians in other specialties.

The growth in health insurance enrollment, the implementation of the Medicare and Medicaid programs for the aged and poor, and the change in reimbursement approaches of insurers from widespread reliance on the indemnity approach to the increasing prevalence of the more generous usual, customary and reasonable approach have contributed to the sharp rise in the physician fee component of the Consumer Price Index. But these factors have actually resulted in additional physician fee inflation that has not been captured by the CPI. Charity care or discounts from customary fees for patients with limited income or insurance coverage were widely prevalent before 1950, especially for high-cost services such as surgery. But as more people acquired health insurance coverage and as the comprehensiveness of insurance changed, the extent of fee discounting diminished. Because the CPI tended to measure changes in the customary fee rather than in the average or "transaction" fee, the gradual increase over time in the ratio of transaction fee to customary fee has resulted in an understatement in the CPI of the true extent of physician fee inflation. This source of bias has resulted in physicians' fees increasing an estimated 20 percent more rapidly per year during the 1950-76 period than the increase reflected in the CPI data.

One major cause of higher physician costs (as well as hospital costs) is the dramatic improvement in the medical care system and the willingness of the American people, with higher incomes and better insurance coverage, to pay for it. Sophisticated and often highly expensive medical services are being used today to treat illnesses and conditions for which treatment may not have been available or was considerably inferior as little as ten years ago. Much of this sophisticated care is being provided by specialists, who increased from less than 40 percent of all physicians in 1950 to about 85 percent in 1976. This increase in specialization has also resulted in greater fee inflation, since specialists tend to charge higher fees than general practitioners for similar services.

In recent years rapidly rising expenses have been cited as a cause of relatively high rates of physician fee inflation. In fact, over the 1971–76 period for which index data on physician expenses are available, physician expenses did rise more rapidly than all consumer prices, but at a slightly slower rate than physicians' fees. The largest input price increase during 1975 and 1976 was the sharp climb in malpractice insurance premiums which, according to one source, rose 84 percent in 1975 and 42 percent in 1976. However, because malpractice insurance costs were not a major cost element for most physicians before 1975, these steep percentage increases cannot explain the large differential between inflation in physicians' fees and overall prices during 1975 and 1976.

The supply of physicians has increased substantially since 1970, from 158 per 100,000 persons to 177 in 1975. The Department of Health, Education and Welfare estimates that, because of continued immigration of foreign-trained physicians and expanding medical school enrollment, the physician supply will increase even more rapidly in future years. The projected supply in 1985 is 222 per 100,000 population. There is some evidence that a substantial proportion of new physicians is practicing, not in areas of short physician supply, but in already oversupplied areas. It has been suggested that, given extensive insurance coverage and lack of consumer resistance to large expenditures for physician services, physicians practicing in these oversupplied areas can, to a certain extent, induce demand for their services and raise their fees. Thus, additional physician and hospital costs may be generated in already high medical care utilization areas, perhaps with little improvement in overall health care.

The study concludes that many of the forces operating in the recent past which caused high physician fee inflation continue to exist: lack of competitive pressures to restrain fee increases, extensive health insurance coverage and insurance reimbursement practices which allow the physician to determine the fee and level of insurer reimbursement. While malpractice insurance costs to the physician seem to have stabilized in 1977, physician fees in that year continued to increase at a substantially higher rate than all consumer prices. In the absence of major insurers altering their reimbursement practices or substantially increasing copayment for physicians' services, there is little reason to predict that physician fee inflation will not continue to outpace price increases in the overall economy.

In terms of consumer outlays for physicians' services, the situation is similar. The combination of extensive insurance coverage removing consumer resistance to the use of high cost services, increasing incidence of physicians providing additional costly diagnostic tests to ward off malpractice suits, and an increasing number of physicians and their evidenced capability to provide additional and more costly services may portend even more rapid rates of growth in consumer outlays for medical services than are currently being experienced.

An additional finding of this report does not relate specifically to physicians' fees, but to a bias in the CPI measure of total medical price inflation. The CPI "basket" of medical care goods and services does not reflect actual medical care expenditure patterns, primarily because it includes only medical care paid for directly by urban employees. Excluded are employer contributions for health insurance. Those items for which health insurance directly pays a greater portion than others would, therefore, have smaller weights in the CPI than they have in actual health expenditures. Because medical services that are underweighted in the CPI—primarily hospital care—have experienced more rapid inflation than overweighted items, medical care price changes, as reflected in the CPI, understate the actual rate of medical care inflation. The extent to which the CPI has understated medical care inflation over the 1967-76 period has been estimated at 27 percent, or 1.3 percent per year. The problem of underweighting hospital care relative to other medical care items is exacerbated in the revised CPI introduced in March, 1978, because employer-paid health insurance has increased in relative importance in recent years.

PHYSICIANS (M.D.s) BY SPECIALTY

Tables 3-2—3-4 provide a breakdown of physicians in the United States and its possessions by specialty and type of activity. These tables are taken from the AMA's report, *Physician Distribution and Medical Licensure in the United States, 1976* (11, pp.49,52,78). The key to the specialty codes on these tables is as follows:

GENERAL PRACTICE

GP   General practice (includes family practice and general practice)

MEDICAL SPECIALTIES

A	Allergy	PD	Pediatrics
CD	Cardiovascular diseases	PDA	Pediatric allergy
D	Dermatology	PDC	Pediatric cardiology
GE	Gastroenterology	PUD	Pulmonary diseases
IM	Internal medicine		

SURGICAL SPECIALTIES

GS	General surgery	OTO	Otolaryngology
NS	Neurological surgery	PS	Plastic surgery
OBG	Obstetrics and Gynecology	CRS	Colon and rectal surgery
OPH	Ophthalmology	TS	Thoracic surgery
ORS	Orthopedic surgery	U	Urology

OTHER SPECIALTIES

AM	Aerospace medicine	PTH	Pathology
AN	Anesthesiology	PM	Physical medicine and rehabilitation
CHP	Child psychiatry		
DR	Diagnostic radiology	GPM	General preventive medicine
FOP	Forensic pathology	PH	Public health
N	Neurology	R	Radiology
OM	Occupational medicine	TR	Therapeutic radiology
P	Psychiatry		
		OS	Other specialty
		US	Unspecified

Distribution among federal agencies of the 27,578 physicians in federal employment, is as follows:

Agency	Distribution
Army	4,574
Navy	4,140
Air Force	3,802
Public Health Service	3,194
Veteran's Administration	10,058
Other Federal service	1,810
	27,578

The VA physicians, and many of the PHS physicians (who provide care on Indian reservations as well as PHS hospitals) are serving the civilian population.

In Table 3-4 the total number of 373,111 nonfederal physicians includes 320,865 whose practices can be classfied, 22,117 who are inactive, and 30,129 whose practices could not be classified. The last two items are not broken down in the table. Not included are 8,757 physicians whose addresses are unknown and not included is any count of the D.O.s.

Of the 320,865 nonfederal physicians, those in the primary-care specialties are:

Specialty	Number of Physicians
General or family practice	53,047
Internal medicine	52,340
Pediatrics	21,108
Obstetrics-gynecology	21,103
	147,598

Nearly half the M.D.s are thus in primary-care specialties that, as noted in the first part of this chapter, is the main focus of public concern as far as physician availability is concerned.

PRIMARY CARE PHYSICIANS

A primary-care physician was defined in 1975 by the CCME (which is sponsored by the AAMC, ABMS, CMSS, AHA, and AMA) as one who provides an individual or family with continuing health surveillance along with needed acute and chronic care, which he or she is qualified to provide, with referral service to specialists as appropriate. General and family practitioners fall within this definition, as do pediatricians, internists, and obstetricians and gynecologists, although not everyone will agree on the latter.

United States and Possessions

Table 3-2. Federal and Non-Federal Physicians by Specialty and Activity December 31, 1976

Specialty	Total Physicians	Major Professional Activity							
		Patient Care				Other Professional Activity			
		Total	Office-Based Practice	Hospital-Based Practice		Medical Teaching	Administration	Research	Other
				Residents—All Years	Full-Time Physician Staff				
TOTAL PHYSICIANS	409,446	318,412	216,533	63,046	38,833	6,935	11,689	8,514	2,893
GENERAL PRACTICE	55,479	54,332	46,628	4,388	3,316	232	628	64	223
MEDICAL SPECIALTIES	99,357	89,213	54,388	24,444	10,381	2,580	2,874	4,191	499
A	1,704	1,571	1,493		78	24	22	83	4
CD	6,769	5,722	4,821		901	300	235	447	65
D	4,817	4,559	3,601	648	310	86	47	103	22
GE	2,374	1,953	1,651		302	140	61	211	9
IM	57,911	52,305	28,170	18,282	5,853	1,179	1,636	2,527	264
PD	22,491	20,520	12,981	5,383	2,156	613	696	552	110
PDA	477	436	333	73	30	13	6	22	
PDC	548	406	231	58	117	64	24	51	3
PUD	2,266	1,741	1,107		634	161	147	195	22
SURGICAL SPECIALTIES	98,667	95,102	68,654	19,079	7,369	1,266	1,138	851	310
GS	32,292	31,119	19,864	8,542	2,713	369	466	237	101
NS	2,985	2,836	2,044	535	257	55	27	53	14
OBG	22,294	21,326	15,995	3,828	1,503	311	375	220	62
OPH	11,455	11,090	8,944	1,616	530	114	61	160	30
ORS	11,814	11,472	8,426	2,061	985	163	69	61	49
OTO	5,864	5,680	4,381	843	456	82	45	37	20

PS	2,351	2,284	1,816	340	128	35	11	16	5
CRS	673	662	602	32	28	1	5	3	2
TS	2,036	1,923	1,414	276	233	42	37	27	7
U	6,903	6,710	5,168	1,006	536	94	42	37	20
OTHER SPECIALTIES	94,940	79,765	46,863	15,135	17,767	2,857	7,049	3,408	1,861
AM	660	384	166	18	200	9	210	32	25
AN	13,182	12,348	9,074	1,737	1,537	523	163	107	41
CHP	2,644	2,186	1,496	309	381	143	222	53	40
DR	3,832	3,547	2,254	555	738	139	28	28	90
FOP	207	107	88	8	11	9	37	8	46
N	4,425	3,707	1,969	1,140	598	227	90	362	39
OM	2,322	1,684	1,582	8	94	7	523	23	85
P	24,432	21,478	12,432	3,959	5,087	509	1,829	450	166
PTH	11,919	9,813	4,272	2,559	2,982	424	455	622	605
PM	1,715	1,544	629	298	617	34	9	16	22
GPM	808	393	236	73	84	46	273	66	30
PH	2,600	756	513	32	211	95	1,498	121	130
R	11,728	10,999	7,028	1,822	2,149	251	123	123	232
TR	1,209	1,150	704	210	236	30	10	18	1
OTHER SPECIALTY	7,638	4,559	2,970		1,589	344	1,252	1,273	210
UNSPECIFIED	5,619	5,110	1,450	2,407	1,253	67	237	106	99
NOT CLASSIFIED	30,129								
INACTIVE	22,117								
ADDRESS UNKNOWN	8,757								
EXCLUDES TEMP. FOREIGN	5,604								

Source: *Physician Distribution and Medical Licensure in the US, 1976.* Copyright 1977, Chicago, American Medical Association, p. 49.

Table 3-3. Federal Physicians in United States and Possessions by Specialty and Activity December 31, 1976

	United States and Possessions	Major Professional Activity							
		Patient Care				Other Professional Activity			
				Hospital-Based Practice					
Specialty	Total Physicians	Total	Office-Based Practice	Residents—All Years	Full-Time Physician Staff	Medical Teaching	Administration	Research	Other
TOTAL PHYSICIANS	27,578	23,682	1,823	4,122	17,737	682	1,756	1,086	372
GENERAL PRACTICE	2,432	2,278	592	205	1,481	13	97	15	29
MEDICAL SPECIALTIES	8,582	7,259	469	1,489	5,301	256	413	574	80
A	74	59	6		53	1	3	11	11
CD	523	388	14		374	44	33	47	9
D	402	351	18	97	236	15	8	19	9
GE	267	186	4		182	31	11	37	2
IM	5,571	4,712	220	1,207	3,285	127	284	408	40
PD	1,383	1,268	194	178	896	17	55	30	13
PDA	17	17	1	4	12				
PDC	24	21	1	3	17	1	1	1	
PUD	321	257	11		246	20	18	21	5
SURGICAL SPECIALTIES	6,442	5,924	181	1,304	4,439	202	205	78	33
GS	2,240	2,044	54	494	1,496	67	90	27	12
NS	192	168	1	36	131	7	7	9	1
OBG	1,191	1,112	61	203	848	21	46	6	6

	C1	C2	C3	C4	C5	C6	C7	C8	C9
OPH	3	17	10	11	351	129	22	502	543
ORS	6	5	21	38	721	186	18	925	995
OTO	2	4	11	19	341	116	10	467	503
PS			3	4	69	17	2	88	95
CRS					12	4	1	17	17
TS	1	6	8	9	113	13	2	128	152
U	2	4	9	26	357	106	10	473	514
OTHER SPECIALTIES	230	419	1,041	211	6,516	1,124	581	8,221	10,122
AM	14	21	185	4	192	15	74	281	505
AN	6	5	12	49	547	111	7	665	737
CHP	1	6	7	5	63	15	11	89	108
DR	12	4	5	18	318	70	11	399	438
FOP	2		3		2		4	6	11
N	7	55	13	24	338	106	14	458	557
OM	7	2	57	3	54	4	110	168	239
P	9	48	203	38	1,732	185	135	2,052	2,368
PTH	27	62	51	20	811	194	23	1,028	1,200
PM	39	1	19	3	227	27	3	257	285
GPM	5	12	47	1	68	21	16	105	172
PH	7	26	154	5	159	8	29	196	409
R	28	18	24	29	710	171	18	899	984
TR	14	4	3	1	67	16	1	84	92
OTHER SPECIALTY	35	135	196	4	339		40	379	749
UNSPECIFIED	24	20	62	7	889	181	85	1,155	1,268

Source: *Physician Distribution and Medical Licensure in the US, 1976.* Copyright 1977, Chicago, American Medical Association, p. 52.

Table 3-4. Nonfederal Physicians in United States and Possessions by Specialty and Activity December 31, 1976

United States and Possessions

Specialty	Total Physicians	Major Professional Activity							
		Patient Care				Other Professional Activity			
		Total	Office-Based Practice	Hospital-Based Practice		Medical Teaching	Administration	Research	Other
				Residents—All Years	Full-Time Physician Staff				
TOTAL PHYSICIANS	373,111	294,730	214,710	58,924	21,096	6,253	9,933	7,428	2,521
GENERAL PRACTICE	53,047	52,054	46,036	4,183	1,835	219	531	49	194
MEDICAL SPECIALTIES	90,775	81,954	53,919	22,955	5,080	2,324	2,461	3,617	419
A	1,630	1,512	1,487		25	23	19	72	4
CD	6,246	5,334	4,807		527	256	202	400	54
D	4,415	4,208	3,583	551	74	71	39	84	13
GE	2,107	1,767	1,647		120	109	50	174	7
IM	52,340	47,593	27,950	17,075	2,568	1,052	1,352	2,119	224
PD	21,108	19,252	12,787	5,205	1,260	596	641	522	97
PDA	460	419	332	69	18	13	6	22	
PDC	524	385	230	55	100	63	23	50	3
PUD	1,945	1,484	1,096		388	141	129	174	17
SURGICAL SPECIALTIES	92,225	89,178	68,473	17,775	2,930	1,064	933	773	277
GS	30,052	29,075	19,810	8,048	1,217	302	376	210	89
NS	2,793	2,668	2,043	499	126	48	20	44	13
OBG	21,103	20,214	15,934	3,625	655	290	329	214	56
OPH	10,912	10,588	8,922	1,487	179	103	51	143	27

ORS	10,819	10,547	8,408	1,875	264	125	48	56	43
OTO	5,361	5,213	4,371	727	115	63	34	33	18
PS	2,256	2,196	1,814	323	59	31	8	16	5
CRS	656	645	601	28	16	1	5	3	2
TS	1,884	1,795	1,412	263	120	33	29	21	6
U	6,389	6,237	5,158	900	179	68	33	33	18
OTHER SPECIALTIES	84,818	71,544	46,282	14,011	11,251	2,646	6,008	2,989	1,631
AM	155	103	92	3	8	5	25	11	11
AN	12,445	11,683	9,067	1,626	990	474	151	102	35
CHP	2,536	2,097	1,485	294	318	138	215	47	39
DR	3,394	3,148	2,243	485	420	121	23	24	78
FOP	196	101	84	8	9	9	34	8	44
N	3,868	3,249	1,955	1,034	260	203	77	307	32
OM	2,083	1,516	1,472	4	40	4	466	21	76
P	22,064	19,426	12,297	3,774	3,355	471	1,626	402	139
PTH	10,719	8,785	4,249	2,365	2,171	404	404	560	566
PM	1,430	1,287	626	271	390	31	80	15	17
GPM	636	288	220	52	16	45	226	54	23
PH	2,191	560	484	24	52	90	1,344	95	102
R	10,744	10,100	7,010	1,651	1,439	222	99	105	218
TR	1,117	1,066	703	194	169	29	7	14	1
OTHER SPECIALTY	6,889	4,180	2,930		1,250	340	1,056	1,138	175
UNSPECIFIED	4,351	3,955	1,365	2,226	364	60	175	86	75
NOT CLASSIFIED	30,129								
INACTIVE	22,117								

Source: Physician Distribution and Medical Licensure in the US, 1976. Copyright 1977, Chicago, American Medical Association, p. 78.

In many countries, specialists rarely provide primary care. In those countries, pediatricians and internists serve primarily as consultants, devoting their time almost exclusively to the practice of their specialty. In the United States and a few other countries, however, most of these two specialties have evolved into primary-care practice; most pediatricians and most internists provide primary care. Relatively few devote their time solely to practice of the specialty. This needs to be qualified in that the pediatrician typically limits his or her clientele to a certain age group; the internist will typically not handle some things that a family practitioner might handle, such as obstetrics and pediatric problems. So, too, with obstetrics-gynecology, which has evolved largely as a primary-care specialty, but in this instance not for general care but for categorical care for obstetrics and/or gynecological problems with female patients going directly to the gynecology specialist without referral.

But the definition developed by the CCME still leaves much to be desired. Other specialties handle a considerable amount of routine primary care that in other settings might be handled by a family practitioner or other health professionals. In this regard, we need note the tendency of many people to self-diagnose and self-refer to a specialist—psychiatrist, surgeon, dermatologist, orthopedist—when, in fact, the family practitioner or other primary-care medical specialist might well be able to handle the problem. We might note the frequent use of ophthalmologists and dermatologists when optometrists and podiatrists might well suffice. And we might also note that the specialties of public health and general preventive medicine do a considerable amount of primary prevention that reduces the need, to some extent, for primary care.

RURAL AND INNER-CITY HEALTH SERVICES

However one chooses to define primary-care physicians, rural areas and inner cities have had considerable difficulty in recruiting and retaining them.

The lack of appeal for rural practice stems from fear of professional isolation—lack of professional interactions, inaccessibility of hospitals, absence of consultation and continuing medical education opportunities, lack of opportunity for spouse, and cultural deprivation (no theater, no concerts, no lectures, limited adult education activities, etc.) The physician today and his or her spouse are urbanites by virtue of their long periods of education and training in urban professional settings, and the adjustment to rural living, while sometimes inviting in moments of idyllic dreaming, has not been successful in most cases. There seems to be greater chance of retention if the physician is originally from a rural area, but no one yet has devised a generally valid formula for the successful establishment of rural practices. Professional as well as personal isolation are factors that are very real, and the former is reinforced to some extent by medical-school faculty and preceptors in residency programs who caution about going to the very rural areas lest a physician get out of date in no time at all. Some also feel that insurance payments, which pay rural physicians less, may also be operative, but the data on this view are sparse.

There is some ambiguity in the word "rural." One federal agency set the definition at a population of 35,000 or 50,000. Other agencies have used other figures, usually lower. It might be noted that rural communities at the 35,000 and 50,000 level, and many even smaller, seem now to be successfully recruiting physicians. The reasons for their successes are at least several: There are more physicians available, and the supply/demand factor operates to secure a more even distribution; the large urban settings are congested and are plagued by high costs and high crime rates; the assets of urban life are not as remote as our road networks improve; the small communities have sought to make their areas attractive to primary-care and other physicians by developing for their communities as optimal hospital facilites as their communities can support and sometimes more than they can support. It is worth noting that when HEW proposed planning guidelines for hospitals, the guidelines would have hit these more rural hospitals because of their tendency for low occupancy; the resulting outcry from rural America forced HEW to backtrack a bit, for these hospitals are not only all that these communities have, but they are also often the needed ingredient to make those areas attractive for professional practice.

The inner-city problems are somewhat different. In large cities, the poor did not always use private doctors. Their needs, historically, were largely handled by the indigent and voluntary-hospital outpatient departments and emergency rooms. As people moved to the suburbs, the physicians went where their paying patients were. Other factors encouraging the out-migration of physicians and discouraging the in-migration of new physicians are the high cost of office and parking spaces, transportation hassles, and crime. In addition, the cities are far more litigiously inclined, and malpractice insurance rates are generally higher. The movement of physicians out of the cities has become a matter of concern because the poor under Medicaid are now entitled to private physician care, but the changed consumer expectations find the cities short of medical manpower. Solving this shortage problem is not easily accomplished.

Part of the concern over the need for primary-care physicians is economic. Rising costs of health care make the principal payers—industry through health insurance premiums and government—want some mechanism to control costs. They look at the need for hospitalization, the length of hospital stay, opportunities to retard hospital expansion, necessity for surgery, and the need for all the specialists. In addition to the items discussed in Chapter 6, two additional approaches are being explored.

The first is to shift to training *more primary-care physicians* rather than specialists who handle, for the most part referred cases. In part, this is designed to create a sufficient supply of physicians so that more will be induced to serve the more rural areas and the inner cities. Also, fearing the truth of the assertion that people do what they are trained to do, by cutting back on specialists, some believe the pressures to undertake the costly specialist services will be lessened. Advocates of this theory note that the British surgical rate is half what it is in this country, and we have twice the number of surgeons, in other words, the more surgeons, the more surgery, and if we can cut the surgical specialties, we can cut the amount of costly surgery. The untested assumptions here are, of course, considerable. Along with this goes efforts to make it difficult for the health system to do the expensive work, cutting back on beds and slowing the acquisition of new equipment. At the same time, there is mounted a great effort to prevent health problems from developing.

The second approach being explored is the use of *second opinions.* Believing that surgeons cut because they are trained to cut, before a patient undergoes elective surgery, there should be a second opinion. If the second concurs, then one can safely assume that the surgery is necessary, particularly since the second party, according to the rules, is ineligible to do the surgery. If, on the other hand, the second opinion is contrary to the first, that does not mean that the first opinion was wrong. What then? A third opinion? Whatever the third opinion is, is the patient any better off than in the beginning? Does one go on to a fourth opinion? Regardless of the opinions, what is the long term effect on the patient? And what happens if the patient chooses to ignore the first or the second opinion? The second-opinion approach is an attempt at prospective quality control, whereas the other measures described in the preceding chapter are retrospective measures.

A number of studies of second opinions are being carried out. Results are yet inconclusive.

FAMILY PRACTICE AND SURGERY

One of the more spirited professional debates now in progress concerns surgery and the family practitioner. Before the time of the ACS and for many years after, the general practitioner did about everything, including general surgery. In many communities in America, particularly in the more remote areas, family practitioners still do a great amount of general surgery-appendectomies, herniorraphies, cholecystectomies, hysterectomies, vein ligations, hemorrhoidectomies, and so on. They have done them for years; they see no reason to give up such surgery; in many communities, in any event, there isn't a board-certified surgeon to do the work. The surgeons, on the other hand, strongly believe that, except in emergencies, surgery should be performed by one trained in surgery.

The AAGP, the predecessor to the AAFP, found, in a 1969 survey, that 39% of its members did major surgery. Estimates in 1973 were that the percentage, including major surgery in their practices, was down to 20 or 25% (12, p.68).

As the number of surgeons grows, and as they spread throughout the country, many are moving into areas in which surgeons had not been before; understandably problems arise. In Kalispell, Montana, a surgeon stated, "I've been here five lovely years, of which three were struggling years. In Kalispell, there's a very good relationship with the family physicians. I'm willing to give them some gallbladders just to get them to be here and provide coordination in family practice (12, p.71).

The varying viewpoints in this Montana town were expressed by others as well. One surgeon said:

A GP should do some surgery. But I don't think he has any business in the belly. A woman who had her gallbladder taken out by a GP developed pain, jaundice, and diarrhea 20 years later. I found a cystic duct remnant with two stones in it. That wouldn't have happened with many surgeons. I'm willing to help a GP with a GP operation, but not a big operation. A GP who feels he's competing with me for hernias will not send me his stomachs, he'll send them to Spokane instead.

Another surgeon observed that "four board-certified surgeons in town are too many."

A general practitioner of long standing in the community said that he gave up surgery "the day a board man arrived." Another GP, who had had some surgical training, observed (12, p.71):

As more surgical specialists have arrived, the GPs have drawn the line on what they do themselves. In my view, we now have to stay out of the stomach and bowel, complicated bile duct surgery, and the more complex orthopedic surgery. But I still do about 85 percent of my own surgery. It isn't just us, but our patients' wishes that have to be considered.

Finally, a family practitioner stated, "In my mind our group is doing some general surgery because it's part of the continuing care we give. Our patients feel confidence in us."

The ACS has, of course, long sought to curb surgery by those not trained to do it, but it allows in its guidelines the possibility for surgery by nonsurgeons, but as the following statement suggests, ACS equivocates (13):

In certain geographically isolated and sparsely settled areas, fully trained surgeons in various fields may not be available. The performance of certain surgical procedures, especially of an emergency nature, by a physician without special surgical training may be in the best interest of the public in that area. The medical staff and the governing body of hospitals in such areas should periodically review the quality, the number, and the variety of surgical procedures being performed, as well as the surgical referral policies of the staff. It is possible that the referral pattern in surgical care is such as to discourage the application of properly trained and qualified surgeons for staff membership.

The content of family practice residencies is expected to cover a variety of specialty areas, "although certain portions may be optional, depending upon the knowledge and skill obtained by the resident in medical school, his interest, and the character of his anticipated practice." Sexist language aside, under the surgical section of the "Special Requirements for Residency Training in Family Practice" in the 1977-1978 *Directory of Accredited Residencies,* it states (14, p.344):

Surgery—The resident should acquire competence in recognizing surgical emergencies and when appropriate referring them for necessary specialized care, an ability to evaluate conditions that require elective surgical management, an understanding of the kinds of surgical treatment that might be employed and the problems that may result form surgical procedures and their management. He should have sufficient knowledge of these procedures to give proper advice, explanation, and emotional support to his patients. He should be trained in basic surgical principles by recognized surgical specialists and acquire from them the technical proficiency required to manage those limited surgical procedures a first contact (family) physician may be called upon to perform. If he expects to include major surgery as a part of his regular practice, he should obtain additional training.

The director of the ACS (C. Rollins Hanlon, M.D.) in the *Bulletin* of the ACS wrote in early 1978 (15):

The College receives a number of letters from Fellows initiated by pressure on them to provide surgical training or surgical privileges for family practitioners or family practice residents in hospitals. The Fellows have properly resisted such pressure for inappropriate surgical privileges.

One can see this pressure as part of a larger movement to downgrade the quality of surgical care, often under the guise of federal cost containment, by abolishing educational standards at various levels in the field of medical care, substituting in their place the vague and dangerous criterion of "tests of competence" . . .

But, it is an even more dangerous delusion to assume that professional expertise, especially in surgery, can be provided by a once-over-lightly type of on-the-job training, or by exposure comparable to an extended rotating internship . . .

His remarks were in response to Family Practice assertions contained in the January 9, 1978 issue of *American Medical News*. Dr. Hanlon went on to attack the aggrandizing efforts of the family practitioners and even rejects the necessity to train them for preoperative and postoperative care. On this he said:

The College has long maintained that leaving the patient in the care of a general practitioner not adequately prepared to recognize and handle post-operative complications is a critical component in the deplorable practice of itinerant surgery. This is the type of care I would be delighted to lose sight of by stamping it out.

One can view this controversy as a professional debate in which the surgeons, following in the tradition of the ACS, continue to stress the importance of strict qualifications for those engaged in surgery, and in which the family practitioners, on the other hand assert that surgery is not the preserve of the surgeons, that the family practitioner, to be a true generalist, must be able to function supportively in this area and in some cases even do the surgery. One can also view this as an attempt on the part of the surgeons to protect their domain both economically and professionally at the very time that residencies are under attack, that the number of surgeons is called excessive, and that public concern increases over the amount and cost of surgery.

An interesting series of questions arise from this controversy that merits answers: To what extent should family practitioners do surgery? If they should not do surgery, and at least 20% are estimated to have surgery as part of their practices, what does this say in terms of the number of surgeons who should be trained? How can one say whether we are "oversurgeoned" or not unless the first question is answered?

THE APPEAL OF SPECIALIZATION

There are many reasons why physicians specialize. Specialists, to begin with, have always been held in high regard by the population. The specialist was something special, a person who could do things that lesser mortals and physicians could not do, a person whose special skills also warranted a higher fee. The very best of these specialists were professors on the faculties of medical schools.

There has always been, of course, a certain aura that surrounded the physician, a mystique that was more pronounced for the specialist who had special knowledge and skills that saved lives, eased pain, and improved functioning.

The lure of specialization is built into our social fabric, and it extends beyond medicine. We ask children, What do you want to be? And we do not expect an answer: just an average person. We expect a child to be something or to want to be, to have expectations that will make her or him distinguishable and distinguished. In the pecking order of our society, specialists are tops.

Reinforcing this social force is the role modeling of medical school faculty. The medical student has to choose how she or he will practice. Many factors may enter this decision process, but since most of the faculty are specialists, the pressure to respond to one of those specialty role models is ever present. But we should not forget that specialization has a certain intellectual appeal. It enables the curious to know more and more about the problems that afflict the human being. But the problems are complex, and the curious have to specialize in order to deal with them.

Other factors may enter. A person's own medical history or that of the family frequently channels a physician's interest. For some specialties, very high incomes are assured, and for some specialties, orderly personal lives are more possible with minimum hassles from emergencies and irregular hours.

Most of the factors that affect the location of primary-care physicians also influence practice-location choice of specialists. Hospital access, however, may be even more critical for the specialist in terms of the supporting services that may be necessary for the effective practice of her or his specialty. Studies have also shown that specialists tend to locate in areas close to the place where the residency is taken. There are some good reasons for this: The new specialist is familiar with the clinicians in the area and tends to know and be comfortable with other specialists for referrals. Conversely, since the new specialist is known by many of the physicians, having interacted with her or him while in residency, the new specialist can anticipate some helpful referrals. To what extent these special factors will affect the new specialty of family practice, it is too early to say. The overall increase in the supply of specialists, the spread of technology, coupled with the disadvantages of urban life, are influencing the movement of new specialists to outlying areas. It is perhaps too early to see any trends in this regard.

REGULATION OF FEES

In recent years, there have been the desire and some attempts by government to regulate physician fees because they were a factor in rising health care costs. By mid-1978, only Maryland had done this but, as we have noted, only with regard to radiology, pathology, and cardiology services in hospitals, and the state's power to do this is being tested in court. A variety of reasons exists for these attempts, and some of the reasons are expressed in "motherhood and God" principles.

The importance of competition as the way to allow the marketplace to set fees is a principle of the FTC. It operationalizes its views by searching for the hidden hand of the AMA in controlling prices and the supply of physicians. In 1977, it asked the U.S. Commissioner of Education to reject the application of the Liaison Committee on Medical Education for recognition as the appropriate accrediting body for medical schools. The FTC felt that the AMA should not be in the position of approving or disapproving schools whose graduates will compete with existing AMA members. The FTC request was rejected. The FTC is also apparently concerned over physician control of licensure and also over the AMA's code of ethics, which serves to restrict competition. In September 1977, it opened an administrative trial of the AMA and Connecticut medical societies on the latter issue. The issue was enjoined over the codes of medical ethics and their prohibition on advertising. It might be noted that in many states the medical codes of ethics allow for advertising but seek to contain it to discourage or prohibit the outright enticement of patients such as exists in some parts of California, where advertising has led to a huckstering for patients by some physicians whose competence and quality of care cannot be judged by the patient. In November 1978, the administrative law judge for the FTC ruled against the medical associations. The AMA stated that it would appeal the finding, contending:

It has been clear throughout the entire proceeding that the AMA is clearly in favor of physician advertising and a free flow of public information about health care services. We are opposed to false and misleading advertising and its adverse impact on the quality of health care available to patients (16).

At various times, officials within HEW have also advocated control over physician fees, suggesting that the rise in fees and physician share of the health-care dollar were moving beyond publicly acceptable limits. Some physicians have suggested that to some extent income envy may lay behind some of the cries for fee regulation. HEW officials in 1977 seemed to be rejecting the FTC notion of opening the health system to meaningful competition, believing instead that the marketplace concepts of industrial competition do not apply to the health field. *Medical World News,* quoting one official, states,

---

Even where there are three times as many physicians in one area as another, demand doesn't get satiated . . . It continues to increase. And prices do not fall—they rise—just the reverse of what economic theory would tell you. There are others who still believe that if we flood the market with enough physicians, prices will drop. There is no evidence for this in any part of the country or in any specialty (16, p.51).

HEW seemed inclined toward direct regulation.

Regulation of physician fees has occurred in the past: Some of the colonial legislatures set the fees that physicians could charge. More recently, there has been a form of fee setting by the health insurance industry. Blue Shield service benefits typically set a ceiling on what a participating physician could receive for care to eligible Blue Shield patients. The schedules of allowances generally reflected the going charges for patients within those income levels. Other insurance companies paid usual and customary fees that normally assumed some kind of assessment of what was usual and customary. Some Blue Shield plans, at least, have in the past conducted fee surveys of physicians that became the basis for their schedules of allowances. In 1978, the FTC criticized the medical profession's domination of Blue Shield boards of directors as contributing to the anticompetition situation that may be against the public's interest.

From 1971 through early 1974, there was control of fees as part of the national wage and price controls effort instituted under the Economic Stabilization Program. Somers and Somers note (17, p.454):

The major effort to contain prices came in 1971 as part of the Economic Stabilization Program, the first peacetime imposition of general wage and price controls in American history. During the first two phases of ESP, August

1971-December 1972, the health industry was treated like the rest of the economy. In Phase III, health care, along with construction, food, and oil, remained under controls while other industries were gradually decontrolled. In the final stages of Phase IV, starting in early 1974, plans were developed for continuing controls on health care, including use as well as price. Hospitals, nursing homes, and physicians declared war on ESP and initiated a series of legal battles. Before the new regulations could go into effect, the battle had been won by the providers. ESP died in April 1974. The lesson may be that any attempt to impose price controls on the health industry alone is probably politically, and perhaps constitutionally, unfeasible.

The question of physcian fees is, of course, intimately tied up with the overall costs of health services. It should be clear that there are no easy answers. The tendency of the government is to look for a quick fix as, for example, its apparent determination to launch a national surgical second-opinion effort for recipients of government-financed care before it receives the findings of studies it initiated to determine whether or not second opinions are really worthwhile. The pressure is on the bureaucrat and the politician, and when pressure is applied, the human tendency is to abandon long-range planning and sacrifice. Ginzburg discusses this complex situation (18, p.211):

As the source of payment for health services shifts from consumers to government, we must anticipate that controversy over the distribution of the dollar will intensify as each organized group of health professionals recognizes that its current income and future prospects will increasingly be determined by the decisions of the bureaucracy which allocates the available governmental funds. If, as has been postulated earlier, the total amount of governmental money entering the system levels off, we must anticipate increasingly acrimonious struggles about decisions affecting relative shares. If foreign experience is any guide, the struggles within the medical profession are likely to be as intensive as those between physicians and those outside.

It would take us too far afield to explore all the ramifications of the approaching struggles over the distribution of the health dollar, but one is worth noting. If physicians feel that they are not properly remunerated, it is likely that they wil trade income for leisure, as many now do when they join group practices, with the result that their hours of effective work per year may shrink by 20 per cent or more. There is some evidence that this is happening in general surgery. When the additional reduction in the hours of work that is almost certain to accompany the rapidly growing proportion of women physicians is taken into account, a further significant shrinking in work time must be anticipated. Here is one more important cost-increasing variable which health planners must take into account.

MALPRACTICE AND PROFESSIONAL LIABILITY

During the 1970s, one of the hot issues in health care revolved around medical malpractice, and the suits against physicians. During the first half of the decade, the number of suits soared, one insurance company stating that the number of claims each year rose by 20%.

Malpractice insurance rates soared, also, particularly for the surgical specialties. For the highest-risk surgery from the point of view of the insurance companies—orthopedic surgery, surgery by obstetrics-gynecology specialists, plastic surgery, cardiovascular surgery, neurological surgery, and head and neck surgery—the insurance premiums went up significantly, particularly in a few of the more litigious urban centers. One heard of insurance premiums running 30,000 and 40,000 dollars a year. Some insurance companies got out of the business. Medical societies formed their own insurance companies (as did some hospital associations for their members).

In southern California and New York, physicians ceased doing nonemergency surgery until the state legislatures came forth with acceptable state programs to get coverage at a reasonable cost.

The surgical areas listed as high risk are high risk in the sense that no matter what the surgeon does, the patient may still be disfigured or otherwise disabled, the case simply being beyond current technology to cure. Physicians argued that lawyers were at the heart of the problem: pushed out of the lucrative automobile cases through no-fault insurance, they cast about and seized on the physician.

A Chicago judge found some support for this. He found not only nuisance cases but poorly prepared cases, cases in which suits were filed before the attorney had satisfied himself or herself that there was medical negligence. By enforcing the court's rules and by not permitting sloppy case preparation and endless continuances, he was able to cut the number of suits. Writing in the AMA News, Judge David Canel said, however (19, p.3):

But if the judiciary and the bar need to clean house and enforce their own standards, I strongly feel that the physicians and hospitals need to do likewise.

I see the evidence for that need in court: one medical specialist involved in 13 suits with settlements from $75,000 to $300,000; another with nine suits, settlements from $75,000 to $100,000. Why do such doctors retain their hospital privileges? Why are they still members of their medical societies?

The rules, the bylaws, the committees, and the review mechanisms which make it possible to get rid of negligent doctors are not lacking. We were revoking hospital privileges 50 years ago when I was the young attorney for a certain hospital in Chicago. The medical societies have had the power to discipline their members ever since those organizations were founded.

If medicine and the hospitals would do a better job of enforcing their own standards, we could substantially reduce the number of meritorious cases that produce big settlements and awards. Until the health care professions take routine, uniform, and effective action to see that their members are doing their jobs the way they should be done, the negligence of some will continue to result in high malpractice premiums for the rest.

In 1976 and 1977, several insurance companies noted a decline in the number of malpractice claims. Whether this is a trend, time will tell. In the mean time, however, physicians in litigious areas are practicing *defensive medicine,* practicing by doing whatever one should do on the assumption that the patient will sue. Translated, this means that physicians will rely less on professional judgment and more on objective tests. But the tests cost money, further driving up health care costs. Moreover, the rising malpractice insurance premiums are written off through increased fees.

MEDICAL DISCIPLINE

Judge Canel raises two important questions: "Why do such doctors retain their hospital privileges? Why are they still members of their medical societies?" Fair questions but difficult ones to answer. To drop a physician—a surgeon—from the hospital is forcing that physician out of the community because he or she would be deprived of livelihood, which, like going to jail, is not decided on lightly but only after the most rigorous trial. If the physician is dropped, the physician simply goes elsewhere and applies for hospital privileges. There is always the risk that the surgeon will sue the hospital either for terminating privileges or for failing to give a good recommendation to the next hospital. More often than not, what happens is that the hospital curtails privileges, restricts them to areas in which the surgeon is less likely to be negligent, or the hospital negotiates: You leave, and we'll praise you. Another form of control exists and operates, but to what extent, it is not known, and that control lies in the fall-off of referrals. If a person's family physician knows that a particular specialist's care is not up to standard in his or her judgment, then the family physician routes the patient to a specialist in whom confidence is held. Until recently, hospitals and their medical staffs were not as diligent as they might have been, in part because they were immune to liability. But now that hospitals may be legally liable under the doctrine of corporate negligence for the malpractice of physicians providing care in their hospitals, the pressure is on to scrutinize matters more intensely. We might note that the shortcomings were not due to desire to cover up or to condone but because challenging a colleague in any field of endeavor is a pretty sticky business, particularly if one has to stick to facts. Often the facts aren't all there, and the case of malpractice is not that clear-cut; much of what is left is judgment, and judgments differ, and these differences are the fuel for litigation. Under the doctrine of corporate negligence, one must have a mechanism for providing consultation to attending physicians when necessary and for assuming that only competent physicians are allowed to practice in the hospital.

Strengthened peer-review mechanisms, including PAS and HUP-type reports, PSRO's, and beefed up JCAH criteria, all contribute to the development of data bases that will enable hospitals and their staffs to monitor and discipline physicians with assured fairness and reduce the likelihood of damage suits by the physician who is called to task.

Another control is developing in the relicensure and recertification procedures being developed by the states and by the specialty boards. There is always the risk, of course, that the disciplined physician might enlist the talents of the FTC, accusing the hospital and medical staff of restraint of trade.

Medical-society discipline has also been hampered like the hospital.

We often hear nonmedical complaints about how physicians cover up for each other, how the medical society serves to defuse situations and to protect the physician. To some extent, this is probably true, but to what extent we simply have no reliable data. In Chicago, Judge Canel reported some interesting figures: Of the 1,100 malpractice suits filed in his court in 1977, most never went beyond the pretrial stage. "Only 97 went on to the trial judges, and 80 of these were resolved in favor of the defendant. The remaining 17 cases were dropped before coming to trial (19, p.3). Whether there were settlements in those 17 cases or in some of the cases disposed of at the pretrial stage, we do not know. The data do suggest, however, how difficult would be the task of a medical society in trying to discipline its members. Discipline by the society, moreover, is largely meaningless if the physician can continue to practice. It is believed that some of the most negligent physicians are not even members of the medical society.

As a nation, we seem somewhat ambivalent about medical societies. On the one hand, we want them to discipline their members, but to be effective at that, they have to have meaningful sanctions, but these they do not have, and we seem reluctant to grant societies those powers. Moreover, as noted above, they have no power over physicians who are not members of their society.

The real power in discipline rests potentially in medical licensure. But the laws in this area are weak. Relatively few states have provisions relating to medical incompetence. And as Somers notes in her book on *Hospital Regulation: The Dilemma of Public Policy* (20, pp.85-86):

Even where incompetence is specified in the law as a basis for disciplinary action, disciplinary procedures in nearly all the states are so weak and so weighted in favor of the doctor that effective action is virtually impossible. In all but seven states—Delaware, Illinois, Louisiana, Maine, Nebraska, Rhode Island, and the District of Columbia—the disciplinary bodies are controlled by the practitioners. The typical pattern is for the disciplinary board to be named by the Governor from nominees submitted to him by the state medical society. In the seven states listed, disciplinary control has been assigned to the courts or some other public body.

Moreover, in most states, discipline is permissive, not mandatory. The word "may" is generally used instead of "shall" in connection with the statutory powers and duty of the board. In such cases, the board may fail to process complaints as it pleases, without any recourse or right of redress by the complainants or the public. Even assuming that a complaint is processed through the investigation, the hearing, and a determination that the stated offense has been committed, there is still no requirement that the board must suspend or revoke the license, or, in fact, do anything more than quietly reprimand the offending physician.

What is more, the boards tend to be underfinanced and understaffed. In an AMA survey in 1960, it was found that while state medical societies felt that disciplinary mechanisms were adequate, in the judgment of the AMA committee, interestingly enough, they were not. Indeed, if one looks at the disciplinary actions taken by the states, one is struck by the statistical inconsistencies.

A number of states are beginning to tighten up as a result of increased concern over the problem. New York, Illinois, and California are known to now have sizable investigative staffs to deal with malpractice and other complaints against the medical profession. In Pennsylvania, the state effort was activated only "after the Pennsylvania Medical Society filed a lawsuit against the State Board of Medical Education and Licensure to force it to spend $2.4 million in license fee collections" (21). With a staff of 12 trained investigators (nurses, former policemen, and military paramedics), backed by three lawyers and seven hearing officers, the program was launched to deal initially with a backlog of 200 cases involving "complaints of unnecessary surgery, excessive X-rays, unexplained hospital and nursing home deaths, and sexual abuse of patients."

The extent to which there is malpractice is not known. We hear of those cases when the patient or survivors sue or complain. We do not hear of the cases in which the patient is never aware of the possibility because of the confidence the patient holds in the malpracticing physician whose bedside manner is a model for patient assurance. One has to be careful in judging malpractice, for like unnecessary surgery, which might be viewed as a form of malpractice, physicians of good faith will differ as to what is and what is not malpractice.

REFERENCES

1. Goodman, L. J.: *Physician Distribution and Medical Licensure in the United States, 1976.* Chicago, American Medical Association, 1977.
2. *Are Enough Physicians of the Right Types Trained in the United States?* GAO (HRD - 77-92), 1978, p. 36.
3. Mechanic, D.: *Public Expectations and Health Care.* New York, John Wiley, 1972.
4. Silver, G. A.: *A Spy in the House of Medicine.* Germantown, Aspen, 1976.
5. Goodman, L. J. Differences in group practice and prepaid group practice, in Henderson S. R.(ed.): *Profile of Medical Practice, 1977.* Chicago, American Medical Association, p.31.
6. Eisenberg, B. S.: Characteristics of group medical practice in urban and rural areas, in Henderson, S. R.(ed.): *Profile of Medical Practice, 1977.* Chicago, American Medical Association.
7. MacColl, W. A.: *Group Practice and Prepayment of Medical Care.* Washington, Public Affairs Press, 1966.
8. *Medical Care for the American People:* Final Report of the Committee on the Costs of Medical Care. Chicago, The University of Chicago Press, 1932; reprinted in 1970 by the U.S. Department of Health, Education and Welfare.
9. Dyckman, Z. Y.: *A Study of Physicians' Fees.* The Council on Wage and Price Stability, Washington, 1978.
10. *American Medical News,* August 1, 1977.
11. *Physician Distribution and Medical Licensure in the United States, 1976.* American Medical Association.
12. *Medical World News,* September 21, 1973.
13. *Bulletin* of the American College of Surgeons, April 1977.
14. *Directory of Accredited Residencies,* 1977-78, "Essentials of Accredited Residencies. Chicago, American Medical Association.
15. Hanlon, C. R.: *Bulletin* of the American College of Surgeons, February 1978.
16. *Medical World News,* October 17, 1977.
17. Somers, A. R., and Somers, H. S.: *Health and Health Care, Policies in Perspective.* Germantown, Aspen, 1977.
18. Ginzberg, E.: Power centers and decision-making mechanisms, in Knowles, J. H., *Doing Better and Feeling Worse.* New York, Norton, 1977.
19. *American Medical News,* April 28, 1978.
20. Somers, A.R.: *Hospital Regulation: The Dilemma of Public Policy.* Industrial Relations Section, Princeton N.J., Princeton University Press, 1969.
21. *New York Times,* July 18, 1978.

4

Nurses, Physician Assistants, Dentists, and Other Health Professionals

NURSES

The nursing profession is undergoing rapid change in the educational and training programs for nurses and in the things that nurses do.

Nursing began as a helping profession in America with training programs associated with general hospitals. The pattern that developed dominated the nursing field until after the Second World War: Nurses were trained for three years in special schools associated with hospitals. On successful completion of the course of study, the graduating student was awarded a diploma, and on passing the state licensing exam, the nurse became a registered nurse, or RN. Most RNs today (approximately 75%) are graduates of *hospital-diploma schools of nursing*. This percentage, however, is changing as diploma programs close due to cost and to professional pressures and as the number of graduates from other types of nurse-education programs rises. This changing scene will be discussed after we first examine briefly the various types of programs.

Hospital diploma school programs typically had a large nursing service component, that is to say, the training was heavily weighted in favor of on-the-job training rather than academic training. From the beginning, these programs served as a form of labor exploitation because so much of the student's time was spent on the wards nursing patients without compensation, save perhaps room and board. As these programs evolved, more and more adopted stronger academic components; in some states, the students took some of their courses at local colleges and universities.

During World War I, a number of university nursing programs were developed that granted, instead of a diploma, a baccalaureate degree. On passing the same state licensing exam taken by the diploma school graduates, the baccalaureate graduate also became an RN. Baccalaureate programs have experienced a rapid rise, and these graduates now constitute over 15% of the total registered nurse population, but because of the growth in baccalaureate programs, these graduates represent over 25% of the total number of nurses completing programs each year. In other words, the total RN population holding baccalaureate degrees is rising.

A third type of nurse training program began to develop during the 1950s in community colleges. These programs lasted two to two and a half years, upon completion of which the student was granted an associate degree; on passing the same state licensing exam as taken by the diploma school and college or university graduate, the student became a registered nurse. About 6% of the total number of practicing RNs hold associate degrees. Over 42% of the new RNs each year are now associate degree graduates.

There are, therefore, three basic pathways to becoming a registered nurse. Each has an academic component; each uses hospital facilities for clinical training; and each graduate becomes registered by taking a common state examination administered by the state board of nurse examiners. It is generally acknowledged that the clinical (on-the-ward) training in the diploma programs is of longer duration than in the other types of programs, that the associate degree graduates frequently do not have sufficient clinical training, and that this must be augmented by in-service training on being hired by a hospital. There are, of course, great variations among programs, with strong and weak programs in each pathway. The baccalaureate approach is distinctive in that it alone has a public-health nursing component. In addition, a baccalaureate degree (in nursing or some other field) is necessary if an RN wishes to pursue graduate training. There is considerable debate over the comparative operational competencies of the graduates from the different types of programs, and there have been attempts to categorize the programs. The data to support the various categorization attempts are far from conclusive because of the great variability among programs within each pathway and the variability of admission requirements by the programs.

There is clearly a movement, however, on the part of nurse leaders to get the diploma schools to close because, they believe, nurse training should be part of an educational system and not under the control of a hospital or of any other profession. Diploma schools are closing, and while professional pressures are operative, the cause is chiefly that of costs. The costs of diploma education can no longer be buried in general hospital costs and covered by Blue Cross and other insurance payments. The views of nurse leaders vis-à-vis diploma education have to some extent spilled over into the classroom, and baccalaureate students frequently are persuaded to view their roles in nursing as professional, that is, as leaders in nursing and as people having a deeper theoretical understanding of nursing practice than the others. Where baccalaureate graduates have not been able to give this perspective in work situations, it has sometimes led to conflict between the baccalaureate and the diploma nurses as well as with hospital administrators, for an experienced diploma nurse is not likely to feel kindly toward a recent graduate from a baccalaureate program who expresses such views, nor is a hospital administrator who is concerned more with nursing and hospital performance.

There is perhaps a deeper issue here, and that is that nursing seems to be a profession in search of identity. Part of this is manifest in the conflict nursing has with the medical profession. Long dependent on medical practitioners, long under their control—and still so in hospitals and doctors' offices—nursing has sought independence. It has sought to define a role that puts it on a par with medicine and not subservient to it. The extremes to which this fight against medicine go are illustrated by the following quote from a recent book on nursing. Referring to the author of the book, the writer of the "Introduction" states (1, p.v.):

Ashley documents how American hospitals were established by men to offer nursing care actually provided by women, women who worked essentially as indentured servants. The male physicians and hospital administrators were preoccupied, as Ashley details, with control over others, profits, and male privileges. The female nurses were committed to service, to health education, and to the welfare of students and patients—important functions often discouraged by medical men.

Part of the search for professional identity has led nursing to give up or to acquiesce in giving up to other groups certain functions that were historically a part of nursing, such as diet therapy, medical social work, medical records, recreation therapy, ward administration, and bedside nursing. A great deal of this giving up was, of course, necessary due to the growing complexity of the health field. No longer could a nurse have all the knowledge and skills necessary to cover these functional areas. Specially trained people emerged to cover those functions. But spinning off those functions raised the question: what is nursing? Bedside nursing was historically a key nursing function. In a very real sense, it was more fundamental to nursing than all the other functions. Now, however, a great portion of bedside nursing is being taken over by the licensed practical nurse (LPN) and the nurse's aide. If bedside care and other things are given up, what is there left to legitimize nursing as a profession?

This question has led nurse leaders to identify different roles. Accepting the proposition that the diploma nurse was a disappearing breed, nurse leaders began to see the associate degree nurse as a technical nurse capable of handling whatever functions remain to patient care in hospital and doctor's office and the baccalaureate nurse as the leader and teacher. Some nurse leaders are even beginning to talk about the professional nurse as being one who is trained at the graduate level with a master's degree as a specialist in a clinical area of nursing (e.g., pediatrics, public health, medical-surgical, intensive care) or as one who holds only a doctorate, not in sociology or higher education but from one of the developing doctoral programs in nursing. Some argue that professional nursing should not be concerned with "sick care" but with "wellness"—with the steps needed to keep from getting sick. Others argue that there is a unique role for nursing that relates to helping people cope with conditions that medicine is unable to cure or help.

However, much of what goes on today in terms of the search for professional identification is also a reaction to domination by physicians. That domination was very real, and it reflected the attitudes dominant in society, attitudes that even Ashley notes were accepted by a large segment of the female population, including the nurses. Although some of the medical rhetoric of the past sounded sexist, to accept that language uncritically would cause one to misinterpret reality. The physician wanted to dominate, to be captain of the therapeutic team, because the physician always was. This domination was not sexually motivated, for even today male lawyers and male health administrators frequently complain of physician domination. Many physicians appear to know it all and to dominate even beyond their areas of competence. But this is, in part, a result of the status of the physician in society and a result of the training process, which creates a positive, decisive person who must often make life-and-death decisions and live with the results of those decisions. Since the physician, by selection and training, is bright, aggressive, and decisive, this makes the physician sometimes hard to deal with, but the imperial-type physicians of 40 and 50 years ago against whom the nurse leaders seem to be fighting have long since passed away. Their successors have some of the same traits, but they no longer demand subservience; they know they have limits; they know that other health professionals exist and have knowledge to which heed must be paid; most will listen; most will compromise and accommodate. It is a changed, and still changing, world.

Change is very prominent in the large teaching hospitals where nurses today are doing things that neither they nor physicians ever thought would be nursing functions. They are doing things that are new as well as things that were once done by physicians. While the *theory* of nursing may not have taken such events fully into account, nursing is being *operationally* redefined. There is, of course, no iron-clad definition of what a nurse or a physician is. The terms and the things they describe are human devices applied to a world that is forever changing. The need for medicine and nursing to reach accommodation at leadership levels is evidenced by the formation in 1972 of the National Joint Practice Commission (NJPC) by the AMA and the American Nurses Association (ANA). Both organizations, and the Kellogg Foundation, provided support grants for its work. At the Third National Conference on Joint Practice, which the NJPC sponsored, it was suggested that "if physicians and nurses can continue to discuss their differences without getting bogged down in semantics, there was hope for progress" (2, pp.17-18).

Nursing Education Approval and Accreditation

Nursing programs—LPN, diploma, associate degree, and baccalaureate degree—must be approved by an agency of state government if graduates are to be permitted to take the licensing exam. The *state board of nurse examiners* is typically the name of the agency in a state that handles this. The National League for Nursing (NLN) provides a mechanism for academic accreditation over and above the state approval process. RNs who are graduates from NLN accredited programs will normally have their licenses endorsed by other states.

Clinical Specialists in Nursing

The complexity of the health field results in large measure from the growth of knowledge. We know more and more today, and health practitioners are able to do more. But coping with this new knowledge has forced specialization in nursing as in medicine. Nurses with a baccalaureate degree may undertake graduate study in a variety of clinical areas to develop the needed special competence for teaching, for supervision, and for advanced practice. Most of these graduate programs included a formalization, in an educational setting, of developments that were occurring in practice, just as diploma and, later, baccalaureate educational programs constituted a formalization, in an educational environment, of what was being learned on the job, on the hospital wards.

In addition to training in such clinical specialties as pediatric, obstetrics, medical-surgical, public health, psychiatric, anesthesia, and midwifery nursing, there have developed a large number of specialized programs, such as transcultural nursing, occupational health nursing, and a number of nurse practitioner nursing programs. Some nurse practitioner programs are geared to training nurses who will work on their own in private practice or as equals on a health care team; other programs are geared to training nurses to provide primary care in rural and other settings.

Graduate programs in nursing can be professionally accredited by the NLN. Approval of graduate programs is usually beyond the scope of state-government authority. In addition to NLN accreditation, specialty subcomponents of a master's program are sometimes also accredited by a nurse specialty body.

Doctoral Programs in Nursing

A growing number of nurses are pursuing doctoral education. In 1973, the American Nurses' Association listed 1,019 nurses with some type of doctoral degree (3, p.138). Considering that there were 815,000 nurses in 1973 (4, p. 187), the number of doctorates is small. Most of these doctorates are in fields other than nursing—sociology, psychology, higher education, and so forth—principally because until very recently there were only a few doctoral programs in nursing. For some time there was question as to whether there was sufficient knowledge in nursing to justify nursing doctorates, but nurse leaders seem to have answered this in the affirmative and programs are developing (5). As yet there is no accrediting process for doctoral programs, but they will probably develop in time under the NLN umbrella.

The American Nurses' Association (ANA) and the National League for Nursing (NLN)

The ANA is a professional organization with a primary focus on nursing practice. It is broadly based and accredits nursing continuing education programs. The NLN focuses principally on educational programs—from LPN, diploma, AD, baccalaureate and advanced degrees. Some disagreement exists between the two groups as to ANA accreditation of continuing education programs.

Licensed Practical Nurse

The licensed practical nurse (LPN) or, in California and Texas, licensed vocational nurse (LVN), is prepared to provide a variety of nursing services to nonacutely ill patients and to assist the registered nurse with those more seriously ill. The LPN is not an RN. The LPN licensing examination is different from the test administered to graduates of diploma, associate degree, and baccalaureate programs. The LPN curriculum is also different, lasting, on the average, 12 months. While some LPN programs are run by hospitals, community agencies, and community colleges, most are part of public vocational schools. Except in a few community college programs there is no upward mobility for an LPN in nursing unless the LPN starts in one of the other nursing programs from the beginning with no transfer credits. LPNs are assuming more and more duties in hospitals, duties formerly assigned to the RN.

Number of Nurses

In 1974, there were 857,000 RNs in the country (647,000 diploma RNs, 51,600 associate-degree RNs, 130,400 baccalaureate RNs, and 28,000 RNs who went on for a master's or doctoral degree). The number of LPNs stood at

492,000 (4, pp.187, 193). By 1975 the total number of RNs had risen to 906,000: 731,500 holding diplomas or associate degrees (this group not broken down), 144,000 baccalaureate RNs, and 30,500 with higher degrees.

PHYSICIAN ASSISTANTS

The physician assistant (PA) movement is a relatively recent phenomenon, beginning in the mid-1960s. Originally, most PA programs were designed to capture hospital corpsmen or medics who were discharged from the armed forces. Since many of these people had had some formal training and usually a considerable amount of experience, it was felt that their talents could be effectively employed in civilian health care. As the draft ended, and the flow of returning corpsmen and medics tapered off, PA programs began to take people who had no previous health training. Some programs found, however, that many nurses wanted to expand their skills by becoming PAs. Schulz and Johnson suggest that among the reasons for the development of PA programs was "a reluctance in nursing to assume more tasks under physician supervision" (6, p.115).

The length of training in PA programs varies. Some lead to a baccalaureate degree and require four or five years. Many last 12 to 15 months. Others are of much shorter duration. Some programs are highly specialized; others are geared to primary care.

The primary-care programs have captured most of the attention because of the potential they offered to make physicians more efficient by allowing them to delegate certain functions and because they offered the possibility for meeting the needs of underserved areas that had not been able to attract physicians.

The *Medex* program is one of the better-known efforts; it began at the University of Washington and later spread to a number of other universities. This program was designed to train PAs as generalist assistants, principally to general practitioners and internists. The University of Colorado pioneered in turning out *pediatric associates* (as well as *pediatric nurse practitioners*). Duke University is credited with having the first PA program in the country.

PA programs are thus training programs run by hospitals and educational institutions to train people with or without previous health experience to do some of the things physicians do and some of the things nurses frequently did as they were trained on the job by physicians. Some nurses resisted the formalization of these educational processes because they were largely physician inspired and controlled (the University of Colorado program an exception, being nurse and physician conceived and controlled) and because some felt that nursing should move away from sick care and whatever physicians do. But the PA programs survived, though current controversy within nursing is concerned with the proper relationship between a PA and a nurse, specifically whether a nurse can or should take an order from a PA (No, say the nurses.) This controversy is not unlike the controversy within medicine vis-à-vis the proper relationship between physicians and chiropractors. Should a physician take a referral from a chiropractor and give a medical report back to the chiropractor on completion of therapy?

The great variability among programs led to a PA-certifying process administered by the National Commission on Certification of Physicians Assistants. The AMA was a major mover in the establishment of the commission. In addition, the AMA, in collaboration with various allied health organizations and medical-specialty societies, moved to establish the Committee on Allied Health Education and Accreditation (CAHEA), which took over from the AMA's Council on Medical Education responsibility for accrediting allied health programs, including PA programs but no nurse programs.

PHYSICIAN-PA-NURSE RELATIONS

The issues that affect the relationships of physicians to PAs and nurse practitioners were highlighted in 1977 in testimony before the Subcommittee on Health of the Committee on Ways and Means of the U.S. House of Representatives. Under consideration was a bill to provide Medicare reimbursement for "physician extenders" who practiced in rural health centers. "Physician extenders" was a phrase designed to cover at least PAs, nurse practitioners, and nurse clinicians.

The subcommittee background material to the hearings, the statements submitted by the American Academy of Physicians' Assistants and by the president of the ANA, and some of the testimony by representatives of the AMA are reprinted from the published hearings (7, p.3-5, 54-57, 61-65, 67-74).

Subcommittee Background Material: Medicare Reimbursement for Services of Physician Extenders Practicing in Rural Clinics

---

I. BACKGROUND

Rural health clinics staffed by physician extenders have developed in many remote, rural communities because of the inability of these communities to attract or retain a physician. Although there is physician backup for the clinics—e.g., availability for consultation and referral of patients, preparation of standing orders, review of patient records—the physician extender functions essentially in an independent setting. The physician extender working in such a clinic may be a nurse, a physician's assistant, or a former medical corpsman who has received extended training and is capable of diagnosing and treating the majority of the community's primary and emergency care needs with only the general supervision of a physician.

Organization of these clinics follows no set pattern and is as diverse as the communities they serve. Some of the clinics are nonprofit while others have developed as profitmaking organizations. They may have been organized by the community they serve and be governed by a community board or they may have been organized by a physician practicing in a nearby urban area. A number of clinics have relied on State and local funding while many were developed with Federal funding under the Office of Economic Opportunity, the Public Health Service Act, or the Appalachian Regional Commission. Their common feature is that they serve rural areas and offer primary care services which would otherwise not be available.

The services provided by physician extenders in such a setting are not presently covered under the medicare program. Medicare law and regulations allow coverage of services provided by physician extenders only: First, when they are provided under the direct supervision of a physician, and second, when they are of the kind traditionally performed as incident to a physician's service. In contrast, the physician extender services provided in rural clinics are customarily provided with only limited physician supervision and are of the type traditionally performed by a physician himself—for example, diagnosis and treatment of a minor infection.

II. SUMMARY OF H.R. 2504 (MR. ROSTENKOWSKI, MR. DUNCAN, MRS. KEYS)

Payment for Rural Health Clinic Services

The bill, H.R. 2504, would provide medicare coverage for services provided by physician extenders in rural clinics. Just as with other organized providers of medical services under part B of medicare, payment for the services would be based on 80 percent of the costs incurred in providing the services and payment would be made directly to the clinic. The allowable costs would include those direct and indirect costs of maintaining the clinic which are reasonable. All the services and supplies which are presently covered under medicare when they are provided by a physician or incident to a physician's service would be covered. Although rural clinics often provide a wider range of services—for example, drugs and dental care—medicare coverage would not be extended to these additional types of services. Just as when covered services are provided by a physician in his office or clinic, the rural health clinic would bill beneficiaries for the medicare part B deductible and coinsurance.

Definition of Rural Health Clinic

In order to assure the quality of the services for which medicare payment would be made, the participating rural clinics would be required to meet certain criteria set forth in the definition of rural health clinic. For example, clinics would be required to maintain clinical records on all patients in accordance with accepted medical standards; to develop policies with the advice of a group of professionals, including one or more physicians and one or more physician extenders, to govern the services provided by the clinic; to provide directly basic diagnostic lab services; and to have available for administering to patients at least those drugs and biologicals that are necessary for treatment of emergencies and which are ordinarily available in a physician's office.

Because the clinics serve as an entry point to the health care delivery system, they would also be required to have arrangements for referral of patients to more extensive medical care services when neccessary. That is, the clinics would have to have arrangements for hospital admission of patients and for access to those diagnostic, laboratory, x-ray, and pharmacy services that are not available from the clinic. In addition, clinics would be required to meet any other requirements the Secretary finds necessary for the health and safety of the clinic patients.

In order to meet the definition of a rural health clinic, a clinic would have to be located in a rural area where the supply of medical services is not sufficient to meet the needs of the residents. This definition would include (but not be limited to) rural areas designated as medically underserved under section 1302(7) of the Public Health Service Act. Since this bill is to address the health care delivery problems specifically resulting from a lack of physician services, only those clinics which are not physician-directed (ie., do not have a full-time physician) would be eligible.

Definition of Physician Extender

The key to the quality of services provided in these clinics is the physician extender who must be capable of performing competently without the immediate supervision of a physician. Because of the diversity of the education and training of physician extenders and the variation in how they are treated under State law, not all those who may be considered physician extenders are suited for providing services in a rural health clinic setting. The bill, therefore, directs the Secretary of Health, Education, and Welfare to determine what specific education, training and experience requirements—or any combination thereof—physician extenders should meet. These requirements would take into account the qualifications necessary to provide primary and emergency care services with the degree of independence from a physician allowed for in the bill.

Requirement for Physician Supervision

The bill also sets forth certain requirements for the degree of physician supervision. A physician would not have to be physically present when the services are rendered. The clinic would, however, be required to have an arrangement with a physician for the periodic review of all services provided by the extender, the supervision and guidance of the extender and the preparation of standing orders for treatment of patients. The physician would also have to be available for referral when necessary and for assistance in medical emergencies.

In addition to these requirements regarding qualifications and degree of physician supervision, physician extenders would also be subject to any relevant State laws or regulations.

III. H.R. 1955 (MR. DUNCAN)

This bill would provide medicare reimbursement for services of physician extenders rendered under the supervision of a physician regardless of where the services are rendered or whether the physician is physically present. Reimbursement for the services provided by the physician extender would be made on the basis of the charge made for the services. No mention is made of what charge medicare should allow for services provided by a physician extender relative to the charge allowed for the same service when performed by a physician.

The term "physician extender" would mean a physician assistant, nurse practitioner, nurse clinician, or other trained practitioner who has successfully completed a program of study approved by the Secretary, who is certified as a physician's assistant by the National Board of Medical Examiners, or who is licensed or otherwise recognized by a State in which the services are rendered.

IV. H.R. 2672 (MR. BROYHILL AND OTHERS)

This bill would provide medicare reimbursement for services of physician extenders rendered under the supervision of a physician regardless of where the services are rendered or whether the physician is physically present.

Reimbursement for the services provided by the physician extender would be made directly to the supervising physician on the basis of the charge made for the service. No mention is made of what charge medicare should allow for services provided by a physician extender relative to the charge allowed for the same service when performed by a physician.

The term "physician extender" would mean a physician assistant, nurse practitioner, nurse clinician, or other trained practitioner who has successfully completed a program of study approved by the Secretary, or who is holding a valid certificate as a physician's assistant issued by the National Commission on Certification of Physicians' Assistants or by any qualified successor to the Commission. The physician extender would also have to be licensed or otherwise recognized by a State as qualified to provide primary health care services in the State in which such services are rendered.

Statement of the American Academy of Physicians' Assistants*

Mr. Chairman and members of the committee: I am honored to have the privilege to testify before the subcommittee once again on the need for legislation to permit medicare (part B) reimbursement for patient care services rendered by physician's assistants; and more specifically, to discuss H.R. 2504 introduced by Mr. Rostenkowski on January 26, 1977.

I am a graduate of the Duke University Physician's Assistant program, and am currently employed by the University of Oklahoma as an assistant professor in the Department of Family Practice and Community Medicine and Dentistry while serving as associate director of the Physician's Associate program. I have also practiced in a rural primary care clinic while employed by the Mayo Clinic-Mayo Foundation. I have been appointed to many DHEW advisory committees and have served on the Board of the National Commission on Certification of Physician's Assistants.

Myths and Misconceptions Regarding the Physician's Assistant Concept

It has been stated that the development of the physician's assistant profession has at best been haphazard and disjointed, with a resultant lack of appropriate standards. Contrary to the opinions of the uninformed, the development of

---

*Presented by Thomas R. Godkins, immediate past president and chairman, Goals and Priorities Committee, American Academy of Physicians' Assistants, to the Subcommittee on Health, Committee on Ways and Means, U.S. House of Representatives, Jan. 28, 1977.

this profession has been done methodically with, in every respect, concern for quality. In September, 1975, I testified before this Subcommittee on the development of this emerging profession.[1] Let me state the myths and counter with the facts.

Myth. Tremendous disparity within the educational process of physician's assistants.

Fact. The American Medical Association's Council on Medical Education in conjunction with specialty medical societies, has developed an accreditation mechanism recognized as an accrediting agency by the U.S. Commissioner of Education.

Myth. No mechanism for quality assurance.

Fact. The National Commission on Certification of Physician's Assistants administers an extremely reliable examination developed by the National Board of Medical Examiners.

Myth. Few States recognize physician's assistants.

Fact. Approximately 40 States recognize and regulate the physician's assistant.

Myth. Poor patient acceptance.

Fact. The literature is replete with descriptive information acknowledging excellent patient acceptance of this health care provider.

Myth. Utilization of P.A.s will decrease the quality of care and increase the inappropriate utilization of diagnostic services.

Fact. Physician's assistants render patient care of an acceptable quality as reported by Record, et al., at the Kaiser Foundation Health Services Research Center in Portland, Oregon, Stanhope at the University of Oklahoma, and Ott at the University of Colorado. In addition, there is evidence that the utilization of physician's assistants does *not* increase the inappropriate use of diagnostic services.

Myth. Physician's assistants increase the risk of malpractice.

Fact. Physician's assistants, by improving the quality and continuity of patient care, reduce the physician's risk of malpractice. Betty Jane Anderson, AMA Assistant General Counsel, has stated, "after looking at ways in which P.A.s perform their services, I feel P.A.s probably hold the potential . . . as . . . one of the best malpractice prevention tools . . . available to physicians."

Myth. Use of physician's assistants will increase the cost of medical care.

Fact. Peterson, et al., at the Baylor College of Medicine, reported an 85 percent reduction in hospitalizations utilizing P.A.s in an ambulatory clinic resulting in a cost savings well in excess of $27,000 (for one year). This data was substantiated by Runyan who also reported cost savings through a

---

[1]"Position Statement on Medicare Reimbursement for Physician Extender Services," presented to the Subcommittee on Health, Committee on Ways and Means, U.S. House of Representatives, by Thomas R. Godkins on Sept. 26, 1975.

reduction in the need for hospitalizations. Most importantly, Record's studies on cost effectiveness of physician's assistants revealed P.A. productivity per clinic work hour compared favorably with physician output rates (for the same office visit categories) and that significant cost savings can be instituted with the utilization of these practitioners.

The development of this profession has not been haphazard and disjointed, but carefully planned by individuals on the cutting edge of medical education.

Congressional Support

The Congress has fostered the growth and development of this profession. Federal funds to support education with subsequent research on the utilization of physician's assistants has been substantial. A reasonable estimate of total federal expenditures for physician's assistant education and research is approximately $47,224,919 in the past decade (exclusive of military expenditures).

In my testimony before this Subcommittee on September 15, 1976 I reviewed the Medicare problem and the legislation submitted before the 94th Congress. The 95th Congress has once again seen the submission of multiple pieces of legislation including: H.R. 2504 by the Chairman of this Subcommittee, H.R. 1955 by Mr. Duncan, H.R. 3635 by Mr. Broyhill, S. 484 by Mr. Pearson, and S. 708 recently introduced by Mr. Clark and Mr. Leahy. All of these bills address the inequity in Medicare Part B which does not allow reimbursement for the patient care services provided by physician's assistants.

The Dichotomy and the Barrier

Title XVIII of the Social Security Act does not adequately authorize Medicare Part B reimbursement for physician's assistant services [Section 1861 (s) (2) (A)]. According to the Social Security Administration, the performance by a physician's assistant of services which traditionally have been reserved to physicians can not be covered under Medicare Part B even though all other "incident-to" requirements are met. This policy of non-reimbursement is the impediment to the optimum utilization of physician's assistants. In 1972 Congress intended to bring resolution to the problem through passage of H.R. 1 (Public Law 92-603, Sec 222) which gave the Social Security Administration responsibility for the implementation of a research study evaluating physician extender reimbursement. This study was intended to be completed in five years, but unfortunately the final outcomes will not be reported until 1979. To add insult to injury, the Bureau of Health Insurance has conducted secretive audits using extremely weak methodology, harassing employing physicians who are attempting to improve patient care and its access. These subversive audits point once again to the need for Congressional intervention to amend the Social Security Act to allow the appropriate utilization of physician's assistants.

The previous administration seems to have had a difficult time dealing with the Medicare problem. I would like to introduce into testimony a copy of an article which appeared in the Washington Post entitled, "Rural Health Care in Appalachia" which ex-Secretary Matthews sent to then Assistant Secretary Theodore Cooper asking, "Is this correct? If so, are we doing the right thing?" The article cited the fact that Medicare regulations prevent clinics from being reimbursed for the services rendered by physician's assistants. I would also like to introduce Assistant Secretary Cooper's response to ex-Secretary Matthews dated May 10, 1976 which in part states, " . . . I do not believe that we are doing the right thing . . . provisions like this inhibit the development of alternative forms of health care delivery, which can provide needed additional access and be of high quality at an affordable cost . . . we are presently studying various legislative and regulatory changes." President Carter and his administration seem sincerely concerned about bringing resolution to this problem and, in his current budget, has requested monies for the continued funding of P.A. programs and to provide for Medicare Part B reimbursement of physician extender services.

Finally, the Comptroller General of the United States in his report to the Congress entitled, "Progress and Problems in Training and Use of Assistants to Primary Care Physicians," concluded:

(1) Physician extenders have generally improved the accessibility and quality of medical care provided in their employer's practices; and

(2) The issue of reimbursing for physician extender services needs to be resolved.

H.R. 2504; Recommendations

In exploring alternative methods and amounts of reimbursement, individuals from the Academy have met with representatives of the American Academy of Family Physicians (AAFP), the American Medical Association (AMA), and the American Nurses Association (ANA). Both the AAFP and the AMA have taken the position that physicians should be reimbursed for patient care services provided by physician's assistants at usual and customary rates of Medicare reimbursement. They oppose suggestions promoting the concept of reduced rates of reimbursement for all physician's assistants. Representatives from these organizations, and our Academy, believe discriminating rates of reimbursement would: (1) increase the administrative costs in implementing the program; (2) connotate "second class medicine" to the consumer (who equates quality with cost); (3) serve as a negative incentive for physician employment of P.A. graduates; and (4) not adequately improve access to care for all Americans. Likewise, the American Nurses Association seems supportive of appropriate legislation which adequately defines the nurse practitioner and the qualifications of these professionals for Medicare reimbursement.

I would like to commend the Congress for introducing substantive legislation: H.R. 2504 by Mr. Rostenkowski, H.R. 1955 by Mr. Duncan, and H.R. 3635 by Mr. Broyhill. All three bills reflect Congressional concern over the potential cost impact of physician's assistant reimbursement on the Medicare program. It is important for this Subcommittee not to overlook physician: P.A. differential training costs which is saving the federal government a substantial amount of money. Likewise, physicians are not "buying" a profit (in a monetary sense) but are employing P.A.s to improve the continuity and quality of care as well as give them time to continue their education. Most importantly, relative to H.R. 2504, Dr. Lawrence at the University of Washington (Seattle) estimates that only 31 of 400 practices utilizing physician's assistants and nurse practitioners in the Pacific Northwest (Washington, Alaska, Oregon, Montana and Idaho) would receive reimbursement under the legislation proposed by Mr. Rostenkowski.

I would like to recommend H.R. 1504 be amended and/or consideration be given toward combining the outstanding components of the legislation submitted in the 95th Congress in the development of a new bill. More specifically, I would like to comment on some of the provisions in H.R. 2504 which warrant further attention:

Proposed. Section 1833, "with respect to rural health clinic services, payment shall be made *** on the basis of costs reasonably related to providing such services ***";

Recommend. "With respect to physician's assistant services, payment shall be made to the supervising physician and/or rural health clinics, on behalf of an individual, at the usual and customary rates of reimbursement";

Proposed. Section 1861, "is located in a rural area *** designated by the Secretary as *** medically underserved ***";

Recommend. Deletion with the adoption of language which provides a consistent reimbursement policy whereby Medicare payment is provided for the provision of services regardless of the location.

Proposed. Section 1861, "is not a physician-directed clinic under direct personal supervision";

Recommend. "The activities and patient care services of physician's assistants shall be provided under the responsible supervision of (a) physician(s). Services of a physician's assistant shall include services performed regardless of whether the physician was actually present and regardless of whether the services were performed in the physician's office or at some other site";

Proposed. Section 1861, "physician extender means *** a physician's assistant, MEDEX, nurse practitioner, or any other such practitioner who performs, under the supervision of a physician *** such services as he is legally authorized to perform in accordance with state law ***";

Recommend. The term "physician extender" and "any other such practitioner" be deleted and the terms "physician's assistant" and "nurse practitioner" be substituted. "Physician's assistants be defined as individuals who have completed an educational program for physician's assistants accredited by the American Medical Association or other recognized accrediting agencies and/or are holders of current valid certificates from the National Commission on Certification of Physician's Assistants"; and the "physician's assistants are recognized as practitioners under the laws of the state in wich the services are provided."

I would like to thank Congress for addressing this important problem. Physician's assistants are improving patient access to care and it seems unfair to deny primary care reimbursement to Medicare beneficiaries. Most importantly, Congress has the opportunity to institute a program which has great potential towards reducing the total cost of health care in the country. Thank you for allowing me to testify.

Statement of President of the American Nurses' Association

I am Anne Zimmerman, president of the American Nurses' Association. With me is Ellen Peach, a nurse practitioner from Idaho and Connie Holleran of the ANA Washington office. I thank you for the opportunity to appear at this hearing today.

We would like to commend the committee for its recognition of the need for changes in reimbursement policies under Medicare that will make possible the continuation of existing rural clinics and the development of new ones. In fact, we speak in support of reimbursing health services such as those referred to in H.R. 2504, regardless of the setting in which they are delivered, rural or urban. Such reimbursement policies should apply for all clinics not just satellite clinics.

Large segments of our rural populations would be without primary health care were it not for such clinics. Established largely in response to a lack of physician services, rural clinics are now to be found in locations throughout the country, many of them operated by nurse practitioners. As you have well recognized, the continued existence of these clinics is threatened by current Medicare regulations which prevent reimbursement unless a doctor is physically present. In light of the millions of federal dollars spent to prepare nurse practitioners, it seems very short sighted to restrict federal payment mechanisms.

We strongly support the move for change in Medicare reimbursement policies and the general approach which the committee is taking in seeking to deal with this problem.

However, we would like to recommend two changes in H.R. 2504 in relation to the role and function of the nurse. These are:

> To exclude nurse practitioners from the umbrella term "physician extenders" and to identify them separately, and
> To remove the requirement of physician "supervision" for the services of nurse practitioners and replace that with physician consultation and referrals, both of whom must also be reimbursable. This would be in conformity with the current practice under Medicare in regards to reimbursement for consultation between physicians.

We not only support collaboration, consultation and referral between nurse practitioners and physicians, but recognize the necessity of this relationship if comprehensive health care is to be provided. Nurse practitioners are ethically, legally and morally committed to the right of consumers to adequate services.

The physician is the recognized expert in medical aspects of health care, the nurse in nursing aspects. The roles of each are complementary and not substitutive.

There is a distinct difference between the nurse practitioner and the physician assistant. The differences between nurse practitioners and, to use the generic term, "physician extenders" (Physician's assistants, medex) are real and not a matter of semantics. These differences relate to (1) definition, (2) preparation, (3) focus of practice, and (4) legal requirements.

1. DEFINITION

In 1970 the American Medical Association Board of Trustees defined the physician's assistant: "The physician's assistant is a skilled person qualified by academic and practical on-the-job training to provide patient services under the supervision and direction of a licensed physician who is responsible for the performance of that assistant." The physician extender performs medically delegated functions.

The nurse practitioner, as defined by the ANA Council of Family Nurse Practitioners, is a primary care provider prepared to give continuous, person-alized care to the patient/client at the point of entry into the health care system and to continue as the individual's care provider. The nurse practitioner is a registered nurse prepared in a degree-granting program or in a post-R.N. continuing education program. The nurse practitioner already possesses a license to practice nursing and is legally liable for her/his own practice and usually carries personal malpractice insurance.

2. PREPARATION

The basic length of preparation for a physician's assistant generally ranges between four months and four years. Admission qualifications range from a minimum of high school graduation to previous training in the military corps. The preparation for nurse practitioners consists of a specialized program of study beyond that required for the R.N. It must meet the ANA Guidelines for Short Term Continuing Education Programs that prepare a nurse to function in an expanded role. Published guidelines include those written for the pediatric, family, adult, school health, college health and the Ob-Gyn nurse practitioners. Programs range from 36-40 weeks in a continuing education program to baccalaureate and master's degree granting programs.

The American Nurses' Association has a certification program for nurse practitioners initiated only last year; already more than one thousand nurses have entered the certification process.

3. FOCUS OF PRACTICE

A conservative estimate of nurses prepared to practice in the expanded role is about 7,000. Although some of these are prepared in specialty practice as geriatrics, school health, Ob-Gyn and pediatrics, there are more than 2,500 nurses prepared as family nurse practitioners. These nurse practitioners are able to provide a broad range of services to all age groups.

The median age of nurses graduating from nurse practitioner programs is 30 years; therefore, many of these individuals have a good practice base behind them. Most nurse practitioner graduates choose settings where maldistribution of health care services exists. Experience to date shows that they tend to reside longer in their respective communities and hopefully will become life long residents.

The nurse practitioner delivers health care which includes not only physical assessment, but also assessment of the emotional and developmental status of an individual and the family as well as an analysis of health behavior.

Nurse practitioners deliver care in a variety of settings including but not limited to homes, ambulatory care centers, HMO's schools, industries, and physician's offices. Statistics indicate that a large number of nurse practitioners are in rural states and the majority practice in clinics providing direct primary care.

Nurse practitioners practice independently and have a collaborative arrangement with a physician. A collaborative arrangement indicates a cooperation in the management of a patient's health care problem, when necessary. It is assumed that a nurse practitioner functioning "interdependently" has a physician available for ready consultation and that she/he can refer patients easily. Such physician services, whether on site or by telephone or other means, must, of course, be reimburseable under all third party payments plans. In this way, the client benefits from both the nursing perspective and the medical perspective. The nurse role and the physician role are not merely greater and lesser degrees of a single role, but are coordinate and complementary in providing high quality primary health care. Each role constitutes a different emphasis of practice. The nurses' emphasis is on the psychosocial needs of patients rather than just the pathological; its emphasis is on preserving wellness, not just curing illness; its emphasis is on the whole patient and on coordinating total health care rather than giving just isolated bits of care.
The scope of primary nursing practice includes:

- Assessment of the physical, emotional, and developmental status of the individual and family;
- Assessment of the environmental status of the community and its impact on health;
- Analysis of health behavior related to personality, life style, and culture;
- Provision of primary care through diagnosis, clinical judgment, and management to restore, maintain, and improve health status;
- Teaching, counseling, and serving as an advocate;
- Collaboration and/or coordination with other health care providers and community organizations;
- Initiation and/or participation in clinical nursing research and in the application of research findings to practice; and
- Evaluation of outcomes of adult and family nursing care.

Practice techniques involve a synthesis of skills from behavioral, social, physical, and health sciences. (Some are more visible than others.)

1. Collection of a data base includes:
   Individual and family health history;
   Systematic physical examination; and
   Appropriate diagnostic studies.
2. Application of clinical judgment from the data base includes:
   Differentiation between normal and abnormal findings;
   Interpretation of diagnostic studies;
   Initiation and management of therapy;

Referral to or consultation with another member of the health care team; Continuous management.

3. Communication skills include:
Record data collection and continuing care in a methodical, concise, easily retrievable, and clear manner.
Application of teaching, learning, and motivational theories to effect therapeutic change in health behaviors;
Ability to interview, listen, clarify values, and problem solve with individuals and families;
Involvement in the organization and teaching of health and health related programs to families and community groups.

4. LEGAL REQUIREMENTS

In most states physician assistants and Medex personnel function under a licensed physician. It is understood that the physician assistant and Medex personnel function under the professional and legal supervision of the physician. Therefore, the physician is ultimately responsible for the care.

In contrast, a nurse is licensed and registered by a state. The law does not place the registered nurse under the direct supervision of any other health discipline. As mentioned earlier, nurse practitioners carry their own malpractice insurance and assume full legal accountability for their individual nursing acts.

In the past few years 31 states have revised their Nurse Practice Acts to clarify the functions of the nurse practitioner in the expanded role.

There must be a system of peer review and other quality assurance mechanisms in operation to evaluate the appropriateness, adequacy and quality of care provided by the nurse practitioner. Standards of care have been promulgated by the profession for each practice area and adherence to these is considered an essential part of professional nursing practice.

Evidence shows there are a number of nurse practitioners functioning as the sole primary health care provider in rural clinics. Some areas where these clinics are located are Kentucky, Tennessee, Idaho, Montana, Vermont, New Mexico, and Washington. Nurse practitioners have brought needed services to people in remote rural communities and underserved urban locations all over the country. Some examples follow.

With the help of an initial federal grant of $27,000, Carolyn Whitaker set up a family nurse service clinic in Red Boiling Springs, Tenn. in 1972. Many individuals of the community had been without any type of health care for 15 years. In the first year of operation, Ms. Whitaker saw over 2,000 patients and had 812 families registered with the clinic.

In July 1971, Wilma Nicholson took over the operation of the SOS Health

Center in Seeley Lake, Montana. The people of the Seeley Lake area had petitioned the state to send in an individual who could act as a para-medical person between themselves and their physicians who were located 60 to 120 miles away. Among her numerous duties, Ms. Nicholson is responsible for seeing to the health needs of one high school and three elementary schools. She operates the ambulance service. Once a month she runs a growth and development clinic for children and once a year she conducts a multiphasic screening program.

Two nurse practitioners provide primary care for the logging community of Darrington, Washington, some 80 miles north of Seattle. With the assistance of a receptionist-clerk, they operate an out-patient clinic providing day-to-day care for the town's 1,100 residents and people in the surrounding area. The nearest physician is 30 miles away over winding mountain roads.

There is no question that the nurse practitioner participates in the medical regime of care through the implementation of appropriate medical orders, and the coordination of the activities and efforts of other health personnel who participate in the patients' care at different intervals.

It is also evident a major portion of care is in the areas of health promotion, prevention activities, counseling and teaching.

Numerous studies document a high degree of consumer satisfaction with the services of nurse practitioners.

At the Harvard Community Health Plan in Boston, an HMO, nurse practitioners see from 30 to 40 percent of the patient population without physician input. The results of a Health Center Survey indicates a greater than 87 percent acceptance of this kind of health care delivery.

The previous material points to the distinct and unique role of the nurse practitioner. It likewise contrasts the differences between nurse practitioners, physicians, and physician's assistants and related personnel. One provider does not and should not substitute for each other. The effective utilization of the skills of each is needed for an effective health team to function.

These differences impact significantly on the rural health care delivery system. Rural America presents a distinctive picture. The very definition of health that is employed in rural health policy proceedings recognizes that health is not solely concerned with medical care but with health in a broader context. This broader context encompasses environmental and preventive health care, nutrition, physical and mental well-being, as well as medical care. More than 70 percent of the health problems in rural America are chronic health problems that limit activity and require continuous health supervision and support in order for the individual to accommodate these within the context of a meaningful lifestyle. Within the rural population itself, these chronic health problems are greatest among middle and older age groups. Nurse practitioners possess the appropriate combination of medical and psychosocial skills to best meet these needs.

In closing, as we stated earlier, we believe that the potential of this legislation will be enhanced by modifying it to exclude nurse practitioners from the umbrella term "physician extenders" and to remove the mandate of physician supervision and substitute reimbursable medical consultation. As you continue your study of this issue, let me point out that a reimbursement system that provides for direct access to professional nursing services could be structured on a fee for service basis for the self-employed nurse engaging in either a solo or group practice. If the nurse is employed by a rural health facility it would be equally appropriate to reimburse the clinic, and we support this concept. Reimbursement based upon a capitation system is likewise acceptable and in some instances more desirable.

In addition, in Sec. (aa) (2) (G) we do wonder just what laboratory services are expected to be on the premises. Are there not options for getting laboratory services that would not be so restrictive yet could control quality of services?

We believe that legislation in this area is vitally needed. We feel that the changes we are requesting are reasonable and important to the future effective operation of many rural clinics and other health care sites where nurses increasingly are functioning in the expanded role. We believe that acceptance of these recommendations will increase the benefit to rural citizens of this bill. We hope that the committee will be able to make the changes we have suggested so that we can actively support enactment of this significant legislation.

Again, I thank the committee for the opportunity to present the views of the American Nurses' Association. We will be happy to supply any additional information and assistance that would be helpful to the committee.

Statement and Partial Testimony of the American Medical Association

Dr. Beddingfield. Thank you very much, Mr. Chairman, and members of the committee. I am Edgar T. Beddingfield, Jr., M.D., a physician in family practice at Wilson, N.C. I serve as chairman of the Council on Legislation of the American Medical Association. Appearing with me today is Harry N. Peterson, director of our Department on Legislation. On my left is Mr. Dan Hill, the assistant director of the Department.

We are happy to be here today to express our views on a subject which we have devoted a lot of time, a lot of thought and, I might add, a substantial budgetary commitment in the American Medical Association—the concern for rural health. We do have some concerns about the bill as it appears before us, but we hope that the hearing today will serve as a focal point, or a catalyst, for continuing discussion of the issue.

The AMA has been at the forefront in supporting the utilization of the physicians' assistants and early recognized their special utility in medical care shortage areas, including rural areas. In the past, we have pointed out the need to support salutary legislation recognizing the role of the physician's assistant in serving to extend the services of a physician into shortage areas.

To this end we support legislation under which medicare would recognize reimbursement to the physician for services performed by him through his supervised assistant and would recognize reimbursement whether the assistant performs services at or away from the physician's office. We believe that this would encourage wider use of the assistant and give proper recognition to the essential nature of the assistant, which is to extend the physician's services. Such provision of service can be of proper quality when the assistant has received sufficient formal training from appropriately accredited training programs, meets any State requirements for provision of services, and remains subject to, and answerable to, the supervision of a physician. The latter qualification makes clear the proper, critically essential role of the supervising physician, which is to assure that his assistant is properly trained and supervised and that the physician responsible for the assistant's actions must remain answerable to, and take responsibility for the proper treatment of, the patient. Failure to retain such a relationship would be detrimental to quality patient care in the long run.

We would emphasize that the physician extender is just that, an extension of and not a substitute for the physician.

While an assistant can be especially advantageous in shortage areas in which no physician is located, caution must be taken to assure that the care provided by the assistant is indeed quality care. In a rush to provide some care to an area which may otherwise have little or no care it would be easy to brush aside proper safeguards. We must preserve for all medicare patients—including those in rural areas—a high standard of care.

The bill before us does address certain of our overall considerations.

EXTENDER REQUIREMENTS

The bill defines the physician extender, in part, as one who performs "under the supervision of a physician * * * such services as he is legally authorized to perform (in the State in which he performs such services) in accordance with State law (or the State regulatory mechanism provided by State law)."

The bill recognize in part the underlying concept, namely, that the extender is actually intended to provide an expansion of a physician's services, with the close and continued supervision of the extender which that implies.

The requirement that the extender meet State requirements is a provision which we have supported, and we believe that such a provision properly recognizes the primary—and exclusive—power of the individual State to determine the qualifications and scope of practice of an extender.

The bill further defines the physician extender, however, as one who also meets such training, education, and experience requirements—or any combination thereof—as the Secretary may prescribe in regulations. We believe that the physician extender should complete a training program or have experience meeting the training program standards of recognized accrediting agencies. Compliance with any standards established in States regulating this category of personnel should be sufficient and proper. The language in the bill authorizing the Secretary to establish standards should be deleted.

I might insert parenthetically here that the Secretary actually has some measure of control over this inasmuch as the U.S. Office of Education within HEW approves the accrediting agencies who in turn set standards for these training programs.

RURAL HEALTH CLINICS

As to the clinics, certain portions of H.R. 2504 recognize concepts on which an extender program should be built. However, other portions of the bill, we feel, are troublesome. While the objective, ostensibly, is to provide payment for services of the physician extender, the bill in fact would add a new payment authorization for rural health clinic services.

Thus, after defining a physician extender and setting certain reasonable—although not sufficiently restrictive—limits on the physician extender and his practice, the bill then goes to great length to set up a new exclusive type of entity under medicare, part B, for purposes of reimbursement. Reimbursable services under the bill—principally those of the extender—would be those services provided only by a "rural health clinic," would be reimbursed only to the "clinic," and would be reimbursed on the basis of "costs reasonably related to providing such services or on the basis of such other tests of reasonableness as the Secretary may find appropriate."

The "rural health clinic" itself would be defined as an entity which complies with all of the following: (1) Provides rural health clinic services, (2) has an arrangement with a physician for review of services provided by the physician extender, for preparation of medical orders, and for referral and for advice and assistance in medical emergencies, (3) maintains clinical records, (4) arranges for referral and admission to hospitals, (5) provides for development of governing policies with advice of a group of professional personnel—including at least one physician and one extender, (6) provides for a physician or physician extender to be responsible for execution of policies, (7) provides directly for routine diagnostic services, (8) complies with State and Federal requirements for storage and dispensing of drugs and (9) meets such other requirements as the Secretary may determine to be necessary.

As a further limitation, such a clinic could only be one which (1) is located in "a rural area where the supply of medical services is not sufficient to meet the needs of individuals residing therein * * * " (2) agrees not to charge for items or services—except for deductible or coinsurance—and incredibly, (3) is not a physician-directed clinic under direct personal physician supervision. The bill would reimburse only the new type of clinic for services of an extender—who could perform what he is authorized to perform under the State law—plus those services which are incident to a physician's services.

A glaring inconsistency is created by the provision limiting payment to a clinic. By what reasoning should a facility be the exclusive entity reimbursed for what must be identified essentially as physician's services? The fundamental concept is that the extender is providing an extension of physician services. The physician character of the services furnished by the clinic is further emphasized since the bill would only recognize, in addition, services "incident to a physician's professional services." We believe that the provisions of the bill in this regard strain logical analysis, in attempting to have medicare pay a specially recognized facility—the rural health clinic—for physician services performed by a nonphysician.

To compound this inconsistency, the definition of a "rural health clinic" specifically excludes a clinic which is "a physician-directed clinic under direct personal physician supervision." Thus, upon close examination, we find the additional anomaly in which the service of the physician extender is not even reimbursed to the clinic if a physician directs the clinic and personally directs the extender. In other words, the nearer the physician comes to directing the extender, the less likely will payment be made under this bill.

It is also interesting to note that of those States having provision for recognition of the physician extender, 36 require the direct supervision and control of the extender by the physician. However, H.R. 2504 would establish a mechanism whereby the extender would not be directly answerable to nor employed by a physician, whereby the employer is a nonphysician, whereby services provided are subject to policies and direction of nonphysicians, and whereby close supervision of the extender by a physician is discouraged.

RESPONSIBILITY FOR EXTENDER

As we pointed out earlier in our statement, we have long supported the use of the physician assistant. However, we believe that this person should be utilized as originally intended, that is, as an extension of and assistant to the physician with the physician remaining primarily responsible for the assistant's patient care functions. We believe that actions of the extender should be viewed as the extension of the physician and therefore the physician should retain sole supervision of the extender.

As the bill is written, however, it is unclear exactly who is responsible for the actions of the extender. Although the definition of the extender requires "supervision" by the physician, the bill in establishing requirements for the clinic, states that policies are developed "with the advice of * * * a group of professional personnel, including one or more physicians and one or more physician extenders, to govern the services" provided by the clinic. Moreover, it provides that a physician or extender may be "responsible for the execution of such policies relating to the provision of the clinics' services."

We must question the adequacy of the limited role of the physician with respect to the provision of medical services by the clinic. Such provisions could allow the extender to be responsible for executing the policies of the clinic in regard to services rendered which are developed only through "advice" of the physician. This language of the bill does not assure sufficient supervision of medical services provided by an extender. This relationship of allowing the nonphysician to assure that he is carrying out the policies of the clinic in regard to medical services is highly inappropriate and could well lead to medicare reimbursement for services which would not be reimbursable under other circumstances. The extender in this case could play a key role in developing policies under which he is carrying out those policies. Thus, the extender could perform medical services under policies developed and carried out by him alone.

PAYMENT INCONSISTENCY

Because payment under this bill is limited to the clinic, the extender's services would be paid in the clinic setting but payment would continue to be denied when services are furnished in another setting.

For example, under present HEW interpretations, the only way in which the extender's services could be reimbursed now would be if they were performed "incident to" a physician's professional service. Furthermore, under the interpretation this

> . . . limits coverage to the services of nurses and other assistants that are commonly furnished as a necessary adjunct to the physician's personal in-office service. Thus, the performance by a physician's assistant of services which traditionally have been reserved to physicians cannot be covered under Part B even though all the other "incident-to" requirements are met.

Now, however, H.R. 2504 proposed to reimburse for such services provided that they are not incident to a physician's services. While we believe that services of an extender should be reimbursed, we do not understand the rationale for allowing such reimbursement to a facility for services performed while those same services are not reimbursable when performed under the direction or supervision of a physician such as in his own office or in a physician-directed clinic.

We believe that the bill as presently written in its attempt to reach a laudable end could create many unintended problems which could adversely affect development of quality care.

AMA ACTIVITIES

The AMA is not unmindful of the needs of shortage areas. We have long advocated increased medical manpower for shortage areas and to that end have strongly supported programs under the manpower law, including the national health service corps program. We have also developed and have had introduced our own bill on rural health care.

We have also long carried out the Project U.S.A. program, designed to fill temporary vacancies for national health service corps personnel temporarily absent for vacations or leaves.

In addition we have also encouraged the development of rural care delivery models with utilization of physician extenders to increase the scope of services and with the use of satellite arrangements in sparsely populated areas. Our annual national conferences on rural health and our extension seminars on health education as well as our publications in the rural health field prepared for public distribution also attest to our support for such developments.

However, while the AMA has provided a leadership role in rural health, we have always adhered to the principle of rural health care equal in quality to that of the rest of the Nation.

As to the physician's assistant, we have also long advocated recognition of their services as part of physicians' services under medicare irrespective of where the extender actually performs the service and irrespective of the physical presence of the supervising physician. We support demonstration projects designed to study the utilization of the physician assistant. The subcommittee is undoubtedly aware of the reimbursement studies now being undertaken by HEW.

I will add one thing to it, however. We do have a legislative proposal of our own which was introduced into the last Congress which never got to hearings. We feel certain it will be reintroduced into this Congress. This proposal is entitled the "Rural Health Care Delivery Improvement Act." We expect to have that introduced again soon and hope that you will give it serious consideration.

CONCLUSION

In conclusion, Mr. Chairman, we are indeed sympathetic with the problem which the committee has before it, and we recognize the desirable objective of the legislation. The bill emphasizes the difficulties which arise when the medicare program is sought to be used and tailored to reach what is perceived to be very limited and special situations. However, once a payment system is provided and an entity created and recognized for payment purposes, proliferation will certainly follow, so it is important that proper medical safeguards be provided. While we recognize also the exigencies that pertain to certain rural situations, we must be careful to avoid a duplication of problems, as recently came to light concerning quality and propriety of services in the so-called medicaid mills, generally identified with urban areas.

We have already pointed out the bill creates many anomalies. If the medicare program is to recognize payment for services of the physician extenders, discrimination should not be created against the fundamental situation out of which the physician extender movement developed. The basic concepts must include: (1) proper supervision and control by the physician of a properly trained physician extender, (2) responsibility in the physician for the services as evidenced by the billing for the services in the name of the physician, and (3) compliance with State requirements. If these are adhered to, the use of physician assistants would be encouraged in shortage areas. To this end, a simple amendment to the medicare law giving recognition to the true nature of the extender's service should be more appropriate than creating the medicare defined rural health clinic in order to recognize the extender's service.

Accordingly, a simple amendment to include the extender's service as an integral part of the physician's service would foster the development of the original concept and help provide quality care in rural areas.

H.R. 2504 in its present form should not be adopted.

Mr. Chairman, we would be pleased to respond to any questions which the subcommittee may have.

Thank you very much.

Mr. Rostenkowski. Any questions?

Mr. Duncan. Dr. Beddingfield, someone suggested here this morning that we might change the name "physician supervisor requirement," to the "physician consultation."

How do you feel about that?

Dr. Beddingfield. We would be against that change, Mr. Duncan. We believe that these physician extenders, be they physician assistants or nurse practitioners, are an extension of the physician; they are acting under his delegated authority and responsibility as it appears in the various State laws. We believe that the physician should maintain the moral, ethical, and ultimate responsibility for the well-being of the patient. The patient looks to the physician, and we will accept that responsibility.

I might add in response—because of the question from the chairman, I believe, to one of the witnesses from the Nurse Association—it is incorrect that nurse practitioners in North Carolina are not dependent practitioners. They are totally dependent practitioners. So her information about the North Carolina act is not correct.

Mr. Duncan. You do disagree with the Governor on his views on the rural health clinics?

Dr. Beddingfield. No; not at all.

As an individual, I am a participant in this program and have worked closely with Governor Hunt during his Lieutenant Governorship. I didn't see anything in his testimony that we could take issue. He did not speak directly to the questions of reimbursement and realized this was controversial.

As to the issue of amending the medicare law to provide payment for services rendered to medicare recipients in rural areas, as long as these extenders meet the conditions that we have outlined in our testimony, we would favor that. I believe that is completely consistent with Governor Hunt's testimony.

Mr. Duncan. Do you agree with his views that something must be done soon or some of the rural clinics may go under, cease to exist?

Dr. Beddingfield. I think that this is a problem. When you say "manage" it depends on what time frame you are talking about. I would like to see action proceed on this. At the same time, we are aware that HEW currently has experiments going on in this area. I happen to be a participant in those experiments. I am a supervising physician for a satellite rural health clinic which is some 17 miles from my principal practice setting. I was selected as one of the participants in this. The experiment was authorized several years ago, it only got off the ground last fall. I think if we are going to examine this method of reimbursement, the time crunch ought not be so that you don't see what the results of the experiments authorized by the Congress are.

Mr. Duncan. Well, as to the clinics that you have knowledge of or some connections with, are the patients receiving quality care?

Dr. Beddingfield. I think they certainly are receiving quality care; yes.

Mr. Duncan. You don't know of any that are not?

Dr. Beddingfield. No; as a matter of fact, in the clinic that I spoke of that I am directly affiliated with, we have been in business for 4 years, 4 years this week. One night this week I had a meeting with the administrator and one of the board members of that clinic, and we reviewed the history of the past 4 years. There has not been a single therapeutic diagnostic misadventure in that clinic in 4 years. The records are reviewed on a very regular basis. They have a superior record and they know when to refer. We think that the experience has been all together a very happy experience.

Mr. Duncan. If these patients didn't receive the treatment that they are receiving now under the present setup with the physician extenders, would they otherwise be able to receive medical attention?

Dr. Beddingfield. A good many of them would not, and certainly access is more directly available. This clinic that I am connected with is seeing now about 30 to 40 patients a day and I would say that probably it would be a great difficulty for over half of those patients—because of lack of transportation and other problems— to get access to a nearby town for the type of problems which they do bring to the clinic.

I think that the others possibly could get there but perhaps at a more advanced stage of their illness. And certainly less conveniently.

ALLIED HEALTH WORKERS

There are 24 AMA accredited allied health training programs. Accreditation is granted by the AMA's Committee on Allied Health Education and Accreditation (CAHEA), which works collaboratively with the various specialty societies, allied health organizations and societies, educational associations, the AHA, and various federal agencies. As with other accrediting bodies, legitimization comes from recognition by the Council on Postsecondary Accreditation (COPA) and the U.S. Office of Education (USOE). Table 4-1 lists the AMA-accredited program areas, and the number of programs accredited in each category. Figure 4-1 shows the types of sponsoring bodies for allied health education and the distribution of sponsorships. It will be noted that hospitals sponsor 57% of the allied health programs and community colleges, 20%. There are, of course, nonaccredited programs in these 24 occupational categories.

There are many accredited allied health programs accredited by bodies other than CAHEA, such as programs in health education, medical dietetics, dental hygiene, graduate programs in health administration, and there are a large number of other allied health occupations for which there is, at this time, no formal program accrediting process except that some of them are parts of regionally accredited academic institutions. There is, for example, no accrediting system for baccalaureate programs in health administration, though nearly all the programs educate students whose degrees are awarded by accredited colleges or universities.

The Bureau of Employment Security of the U.S. Employment Service in the U.S. Department of Labor issued, some years ago, a *Health Careers Guidebook* that describes a great many of the occupational roles in the health field. The AMA has also issued a handbook describing some of the allied health occupations—*Horizons Unlimited*.

Table 4-1. Student and Statistical Data for Each Accredited
Allied Health Profession

Occupational Title	No. of Programs 7/18/78[a]
1. Assistant to the primary care physician	50
2. Cytotechnologist	96
3. Electroencephalographic technician	1
4. Electroencephalographic technologist	11
5. Emergency medical technician-paramedic	. . .
6. Histologic technician	36
7. Medical assistant	116
8. Medical assistant in pediatrics	2
9. Medical laboratory technician (*associate degree*)	72
10. Medical laboratory technician (cetificate)	109
11. Medical record administrator	44
12. Medical record technician	70
13. Medical technologist	666
14. Nuclear medicine technologist	142
15. Occupational therapist	53
16. Ophthalmic medical assistant	1
17. Physical therapist	79
18. Radiation therapy technologist	94
19. Radiographer	836
20. Respiratory therapist	159
21. Respiratory therapy technician	131
22. Specialist in blood bank technology	65
23. Surgeon's assistant	2
24. Surgical technologist	68
Total	**2,903**

[a]*Essentials* adopted by the AMA Council on Medical Education Sept 8, 1978. *Essentials* are being drafted for the anesthesiologist's assistant, cardiovascular perfusionist, and diagnostic medical sonographer.

Source: JAHA, Dec 22/29, 1978-Vol. 240, No. 26

DENTISTS, OPTOMETRISTS, PHARMACISTS, PODIATRISTS

These four professionals play a major role in providing health services to people, but their linkages to the rest of the health system are not as complex as medicine and nursing.

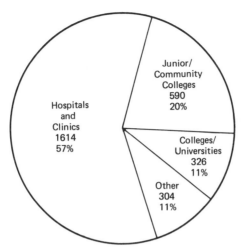

Figure 4–1. Distribution of sponsors of allied health education programs: hospitals and clinics, **57%**; junior/community colleges, **20%**; colleges/universities, **11%**; medical schools, **5%**; U.S. government institutions, **2%**; special schools, **2%**; proprietary schools, **1%**; and blood banks, **1%**. (Source *JAMA*, Vol. 240; Dec. 20/29, 1978.)

Dentists

Dentistry is one of the oldest of the health professions, and the training of dentists today is very similar to that of medical doctors in terms of undergraduate predental education and the first two years of the four-year undergraduate dental school. Most dentists are in private practice—working alone or in groups. There are eight dental specialties (8, p.85):

- Endodontics (root oral treatment)
- Oral pathology (diseases of the mouth)
- Oral surgery (surgery of the mouth)
- Orthodontics (teeth straightening)
- Pedodontics (children's dentistry)
- Periodontology (treatment of the tissues or gums supporting the teeth and the underlying bone)
- Prosthodontics (making of artificial teeth or dentures)
- Public health dentistry

Graduates from American dental schools receive either a DDS (Doctor of Dental Surgery) or a DMD (Doctor of Dental Medicine). The degrees are equivalent, a school opting for only one of them. Licensure comes from the state. A national test, prepared by the National Board of Dental Examiners, is used by most state dental boards. Dental schools are accredited by the Council on Dental Education of the American Dental Association. There were 59 schools of dentistry in the United States at the end of 1978.

Optometrists

An optometrist is a doctor of optometry (O.D.). The O. D. should not be confused with the D. O., the latter being a doctor of osteopathy, nor should the O. D. be confused with the ophthalmologist, who is a medically qualified physician with a specialty qualification for diagnosis and treatment of eye conditions. The optometrist is trained and licensed by the state "to examine eyes and related structures to determine the presence of vision problems, disease, or other abnormalities ... prescribes and fits eyeglasses, contact lenses, or other optical aids, and utilizes his (or her) training to preserve, restore, and enhance the efficiency of vision (8, p.233). There are 13 schools of optometry approved by the Council on Optometric Education. The length of optometric training is four years. While most schools require at least three years of pre-optometric study in a college or university, most optometric students (over 70%) begin professional studies after completion of a baccalaureate degree. Most state licensing boards now accept for licensure the results of a national board exam.

Pharmacists

" ... the pharmacist is more than a dispenser of drugs and health supplies, important though that function is. The pharmacy is actually a community center for information on topics related to health" (8, p.189). It is not uncommon, particularly in small towns, for the local pharmacist to be known as "doc." Rare is the person who hasn't consulted the pharmacist about some problem and asked for advice as to an appropriate medication that might be had without prescription. Rare, too, is the pharmacist who doesn't give the advice, though the pharmacist is usually careful not to diagnose.

Pharmacy is, of course, an ancient profession. Certainly it was prominent in seventeenth century England; the practitioners were apothecaries who ran shops and compounded various drugs and medications. The pharmacist today, however, is rarely called on to compound a drug or medication since they come packaged from the manufacturer. The chief function of about 80% of the pharmacists is that of dispensing medications prescribed by physicians, dentists, and other practitioners who are legally entitled to prescribe. They carry out this function in retail pharmacies. Most of the remaining pharmacists (20% of the total) work in hospital and health center pharmacies, research institutions, and with pharmaceutical manufacturers. Hospital pharmacy is now considered a specialty within the profession.

Pharmacy schools are accredited by the American Council of Pharmaceutical Education. Some schools now require two years of pre-pharmacy study and four years of pharmacy school study and award a Doctor of Pharmacy degree. Other schools grant a Bachelor of Science degree for a lesser period of study, usually five years. There are 72 accredited schools. Licensure depends on a successful pass of the state licensing exam. There is at present no national exam.

Podiatrists

The podiatrist is a D. P. M. (Doctor of Podiatric Medicine). The podiatrist diagnoses and treats diseases and deformities of the feet. Most podiatrists are in private practice, and they commonly are called on to treat patients in hospitals and nursing homes.

Training normally entails three or four years of pre-podiatry study in a college or university (over 90% of the students hold a baccalaureate degree by the time they begin professional studies), followed by four years of professional training in one of the nation's five accredited colleges of podiatry. Schools are accredited by the Council on Podiatry Education. The national exam, prepared by the National Board of Podiatry, is accepted for licensure by a growing number of states.

CHIROPRACTORS

Chiropractors are licensed in all states, and some of their services are covered by Medicare and Medicaid. Despite the fact that some of their services are covered by Medicare and Medicaid and some other health-insurance policies, it is a "profession" that is at the center of a political storm. Chiropractors are not medically qualified. At the heart of their practice is the belief that many physical conditions are caused by misaligned (subluxated) vertebrae and that treatment by manipulation can successfully relieve a patient's symptoms and can, in fact, cure.

Chiropractors have been labeled "quacks" and "unscientific" by the medical profession. *Medical World News* (December 11, 1978), in a lengthy report on chiropractors, quotes the report of the New Zealand Medical Association's assessment:

The available scientific evidence suggests that the benefit of chiropractic—if benefit there be—is largely due to the transference of confidence from chiropractor to patient, the sharing of *faith* in manipulation as a form of therapy, the placebo effect of the laying-on of hands, and the fact that the minor musculoskeletal disorders that fall into the province of chiropractic are themselves self-limiting or subject to spontaneous remission.

There are some 18,000 chiropractors (D. C., Doctor of Chiropractic) in the United States, nearly half located in California, New York, Missouri, Texas, and Florida. There are currently 16 chiropractic schools in the United States. The length of chiropractic training is four years, and at least two years of college are required for admission. Critics of chiropractics argue that scientific evidence as to the curative powers of its methods is lacking.

What makes this "profession" the eye of the storm is its militancy in demanding that its services be covered by health insurance policies and government programs, the pressures it is exerting to secure hospital privileges to treat patients, and its successful lawsuit against the AMA, AHA, JCAH, and others, securing their agreement not to restrain chiropractic access by prohibiting their members from accepting chiropractic referrals. At issue was the refusal of a hospital in Pennsylvania and of its radiologists to accept a chiropractic referral for x-ray studies. The American College of Radiology was unhappy over the agreement of other defendants to settle the suit, believing that the settlement left the radiologist at risk of violating the AMA's ethical code. Either the radiologist who accepted the referral was in violation because he or she was cooperating with the practice of unscientific practitioners or, if referral was accepted, guilty of abandoning the patient after reading the x-ray film (*Medical World News*, December 25, 1978). Similar suits are pending in other states. At the August 1979 meeting of the AMA House of Delegates, the delegates agreed to cease referring to chiropractic as an unscientific cult, and to remove from its code of ethics the prohibition of physician association with chiropractors. The delegates' action was clearly a defensive response to the lawsuits, although the AMA position is still one of wanting to see supporting scientific evidence as to the value of spinal manipulation.

HEALTH ADMINISTRATORS AND HEALTH PLANNERS

The health industry is large and complex. It is labor intensive, a heavy user of people, and the industry requires a large amount of money to fuel its operations. Skilled health administrators are much in demand to run the hospitals, nursing homes, primary care centers, health departments, mental health centers and hospitals, home care agencies, and so on. "To run"—by which is meant to plan the activities, to assemble or secure the resources, and to manage the use of those resources so that the purposes of the organization are fulfilled. Planning is, of course, an essential part of every administrative job, but in the larger organizations, the planning function is frequently delegated to someone whose planning skills are well developed, to allow that person to focus on planning only and to advise the administrator as to what he or she should adopt as the planned course of action for the enterprise. In recent years, because of the complex interrelationships and dependencies between health agencies and government, there have developed specialized health agencies whose principal purpose has been to plan, still in an advisory capacity to the community at large as well as to the many health service agencies in the community and state.

Historically, the top administrator in most large health institutions was a physician or a nurse. Few were trained for their administrative roles. Even today, one finds health administrators and health planners who grew or fell into their jobs, whose academic preparation was not geared to either of these roles. In recent years, however, health agencies have turned increasingly to people who have academic training in health administration or health planning. The necessity for specially trained *health* oriented people and not just any business-administration or planning program graduate stems from the complex nature of the health industry and the historical context within which the agencies and health professions operate. Needed are people who understand not only planning and administration but also the special aspects as they apply to the health field—the importance of knowing, in other words, the sociology of medicine and of the various health professions, of knowing about health and sickness and how the professions deal with them, of understanding the constraints under which the health professionals operate—for the administrator and planner have to apply their skills and adjust to a milieu that is professionally dominated, indeed, professionally controlled. This finds expression in the time-honored doctrine of the doctor-patient relationship, into which there should be no interference. Increasingly, there is interference, and some of it necessary due to the growing complexity of medical practice, but the good health administrator and health planner must know how to orchestrate that intercession without prejudicing the confidentiality of the doctor-patient relationship and without prejudicing the ability of the physician to render the best care for the patient. Well-trained health administrators and health planners are sensitive to these special circumstances and are able to apply their administrative or planning skills in that context so that the aims of the agency are achieved in terms of seeing to it that the highest quality service is delivered.

The academic training of health administrators and health planners takes place in a number of settings. Until recently, most were trained and awarded a master's degree by a school of public health or a school of health administration. The course of study usually lasted one or two years, depending on the school. Initially, the *schools of public health* were geared to train a variety of public health workers, public health administrators being only one. Most of the public health administration graduates went to work in public-health departments, though in the last few decades graduates have been moving into other health administration areas, also. The *schools of health administration* were primarily geared to the training of hospital administrators. In fact, until about 1970, most of these schools were known as schools of hospital administration. The name change was designed to reflect the recognition by the schools that they were training not only hospital administrators but also administrators for other kinds of health agencies. Some of the schools of health administration were administratively part of schools of public health. Others were associated with schools of business administration. Some were in other organizational units of a university. In recent years, there has been some rivalry between the public health and health administration schools relating to disagreements over access to federal training grant monies and to accreditation.

The late 1960s witnessed the development of a number of baccalaureate programs in health administration and health planning, and during the 1970s the number of programs grew rapidly. Some programs were geared to hospitals, some to long-term care, some to training generalist health administrators or health planners. During the early development period of the baccalaureate movement, the undergraduate and graduate programs clashed but worked out, over time, most of their differences. Most baccalaureate programs at this time are free standing in that they are baccalaureate programs only, and the faculty do not teach in a graduate program. There are a number of exceptions to this. There is not an accrediting process for baccalaureate programs at this time.

There has developed a small number of associate-degree programs in health administration. The academic setting for these efforts is limited by the nature of professional resources available to these programs. They are too few in number and too small in student body to determine, at this time, what their future role will be.

REFERENCES

1. Heide, Wilma Scott: Introduction, in Ashley, Jo Ann: *Hospitals, Paternalism and the Role of the Nurse.* New York, Teachers College Press, 1976.
2. Hospitals, JAHA, 52; 1978.
3. Notter, Luceile E., and Spalding, Eugenia Kennedy: *Professional Nursing, Foundations, Perspectives, and Relationships,* ed. 9. Philadelphia, Lippincott, 1976.

4. *National Health Insurance Resource Book*, rev. ed. Committee on Ways and Means, U.S. House of Representatives, 1976.
5. Schlotfeldt, Rozella M: The professional doctorate: rationale and characteristics. *Nursing Outlook*, May 1978.
6. Schulz, Rockwell, and Johnson, Alton C: *Management of Hospitals*. New York, McGraw-Hill, 1976.
7. *Medicare Reimbursement for Physician Extenders, Practicing in Rural Health Clinics*, Serial 95-8. Hearings before the Subcommittee on Health of the Committee on Ways and Means, House of Representatives, 95th Congress, First Session, February 28, 1977.
8. *Health Careers Guidebook*. Washington, U.S. Department of Labor.

5
History of Hospitals

EARLY HOSPITALS

The hospital has become an essential public service agency. It is as necessary to man's physical well-being as the church is to his spiritual welfare and as the school is to his intellectual development. No other agency that serves the public has had to make greater efforts in overcoming popular prejudices, in adjusting its organization and functions to changing conditions, and in establishing its value to society in so short a period of time. Courts of justice depend upon centuries-old codes of law to control human behavior. Education is based on the transmission of ideas and knowledge from one culture to another through spoken, written, and printed language. Hospitals deal with life itself. They reflect the rapid strides in the biological sciences in the last hundred years. They are created and maintained through the power of humanitarian and religious forces. Herein lies the secret of progress in the development of hospitals.

As medical science determined the causes of disease, disclosed the means of transmission, and established methods of prevention, the hazards involved in assembling large numbers of the sick and injured in one place were gradually removed. The development of instruments of precision and of many laboratory aids to diagnosis and the discovery of more effective measures of treatment greatly enhanced the role of the hospital in the over-all program of medical care. The public responded slowly at first, but with ever quickening pace as knowledge of the benefits conferred by modern medicine became known.

Up to this century hospitals were not objects of public esteem. They were

This chapter reprinted by permission of the publishers from HOSPITAL CARE IN THE UNITED STATES, A Study by The Commission on Hospital Care, A.C. Bachmeyer, Director of Study, Cambridge, Mass.: Harvard University Press, Copyright © 1947, 1975 by The Commonwealth Fund.

founded as shelters for the aged and infirm, orphans, vagrants, and the maimed; as part of the charitable program of religious and welfare organizations; as protection for the inhabitants of a community from communicable diseases and from the dangerously insane; and as emergency quarters to accommodate wounded and sick soldiers, sailors, and marines during wartime.

The earliest American hospitals were crowded and unsanitary; medical care was meager and largely ineffective. Their poor reputation deterred people from entering them voluntarily. The hazards to health were usually greater in the hospital than in the home. Admission to these institutions was frequently regarded as a disgrace.

The development of the hospital during the past hundred years as a health and social agency is one of the outstanding achievements marking the advance of civilization. Except for the underlying motive, which was the care of the sick, the pesthouses, almshouses, and infirmaries of a hundred years ago offered little to compare with the efficiently organized, complex, and coordinated facilities and services of the modern hospital. The index of progress, however, is never measured purely by the finger of time. With hospitals, such an index would be entirely misleading because they were highly developed in earlier times, but retrogressed due to ignorance, prejudice, lack of financial support, and the absence of public interest. Religion has greatly influenced the development of hospitals through all ages and was chiefly responsible for their first establishment and maintenance. War, too, though usually considered a destructive influence, has been the means of advancing these institutions rapidly and importantly in times of duress.

The hospital of the present day is the central agency wherein the benefits of modern medical knowledge and skill are made available to every individual in the community. It is a philanthropic and scientific organization in which are concentrated the skilled personnel and the facilities required by the modern physician for competent professional practice. In it medical and social science is applied to the problems of sickness and health. In it are educated and trained the professional staff and the nonprofessional personnel whose services are requisite for effective medical care. In many modern hospitals provision is made for the conduct of research in order to continue the advance of medical science. The successful conduct of these functions has developed public interest and confidence in modern hospital service.

During the last century the science of preventive and curative medicine has been so greatly advanced as to make necessary the development of a system of hospitals throughout the entire nation. Hospital facilities have improved and services have been extended as a direct result of advances in medicine, medical education, and nursing and the expansion of public health activities. The urbanization of the population, the extension of general education, the modernization of transportation and communication, the establishment of huge industrial enterprises, the development of natural resources, periods of prosperity and economic depression, two world wars, nation-wide movements for social reform—these factors and the influence of the basic principles of American democracy have contributed to the status of the modern hospital.

The development of hospitals in the United States can best be traced by a brief résumé of the history of hospitals from the earliest times through the Renaissance and a broader review of their establishment on the North American continent.

Ancient and Medieval Hospitals

The profession of medicine arose out of the ancient civilizations of Egypt, Babylonia, Persia, India, and Greece. Medicine was closely associated with religion, and medical care was provided through the temples. Later, particularly in India, many hospitals for the sick poor were established and systems of medical practice were developed by the Buddhists.

The advent of the Christian religion with its emphasis upon man's responsibilities toward his fellowmen gave great impetus to the humanitarian and altruistic care of the sick. By the Fourth Century A. D., through the efforts of Christian church members and officials, hospitals were beginning to be founded for lepers, famine victims, and other stricken by a variety of scourges in most of the cities of the Byzantine Empire. In Rome, wealthy Christian women organized and supervised hospitals in their palaces. Hospitals were built for acute, infectious, and incurable cases; some were established for members of various trades; and there is also a record of some convalescent homes. Eventually there were specialized institutions for the care of the sick, the blind, the crippled, the foundlings and orphans, the helpless poor and the aged, and poor and infirm pilgrims.

Hospitals began to appear in western Europe in the Fifth Century. Hotel Dieu of Lyons, founded in 542, and Hotel Dieu of Paris, established in 650, were charitable organizations embracing every form of aid to the poor and needy—inn, workhouse, asylum, and infirmary. Hospitals in the huge Arabian kingdom, extending from Spain through North Africa into western Asia, were numerous and well equipped, with medical and nursing staffs.

Religious communities became outlets for the spiritual inspiration men and women had for securing salvation through good works. Several Sisterhoods and Brotherhoods, whose many activities included nursing, originated in the Sixth Century. Charlemagne ordered his canons to contribute a tenth of their revenues to maintain the sick poor; and in order that the clergy might more easily visit the sick, hospitals were built close to or were integral parts of monasteries. These monastic infirmaries were really hospices or resting places for pilgrims as well as for the sick. The first purely nursing order, founded about 1155, was the St. Augustine nuns. They carried the heaviest burden of hospital care during these times. St. Bartholomew's Hospital, the first English institution worthy of the name hospital, was started in 1123 by a court jester turned monk. St. Thomas' Hospital in London, which later became famous for the Nightingale School of Nursing, was built in 1213.

The religious and military enterprises of the Twelfth and Thirteenth Centuries known as the Crusades greatly influenced the extension of hospitals, for all along the routes of pilgrimage hospitals were established to aid those who would follow. Those built at Malta and Rhodes by the Knights of St. John of Jerusalem are still in existence. Leprosy, which appeared in Europe in the Sixth and Seventh Centuries, became widespread during the Crusades. This scourge was unparalleled before or since in intensity and devastation. Numerous lazarettos, built for segregation purposes, aided greatly in controlling the dread disease.

Most medieval hospitals—some 19,000 were scattered throughout Europe in the Thirteenth Century—were church institutions with blocks of wards surrounding a chapel. Nursing by monks and nuns and seclusion were emphasized. This system contributed to an economical and convenient administration. Healing the soul, however, took precedence over healing the body. In the Fourteenth and Fifteenth Centuries the enthusiasm for religion and charity waned. The church became very wealthy, politically powerful, and corrupt. Revenues formerly allotted to hospitals were diverted from their original purpose to the clergy and laymen. Religious nursing groups gradually became subordinated to the clergy and finally found themselves forced into supervising ignorant women who knew nothing of nursing procedures. After the ecclesiastic law forbade the clergy to shed blood or perform dissections, a new profession of tonsors—barbers and bloodletters—came into being.

Hospitals in the Renaissance and the Reformation

The Renaissance was a period of great intellectual activity with the revival of study of the ancient scientists and philosophers and the formulation of new ideas in science and philosophy. Botany and anatomy were emerging as new sciences; chemistry and physics were further developed.

During the Reformation, church property was confiscated and many religious organizations were disbanded in the newly Protestant countries. In the course of Henry VIII's contest with the Catholic church, he suppressed the monasteries and appropriated their revenues because the monks and friars in England were the most ardent advocates of papal authority. The immediate result of monastic dissolution was the discontinuance of hospitals and refuges upon which the poor depended for charity. Henry VIII finally restored St. Bartholomew's Hospital as a secular institution and endowed it with what had been its own revenues on condition that the people would provide an equal income. The Hospital of St. Mary of Bethlehem (Bedlam) was converted from a monastery to an asylum for the insane in 1547, and Christ's Hospital, also a monastery, was chartered for orphans in 1553.

The wars of the Sixteenth Century influenced the establishment of hospitals for those who became sick or were wounded in battle. However, these hospitals and refuges were municipal in authority and bore all the disadvantages and abuses inherent in political control. The religious motive was absent in the lay persons employed in these institutions, and people refused to do the menial work required of those who nursed and cared for the sick poor.

Rich and poor alike were plagued by a variety of epidemic diseases. Since no scientific explanation was vouchsafed, their cause could only be attributed to mythological and superstitious ideas of the physical and metaphysical. Many factors contributed to the havoc disease played on human life: walled medieval towns were crowded, squalid, and unsanitary; antagonism and strife between principalities led to social and economic oppression; soldiers, students, and vagrants spread disease in the course of their travels; the important role of personal hygiene in the maintenance of good health was unknown.

Ambitious kings and queens of the Sixteenth Century, inspired by the discovery of new lands, visualized the building of great empires with the expansion of foreign trade and commerce. Adventurers were commissioned to participate in exploring expeditions to find and conquer new worlds or lay claims to rich foreign countries.

Cortez, arriving in Mexico in 1519, found an advanced civilization among the Aztecs, which included physicians and nurses, a wide knowledge of herbal medicine, and a systematic provision for care of the sick. In gratitude to God for his victory and to expiate his sins, Cortez built in 1524 the Hospital of the Immaculate Conception in Mexico City to provide a refuge for the sick poor and entrusted it to a nursing Brotherhood. In his will he endowed this institution permanently and charged his descendants with its maintenance. In 1663 the name was changed to the Hospital of Jesus of Nazareth and thus it is known today, the oldest hospital on the North American continent with a continuous history of service.

Religious orders of the Catholic church accompanied the Spaniards to the Americas to teach the principles of Christianity to the pagan Indians and thus promote colonization. From Mexico they traveled northwest through what is now New Mexico, Arizona, and Lower California. Instead of establishing institutions like the monasteries in Spain, they set up a monastic type of organization called a mission where the padres and friars valiantly and diligently taught and dispensed nursing and medical care to the Indians. Well-organized hospital service was impossible in these missions, but their services were such that they may be called the forerunners of the earliest hospitals in the southwest.

Seventeenth Century Hospital Development

Whereas Renaissance physicians commonly followed special lines of investigation in anatomy and botany, Seventeenth Century physicians distinguished themselves as mathematicians, astronomers, microscopists, and chemists. During this era, universities and scientific societies were founded and periodic literature began to appear.

William Harvey made one of the greatest contributions to medical science by coordinating the findings of his predecessors with his own experiments in the publication in 1628 of his book on the circulation of the blood. Intravenous injection of drugs was successfully performed in 1656 and the transfusion of alien blood was accomplished in the next decade. About this same time, Sir Thomas Sydenham, whose methods of observation were copied by many physicians after him, became famous as a clinician.

EUROPEAN HOSPITALS

Well-managed hospitals, organized nursing, and the charitable care of the sick had largely disappeared in the Protestant countries. There was a definite shift from monastic beauty toward utility in the newly built hospitals. Unsanitary conditions caused frequent outbreaks of epidemics within their walls. Nursing changed from centuries of gratuitous service to a paid service by a secular riff-raff of illiterate and drunken women who were not acceptable in other kinds of work. Hospital nursing became so involved with the domestic duties of scrubbing and laundry that mismanagement, understaffing, and deliberate exploitation were inevitable. The administrative staff of women was clothed with the meaningless though dignified title of Sister, a carry-over from the days of the sympathetic and understanding religious Sisters.

In the countries where Catholic orders still existed, nursing had not been so debauched. However, visiting the sick poor in their homes was imcompatible with the cloistered seclusion of the nuns. In Paris, early in the Seventeenth Century, St. Vincent de Paul laid the foundation of modern social service by establishing municipal homes and trade schools for beggars, thousands of whom were overrunning Europe at the time. Also, with the help of St. Louise de Marillac, he developed an organization known as the Sisters of Charity to carry on a humanitarian program including nursing. These laywomen attended the poor in their homes and provided some nursing service in hospitals. This new type of nursing, less restricted than formerly, soon spread through all the Catholic countries of Europe and reached America in the early Nineteenth Century.

NORTH AMERICAN HOSPITALS

From the beginning of the Seventeenth Century to the American Revolution the Old World was in a state of physical, intellectual, moral, religious, military, economic, and political turmoil. Despite a fierce resistance to change, the feudalism of the Middle Ages disappeared. The territorial discoveries of the preceding century provided not only a good source of investment for the countries which had staked their claims in the New World, but also a refuge for those unhappy people who suffered from religious persecution, extreme poverty, military service, political disputes, and adverse social legislation. Religious clashes were associated with the political interests of Catholic and Protestant kings and queens, with the conflicts of nations over commerce and empire in the Old World and beyond the seas, and with class struggles.

Jesuits, Franciscans, and Dominicans came to New France to carry on religious, charitable, and educational work among the Indians and white settlers. Father Paul le Jeune in importunate letters to friends and relatives in France concerning the necessity for a hospital aroused the interest of the Duchesse d'Aiguillon, who sought assistance from the Sisters of St. Augustine, and Mme. de la Peltrie, who enlisted the aid of the Ursuline nuns. Three nuns from each order sailed together from France in 1639 in response to Father le Jeune's call. Immediately upon arrival in Quebec, they set up an emergency hospital in a cottage to care for the victims of a smallpox epidemic, many of whom were Indians. Thus they established the second hospital on the North American continent. The Sisters faced almost insurmountable hardships—epidemics of typhus, smallpox, and yellow fever, Indian massacres, famine, fires, floods, poverty, and war. But their ultimate success is mirrored in the service that the Hotel Dieu in Quebec maintains to this day.

Those who promoted the colony of Montreal included a hospital and a school in their original plans. However, it was largely through the efforts of a nurse, Jeanne Mance, and a benefactress, Mme. de Bouillon, that the Hotel Dieu de Montreal was established to care for sick colonists, Indians, and wounded soldiers in 1644.

The General Hospital of Quebec was opened for service in the last decade of the Seventeenth Century and is accordingly one of the earliest hospitals in North America.

The English had no organization comparable to that of the French and Spanish missionaries to help them colonize the New World. Most of the English colonists were from the middle classes, embracing the agricultural, mercantile, and artisan groups. They were also predominantly religious dissenters from the Church of England. About two-thirds of the emigrants were able to finance their own passage across the Atlantic Ocean; the remaining third worked off their debt of passage money by becoming indentured. The practice of medicine and nursing was left to individuals, many of whom were untrained. Few places that could be called hospitals were built, but shelters were occasionally provided for the sick disembarking from ships. Such was the hospital at Henricopolis (Dutch Gap, Virginia), which accommodated about eighty medical and surgical patients and afforded some nursing care. This first colonial hospital served the people coming to Virginia only a short while, for it was destroyed by fire in the massacre of 1622.

In most places, however, if there was need to care for sick soldiers and sailors, they were billeted with private families. When the English took New Amsterdam in 1664, they found that a small hospital had been established for soldiers and Negroes by the Dutch West India Company. In 1679 this hospital consisted of five houses.

Except, therefore, for those in Quebec and Montreal, no enduring hospitals were founded during the Seventeenth Century on the North American continent.

DEVELOPMENT OF HOSPITALS, 1700–1840

The best scientific work of the Eighteenth and early Nineteenth Centuries was done in chemistry, mathematical physics, and applied science. A monumental step in physiology was the development of the modern theory of respiration, based upon the identification of carbon dioxide, nitrogen, hydrogen, and oxygen. Surgery and midwifery in England developed under the influence and teaching of John and William Hunter. The pulse watch, the stethoscope, and the use of percussion were introduced in this period.

The medical highlight of the Eighteenth Century was the introduction of preventive inoculation for smallpox. The idea was old, but its use did not become widespread until after its introduction in England and America. Smallpox was much more readily accepted than inoculation; in fact it was recognized as a necessary evil and was so commonly taken for granted that only the worst mortality experiences were recorded. In 1796 Edward Jenner, from his observation of certain farm conditions, developed vaccination, the most effective measure ever devised for controlling smallpox.

European hospitals reached the lowest level of service in history in the Eighteenth Century; the notoriety for their uncleanliness, mismanagement, and slovenly, incompetent nursing care lasted well into the Nineteenth Century. Only a modicum of improvement in the internal management of hospitals resulted from the treatises on sanitary science that appeared at this time.

Bad as was the management of hospitals, the treatment of the insane was worse. When kept in confinement, they were either chained or caged and it was not unusual for the public to pay admission fees to view their abnormal behavior. Insanity was regarded as a disgrace, not an illness. Few people realized the extent of the degradation of hospitals and fewer persons devoted efforts to bettering the conditions.

Hospital Reform in France

One of the most important influences in the reform of the construction of hospitals resulted when part of the Hotel Dieu in Paris burned in 1772. A committee headed by M. Tenon was appointed from the Academy of Sciences by Louis XVI to investigate the conditions and to recommend a plan of improvement. At the time there were about 5,000 inmates; 486 beds were single and 1,220 beds were occupied by four to six patients at times. The segregation of patients was limited to one smallpox ward, two surgical wards, and one obstetrical ward, while the remaining insane, contagious, and fever victims were thrown indiscriminately together, convalescents with the dying, mild cases beside those seriously ill. Sanitation was badly neglected; the halls were obnoxiously filthy and verminous; there was no ventilation; and pails of live coals distributed throughout the building provided not only the sole source of heat but also a serious fire hazard. Septic fevers, infections, and scabies were added to the patients' ailments. The average mortality was 25 percent and recovery from surgical operations was a rarity.

The committee in its report in 1786 proposed to replace Hotel Dieu with four hospitals of 1,200 beds each. The wards for the sick were to be detached from other buildings with their walls exposed to sun and wind. In 1787 the government accepted the proposal, but the French Revolution prevented the execution of the project. In 1803, after the state assumed control of hospitals in France, reforms were instituted in the Parisian hospitals in respect to cleanliness, nursing and management. However, the recommendations of the committee played little part in the establishment of hospitals. They continued to be large, solid, multiple-storied structures with wards and administrative offices all in one building. Not until 1854 was a hospital built in Paris which followed Tenon's plans.

Hospital Improvement in England

Between 1789 and 1793 John Howard, an Englishman, made several tours of investigation of the prisons, hospitals, and lazarettos of England and the continent with a view toward their improvement. He drew public attention to the conditions prevalent in all these institutions and recommended changes which would, if put into effect, decrease the epidemic fevers that ran riot in the crowded quarters. He advocated perfect cleanliness within hospitals and felt that they should be situated outside the city and should consist of no more than two stories with large windows built opposite each other for ventilation.

The exhaustive studies made by Howard and Tenon disclosed the deplorable conditions existing and started the movement for hospital reform. In the late Eighteenth Century, the increasing emphasis on the rights of man leading to democratic advances in English factory laws and to the American and French Revolutions was accompanied by a growing awareness of the necessity of providing care for the dependent and unfortunate. To provide humane treatment of the insane, William Tuke in 1794 founded the Quaker Retreat at York, England. Another attempt at reform appeared when Philippe Pinel, with the consent of the French National Assembly, had the restraining chains struck off 49 mental patients at Bicêtre in 1798.

Developments in America

In 1700 Boston had approximately 7,000 inhabitants and was acclaimed the largest city in the colonies; Philadelphia and New York each had about 4,000 population; Newport had 2,600, and Charleston, 1,100. As these seaport towns grew, it became increasingly necessary to provide some kind of refuge for shipboard victims of contagious diseases. Pesthouses, isolation hospitals, and quarantine stations were organized purely for segregation purposes to prevent the contagion from spreading to the inhabitants. Usually these buildings were located outside the city or on islands to give them as complete isolation as possible. In 1717 the Boston Selectmen were authorized to lease an acre of land for a contagious hospital. Fisher's Island was purchased in 1743 for the Philadelphia pesthouse; Charleston built an isolation hospital on Sullivan's Island, but it was carried away in the Cooper River flood in 1752; New York also had a contagious unit. These institutions were not used by the inhabitants of the towns near which they were located.

In many communities, private hospitals were set up by their physician or surgeon owners for people recovering from the effects of inoculation, for surgical cases, or for maternity patients. One method used in providing for the mentally ill and the poor was to sell them at auction to the lowest bidder who would take them and care for them for a period of one year at a stipulated fee. Sometimes the town board would order relatives or friends to build small strong houses or fix cells in basements or attics for the insane. These practices were carried out in rural areas more than in cities where almshouses and jails were established as abodes for the indigent and insane. Provisions for the care of the latter in these city institutions were beyond description. Handcuffs, iron collars, and leg irons were commonly used, and confinement in unheated cells under filthy living conditions and with inadequate nourishment was the usual practice.

ALMSHOUSES

Philadelphia Almshouse. William Penn is reported to have founded the first almshouse in Philadelphia in 1713. It was supported by and was open only to Quakers. In 1728 the Philadelphia Overseers of the Poor petitioned the Provincial Assembly for assistance in providing institutional facilities for the care of increasing numbers of the poor from foreign ports and neighboring provinces as well as insolvent debtors and their families. When the petition was granted, £1,000 was made available to purchase land for the erection of an almshouse. Special quarters were arranged for the insane poor until the Pennsylvania Hospital was built, at which time the overseers paid the managers of that institution to take care of the more violent mental cases. In 1767, a building was erected at a different location and opened as an almshouse, infirmary, and workhouse. Soon after the turn of the century, cells were fitted up in the cellar of one part of the almshouse and about ten insane patients were returned to it from the Pennsylvania Hospital. In 1833, the establishment was moved from the central part of the city to Blockley Township, and it was known as the Philadelphia Hospital and Almshouse until the name of the department reserved for the sick became the Philadelphia General Hospital in the early Twentieth Century.

Bellevue Hospital. Bellevue Hospital traces its origin to the Poor House of the City of New York, established in 1736 to house the poor, aged, insane, and disreputable. Five years previously, the New York census listed 1,400 houses and about 8,600 inhabitants. There were no organized resources for furnishing food and clothing and shelter to the beggars, vagabonds, and criminals of the city. Their extreme suffering during the winter months finally induced the Common Council to take definite steps to erect a public workhouse and house of correction. It was a two-story building with a cellar for those sentenced to hard labor and a cage for the refractory; an infirmary with six beds was accommodated on the second floor. At the time of the Revolution, the inmates were transferred to Poughkeepsie and the British took possession. Patients and prisoners were returned in 1783 and almost immediately the facilities were strained by the need for isolating yellow fever victims. A new building was erected in 1796 and a third almshouse was built in 1811, from which time the hospital became the most important department of the institution. In 1794, six acres of land on the East River, called Belle Vue, were purchased, but it took another two decades before the Bellevue Establishment was completed and ready for occupancy.

Charleston Almshouse. Public charity in South Carolina, dating back almost to the first permanent settlement of Charleston, was based on the poor laws of England. In 1722, the Assembly passed an act authorizing wardens and vestrymen to levy assessments for the maintenance of the poor who had been residents of the parish for a year. The parish officers were responsible for taking care of the sick in their homes or placing them with private families and paying for their care out of parish funds. When this condition became too burdensome, the Vestry of St. Philip's Parish in 1734 petitioned the governor for permission to build a hospital, workhouse, and house of correction. A combination refuge for prisoners and paupers was opened in 1738, chiefly for chronic cases; the meager records indicate that this institution had only a brief existence.

Charity Hospital. In 1736, a French sailor, Jean Louis, left an endowment of 12,000 livres to found a hospital and to provide necessities to succor the sick of New Orleans. L'Hôpital des Pauvres de la Charité, as it was known in legal records, was completed in 1737 and named St. John Hospital. It served not only as a hospital but as an asylum for indigents. In 1779, the building was wrecked by a hurricane, whereupon a Spanish nobleman gave 114,000 livres for rebuilding the hospital on condition that salvage material from the ruined building be used. The new brick structure in 1786 accommodated twenty-four beds and a chapel. This institution was built for the use of the destitute, but those not in dire need were admitted on a fee basis. Fire destroyed the hospital in 1809 and it was replaced six years later with a 120 bed hospital and asylum for children; in 1820 the legislature passed an act providing for a separate annex for the insane. The new Charity Hospital in 1832 had room for 400 patients; and soon after the Sisters of Charity from the motherhouse in Maryland were invited to assume the management of the interior economy of the hospital.

It will be noted that these institutions have been classified as almshouses rather than hospitals for the obvious reason that they were all founded primarily to aid the poverty-stricken who had no place to go and no one to administer to them. They were havens of refuge for the indigent, criminals, the physically handicapped, foundlings, and the mentally unbalanced. Some were sick upon admission and others became ill on the premises. There were no hospitals to which the ill could be sent and thus the need arose for the almshouse authorities to provide some kind of bed care. As more people were crowded into a city's almshouse, it became necessary to provide separate floors or departments and even buildings within the establishment for each category of inmate. The original function of housing the heterogeneous derelicts of society was gradually overshadowed by the enlarging hospital department as more services were required and made available to mental and surgical patients. These departments eventually became public hospitals independent of the other divisions of the almshouse. Finally, the orphans, criminals, blind, and deaf were transferred to institutions established especially for them, and the almshouse was dedicated solely to the care of the poor.

By tracing the development of the almshouse as it related to hospital care, we can easily see that it was a means of furnishing public assistance at a time when hospitals did not exist. But almshouses offered nothing to those who might require institutional care exclusively for illness and who could afford to pay for such service. A new social agency, the voluntary hospital, would come to serve these people as well as the indigent.

VOLUNTARY HOSPITALS

Pennsylvania Hospital. An attempt to found a hospital in Philadelphia in 1709 failed and the need became less urgent after the opening of the almshouse. Therefore, when Thomas Bond returned in 1750 from Europe equipped to practice surgery and midwifery, he found no suitable hospital facilities in Philadelphia, the richest, most populous city and the center of culture in the colonies. Dr. Bond tried to enlist the interest of his friends and colleagues in the hospital project, but he was unable to make much progress until he obtained the cooperation of Benjamin Franklin. The latter subscribed generously and publicized the need for such an institution. Some contributions were received, but not enough to start building.

Therefore, the contributors organized and appealed to the Provincial Assembly of Pennsylvania in January 1751 for assistance. The immediate reaction was opposition to an outright grant. No one considered it essential to have a hospital for private patients. It was felt that such an institution should serve only the poor and homeless, and Philadelphia already had an almshouse. With clever ingenuity Franklin appealed to the charitable and philanthropic instincts of the assemblymen and enhanced the proposition with the idea that a hospital would protect them from sickness. He had a bill drawn which provided that, if the contributors could secure from subscriptions the total amount of £2,000, the Assembly would provide a similar sum in two yearly payments for founding, building, and finishing the hospital. The bill passed, not because the assemblymen were convinced that the city needed a hospital, but because they had no faith that the contributions would ever reach £2,000. That everyone's donation would be doubled captured the popular imagination and soon subscriptions exceeded the required sum, making it possible for the contributors to claim the public gift to carry their plan into execution.

Thus the Pennsylvania Hospital, chartered by the Assembly of Pennsylvania in 1751, became the first institution incorporated solely for the care of the physically and mentally ill, regardless of economic status, race, or creed. This marks the beginning of voluntary hospitals in the United States.

New York Hospital. In May 1769, Samuel Bard, a twenty-seven-year-old professor of medicine in New York, delivered the graduation address at Trinity Church for the first two graduates of the King's College Medical School, founded in 1767. In his speech he emphasized the extreme necessity of establishing a public hospital, not only as a place in which to give care to the sick but also as a source of instruction to medical students. The interest of the audience was thus aroused and at the suggestion of the governor a subscription fund was started with the campaign extending from the city's seven wards and the clergy to merchants in England and Ireland. A charter was granted to the Society of the New York Hospital, and the cornerstone for the second voluntary hospital in this country was laid in September 1773. Plans were drawn by Dr. John Jones, also a member of the King's College faculty. It was his belief that architects always tried to plan for the greatest number of people in the least space whereas physicians desired room enough in hospitals for the use and convenience of the sick. Fire destroyed the nearly completed building early in 1775, but more funds were secured and the hospital was rebuilt in time for the New York Committee of Safety to order the governors of the hospital to admit colonial troops. Shortly thereafter, the British and Hessians took over the hospital and used it as a barracks and military hospital for seven years. When the soldiers were withdrawn, the buildings were used for medical instruction and meetings of the state legislature, so that it was not until 1791 that civilian patients were admitted to the 500 bed hospital. The medical staff then became a medical faculty and organized clinical lectures and instruction for students.

Massachusetts General Hospital. In 1810, two Boston physicians sent a circular letter to influential citizens to interest them in establishing a charitable hospital in that city. The legislature of the Commonwealth of Massachusetts granted the charter in 1812, incorporating 56 distinguished inhabitants of the various towns of the state in the name of the Massachusetts General Hospital. The governor, lieutenant governor, president of the senate, speaker of the house, and the chaplains of both houses constituted a board of visitors, who chose four of the twelve trustees placed in charge of the institution. The Commonwealth also donated the Province House, a mansion previously used as a residence by governors of the state, with authority to sell it and use the proceeds for the construction of a hospital, provided that within five years an additional sum of $100,000 should be obtained by private subscription and donations. The charter obligated the corporation to support thirty sick and lunatic persons who were charges of the state. Later this was modified to make the number of patients thus supported depend on the actual income from Province House. This provision, however, tended to make the institution a pauper establishment and it was invalidated in 1816, when authority was given to sell Province House on condition that the proceeds of the sale be paid into the state treasury unless within one year from the date of the sale the additional sum of $100,000 should be obtained.

The War of 1812 delayed the plans for building the hospital, but in 1816 the trustees instituted a house-to-house canvass and received such liberal gifts from the 1,047 subscribers that within a week $94,969 was collected. On July 4, 1816, a cornerstone was laid by the Grand Lodge of Free Masons of Massachusetts. When the hospital admitted the first patients in 1821, it became the third voluntary general hospital in the United States.

New Haven Hospital. The fourth voluntary general hospital was incorporated as the General Hospital Society of Connecticut in New Haven in 1826. Four professors in the Medical Institution (later the Yale School of Medicine) pledged their professional services as well as ten per cent of their incomes from the school for five years; in each case the sum was not to exceed $100 a year. The state medical society, also eager to aid in the erection of a hospital, lent financial assistance and voted that the hospital be located where it would best serve the interests of the medical school.

Other Voluntary Institutions. Few other voluntary general hospitals appeared before the middle of the century. It is believed that the Warren A. Candler Hospital in Savannah, which is now owned by the Methodist Episcopal Church, South, was started as the Savannah Hospital in 1830 by two philanthropic gentlemen who wished to help the poor of the city. The Lowell Corporation Hospital was established by the cotton manufacturers of Lowell, Massachusetts, for their employees in 1836. Several years later it was opened to the community and as recently as 1930 was transferred to a Brotherhood of the Catholic church. The establishment of Rex Hospital in Raleigh, North Carolina, was made possible through a bequest of $10,000 in the will of John Rex in 1839, although reports indicate that the trustees did not actually operate a hospital until 1892, when they took over a small Episcopal church hospital which had been functioning for several years. Two institutions for aged and afflicted Negroes were incorporated: (1) the Georgia Infirmary, Savannah, in 1832 and (2) Lincoln Hospital, New York City, which started with weekly home visits and became a hospital in 1840.

Voluntary hospitals for special types of illness were limited in number. The Boston Lying-in Hospital was founded in 1832 by the Massachusetts Humane Society and the Massachusetts Charitable Fire Society; lack of funds necessitated its being closed temporarily between 1857 and 1873. In Philadelphia a small maternity hospital, now called the Preston Retreat, opened in 1836.

James Wills, who died in 1825, left money in trust to the city of Philadelphia to found a hospital for the relief of the indigent blind and lame. The Wills Hospital was completed in 1832 and gradually its service came to be devoted entirely to ophthalmology.

In 1801, Captain Robert R. Randall of New York willed a large portion of his estate to found and permanently endow the Sailors' Snug Harbor Hospital; this hospital for aged and decrepit sailors was built on Staten Island in 1833.

Voluntary Mental Hospitals. After 1800, several groups of charitable citizens promoted the establishment of hospitals for the insane. Benjamin Rush worked for reform in the treatment of the insane and was the first to utilize occupational therapy in the United States. Influenced by the management introduced by the Tukes at the York Retreat in England and the humanity of Pinel in France, philanthropists directed their efforts toward devising occupations and diversions, regulating meals and exercise, encouraging work and play, and discarding restraints.

The Society of Friends in Philadelphia proposed in 1811 to provide for its members who might be deprived of their reason. Six years later the association formed by the contributors opened the Friends Hospital on its present site. Admittance was restricted to Quakers until 1834, when the hospital's facilities became available to anyone requiring mental treatment.

At the time funds were being raised to build the Massachusetts General Hospital, some of the money collected was specifically designated for a mental hospital. The urgency of providing an asylum took precedence over the construction of the general hospital and McLean Hospital was ready for occupancy in 1818, three years before the Massachusetts General.

In 1792 the first mental patient was admitted to the Society of the New York Hospital. Though a separate building was set aside for mental patients in 1808, it soon became inadequate. Therefore, land was purchased in upper Manhattan, where the Bloomingdale Asylum was built in 1821 as the mental division of the New York Hospital. It was later moved to Westchester County.

The Medical Society of Connecticut became interested in care for the mentally ill in 1812, and a committee was appointed to study the problem. In 1821, under the guidance of Dr. Eli Todd, the project began to mature. A canvass of the number of insane in the community revealed the need for such an institution. By the following year enough money had been subscribed to start building, and additional funds were secured from special contributions in churches over a period of the next five years. The first patients were admitted to the Hartford Retreat in 1824.

The Brattleboro Retreat in Vermont is also one of the oldest mental hospitals in the United States. A bequest in 1834 made possible the opening of the hospital in 1836.

The initial step in the development of hospitals in the United States was distinguished by the inception of voluntary hospitals to serve the sick and injured regardless of economic status, race, color, or creed. Not only were they the first institutions devoting their services solely to the sick, preceding church and public hospitals in chronological time of founding, but they were also a departure from the contemporary English pattern in two respects: in the admittance of paying patients and in the method of financing operations. Voluntary hospitals were a form of charitable agency not connected with church or state. They were founded by gifts and subscriptions collected from donors who had an interest and pride in civic affairs and a desire to participate in philanthropy. They maintained by these funds and also by payments received from patients who could compensate the hospital for services rendered.

The foregoing brief histories of the earliest voluntary hospitals indicate that one was an outgrowth of a surgeon's desire to have a place suitable for the practice of surgery and obstetrics; two were established in order to provide clinical instruction for medical students. They were not all general hospitals; some limited their service to maternity patients, to the blind and lame, or to chronic and convalesccent sailors. The significance of the voluntary mental hospital movement lay in the number that were founded in a relatively short period time and in the type of management that was introduced in an attempt to provide humane treatment. The underlying motive in each of these instances and of all future voluntary hospitals was the recognition of community responsibility toward the members of society.

The pattern begun with these first voluntary hospitals has been influential in shaping the functions and administration of all the hospitals that have followed. The fundamental features that set them apart from public, and proprietary hospitals are unique in the history of the world's hospitals.

STATE MENTAL HOSPITALS

Throughout the Eighteenth Century little attention was paid to the care of the insane. Dangerous individuals were confined in almshouses and jails for the protection of the rest of the community. Those who were not violent were free to roam at large. The first attempt on the part of a state to provide proper care and legal confinement for the mentally ill was the founding of the Public or Lunatic Hospital or Mad House by the Virginia House of Burgesses at Williamsburg in 1773.

Concurrent with the voluntary mental hospital movement of the early Nineteenth Century, many of the states gradually realized their responsibility toward the mentally ill and found it necessary to take some action in respect to special institutions for them. Kentucky opened a state hospital for the insane at Lexington in 1817, South Carolina at Columbia in 1828, Maine at Augusta in 1834, and New York at Brooklyn in 1838. Virginia located a second hospital at Staunton in 1828. McLean Hospital, situated outside Boston, did not have space enough to care for all the pauper insane of Massachusetts and therefore a state hospital was built at Worcester in 1832; in 1839 Boston provided a municipal hospital, which subsequently became a state institution for the insane. In Cincinnati the insane were transferred from the Commercial Hospital and Lunatic Asylum of Ohio to a state institution in 1838. Georgia, Indiana, Tennessee, New Hampshire, New Jersey, and New York authorized the establishment of state insane asylums in the 1830's, but the buildings were not completed and ready for occupancy until during the next decade.

The Public Hospital of Baltimore was established for the pauper sick, the insane, and seafaring persons of the state of Maryland in 1789 but was not completed until 1798; it was used exclusively as an insane asylum after 1839. When more space was needed a few years later, a site was purchased at Catonsville. The construction of the Spring Grove State Hospital was interrupted by the Civil War and not resumed until 1864, when the board of visitors sold the old buildings to Mr. Johns Hopkins for $150,000. This property was released to Mr. Hopkins in 1872, when the patients were moved to the new establishment, and became the site of Johns Hopkins Hospital in 1889.

This period witnessed not only the founding of the voluntary and state insane hospitals but also the combination of lunatic asylum and poorhouse which was developed by county authorities. The system was generally adopted, as it seemed much more humane than the use of the jail and it was admittedly a cheaper method of caring for the mentally ill. Eloise Hospital, which was started in 1835 in Wayne County, Michigan, with service to the old and young, the deaf, dumb, and blind, the insane, and the destitute, is maintained today as one of the largest county institutions in the country. It has approximately 6,000 beds and separate departments for acute and chronic illness, mental diseases, and domiciliary care for the indigent.

County and state authorities were so thoroughly imbued with these trends— one toward county poor farms, the other toward state insane asylums—that the practice has continued and spread through every state. Variations and improvements have been suggested from time to time, but essentially these trends still continue.

THE WESTWARD MOVEMENT OF HOSPITALS

Hospitals accompanied migration as the frontier moved westward. The dangers, illnesses, and injuries encountered in navigating the Mississippi River and its tributaries made hospitals a vital necessity. The geographical location of Cincinnati and the growing Ohio River trade greatly influenced the increase of both the permanent and transient population in that city. Hospitals for cholera and smallpox victims were often opened at the time of an emergency and closed again as soon as the epidemic abated. In 1815 the township trustees of Cincinnati rented a house in which to provide care for the sick and indigent. Daniel Drake, for forty years the most influential medical figure in the Ohio Valley, founded the Medical College of Ohio in 1817 and from that time promoted the establishment of a hospital in Cincinnati to provide clinical instruction for medical students.

In 1819 the legislature of Louisiana proposed that the states bordering on the Mississippi River and its eastern tributaries establish hospitals and give to travelers reciprocal benefits of this hospital service. In New Orleans the already established Charity Hospital furnished facilities to comply with this proposal. Louisville and Cincinnati both founded hospitals, assisting people in their respective areas. But the project failed because of lack of coordination between the states.

Cincinnati General Hospital. Motivated by a desire to provide hospital facilities for the sick poor and for boatmen on the Ohio River as well as education to medical students, the Ohio legislature established the Commercial Hospital and Lunatic Asylum of Ohio in 1821. The law provided a dual system of control by giving the trustees of the Township of Cincinnati power to appoint a steward, a matron, and other necessary servants with the exception of the apothecary or house surgeon who was to be appointed by the faculty of the Medical College of Ohio. The hospital was completed in 1823 and served as hospital, insane asylum, orphanage, and almshouse for twelve years. In 1835, the orphans were removed and subsequently both insane and paupers were transferred to other institutions. The name was changed to Commercial Hospital in 1861 and a separate board of trustees was established. In 1869 it became the Cincinnati Hospital, continuing as such until 1915, when the present buildings were occupied and "General" was added to the name. It remains under municipal control except that since 1926 the University of Cincinnati has been responsible for the medical work, nursing, and teaching in the institution.

Louisville General Hospital. A smallpox epidemic in 1817 forced the 4,000 inhabitants of the city of Louisville to open an unused hemp factory for a temporary hospital. In the same year the state of Kentucky incorporated the Louisville Hospital Company and granted it authority to procure a site for a hospital and to raise a sum not exceeding $50,000 for its construction. In 1821, $10,000 was appropriated by the state to erect a building on donated land. With an additional $6,000 the hospital was completed in 1823. The hospital was supported by a two per cent tax levied on all auction sales, except on articles grown or manufactured in Kentucky; the annual revenue amounting to approximately $3,000 was augmented by a yearly grant-in-aid of $500 from the Federal Government. Since 1836, when the management of the hospital was turned over to the city of Louisville, the hospital has continued as a municipal institution. The control is now vested in the Board of Health of Louisville and Jefferson County, and by agreement the University of Louisville is responsible for the medical service.

These were the first hospitals in the Ohio and upper Mississippi Valleys and west of the Allegheny Mountains. Both are under municipal control and both are affiliated with the only municipal universities which conduct schools of medicine.

OTHER EARLY HOSPITALS

It may be assumed from available historical records that almost every city of any size had a pesthouse in which to isolate patients at the time of an epidemic. However, once the contagion subsided, townspeople seldom felt it necessary to continue the hospital service. Most cities also provided an almshouse for the poor and if a pesthouse was not available, an infirmary might be added to the city almshouse. The facts are so meager that it has been difficult to determine just how much hospital service was available in these institutions. Many have changed names, administration, and control, and through the various transactions continuity of records has been lost and the facts are incomplete. Many a county or municipal hospital of today was originally a combination of almshouse and infirmary. The leading examples are Bellevue and Philadelphia General Hospitals. In addition, it is known that Kings County Hospital in Brooklyn was organized in 1830 as the Kings County Almshouse and Infirmary; the Cleveland City Hospital was in 1837 a shelter for the aged and infirm; and the New York City Hospital began as a hospital ward of the penitentiary located on Blackwell's Island in 1832. It is possible too that the Baltimore City Hospitals and Jersey City Medical Center were outgrowths of almshouse-infirmaries and pesthouses in those cities.

Some cities founded institutions solely as hospitals and arranged for Catholic nursing sisters to attend to the internal management. The authorities of Mobile, Alabama, established a hospital in 1830 which has always been owned by the city and always managed by the Daughters of Charity. Likewise the city of Augusta, Georgia, built a hospital in 1834 which was operated for many years by a Catholic Sisterhood. The city finally assumed management and replaced the old physical plant with the University Hospital.

There were also two instances of established hospitals being taken over by state governments. Early records of the Natchez Charity Hospital in Mississippi indicate that both the city of Natchez and the hospital were incorporated in 1805. Service was maintained for the indigent sick of the community in buildings erected on Hospital Hill until 1840, when the Federal Government closed the marine hospital at Natchez. At that time the state decided to use the marine hospital buildings to house the city hospital.

University Hospital, Baltimore, resulted from the necessity of having an infirmary in which the students of the Maryland Medical and Chirurgical Faculty could be instructed in the practice of medicine and surgery. In 1823, when this hospital was established as the Baltimore Infirmary, it was under the immediate control of the college faculty; the nursing service was controlled by the Sisters of Charity of Emmitsburg. Shortly thereafter the legislature of Maryland took charge of the hospital and received about $4,000 a year from the Federal Government for service to maritime seamen.

CHURCH HOSPITALS

De Paul Hospital, St. Louis. The first hospital west of the Mississippi River and the oldest extant Catholic hospital in the United States was called, at the time of its inception in 1828, the St. Louis Hospital. Generous gifts of land and money from John Mullanphy and the efforts of the Bishop of St. Louis in securing the services of the Daughters of Charity of St. Vincent de Paul made possible the opening of this hospital in a two-room log cabin. The illnesses, hardships, and fatigue of emigrant families seeking new homes and fortunes in the west brought the first patients. Larger quarters were acquired in 1832, but that was the year that Asiatic cholera struck St. Louis and the hospital was immediately crowded to capacity with victims of the plague. Until separate institutions were established, the city authorities sent orphans, the insane, and the destitute in addition to the sick to De Paul Hospital for care.

St. Joseph Infirmary, Louisville. The Sisters of Charity of Nazareth, who opened a shelter in Louisville to the orphans of plague victims, added emergency hospital service to their duties in 1836. This was the beginning of St. Joseph Infirmary, the second Catholic hospital.

Mt. Hope Retreat, Baltimore. A plague epidemic in Baltimore in 1840 was responsible for the founding of Mt. St. Vincent's Institute by the Sisters of Charity. After the epidemic, city officials requested that general hospital service be continued for the sick and insane. Since 1857, it has been a nervous and mental hospital known at Mt. Hope Retreat and is still under the control of the Catholic church.

These three Catholic hospitals were the only church hospitals founded prior to 1840 that are still in existence. Records would indicate that no other hospitals were established by Catholic or Protestant churches before 1840. In the latter half of the century churches gained in strength and to no small degree were responsible for the tremendous growth of hospitals in that period.

FEDERAL HOSPITALS

To fill an immediate need, the Continental Congress provided emergency temporary hospitals for soldiers participating in the Revolutionary War. When the Federal Government had been established at the end of the Eighteenth Century, provision was made by Congress for temporary and permanent army hospitals and for permanent marine and naval hospitals.

Army Hospitals. In themselves, the hospitals provided for the army during the Revolutionary War play an unimportant role in the history of hospitals, but they do illustrate what was done at that time of disorganized emergency. They were the first attempt at what was to become a highly developed permanent system of army hospitals.

At the outbreak of the war, the colonists were completely lacking in medical or military organization. So great were the poverty of the colonies and the exigencies of the army and so frequent were its movements that it was impossible to devote any time to building general hospitals or to training and organizing a medical staff. The wounded were cared for in all kinds of houses and shelters. Dr. John Morgan and Dr. William Shippen, the first directors general of the Revolutionary War hospitals, and several other surgeons favored general hospitals, but there were many who supported the small regimental hospitals used by the British.

The only accessible literature on military medicine was a book published in 1776 by Dr. John Jones, who had drawn the plans for the New York Hospital. It was entitled *Plain, concise, practical remarks on the treatment of Wounds and Fractures to which is added an Appendix, on Camp and Military Hospitals; principally designed for the use of young military and naval surgeons in North America.* Dr. Jones recommended that milder cases be treated in camp where there were better chances for recovery; that in no case should private houses be occupied for hospitals, but that churches, barns, or houses open to the rafters should be employed to one-third of their capacity. These directives, however, were not followed in the campaigns of the continental army. Private homes and tents continued to be used and were too crowded to keep disease from spreading.

When Dr. James Tilton was in charge of the general hospital at Trenton, he initiated a system of hospital huts which helped diminish sickness resulting from "crowd poisoning." He abandoned hospital tents and private houses and erected log huts, each of which would house five or six men. Each hut had a hard dirt floor, air could penetrate the crevices, and a hole in the roof furnished an exit for smoke from the center fireplace. The mortality from typhus diminished appreciably and the general results were excellent. He presented his theories of construction of military hospitals to Congress in 1781 in an attempt to get them adopted for general use by the army. In his report he indicated that half the army during the years 1777-1779 died from the effects of admitting all the sick into general hospitals; he also proved that more surgeons died in service than officers of the line as a result of infection. In 1812 his experiences during the war were published in a small volume entitled *Economical Observations on Military Hospitals and the Prevention and Cure of Diseases incident to an Army.*

For a time all affairs of the hospital department of the army were referred to a special Medical Committee of Congress. This body was terminated when the Board of War was founded. The hospital department was virtually disbanded in 1783 when furloughs were granted to the medical staff. Consequently no provision was made to care for those maimed and disabled in the war. In March 1799, Congress passed an act giving the physician general power to set up temporary hospitals with the approval of the commanding general in the district and permanent hospitals with the approval of the President of the United States.

Medical and hospital facilities for soldiers during the War of 1812 were considerably improved under Dr. Tilton's direction. Temporary hospitals were organized wherever they were needed in whatever buildings could be appropriated. At Burlington, Vermont, the hospital had 40 wards which contained about 750 patients segregated by type of disease and injury.

The modern history of the medical corps of the army dates from regulations formulated in 1818, which provided for the appointment of a surgeon general and his direct authority over medical officers. After the reduction of the army in 1821, the medical corps became sufficiently well organized to function effectively. Thereafter hospitals were established, chiefly for emergency purposes, at the army posts along the frontiers of the Northwest Territory and gradually moved westward to the Pacific coast. Some of these early station hospitals became permanent general military hospitals.

Marine Hospitals. Although the facilities in small contagious hospitals for passengers disembarking from ships at Atlantic coastal ports were available to seamen, the need for the establishment of hospital service specifically for sailors was voiced. It was not until 1787, however, that the Virginia legislature passed the first act to found a marine hospital for aged and disabled seamen at Washington, County of Norfolk. In 1791 the Boston Marine Society petitioned Congress for assistance in erecting a hospital for American seamen in that area. Seven years later an act of Congress provided that after September 1798 the master of every American ship arriving from a foreign port should pay to the Collector of Customs the sum of twenty cents a month for each seaman, such sum to be deducted from the seaman's wages. The President was authorized to use this money to provide temporary relief and maintenance for sick and disabled seamen in existing hospitals, to accept buildings, grounds, and donations for hospitals, and to appoint directors of marine hospitals in various ports. Each director was to supervise expenditures in the port assigned to him, to provide accommodations and govern the hospital under the general instructions of the President, and to render a quarterly account to the Secretary of the Treasury. This was the first attempt on the part of the Federal Government to provide medical services and hospitalization to certain persons under a scheme of compulsory sickness insurance.

After this Congressional action and because of inadequate state operating funds, the Virginia legislature in 1798 offered the Norfolk hospital to Congress for the sum of money still due the contractors. The transaction was completed in 1801 and the United States acquired its first marine hospital. In the act of 1802, which provided for an appropriation of $15,000 for the Boston marine hospital, the money collected for the benefit of the sick and disabled seamen was constituted a "Marine Hospital Fund."

For a number of years after the establishment of the service, expenses had to be met out of the fund created by the tax upon seamen and, as the amount collected proved insufficient to meet demands, restrictions were necessary from time to time to keep expenditures within the available fund. An arrangement was made to provide medical and hospital services through the utilization of local facilities, but marine hospitals might be built if no local hospitals existed. Chronic and incurable cases were excluded and relief was allowed for no longer than four months. In places where there were no hospitals, medical charges were restricted to twenty cents a day with board, lodging, nursing, and washing fixed at $2.50 per week.

Increasing use of the Mississippi River and its tributaries made necessary the provision of hospital facilities for those engaged in commerce on the inland rivers. The act of 1802 provided not only for the establishment of a marine hospital at New Orleans, but also thereafter the master of every boat or raft used on the Mississippi was required to deduct twenty cents a month from each seaman's wages and pay that amount into the Marine Hospital Fund. The first marine hospital at New Orleans was not erected for several years, but seamen were admitted to Charity Hospital as early as 1804 and a physician was appointed to attend them.

The settlement of the Louisiana and Northwest Territories and the development of transportation facilities on the Great Lakes and western rivers required hospitals in those regions. In 1837, the President was authorized to purchase up to three sites for hospitals on the Mississippi River, three on the Ohio, and one on Lake Erie. Several other sites were authorized for purchase subsequently on the navigable rivers and Great Lakes.

Naval Hospitals. In March 1799, the Congressional act of 1798, which referred only to merchant seamen, was extended to include governmental naval service, and twenty cents a month was henceforth deducted from the pay of each sailor and officer of the navy. The money was paid into the Marine Hospital Fund, and members of the navy were accorded the same benefits as were the crews of merchant vessels.

For several years much dissatisfaction prevailed with arrangements for navy sick relief. In 1810 at twenty-four of the chief seaports of the Atlantic and Gulf states some effort was made to afford relief, but it seemed to accrue chiefly to men who manned the merchant vessels. Norfolk and Boston maintained hospitals. New York, Philadelphia, Savannah, and New Orleans made provision for the sick at local hospitals, while at several other ports board was provided in private houses at the expense of the government.

In January 1811, the Marine Hospital Fund amounted to $73,288.38, of which $55,649.29 had been accumulated from deductions from the pay of naval officers and seamen. A separate Naval Hospital Fund was then established; the Secretaries of the Navy, Treasury, and War were appointed commissioners of naval hospitals and the hospital tax accruing from the navy was paid to them. The fund was augmented by $50,000 appropriated from the unexpended balance of the Marine Hospital Fund, which was considered the amount belonging to the navy from payments made prior to the passage of the act. The commissioners were authorized to procure sites for hospitals and to erect buildings with at least one permanent asylum for disabled and decrepit naval officers, seamen, and marines. But it was fifteen years before any serious attempt was made to erect substantial hospitals for the navy.

Crude temporary structures were provided as early as 1811 at the Philadelphia and Norfolk navy yards. New sites were purchased in 1826 and construction was started. One wing of the Norfolk hospital was completed for occupancy in 1830 and parts of the Philadelphia Naval Hospital and Asylum were occupied in 1833. Hospital facilities were subsequently made available for naval officers and seamen at several other ports.

In June 1832, Congress gave full jurisdiction over naval affairs to the Secretary of the Navy, after which hospital building progressed more rapidly. In August 1842, the Navy Department was reorganized. The management of the medical department was vested in the Chief of the Bureau of Medicine and Surgery, chosen from the surgeons of the navy.

These were the earliest army, naval, and marine hospitals. The service rendered in them was no better and no worse than that provided in any hospital of the period. Their importance lies in the fact that they laid the basis for future hospitals of the army, navy, and Public Health Service.

There are no accurate figures available to tell the extent of hospital service in 1840. A survey based on the 1945 listed data of hospitals in the *American Hospital Directory, 1946* reveals from the gathered dates of establishment that 52 hospitals had been founded before 1840. The majority of these were voluntary institutions. This is an approximate figure, as it includes only those that are still in existence. There undoubtedly were other hospitals founded and subsequently closed for which there is no record extant.

EXPANSION OF HOSPITALS, 1840-1900

The social, economic, and scientific progress made in the sixty years prior to 1900 laid a firm groundwork for the great Twentieth Century growth of hospital facilities and the concomitant improvement of hospital service. The principles of American democracy engendering the spirit of equality, the spread of popular education, and the opening of many and varied opportunities to all classes of society were the inevitable accompaniment of political and economic independence. Distances were overcome by means of improved transportation and communication; thousands of immigrants from Europe and the migration of native inhabitants rapidly pushed the frontier westward and also brought about the concentration of people in urban areas. The inventions of time-saving and labor-saving machines and the development of electrical power and light resulted in many advances in industry; at the same time, powerful interests forced the development of the country's rich natural resources. Vigorous intellectual activity led the way to a vast interchange of ideas between individuals and countries. All these factors were influential in evolving better living conditions, but paramount in the expansion of hospitals were the advances in nursing and the medical sciences.

Influence of Reform Movement upon Mental Hospitals

Early in the 1840's, Dorothea Lynde Dix became interested in the welfare and treatment of Boston's insane after she had conducted Sunday School services among the female inmates of the Cambridge jail. With the zeal of a true reformer, she made a systematic investigation of all the Massachusetts jails and almshouses and carefully recorded her observations. When she revealed to the state legislature in 1843 that insane persons were "confined in cages, closets, cellars, stalls, pens: chained, naked, beaten with rod and lashed into obedience," great interest was aroused among sympathetic citizens who were totally unaware of the disgraceful situation and consternation was created among the keepers who could see their livelihoods and reputations tottering. Her revelations resulted in the enactment of legislation in 1843 providing for enlarged quarters at the Worcester State Hospital.

News of the survey in Massachusetts spread to other states and Miss Dix was asked to investigate similar conditions in Rhode Island. Her report for that state resulted in the endowment of Butler Hospital in 1844, an institution for the indigent insane.

From these two New England states, Miss Dix extended her work south and west to the Mississippi River, traveling more than 10,000 miles to study prisons, poorhouses, county jails, and houses of refuge. She assisted individuals and committees to prepare bills for state legislatures that would bring about appropriations for founding state mental hospitals. She also showed her ability in conducting campaigns for funds for voluntary establishments.

Miss Dix was instrumental in the creation of the first federal hospital for the insane (St. Elizabeths Hospital) in Washington, D. C., in 1855. It was essentially a military institution, but it also admitted patients from the District. During the Civil War one building with 70 beds was set aside for wounded seamen of the Chesapeake and Potomac fleets and several wards in the main building were prepared to receive 250 sick and wounded soldiers. After the war it became the official hospital for governmental beneficiaries who were insane.

During President Franklin Pierce's administration (1853-1857), Miss Dix attempted to carry a bill through Congress providing for the setting aside of 5,000,000 acres of public lands for the benefit of the insane. When this was defeated, she increased the demand to 12,500,000 acres and succeeded then in getting the legislation passed by both houses of Congress. However, President Pierce vetoed the measure, saying, "Begin with doing anything for the insane and soon will the Federal Government have on its hands the support of every sick man, every vagabond, every drunkard in the land." Undaunted, Miss Dix traveled widely during the five years before the war, soliciting funds, recommending personnel, and seeking to improve the conditions in mental hospitals. The war interrupted her work, but before her death in 1887 she was directly responsible for founding or enlarging thirty mental hospitals. The changes she wrought in thought and practice regarding the insane and her theories of prevention of mental illness through study and proper mental hygiene form the basis of the present system of mental hospitals under governmental control.

By 1870 there were about fifty public and sixteen private mental hospitals with capacity for 17,000 patients. There was a definite attempt by this time to give humane care, though scientific treatment was unknown. Most institutions were asylums in deed and name, places for the custodial care of the mentally deranged. Few records were kept and any improvement in the patient's condition could only be attributed to factors other than planned therapy. The large hospitals, which were built as a result of Miss Dix's crusade against the brutal treatment of mental patients, soon became overcrowded, however, and conditions at the end of the century were just as bad as at the time she undertook her campaign for reform.

Influence of Advances in Nursing

Most of the hospitals in the United States in the early Nineteenth Century were disgraceful in their degradation; they were dirty, unventilated, and contaminated with infections. The spread of disease was facilitated by such conditions. The only lay nurses who could be obtained were aged inmates or women who could get no other employment and were willing to include menial tasks with nursing. Their work was not subject to inspection or discipline. There was practically no nursing service at night except for childbirth or in case of impending death, at which time a "watcher" would be hired. The general public knew little of these conditions. Because of restricted visiting hours or lack of friends, patients were often cut off from the outside world. Tours of inspection by boards of management revealed only superficial phases of internal management and failed to disclose actual conditions. The neglect and ill-treatment of patients and the high death rate created a popular prejudice against hospitals.

CATHOLIC SISTERHOODS

The only kindly and humane nursing was done by the Catholic religious orders whose members were fairly well educated, earnest, and devoted in their endeavors. Members of the American branch of St. Vincent de Paul's Sisters of Charity, founded at Emmitsburg, Maryland, by Mother Elizabeth Seton in 1809, were occasionally secured for emergency nursing by the city authorities of New York, Philadelphia, and Baltimore. In the decade before 1850 they were also responsible for founding hospitals in Detroit, Philadelphia, Buffalo, Milwaukee, and New York City. By 1860, they had established hospitals in Norfolk, Mobile, Rochester, Troy, Cincinnati, New Orleans, St. Louis, and even as far west as Los Angeles.

Other Catholic orders also sent members to America for missionary work, and they organized several hospitals, especially throughout the middle and far west. The Catholic hospital movement, which began with the foundation of these religious communities in the larger cities and the first Catholic hospitals where simple nursing procedures were performed by the Sisters, gained even greater impetus after schools of nursing were started.

DEACONESS MOVEMENT

The institution of Protestant Deaconesses, incorporated under the state laws of Pennsylvania in 1850, was initiated by the work of Pastor Theodore Fliedner and his wife Fredericke at Kaiserswerth, Germany, in 1833 with visiting the sick in their homes. In 1836 at Kaiserswerth the Fliedners opened the first school for deaconesses and a hospital for patients who could not be cared for by the visiting nurses. The organization of the hospital, the selection of women applicants, and their instruction were Mrs. Fliedner's responsibility. Their training was designed to fit them not only for nursing and religious duties but also for teaching other deaconesses. The success of the Fliedner establishment was so apparent and answered the need so efficiently that within ten years of its founding, the motherhouse had trained more than a hundred deaconesses. The deaconess movement changed the concept of nursing both in Germany and far beyond its borders. Fliedner finally gave up his pastorate in order to establish branch homes, to assign graduates to teaching, prison, or relief positions, and to introduce nursing staffs in hospitals.

Elizabeth Fry, who was continuing John Howard's work in English prisons, visited the deaconess motherhouse in 1840 to learn the details of general management, curriculum, and student practice from the Fliedners. She then returned to England and established the Protestant Sisters of Charity, later called the Protestant Nursing Sisters. Their training, however, was slight, as they had no school, but they learned a few procedures from visiting at Guy's Hospital, London.

The Rev. Dr. William A. Passavant, pastor of the first English Lutheran Church of Pittsburgh, visited Kaiserswerth in 1846 and was so impressed with the practical services of the deaconesses that he immediately made plans to introduce the same system in this country. Before he left Germany, he arranged with Pastor Fliedner to send some deaconesses to him in Pittsburgh to help him start a hospital. Before they arrived, however, Dr. Passavant opened the Pittsburgh Infirmary to care for cholera patients. In 1849, Fliedner brought four deaconesses to Pittsburgh to take charge of the first Protestant church hospital in the United States. Under Dr. Passavant's leadership, deaconess hospitals were also founded in Milwaukee in 1863, Chicago in 1865, and Jacksonville, Illinois in 1875.

Several deaconess motherhouses and hospitals, all planned according to the Kaiserswerth motherhouse, were also started in connection with the German, Norwegian, Swedish, and Danish Lutheran Synods.

The Rev. W. A. Muhlenberg, rector of the Protestant Episcopal Church, New York, introduced the deaconess movement into the Episcopal Church of America by organizing its first Sisterhood and opening a dispensary in connection with the Church of the Holy Communion in 1852, which became St. Luke's Hospital in 1858. Several dioceses of the Protestant Episcopal Church followed Rev. Muhlenberg's example and created Sisterhoods and hospitals in eastern and middle western cities. In addition, on the west coast Bishop Wistar Morris founded the Good Samaritan Hospital in Portland in 1875 and the Sisters of the Order of the Good Shepherd founded the Los Angeles Hospital of the Good Samaritan in 1887.

A training school for Methodist Episcopal deaconesses was started in Chicago in 1885 and led to the establishment of the association by the General Conference in 1887 at the request of the women of the church. The German Central Deaconess Board was organized in 1897 to supervise deaconess work within the German Conference of the Methodist Episcopal Church and established Bethesda Hospital in Cincinnati.

The Evangelical Synod of North America and the Evangelical Church both contributed to the establishment of hospitals in the middle west by the foundation of deaconess societies.

The worthy efforts of the Fliedners thus brought about better nursing service and influenced the growth of hospitals among the Protestant denominations where the deaconesses could be trained and could work.

FLORENCE NIGHTINGALE

The reputation of Kaiserswerth also became known to Florence Nightingale. Following a two weeks' visit in 1850, she spent four months in training there in 1851. She then went to Paris and worked in hospitals with the Sisters of Charity and the French surgeons. In 1853 she took charge of the Establishment for Gentlewomen during Illness in London and had just accepted the position of superintendent of nurses at King's College Hospital when she was sent officially by the British government to the Crimea to take charge of the care of the war wounded and sick. Her staff, composed chiefly of practical nurses, also included a few Catholic and Protestant nursing sisters. There she found thousands of sick and wounded soldiers suffering under filthy and chaotic conditions from lack of nursing service and supplies. Wooden barracks or huts, raised from the ground with double walls as protection from heat and cold, with ridge ventilation and heated by means of open fires or stoves, were installed and proved far more satisfactory as hospitals than other buildings. Against the opposition of the medical officers she organized the hospital work in an orderly way and was successful in reducing the death rate from 42 to 2 per cent. This work marked the beginning of a career that completely changed the concept of nursing service and education. Miss Nightingale subsequently was responsible for fundamental reforms in hospital organization and administration, in construction, sanitation, and dietary service.

When she returned to England, the Nightingale Fund was established to provide for the training of nurses. The Nightingale School was organized at St. Thomas' Hospital, London, in 1860. This school for nurses emphasized the authority of the matron superintendent, good living conditions for students, classroom teaching, the teaching supervisor, and the need for intelligent and refined students.

Miss Nightingale's prolific writings revealed to the world her sound theories of health organization. Her books were the first to acquaint the people concerning the problems of hospitals and nursing. *Notes on the British Army* marked a turning point in the history of military medicine. *Notes on Hospitals,* published in 1858, is considered a most valuable contribution and revolutionized hospital construction, emphasizing sanitation rather than beauty. Her suggestions based on the Crimean experience were accepted by the British authorities and the barrack-hospital plan for military hospitals was adopted. She also advocated that all old civil hospitals should be replaced with new ones and that large city hospitals should be supplanted by small cottage hospitals outside the city limits.

Notes on Nursing appeared in 1859 and remains a classic to this day, for the principles she laid down are still followed. The practical application of her ideas proved the value of a definite plan of education for nurses. She had found a way of providing efficient nursing service outside the control of any religious group and also a suitable and useful occupation for women seeking to use their talents outside the home.

Her fame spread far. In the United States her nursing procedures were practiced during the Civil War, but her principles of nurse training were not adopted until about 1873, when the first schools of nursing were opened. In these early schools there was a concentrated effort on the part of the founders to follow Miss Nightingale's advice and counsel.

THE CIVIL WAR

When the Civil War started, the governmental medical service was better organized than in any previous war in which the United States has been involved. However, scientific medicine and bacteriology were still unknown, trained nurses did not exist, and medical supplies were insufficient or unavailable. President Lincoln, knowing of the good services being rendered by the Catholic Sisterhoods, called on them to undertake the nursing of the wounded soldiers. Sisters of Charity, Sisters of Mercy, Holy Cross Sisters, and Ursulines cared for soldiers in their own hospitals, in army hospitals, and on the battlefield and assisted in establishing field and permanent army hospitals.

Yet there were not enough Sisters to care for all of the sick and wounded soldiers. Hundreds of lay women were also needed. Within thirty days after the call to arms, the Women's Central Committee of New York had selected a hundred women for army service and had admitted them to Bellevue, St. Luke's, and other hospitals in the city for a month's preparatory training, which though inadequate was better than none at all.

In June 1861, Dorothea Dix was appointed Superintendent of Female Nurses for the Union Army by the Secretary of War. Women in the northern states offered their services, so that the Civil War nurses outside the Sisterhoods numbered about 2,000. Many men, ex-patients and those unfit for active service, were also used as nurses. In the south, likewise, the women met the emergency by contributing nursing service in the temporary hospitals, in homes, and in tents provided for Confederate soldiers.

The Civil War brought to light the glaring deficiencies of nursing service both within and outside hospitals. The role women played as nurses acted as an opening wedge for the continuation of that work in peacetime. In general, their service was most enlightening to the men who received their ministrations, to the physicians and surgeons who accepted their assistance on the battlefield and in the war hospitals, to relatives and visitors of the sick and wounded who, for the first time, encountered women as nurses outside their own homes and families, and most of all to the women themselves who saw that nursing could become a career.

THE RED CROSS

Inspired by Miss Nightingale's work in the Crimean War, Jean Henri Dunant originated in Switzerland in 1863 a plan for organizing in every country an independent society for relief to serve not only in time of war but also at times of disaster from wind, fire, or flood. Personnel and supplies were to be guaranteed neutrality under the symbol of the Red Cross. The Geneva Convention stipulated that each country which ratified the Red Cross idea should have a national committee, civilian in character and function. The United States was invited to join after the Civil War, but signature was withheld until 1882. Since the formation of the national society, both men and women have been given first-aid instruction to mitigate and prevent suffering in time of dire need. Also, since 1900 the American Nurses' Association has constantly solicited the enrollment of professional nurses in the Red Cross in order that they may be available in times of disaster. This was a radical departure from the plan followed in most European countries where Red Cross nurses were prepared through short courses of training for war service.

NURSING SCHOOLS

The provision of training for a superior type of nursing was one of the principal objectives in incorporating Woman's Hospital of Philadelphia in 1861. The first permanent school of nursing provided a six months' course and one graduate was reported in 1865, but the school did not begin to flourish until 1872.

The New England Hospital for Women and Children included a school for nurses in its 1863 charter. Before the one-year course was started in 1872, about thirty nurses were trained in maternity service but were not called graduates.

The year 1873 is notable in the history of nursing for the establishment of nurse training schools in three outstanding hospitals, Bellevue, New Haven, and Massachusetts General. These three schools were the beginning of formal nursing education in the United States. Not one originated within the hospital, but each was implanted by the efforts of outsiders who were inspired to do something concrete about the inadequacy of care rendered the sick. Although they were patterned after the Nightingale School in London, there were a number of dissimilarities which reflected the differences in hospital operation in Europe and America.

In an attempt to start a nurse training school, the New York State Charities Aid Association, consisting of a group of women who had served during the war, appointed a visiting committee to investigate conditions at Bellevue Hospital. The committee, in spite of the disapproval of the medical board, pursued its survey and found inefficient management, bad nursing, and neglected patients. The nurses, attendants, and general helpers were incompetent, ignorant, indifferent, and dishonest. There were only three night watchmen to make rounds among 800 patients.

While Dr. Gill Wylie, a former intern at Bellevue, went abroad to consult Miss Nightingale about opening a nurse training school, the ladies secured funds by public appeal and succeeded in getting six wards set aside for the experiment. Sister Helen, a graduate of University College, London, and a member of the All Saints' Sisterhood in Baltimore, became superintendent in 1873 and the school was officially opened.

Conscientious, intelligent women were selected for the first class and of the original twenty-nine accepted for the course, six were graduated in 1875, having completed a two-year course. Miss Linda Richards, who had had some previous training at the New England Hospital in Boston, served as night superintendent for a few months and started the practice of keeping records and writing orders. There was no class work and lectures were irregular during the first years, but teaching on an individual basis was conducted in the wards. The results within the hospital were obviously so much better than ever before that within a short time the doctors approved of the school.

New Haven Hospital appointed a committee of three doctors in 1872 to consider the practicability of training nurses. They decided it would be inadvisable for the hospital itself to undertake such work, but they recommended a separate school with the hospital as its practice field. The Connecticut Training School under the supervision of a graduate of Woman's Hospital, Philadelphia, opened in October 1873 with three students.

The Boston Training School, which opened in November 1873, developed in the Massachusetts General Hospital. The organizing committee was made up of a group of socially prominent men and women who had to contest the disapproval of the trustees and medical staff to promote the training school. Finally two wards were allotted for the experiment and subscriptions were obtained for the school. Linda Richards became superintendent of the school and by the end of the first year she had convinced the doctors of the value of the new school and it was accepted by the trustees as part of the hospital.

The need for intelligent women to be trained as nurses had been felt during the Civil War. Women nurses in the war felt the touch of independence, and nursing as a career outside the home beckoned to them. It was soon discovered that student nurses were better disciplined, performed better service, and were less expensive than untrained hired women. Hospital managers generally opposed the innovation. The early demonstration of greatly improved nursing service won public support and this together with the economies effected overcame all opposition. From 22 schools for nurses and about 600 graduates in 1883, the schools increased to 400 with approximately 10,000 graduates in 1898.

Influence of Advances in the Science of Medicine

It may be said that the transition to modern medicine through the application of exact science to the practice of the healing art took place during the latter half of the Nineteenth Century. The many discoveries in the biological sciences and the development of many technical appliances which physicians found useful in diagnosis and therapy gave marked impetus to the change. As investigators discovered the causes of disease and devised means of prevention and cure, the practice of surgery and medicine was revolutionized.

ANESTHESIA

American surgeons of the early Nineteenth Century had sufficient knowledge of anatomy and physiology to perform many operative procedures. Modern operative gynecology was founded by McDowell and Sims. Patients, however, suffered great agony from the pain of surgical procedures and surgeons were at a serious disadvantage because of the speed with which it was necessary to work. Almost all wounds became infected and the mortality frequently ran as high as 90 per cent.

In England, Germany, and America, opium, wine, brandy, or henbane with lettuce was administered in large doses the day of the operation; mesmerism, strapping the limb above the point of operation to numb the nerves, noise, and other means were employed to divert the patient's attention. Therefore, it was considered miraculous when ether completely deadened the pain of a surgical operation performed by Dr. Crawford W. Long in 1842 in Georgia. However, Dr. Long did not make known his discovery until after Horace Wells, a dentist in Hartford, Connecticut, in 1844 had used nitrous oxide when extracting a tooth and William Morton, a Boston dentist, administered ether in an operation for a tumor, performed by the senior surgeon at Massachusetts General Hospital in 1846. The effects of ether were so remarkable in producing insensibility that Dr. Oliver Wendell Holmes gave it the Greek name of anesthesia. Sir James Simpson in England tried in 1847 to deaden labor pains with ether, but found chloroform more successful. Who deserves the credit for discovering anesthesia is of far less importance than the fact that it was discovered. The innumerable operative procedures that have been devised and performed in the last century would have been quite impossible without the aid of anesthesia.

PUERPERAL FEVER

Oliver Wendell Holmes, after observing a great many maternity cases in Boston, concluded that childbed fever was a contagious disease transmitted from patients with puerperal fever, erysipelas, and infected wounds to women in labor through the medium of the hands and clothing of doctors and midwives. In his paper *On the Contagiousness of Puerperal Fever,* published in 1843, he advocated the careful cleansing of the physician's hands and a change of clothing before attending deliveries.

In the same decade Semmelweiss was making a study of post-mortem tissues of women who had died from puerperal infection in Vienna hospitals. He believed that medical students working on dissections prior to attending obstetrical cases were responsible for the high mortality rate. He reached the same conclusions as Holmes, adding to unclean hands and dirty clothes the unsanitary conditions in hospitals as factors in transmitting puerperal fever. His book on *The Aetiology, Concept and Prophylaxis of Childbirth Fever* gave to the world his theories and methods of treatment, which he had proved when he reduced the death rate in the maternity wards between 1846 and 1848 to one-tenth of the previous rate through the simple expedient of cleanliness.

Both Semmelweiss and Holmes, in advocating antisepsis, indicated the way to a great reduction in maternal mortality, but for a long time professional approval was withheld and their ideas were ridiculed in both America and Europe.

LOUIS PASTEUR

The French chemist, Pasteur, demonstrated the scientific basis for Semmelweiss' theory when he proved that bacteria were living microorganisms which increased through reproduction, not by spontaneous generation, and that they could be destroyed by heat and chemical action. His work laid the foundation for the science of bacteriology and for the subsequent advances in this field. The application of his discoveries to chicken cholera, anthrax, and rabies introduced the practice of inoculation for the prevention of disease.

LORD JOSEPH LISTER

Recognizing the significance of Pasteur's theory of the causation of disease, Lister sought a way to destroy germs on the hands, instruments, and dressings in the operating room. His success with carbolic acid sprays as an antiseptic in surgical operations after 1865 not only hastened wound healing, but reduced the mortality rate in his hospital from 45 to 12 per cent. Antisepsis was the forerunner of aseptic surgery, which could be deliberately planned, thus greatly increasing the number and extent of operative procedures and the treatment of conditions amenable to surgery.

The transition from chemical to physical sterilization was promoted by Merke's investigation of the effects of steam on living organisms. In 1881, Koch and his associates perfected Merke's idea of steam sterilization. It was von Bergmann, however, who introduced steam sterilization in surgery in

1886 and established in 1891 the present standardized procedures of boiling and exposure to steam under pressure.

THE MICROSCOPE

Though the achromatic lens had been developed for the microscope in 1810 and Johannes Müller first used the instrument for studying tissues in 1830, Virchow made the greatest contribution to pathology with his cell theory as the basis for the analysis of diseased tissues. His development of methods of scientific diagnosis made the microscope and the laboratory indispensable in medical and surgical practice.

ROBERT KOCH

Contemporary with Pasteur's efforts to prevent disease was the development of Koch's theory of specific infection. Using Perkins' discovery of aniline dyes to devise a laboratory technique for staining specimens for identification and culture methods to separate bacteria one from another, Koch was able to identify the anthrax, tuberculosis, and cholera bacilli. When research revealed that tuberculosis was transmitted from person to person and that the bacillus would not develop in pure, dry air and sunshine, open air sanatoria were established wherever the climate was favorable.

OTHER ADVANCES

Progress in the field of immunity with the production of vaccines, antitoxins, and immune serums paralleled the development in bacteriology and pathology. In 1883 the microorganism causing diphtheria was isolated by Klebs and Loeffler, and in 1894 von Behring introduced the principle of using serum from immunized animals to prevent the disease. The typhoid bacillus, discovered in 1880, was found in contaminated food and water, and vaccination with killed bacilli was undertaken as a prophylactic measure against typhoid fever in 1896. In 1897 Ehrlich established his side-chain theory which explained the mechanism of immunity and allergy.

The study of circulation advanced more in the hands of the physiologist, Karl Ludwig, than it had since the work of Harvey. Claude Bernard's and Brown-Sequard's study of digestion, nutrition, metabolism, and the ductless glands was the beginning of the sciences of biological chemistry and endocrinology.

A large number of precision instruments were invented in this period which assisted in the determination of more accurate diagnoses. Among these were the clinical thermometer, ophthalmoscope, and laryngoscope developed before 1860; the gastroscope, the sphygmomanometer, and the cystoscope before 1883; and the bronchoscope in 1898. Edison's invention of the incandescent light made the visual instruments even more useful.

High frequency currents were introduced by d'Arsonval in the late 1880's and were later used in diathermy. In 1893 Finsen introduced light therapy for the treatment of skin diseases, and in 1896 he published the results of his work on the use of ultraviolet rays. Roentgen's discovery of x-rays in 1895 revealed a new kind of radiation which would pass through many substances that are opaque to ordinary light, would affect photographic plates, and would produce fluorescence in certain salts. Subsequent research proved the value of x-rays in diagnosis and in the treatment of skin diseases and some malignant tumors. In 1898 the Curies isolated radium. Three years later its action on tissues became known by chance when the Parisian Professor Becquerel received a severe skin burn from a tube of radium he was carrying in his pocket.

Public Health

The foundations of voluntary and official public health agencies were laid at the end of the Eighteenth Century with the establishment of the first dispensaries and the first local boards of health. In the latter part of the Nineteenth Century health laws were enacted by many cities, state departments of health were founded and the federal health service was reorganized.

When the Constitution of the United States was formulated, the states retained the function of the preservation of health within their respective borders and were responsible for all except interstate and international health activities. However, state authorities took no action in respect to health problems until pressure was exerted by the public in several localities which shared the common problem of an epidemic.

The first local court order was passed in Massachusetts in 1647 as a precaution against the importation of yellow fever. Ships arriving in Boston from the West Indies were not allowed to land passengers or discharge cargo without permission from the city council. This order was repealed two years later when the danger from yellow fever had subsided. Petersburg, Virginia, was the first locality to establish a board of health in 1780. New York followed in 1796 and Baltimore in 1798. In 1797 Massachusetts passed an act making it possible but not obligatory for certain well-populated communities to have boards of health and as a result one was founded in Boston in 1799. The establishment of public health departments by local communities was prompted by the need to meet emergency situations. It was not contemplated in most instances that these departments would have continuous operation.

About the same time a voluntary health movement developed and proved more effective than the local governmental agencies. Poverty incurred by the destruction of property during the Revolutionary War and the large number of war wounded in all the cities, especially among people who had always maintained themselves and their families before the war without the aid of charity, brought about the formation of a new type of agency, the dispensary, to care for health needs. The Philadelphia Dispensary originated with the Society of Friends in 1786; the New York Medical Society in cooperation with the governors of the New York Hospital opened a dispensary in 1795; the Boston Chamber of Commerce started the third dispensary in the United States in 1796; and the Baltimore General Dispensary was established in 1801 under the auspices of the leading clergymen and citizens of that city. These first four dispensaries had several features in common: They were all independent of hospitals; they were all private institutions financed by bequests and voluntary subscriptions; their original purpose was the dispensing of medicines and drugs to ambulatory patients at a given time and place. Gradually physicians were employed to visit in their homes those who were unable to go to the dispensary. The movement spread to many cities and in some more than one dispensary was established. Special dispensaries or infirmaries for ailments of the eye and ear were opened in New York in 1820 and in Boston in 1826. Other dispensaries were established by physicians who wanted to specialize in a certain phase of medicine and realized they could advance their knowledge and skill through the study and care of large numbers of dispensary patients.

Throughout the Nineteenth Century public health work in cities and towns was concerned primarily with the quarantine of communicable diseases, environmental sanitation, and vaccination for smallpox. The mortality rates of ordinary diseases, especially among children, did not cause any activity on the part of the local authorities. Epidemics of cholera occurred in several cities in 1849 and again in 1854. Each time, people sought refuge outside the cities, but no official measures were taken to control the disease.

Against the opposition of property owners and politicians, Dr. Stephen Smith revealed the status of sanitary conditions in New York City and with the aid of a group of citizens effected the passage of the Metropolitan Health Law in 1866, which led to the founding of the New York City Health Department. When cholera broke out again, the authorities had it quickly under control. Other cities became interested in the results obtained in New York City and used the New York law as the basis of their municipal legislation. Even so, the growth of local health administration was slow. There were still only 37 local health departments in the United States in 1873.

The most notable event in the progress of public health and the development of public health laws was the report of the Massachusetts Sanitary Commission in 1850. A publisher and statistician, Lemuel Shattuck, was appointed chairman of the Commission to make a sanitary survey of the state in 1849.

Shattuck's comprehensive report recommended that the public health laws of the state be improved and that a general board of health be established with a full-time salaried secretary and members representing medicine, law, engineering, natural philosophy, and two other professions or occupations. His extensive survey revealed that action should be taken with respect to housing, streets, schools, public bath houses, vital statistics, inquests, cemeteries, quarantine of contagious disease, tuberculosis, the insane, smoke and other nuisances, patent medicines and nostrums, adulterated food, drink, and medicines, water, excreta disposal, the formation of sanitary associations, and the establishment of schools to educate nurses. He upheld the theory that all persons should be educated in sanitary science and individually should do everything possible to promote personal health and prevent disease. The Commission's report was considered outstanding and even daring at the time it was submitted, but it was not put into effect. In fact, it was neglected until after the Civil War had made people more health conscious. Then the report was revived and action was taken.

Yellow fever was responsible for the establishment of the first state board of health in Louisiana in 1855. However, when the epidemic which prompted the state action abated, the board became dormant; it was revived late in the century. Actually, the Massachusetts State Board of Health should be accorded first place, since it has operated continuously and effectively since its founding in 1869. Several other states shortly thereafter established state boards of health: California in 1870, Minnesota and Virginia in 1872, Michigan in 1873, Maryland in 1874, and Alabama in 1875. By 1878, sixteen such departments had been organized.

The federal marine hospitals about the middle of the Nineteenth Century were greatly hampered because of various restrictions. Political pressure forced the building of hospitals in certain favored locations regardless of the needs of beneficiaries. Sites were purchased in unsuitable places and had to be abandoned. Hospitals were built and never occupied.

In 1869 the Secretary of the Treasury arranged for Dr. John Shaw Billings to investigate the marine hospitals and to make recommendations for their improvement. As a result, the Congressional Act of 1870 brought about a reorganization of the service on a national basis. Dr. John M. Woodworth, who had been in health work in Chicago and had served with the Union Army, was appointed to reorganize the Marine Hospital Service and its procedures along military lines. In 1884 the beneficiaries of the Service (whose wage deductions had been raised from twenty to forty cents a month) were no longer compelled to contribute to its support. A special tonnage tax was instituted to share the expenses with general taxation. The Service became strongly centralized under Woodworth's direction and careers as full-time medical officers in the Service were opened for the first time to physicians.

In 1878 the Federal Government enacted a national law which directed the Marine Hospital Service to prevent the introduction of contagious and infectious diseases into the United States. In the following year provision was made for the establishment of a National Board of Health to take charge of interstate and foreign quarantine. However, opposition to the board was so severe that it ceased to function after four years and quarantine duties were returned to the Marine Hospital Service. In 1893 Congress passed a law forbidding the entrance of any vessel from a foreign port except in accordance with the national quarantine law.

Up to 1900 the local, state, and federal health services were chiefly concerned with problems of quarantine. In addition, local and state departments made more or less ineffective attempts to improve sanitation. Some departments supported vaccination against smallpox. The only other activity of the Marine Hospital Service was the care of the government's beneficiaries for whom the service had been originally organized.

Hospital Progress

The years 1840 to 1900 are most significant in the history of American hospitals. It was during this period that hospitals underwent a drastic evolution in purpose, function, and number. From supplying merely food, shelter, and meager medical care to the pauper sick, to armies, to those infected with contagious diseases, to the insane, and to those requiring emergency treatment, they began to provide skilled medical and surgical attention and nursing care to all people. Many church hospitals were founded during this period. Roman Catholic Sisterhoods established the first church hospitals at centers of colonization. The various Protestant denominations followed with the organization of hospitals in all parts of the country. Hospitals were established by Jewish philanthropic organizations in order that Jewish patients might observe their dietary laws more faithfully and to provide educational and work opportunities for Jewish physicians. A few women's and children's hospitals were established under the management and control of women; in several instances these were founded to provide hospital facilities for women physicians. Churches, missions, fraternal and trade societies, and other nongovernmental associations organized dispensaries to assist their members and to some of these were added hospital wards for people requiring surgical operations or other in-bed care.

The principal influence in this hospital development came from the advances in medicine and nursing in European countries which filtered into the United States after the Civil War. Progress was gradual. For generations faith had been placed in traditional methods. Adherence to old beliefs had to be overcome before the benefits of anesthesia, antisepsis, and the laboratory sciences were wholeheartedly accepted and applied to the improvement of hospital service. Both the public and the medical profession had to be convinced that general cleanliness was necessary, that asepsis was efficacious, and that the new methods of examination, diagnosis, and therapy were better than the old.

Up to the time of the Civil War American army units were located at small garrisons along the coast and the Indian frontier. Each station provided a small hospital for emergency care of the sick and wounded. During the war each regiment established a regimental hospital. As regiments were grouped into brigades and brigades united to form divisions, the hospitals followed the troop movements. The sick and wounded who could not be moved were left behind the line of battle in civilian hospitals which provided more comfort and convenience than the hospitals that moved with the army.

The United States Sanitary Commission, founded by the Rev. Henry W. Bellows of New England, was established early in the war to advise the Medical Department of the Army. The Commission collected and distributed supplies, planned camps and their sanitation, tended the wounded on the field and in hospitals, and equipped a hospital train. The committee on hospitals based their recommendations to the government on Miss Nightingale's suggested system of military hospitals. Instead of using old buildings for general hospitals, they advocated the erection of wooden barracks with ample ventilation and space enough to accommodate from thirty to sixty men. The government at once commenced the erection of two temporary model hospitals in Washington to conform with the plans of the committee.

The war hospitals for both the Union and Confederate armies followed the same principles of construction: (1) the hospitals were placed on a large area of ground so that the barracks might be widely separated from the administration building and from each other; (2) the wards connected by a corridor were only one story in height, were ventilated by openings along the ridge of the roof, were heated with stoves, and were temporary in character. The first hospitals were for 250 beds with the wards varying in size from 25 to 50, but later they were greatly enlarged. At one time these governmental hospitals had as many as 134,000 beds.

So great was the success in treating the wounded in these hospitals that many of the methods followed were adopted by civilian hospitals. The Germans also during the Franco-Prussian War not only constructed military hospitals on the American plan but also applied the principles to civilian hospitals after the war.

The Civil War increased the number of military hospitals throughout the battle areas, but interrupted the building of governmental and voluntary hospitals for public usage. During the war a large contraband camp for escaped Negro slaves was established in Washington. On March 3, 1865,

Congress created the Freedmen's Bureau for the relief of unemployed, ill, and infirm Negroes. No provision was made for medical or hospital service for these people, but the powers of the Bureau were broad and a medical division was organized to provide care for sick, injured, and refugee freedmen. By September 1867, the Bureau was operating 46 hospitals with 5,292 beds. The hospital and asylum in Washington was continued under Bureau management until June 30, 1872, when its administration was transferred to the Department of Interior.

The defects brought to light during the wartime emergency emphasized the need for better civilian hospital construction. Pasteur's theories concerning the relation of bacteria to disease and Lister's principles of antisepsis were not at once thoroughly understood. Many people, including the medical profession, supposed that diseases were produced by emanations from the soil and that the air surrounding patients in hospitals was poisonous and dangerous. Such speculation greatly influenced hospital construction and a solution was presumed to be found in treatment in the open air, in tents, or in destructible pavilions. These were classified as the barrack system and consisted of temporary one-story wooden structures which provided ample light, air, and space but were difficult to heat and maintain. The only known method of coping with a situation in which hospital buildings were saturated with infections was to destroy and replace them from time to time. However, a compromise was introduced in the form of pavilion hospitals. They were permanent units of two or more stories, built of brick or stone, not connected with any other pavilion or with the general administrative office except by covered walks. This method divided the hospital into separate units of varied sizes having only administration in common. The first examples of detached pavilions in the United States were Roosevelt Hospital, New York; Presbyterian Hospital, Philadelphia; two wards at Boston City Hospital; and one ward at Massachusetts General Hospital, Boston.

Throughout the Nineteenth Century the status of many of the medical schools was deplorable. Proprietary schools flourished. Standards of admission were low, sessions short, courses ungraded; instruction consisted in dogmatic, theoretical, and repetitious lectures. Many of the teachers were mainly interested in private practice. The few laboratories that existed were almost useless for lack of equipment. There were very few libraries. Most of the medical schools had no hospital facilities. Only 5 per cent of the graduates of the American medical schools of the period had the advantage of clinical study and experience before they encountered their first patients. Practical instruction was usually obtained through an apprenticeship under the direction of a preceptor. In only a few instances were the schools integral parts of universities and conducted in accordance with the standards of higher education. The best training in medicine was secured only at great cost in

European medical centers. The value of research and experimental medicine was realized in Europe, but there was comparatively little effort to introduce these procedures and techniques in this country.

This was the situation until after the Civil War. Attempts at improvement were beginning to be made, but no great changes developed until Johns Hopkins Hospital was completed and in operation. A new era of hospital development began when the plans for Johns Hopkins Hospital and Medical School were formulated. These envisioned the coordination of medical science, medical education, and hospital service.

JOHNS HOPKINS HOSPITAL

Several years before his death, Johns Hopkins, a multimillionaire of Baltimore, divided $7,000,000 equally to found a hospital and a university. Separate corporations, each having a board of trustees and its own funds, were formed in 1867. Nine of the trustees on the hospital board were also members of the university board, thus ensuring liaison between the two institutions.

In Mr. Hopkins' letter of instruction to the trustees in March 1873, specific directions for the future hospital were made. The buildings should accommodate up to 400 patients, most of whom were to be indigent sick of the city admitted without charge, without regard to age, sex, or color. Patients should be so disposed as not to endanger the other inmates; a limited number of patients might also be admitted who were able to pay for their care. The trustees should secure surgeons and physicians of the highest character and the greatest skill for the hospital. A training school for female nurses should be established. A convalescent hospital should be affiliated with the main hospital to hasten the recovery of the sick and ensure the availability of rooms for those requiring immediate attention. Though the influence of religion should be present, the administration should not yield to any sectarian discipline or control. Above all, the hospital should ultimately form part of the medical school of the university.

The trustees were business men familiar with the management of men and money, but they were uninformed concerning hospital problems. There was much discussion in medical circles over the best way to build hospitals at this time and the authorities differed widely because of the prevailing opinions concerning disease and infection. The trustees recognized the desirability of building a hospital that would embody the newer conceptions of medical progress.

Francis T. King, the first president of the board of trustees of the hospital, asked for assistance from five physicians who were recognized as authorities on hospital construction and management. In his letter to these experts, Mr. King inquired as to the best system of hospital construction with special reference to the relative merits of the pavilion system and the barrack system;

whether the accommodations needed for a training school for nurses should be within the hospital building or separate from it; what accommodations would be necessary for the medical classes of the university to be held in the hospital; whether the buildings of the school of medicine should be in close proximity to the hospital or erected with the other buildings of the university some distance away; what provisions should be made for accident cases and for out-patients to be treated in the dispensary; the best methods of heating and ventilating hospital buildings; and finally the details of management.

Each man prepared a plan for the future hospital and submitted schemes for the organization, equipment, and general management. The essays differed on many points, but there was general agreement that the permanent pavilion type of structure excelled temporary wooden buildings.

The essay of Dr. John Shaw Billings, an officer of the United States Army Medical Corps, was the most acceptable and revealed his wide experience and knowledge of hospital construction and his interest in medical education. He indicated that the plan of the hospital must depend upon the extent and the manner of its connection with the medical school. He advocated small classes, high standards of preliminary education, a four-year medical course, rigid examinations, and practical work in the various departments of the hospital. He recommended a permanent type of hospital with a separate building for nurses and emphasized the need of proper provision to prevent the spread of infectious diseases within the hospital.

Dr. Billings was retained to supervise the construction of the hospital. Plans were finally approved and construction was started in June 1877. Building proceeded very slowly, as the cost of construction had to be met out of endowment income and only $100,000 was available each year. When the hospital, consisting of seventeen buildings, was formally opened in May 1889, it had a bed capacity for about 250 patients (see Fig. 5-1).

The medical school did not open until 1893, four years after the hospital had thoroughly established its clinical methods. These methods inaugurated a new era in this country in teaching and in the promotion of scientific inquiry in medicine, surgery, gynecology, obstetrics, pathology, and the clinical laboratory.

The keynote of the whole building program was that the hospital was an integral part of the medical school, ensuring the accessibility of hospital facilities to students. Patterned after the great European hospitals connected with medical schools, the hospital was to teach students the best known methods of caring for the sick and also serve as a great laboratory to advance the knowledge of the causes, processes, and treatment of disease.

The changes in the nurse training school at Hopkins were as radical for nurses as the medical school was for physicians. Many of the innovations were proposed by Miss Nightingale, with whom Dr. Billings conferred concerning both nursing education and hospital construction. The one-year

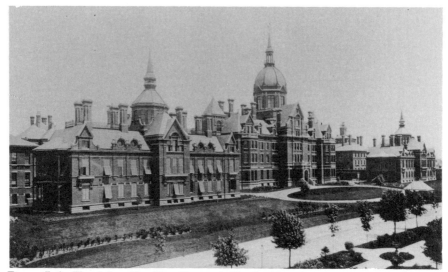

Figure 5–1. The Johns Hopkins Hospital. The building behind the oval in this old
photograph still stands and continues to serve as the main entrance to
the hospital. (Courtesy of The Johns Hopkins Medical Institutions.)

course of training followed by a second year of experience with private
families was replaced with amplified, systematized, and graded instruction
extending through two years. Students were no longer sent to private homes
during the second year. Graduate nurses rather than students were placed in
charge of departments. The nurse training school at Hopkins attained educational status by means of a new curriculum, required attendance at lectures,
and periodic examinations.

So much thought and care were given to planning Johns Hopkins Hospital
that before a single patient had been admitted, the hospital had achieved a
nation-wide and world-wide reputation. It was looked to for all that was best
in medical and nursing education, for liberal and progressive ideas and
methods. A standard was set whose excellence forced other schools and
hospitals to make radical changes as a matter of self-preservation.

In the terminal decades of the century the value of the hospital as an
educational institution for medical students, nurses, and physicians was well
recognized. The public came to realize that certain forms of disease and injury
could be better treated in hospitals than in their own homes. By the end of the
century, hospitals were admitting increasing numbers of paying patients in
special wards and rooms set apart from those for the destitute. Advances in
medical science and nursing care gave infallible proof to the public that
hospitals were essential to the health of the community.

6
Hospitals

MacEachern, in his classic text *Hospital Organization and Management* writes that "the primary function of the hospital, the one which has been constant throughout the whole of its evolution, is to care for the sick and injured. While other important functions have developed, they are all subordinate and are recognized as part of the responsibility of the hospital because they contribute to the care of the sick." (l, p.29).

Later, MacEachern states: "Its single purpose is to receive the human body when for any reason it has become diseased or injured and to care for it in such a manner as to restore it to normal or as nearly normal as possible." (1, p.83). As one looks at the health field, however, one finds all kinds of hospitals, large and small, teaching and nonteaching, nonprofit and for profit, church and community owned, as well as hospitals for special purposes. This complex scene is the result of a long evolutionary process.

GENERAL HOSPITALS

The *general hospital* is the one with which we are most familiar. It provides a variety of diagnostic and therapeutic services for both medical and surgical cases. It is usually thought of an an acute, short-term (30 days or less) institution. At its most advanced development, it handles most every kind of case; it is truly a *general* hospital. But there are, and have always been, compromises on this ideal. In the early part of this century, it was easier for a hospital to approach the ideal, as the ideal was then defined, because the limits of our knowledge and technology did not suggest or permit the sophisticated differentiation that we now find. In those days, there were no antibiotics, no open heart surgery, much less sophisticated radiological and pathological technology, nor were there any of the monitoring devices that one finds today in an intensive-care or coronary-care unit. In those days, the general hospital did do about everything except where tradition, clinical considerations, and/or chronicity dictated that it not handle certain types of cases. The mentally ill represent a good example. With few exceptions, they were relegated to special hospitals. By tradition, they were outside the mainstream of medical care, in large part because the problems those cases presented were beyond clinical competence; the medical doctors simply didn't know enough about the problem to know how their skills could be effectively applied. As a result, the problem of mental illness was essentially a chronic disease, although the symptoms were often acute.

Tuberculosis (TB) patients were similarly separated, and if one goes back far enough, one finds contagious diseases similarly isolated in special hospitals-isolation hospitals, fever hospitals, contagious disease hospitals. In some communities, obstetrical and gynecological cases were reserved for special women's hospitals, as were eye, ear, nose, and throat (EENT) cases; nor should one forget the chronic disease hospitals for children with their special services for the severe cardiac and orthopedic problems. Frequently, some of these special hospitals were started by individual physicians who needed a few beds for their own convenience or to minimize risk of infection from other kinds of cases. Maternity (lying-in) hospitals and EENT hospitals are examples of these. As we shall see, many of these kinds of private hospitals evolved, over time, into larger proprietary hospitals and, in some cases, community hospitals.

The compromises today on the ideal model of a general hospital are very different. No longer is there the need or justification for separate hospitals for TB and contagious disease cases. These can now be prevented or handled on an ambulatory basis: when hospital care is needed, the services of a general hospital are usually more appropriate. Nor is there need for short-term segregation of the mentally ill, though tradition and limited knowledge still keep these patients out of most general hospitals. Today the differentiation and the compromises on the ideal model of a general hospital are dictated, however, largely by technology and cost. Some kinds of cases require highly trained clinicians whose skills cannot be maintained unless they are employed in a large hospital with a high volume of cases. Open-heart surgery would be one example. One would hardly want to be operated on by a cardiac surgeon whose skill is maintained solely in a rural 25-bed general hospital. But cost is another issue, and a related one, for highly specialized services typically require extensive support from other hospital services. An open-heart-surgery team requires, among other things, a good kidney service and sophisticated laboratory support. Neither of these could be justified clinically or economically in a 25-bed general hospital. Thus, general hospitals today are almost always compromises on the ideal, the smaller hospitals tending to compromise more on the ideal than the large ones.

General hospitals today may be sponsored or owned by the community, a church, or simply people belonging to that church, the government, a university, a cooperative, an individual physician or group of physicians, or by investors. The nature of sponsorship may change over the years: some physician-owned and church-sponsored hospitals, for example, have, over the decades, become community sponsored. Some of the latter have retained their original names, thus revealing their church origins. The owners of hospitals do not always operate them. One occasionally hears, for example, of a community general hospital run by one of the Catholic nursing orders, and one hears increasingly of community and church general hospitals that are managed under contract with a professional hospital-management firm.

A *community general hospital* is by definition nonprofit and voluntary. It is nonprofit (some use the phrase not-for-profit) in that it is not required to pay taxes on its income or property, nor does it distribute any leftover monies to any individual as profit. It is voluntary because the development and financial backing of the institution is done voluntarily by citizens without governmental coercion. Responsibility for a community general hospital rests with a board of trustees, members of which are elected. Trustees receive no pay for their services as trustees; are responsible for determining the policies of the institution, the hiring of senior administrators, and the appointment of physicians to the medical staff; act as trustees for the assets that as a board they hold in trust for the community.

Election methods for trustees vary. Some boards are highly restrictive and almost self-perpetuating. In many cases, the trustees are elected by voting members of the hospital corporation, voting members typically securing the privilege of the ballot by having contributed to the hospital. The hospital's charter will define the manner of election. Though the electorate may be nonrepresentative of the total community because the eligible voters may be nonrepresentative (trustees tend to be drawn from the business, banking, industrial and professional leaders in the community), the general view is that the trustees are nonetheless trustees for the total community served by the hospital.

Wing puts this in perspective when he writes (2, pp.147-149):

Because of the considerable amount of trust or reliance being placed in the trustee and the ease with which a trust can be abused, the law holds a trustee to a strict standard of care. Unlike the legal concept of negligence . . ., which requires that each person act reasonably or "nonfoolishly", the actions of trustees are examined much more closely to see if the beneficiaries' interests are actually being served. This special relationship between the beneficiary of a trust and the trustee is called a fiduciary relationship and carries with it this strict basis for liability. The only major difference between a simple trust and the slightly more complex concept of a charitable trust is that a charitable trust can only be formed for designated purposes that the law has defined as benefiting the general public. This would not be satisfied by providing food and shelter to one individual or even several people, but must benefit a sufficiently large group of persons to be serving the public interest . . . The general public can enforce a breach of a fiduciary duty by the trustees through the public's lawyer, the attorney general.

Wing goes on to note:

Most hospitals that were set up originally as charitable trusts have taken advantage of the corporate form of business. Many have organized under special statutes allowing for nonprofit or charitable corporations. As with charitable trusts, this allows donors to give to the corporation and deduct the gift from their federal and state income tax and also allows the corporation to be exempt from state and federal tax on the corporation's income. One important difference between charitable trusts and charitable or nonprofit hospitals is that charitable or nonprofit hospitals are allowed by law to serve the entire public, not just the poor or other "deserving" classes of people.

The reliance on community business, industrial, and professional leaders on hospital boards has long standing historical roots. These people were the very ones who could provide leadership in raising funds to support the hospital, and in a great many cases they underwrote hospital deficits with personal checks. Though the latter practice has declined sharply, these community leaders tend still to dominate the boards because of their ability to exercise influence on behalf of the hospital, because of their valued entrepreneurial skills that are engaged in hospital work without cost to the hospital, and because these people are in positions in which they can readily allocate some of their working time to hospital activities.

The community general hospital, like most general hospitals, may be large or small, teaching or nonteaching. The size of the hospital, typically indicated by the number of beds, depends on the size of the population served, the range of services provided, and whether or not it is used as a referral hospital. A small community may only be able to justify a small general hospital, just large enough to support financially the general run of cases. Depending on the community, this may mean only six or 20 beds, or 75 beds, or 100 beds.

Smaller communities must also limit the range of services provided because the volume of patients may be so small in a specialized area of medicine that not enough patients will use the service to justify the expense of developing and maintaining it. Similarly, in such cases, there would not be enough cases to enable the specialist to maintain his or her skills. In these instances, the more specialized services needed by a patient would be secured by referring the patient to another facility that has been able to put together and maintain that service. As one looks around the country, one can find a number of large community hospitals in relatively small communities whose hospital sizes and complexity are justified by the fact that they are referral hospitals. Generally speaking, however, the larger the community served, the larger the hospital, larger in terms of number of beds, range of specialists, and range of supporting equipment and services.

A community general hospital, like most other general hospitals, may also be a *teaching hospital*. Teaching hospitals were defined by the presence in the hospital of an approved residency or internship program. With the demise of the free-standing internship, the criterion now rests solely on the presence of an approved residency program. It should be emphasized that the presence of nursing or other health professional programs in a hospital does not define whether or not it is a teaching hospital.

It might be noted that historically most teaching hospitals were either public general hospitals for the poor or other types of general hospitals with a large number of indigent patients. These indigent patients were the ones on whom the medical students, interns, and residents learned. The patients, in a sense, paid for their care by allowing their bodies to be used for medical training purposes. The poor frequently resented this form of payment, and they often looked upon the hospital as the place where "they" experimented on patients. It was, in part, this perception by the poor that contributed to the development of Medicaid, under which all people were entitled to private care, but by that time (1966), teaching hospital practice had changed, and all patients—paying as well as indigent—were teaching patients.

The nomenclature is somewhat imprecise, for one often hears a *medical-school hospital* referred to as a teaching hospital. It is, for medical-school hospitals have in training not only undergraduate medical students working for the M.D. or D.O. degree but also residents. On the other hand, many teaching hospitals do not have a significant number of medical students being taught in their hospitals but mainly residents. While there is a developing trend for university medical-school control of graduate medical education in outlying hospitals, the flow of undergraduate medical students to such institutions is small enough to justify the definition of a teaching hospital as one in which there is one or more approved residency training programs. Where a teaching hospital has a major commitment to undergraduate medical education, then that hospital might be called a medical-school hospital. Where the affiliation of a hospital with a medical school is nominal, one can determine whether it is teaching or nonteaching and argue (if one chooses) as to whether or not it even ought to be called a medical school affiliated hospital.

Church general hospitals are almost identical to community general hospitals. They may be small or large, teaching or nonteaching, or medical school. They are different only in that they are owned or heavily influenced by the churches or church groups that sponser them. A large number of Protestant denominations and Catholic orders and dioceses own and operate hospitals. Their roles in this field have deep historical roots. Though rooted in a religious denomination, none are discriminatory in terms of access to care (save the limitation dictated by whether or not one's physician has admitting privileges), although a church hospital may be sensitive to the special spiritual or dietary needs of the denomination that sponsors it. While a Lutheran or Catholic hospital may make heroic efforts to meet the dietary needs, for example, of an Orthodox Jew, a Jewish hospital will be geared to meet such needs routinely. It might be noted, with regard to Jewish sponsored hospitals, that the sponsorship is not by the synagogue or other official body but by the Jewish community.

As suggested earlier, there is a tendency for the churches to lessen the extent of their control of the hospitals. This is reflected in the makeup of their boards on which nonchurch members serve and on which fewer and fewer church officials and ministers serve. This may be a reflection of the increased secularization in American society as well as recognition of the need for many other talents for the successful direction of a hospital.

Government general hospitals are of many types. The federal government owns and operates general hospitals for clientele for whom it is responsible. Specifically, the federal government, through the Department of Defense, has a large number of army, navy, and air force hospitals. While some of these hospitals specialize—mental illness being the most common type of specialized facility—most are general hospitals. The Veterans Administration (VA) also has a large number of hospitals throughout the country to care for veterans with service connected disabilities as well as nonservice connected disabilities when the veteran cannot afford private care. Some of its hospitals are psychiatric, but most are general, with strong rehabilitation medicine services. HEW maintains two types of general hospitals. The first group is administered by HEW's Indian Health Service, with approximately 50 hospitals located on various Indian reservations. The second group of HEW general hospitals are the eight Public Health Service (PHS) hospitals. These hospitals were established in some of our larger seaports and serve merchant marine employees, coast guard employees and their dependents, as well as a number of other federal employees and dependents who are entitled to government care. Several presidents have sought in recent years to turn these hospitals over to the communities in which they are located but have been frustrated in this effort by Congress. Closing a PHS hospital is like closing a military installation: It cuts off federal paying jobs and the general flow of federal monies into that community. Congressmen from the states in which these hospitals are located understandably resist their being closed. General hospital services are also provided by the U.S. Department of Justice for inmates of federal prisons.

State-government general hospitals are of three types. First is the hospital owned and operated by the state as part of the state university medical school operations. These hospitals are more or less under the control of the university medical school. The second type of state general hospital is part of the state penal system. The third type is found in some states—general hospitals to serve poorer sections of the state. Pennsylvania, for example, has a number of state general hospitals serving communities like a community general hospital, that is, with paying patients, except that the governing board is politically appointed, some staff change with changes in the state administration, and the hospital budget is based on state appropriations. Not all states with such hospitals are as patronage oriented.

County and city general hospitals exist in many parts of the country. In the large urban areas, these tend to be indigent hospitals, although since the advent of Medicare and Medicaid and the growth of private health insurance, some of the predominantly indigent hospitals are beginning to take in private patients. The governance of these hospitals by local government will vary from the highly political to the highly professional, depending on the style or pattern of political practice in that area. In the larger cities, these are frequently teaching hospitals and also hospitals with strong medical-school ties. Some famous hospitals are in this group, including Bellevue in New York, Cook County in Illinois, D.C. General in the District of Columbia, Boston City Hospital, and Baltimore City Hospitals.

One other type of governmental general hospital is one established by a special governmental hospital district or authority. Like school districts, these special governmental authorities typically have certain taxing powers as well as authority to establish and run the hospital. These hospitals tend to be similar to community general hospitals.

University general hospitals are controlled by most, but not all, university medical schools. As noted earlier, state universities usually have de facto control of the university medical school hospital, although ultimate ownership is by the state government. Other medical schools control their hospitals in similar ways except that ultimate control may rest with the university board of trustees. There are, of course, many variations and gradations vis-à-vis ownership and control. Some medical schools do not have their own hospitals but rely, instead, on affiliated institutions. Tradition, along with the affiliation agreements, may give the medical school considerable control of the institution even though it does not own or manage it.

Cooperative general hospitals are very similar to community general hospitals except that they are generally organized with strong consumer control, and medical services are provided by physicians in group practice.

All the above are either government or nongovernment hospitals, and all are nonprofit by virtue of their governmental status or their having met the state's requirements for nonprofit standing.

Another type general hospital exists, however, and that is the *for-profit* or *proprietary institution*. These are *investor-owned hospitals*—owned by one person or a group on a partnership basis or a corporation. In the United States, these hospitals are often called private hospitals. The word "private," however, can be misleading, for in some other countries "private" refers to nongovernmental, and a private hospital in those countries can be either nonprofit or for profit.

Over the decades, the picture with regard to these hospitals has changed considerably. At the time of Flexner, it was estimated that 56% of the hospitals in the nation were proprietary (3). Since then, there has been a steady decline to 25% in 1941, and 11% in 1968. In recent years, the number of proprietary hospitals and their beds have increased to nearly 13% of the nonfederal hospitals and nearly 8% of the nonfederal beds. These figures (13% and 8%) were derived from AHA data (4) and indicate that proprietary hospitals tend to be smaller than nonprofit hospitals.

Most of the proprietary hospitals were originally set up by physicians to meet local needs. As one leafs through the AHA *Guide to the Health Care Field*, which is issued annually and lists all hospitals, one can hypothesize that those very small 10 and 13-bed general hospitals today that are owned by individual physicians continue in that tradition. Generally, however, the individual physician owned hospital has given way to the larger institutions because of population shifts, increased costs, and the necessities of modern clinical practice. Some of the very small institutions that continue to exist undoubtedly have a very limited range of services, in many cases they may be nothing more than facilities for relatively minor cases, holding beds for the eventual transfer of the more acutely ill patient.

Among the proprietary general hospitals are a number that are controlled by a partnership. These are very similar to the single-ownership hospitals. One finds the partnership arrangement relatively common among the proprietary, nongeneral, or specialized hospitals.

It might be noted here that *doctors'* hospitals, in which the words *doctor* or *doctors* appear, may be profit or nonprofit. Some were established, as noted two paragraphs above, to meet community needs, there being no alternative. Some were established as a result of professional conflicts within an existing hospital, one group breaking off to establish its own institution. Some were established by physicians who were unable to secure hospital privileges in existing institutions. Some, as noted with ENT hospitals, may have developed as institutions in which specialized therapy could be administered in what the physician felt was a more controlled environment. Some came about because of physician frustration with lay administration—how the institution was run and what was and was not purchased. Some were developed as a vehicle for making money over and above the income from professional practice. These reasons apply, of course, to all physician owned hospitals whether they use the word *doctors* or not. There is a tendency for all of these hospitals to evolve into nonprofit institutions, though this is not without its problems: in mid-1978, in northern Virginia, one such hospital wanted to become a nonprofit institution, but the move was opposed by local government because of the adverse effect this would have on the tax base of local government.

Among the proprietary hospitals, the corporately owned hospital is perhaps the most important. There have developed a number of corporations that build, own, and/or operate general and special hospitals. American Medicorp of Bala Cynwyd, Pennsylvania owns 41 hospitals, manages eight other proprietary hospitals, manages eight nonprofit hospitals, and has three hospitals under construction. Hospital Affiliates International of Nashville, Tennessee, owns 43 hospitals, manages nine proprietary hospitals, manages 59 nonprofit hospitals, including one that is overseas, and has under construction nine other hospitals (six of which are nonprofit). Hospital Corporation of America, also Nashville based, either owns, manages, or has under construction 111 hospitals. Humana Incorporated of Louisville, Kentucky has 58 hospitals. There are, in addition, some 30 other corporations that own or manage hospitals. That this is business is perhaps best illustrated by the Ramada Medical Corporation, which is a wholly owned subsidiary of Ramada Inns, Inc. For further information on these companies, one can consult the annual *Directory of Investor-Owned Hospitals and Hospital Management Companies*, which is issued by the Federation of American Hospitals, the federation being their organization. It should be noted that not all investor-owned hospitals are owned by the multihospital management corporations.

Many of the investor-owned hospitals are also members of AHA and are accredited by the JCAH. Not all the investor-owned hospitals are general hospitals; many are psychiatric institutions. In Maryland, for example, of the six investor-owned hospitals, three are psychiatric hospitals that have been in operation for quite some time. Each has permitted a group of psychiatrists to carry out psychotherapy in what they felt was the most appropriate setting.

Sometimes these kinds of hospitals, which were started by physicians, provided the optimal therapeutic milieu as they saw it.

Some of the community and church general hospitals have turned to these management corporations for management for a fee. Some, as we noted from the data cited above, have turned to these corporations to build their hospitals as well. Some *investor-owned* hospitals have also turned to these corporations for management. Of the 986 operational general and special investor-owned hospitals in the United States that are listed in the 1978 directory, only 438 are owned by the management corporations. Of the remaining 548, 62 turned to the management corporation for management; the others were self-managed. The management corporations also managed 179 nonprofit hospitals in the United States. Some of the corporations owned or managed hospitals in foreign countries, but they are not counted in the above figures, nor are the hospitals under construction.

The investor-owned hospitals are controversial. To appreciate the controversy, one needs to recognize that they labor still under the shadow cast by the very large number of proprietary hospitals that existed before the national hospital accreditation program began in 1952, a shadow that raised many questions about quality of care in proprietary hospitals in terms of the qualifications of the doctors and nurses and the appropriateness of their services, the cleanliness and overall safety of the facility, and so on. The situation is different today in that most of the hospitals are accredited by JCAH and are further monitored by the Professional Standards Review Organization (PSROs). There are, in other words, insufficient data to support the assertion that quality of care or efficiency of care is below the average standard of the other general hospitals.

The investor-owned hospitals suggest that it is possible to provide quality care, with efficiency, at costs comparable or below those of other general hospitals and make a profit as well. The nonprofit hospitals contend, on the other hand, that the proprietary hospitals tend to be small and are thus able to handle the easy cases, leaving the tougher and more expensive kinds of care to the nonprofit institutions. This, the non-profits argue, forces their average costs up. The proprietary hospitals, they also argue, make a profit on the easy cases, which "profit" in the nonprofit hospitals would be an offset against the more expensive cases.

The answers in this debate are not available. It is true that 57% of the 986 investor-owned hospitals have less than 100 beds and that 85% have less than 200. The economics of the health field dictate that these hospitals can only handle a limited range of cases and cannot justify much of the very sophisticated equipment and services. Significantly, 58% of these hospitals are located in five states: California, Florida, Tennessee, Texas, and New York. Stewart suggests a partial reason for this(3):

In New England, where churches were established with broad social base, voluntary institutions were readily made available. In other areas of the United States, like California, charitable institutions did not have the capacity to establish enough hospital facilities. Consequently, the responsibility was frequently left to the physician; or in keeping with Mexican-American attitude of individual paternalistic social responsibility, to a wealthy benefactor.

In support of this notion, it is worth noting that California, Florida, and Texas have been high-population-growth states. Other factors have undoubtedly been operative.

As a final note on the definition of different types of general hospitals: The description of general hospitals applies to both *allopathic* and *osteopathic* institutions. While the allopathic (M.D.) oriented institutions predominate in this country, the same types of hospital control apply also to the hospitals that were established to serve osteopaths. The separation has historical roots—when neither would relate to the other school of medicine. But times have changed, and now D.O.s serve on the staffs of allopathic institutions and M.D.s on the staffs of osteopathic hospitals. In some communities, mergers of the institutions have been talked about and consummated.

Before considering the organization of the general hospital and factors affecting its operation, we might digress briefly to describe some of the other kinds of hospitals that exist.

SPECIAL HOSPITALS

Sponsorship of the special hospitals will vary from community to church to government to investor-owned to university. Government control, as we shall note, is particularly prominent in the areas of mental illness and mental retardation.

Maternity or lying-in hospitals are declining in importance. At one time, they were very sensible types of institutions, segregating a relatively simple condition from the general hospital-type patient and minimizing thereby the risks of infection. They provided, moreover, a setting for delivery and for care of the newborn child that many felt was an improvement over home delivery. The costs of maintaining such specialized facilities, particularly with the support services needed to handle the more complicated deliveries, have militated against their survival. While some continue to exist, they tend to merge with other institutions to achieve economies of scale and the resources for survival.

Womens' hospitals are very similar. They generally handle deliveries as well as gynecological cases. In some instances, they have become general hospitals for female patients either out of economic necessity for survival or to provide, in the old days, that type of care fit for ladies. These hospitals, as they face the rising cost demand and the need for more complete support services, are finding it difficult to go it alone, and there is a tendency for them to merge with other institutions. Some of these hospitals also handle pediatrics.

EENT, ENT, and *eye hospitals* are specialized facilities that frequently were developed by one or a few doctors to deal with those problems in a special setting. They still exist but, like the others, often have difficulty in maintaining their independence both financially and technologically. Survival of special hospitals such as are described above and below can sometimes be achieved by affiliation—as distinct from merger—with other institutions.

Children's hospitals are typically special facilities dealing mainly but not exclusively with chronic and congenital cardiac and orthopedic-pediatric problems. Whether needed surgical care is performed in these hospitals or in other institutions will vary. Advances in technology and scientific medicine generally dictate a close affiliation with other hospitals in order to benefit from the latest instrumentation and the now essential supporting specialties and services. Typically, these hospitals will have a strong service in rehabilitation medicine.

Rehabilitation hospitals have developed to rehabilitate the chronically ill to a maximum level of functioning, the patients for whom cure is probably not possible but whose level of functioning can be improved. These include amputees, spinal-cord injuries, stroke victims, and so forth. These are generally long-term care facilities in which, by definition, the average length of stay for all patients is more than 30 days. As might be expected, these institutions are strong in the physical medicine and rehabilitation specialty.

Chronic disease hospitals are difficult to describe because they vary so much from each other. Clearly they are, by definition, long-term care, that is, average length of stay is more than 30 days. Generally, they do not include the mentally ill or mentally retarded. Beyond that, one has to look at each institution. Some are simply convalescent facilities; some are repositories for the incurably ill, both chronic and terminal; some are rehabilitation facilities; some are homes for the aged with perhaps a few infirmary beds.

Hospices are beginning to develop as specialized facilities to care for the terminally ill, giving special attention to the relief of pain and spiritual support for both patient and family. While many hospices are facility based, some function as community service agencies visiting and caring for patients in their homes and in other facilities.

Mental hospitals, like general hospitals, are controlled by different groups. State governments and, in some instances, local governments have been primarily responsible for establishing facilities for the care of the mentally ill.

The *state mental hospitals* have tended to be remote facilities in the countryside and underfinanced. Patients were frequently there for extended periods of time, sometimes for decades. In recent years, governments have sought to close these facilities since current theory holds that most of the mentally ill can be dealt with in community settings, either community facilities or on an outpatient basis. Like all hospitals, and particularly like the chronic disease hospitals, the patient mix is not always as the institution's mission dictates. The mental hospital in the United States, as in many other countries, has been called on to deal not only with the mentally ill but also to shelter many aged persons for whom there is no appropriate community facility or home. In government mental hospitals, moreover, one frequently finds mentally retarded patients who were inappropriately placed and sometimes other patients who suffer primarily from chronic physical illnesses.

As large institutions, the need exists for full medical and surgical services as well as psychiatric services. In some hospitals, the surgical services are on the grounds; in other hospitals, the patients are transferred to a general hospital for surgery and, as necessary, for more specialized medical consultation and testing. Because these institution are underfinanced and consequently understaffed, they have attracted a large number of FMGs whose native language is not English and who are not fully licensed. Since care of the mentally ill requires extensive verbal interaction with the patient and understanding of the patient's values and social milieu, the FMG staffing patterns are cause for considerable concern. The concern is heightened when so few of the FMGs pass the state licensing exams. The understaffing of these hospitals has frequently led to a backup of patients in the admission wards with resulting delays in diagnostic workups, delays sometimes lasting more than a month. The understaffing has also led many hospitals to warehouse patients, to store them without providing an active treatment program. This has been the subject of some litigation, and courts have been ordering states either to provide treatment or release the patients.

Nongovermental mental hospitals have been developed by church groups, by the community, and by individual or groups of physicians. The sponsorship implications are the same as for general hospitals. The nongovermental hospitals are generally better staffed, providing prompt diagnostic workups and active treatment programs for all patients. The cost is much more than in government institutions. Supporting medical and surgical services are as in government hospitals except that since these hospitals tend to be smaller, the range of resident services tend to be less, and rarely are major surgical services provided.

There is a slight nomenclature issue that ought to be noted. In the general hospital setting, "private" hospitals in the United States are usually equated with "investor owned" or "for profit." While this use of "private" is imprecise, it is still used commonly. In other countries, "private" typically refers to nongovernmental institutions that may be nonprofit or for profit. The word private, when applied to mental hospitals in the United States, conforms to the foreign practice and refers to "nongovernnmental"—church, voluntary, and investor owned.

Turning from the mentally ill to the mentally retarded, we find a similar situation, that is, most hospital care is provided in government institutions that tend to be located in remote settings and to be understaffed and underfinanced. Most of these institutions are typically known as *state schools and hospitals*. Training and education are an important part of the work with the mentally retarded; hence, the coupling of "state school" with "hospital."

We have dealt previously with *TB hospitals* and *contagious-disease hospitals*, noting that they are disappearing. There are many other kinds of special hospitals for special diseases or conditions—cancer, leprosy, alcoholism, orthopedics, burns, epilepsy, cardiac ailments, geriatrics—as well as for research. For research, one can cite the Rockefeller University Hospital (40 beds) in New York City or the Clinical Center (541 beds) of the NIH in Bethesda, Maryland, or St. Jude Children's Research Hospital (48 beds) in Memphis. Or one could cite the National Jewish Hospital and Research Center (200 beds) in Denver, which focuses on asthma, clinical immunology, tuberculosis, and chest diseases. Some examples of other special hospitals: For orthopedics there is, in Los Angeles, the Orthopaedic Hospital (162 beds). For heart disease, one can site the Miami Heart Institute (258 beds) in Miami Beach. For alcoholism, there is the Caron Hospital, which is part of the 83-bed Chit Chat Farms in Wernersville, Pennsylvania. One should not forget the college and university infirmaries. Leafing through the AHA *Guide to the Health Care Field* can be a rewarding experience in terms of the variety of institutions, their origins (as indicated by their names as well as by type of control), their sizes, their services, and their mergers.

One should bear in mind that the definitions that apply to the various hospitals are not rigid. As noted at the outset, all hospitals, general and special, are in a sense compromises on the concept of total hospital. Not only do hospitals in each category differ from each other in scope of services, but also they differ in patient mix. Whereas a special hospital may exist in one community, the same kind of hospital in another community may be part of a broader based institution. Specialized hospitals sometimes developed because of the presence of a benefactor, sometimes because a physician had a unique therapeutic approach that could best or easily be handled separately. What is clear, however, is that rising costs, coupled with new technology and the interdependency of the various specialties, are dictating affiliations and mergers. Completely free-standing institutions, including the very small general hospitals, are dying breeds.

HOSPITAL STATISTICS

The most reliable source for data about hospitals is the AHA. The AHA conducts each year a survey of all hospitals that are registered with the association. Not all registered hospitals are accredited institutions or members of the AHA. All registered general hospitals do have, however, at least six inpatient beds, an organized medical staff, continuous nursing services, a pharmacy service supervised by a registered pharmacist, a governing authority and chief executive, up-to-date and complete medical records on each patient, food service, clinical laboratory and diagnostic x-ray services, an operating room, and control of patient admission by the medical staff. While anatomical pathology services need not be present, they must be regularly and conveniently available(5, pp.5,6). Comparable requirements are listed by the AHA for registration of special hospitals. The listings are as complete as one can find. (It includes both allopathic and osteopathic facilities.) It might be weak at the interface with nursing homes, some of which are listed but most of which are not.

The results of the AHA annual survey are published in two volumes each year. One volume, *Guide to the Health Care Field*, lists all registered hospitals, their addresses and telephone numbers, the names of the administrators, and for each hospital, information about its control, type of services—and specific services, whether it is a long-term or short-term stay hospital—as well as data on its admissions, expenses, and personnel. The *guide* also lists the names, addresses, telephone numbers, and chief executives of a large number of international, national, and state health organizations and agencies. It also lists many of the educational programs in the health field.

The companion volume to the *Guide to the Health Care Field* is *Hospital Statistics*, which provides a composite statistical profile of all registered institutions. It does it nationally, by region, and by state. It does it by hospital size and hospital sponsorship. One can quickly ascertain how many hospitals there are in the United States (7,082 in 1976), how many beds they had (1,433,515), how many admissions there were (36,776,000), what the average occupancy was (76%), and how many outpatient visits there were (270,951,000). One can get information on births, the number of bassinets, the number of employees, payroll expenses, costs, revenues, total assets, and average length of stay. There are data on the number of nurses, physicians, dentists, and LPNs employed by the hospitals, the number of residents and other trainees, the number of surgical operations, and a breakdown on the outpatient visits in categories of emergency, clinic, and referred. There are data on the number of postoperative recovery rooms, intensive-care units for cardiac care only, intensive-care units for mixed patients, open-heart-surgery facilities, pharmacies and how staffed, x-ray therapy, cobalt therapy, radium therapy, diagnostic radiois-otope facilities, therapeutic radioisotope facilities, histopathology laboratories, organ banks, blood banks, electroencephalographic services, respiratory ther-apy departments, premature nurseries, neonatal intensive-care units, self-care units, skilled nursing or long-term care units (many general hospitals have or are developing these units as part of their complexes), hemodialysis services, burn-care units, physical therapy departments, occupational therapy depart-ments, rehabilitation services, psychiatric services (including inpatient, outpa-tient, partial hospitalization, emergency, foster care and/or home care, consul-tation and educational), clinical psychology services, outpatient departments, emergency departments, social work departments, family-planning services, genetic counseling services, abortion services, home care departments, dental services, pediatric services, speech pathology services, hospital auxiliaries, volunteer services departments, patient representative services, alcoholism/chemical-dependency services, and TB and other respiratory disease units.

Other useful reports are issued periodically by HEW. Among these is *Health-United States*, an annual report by the secretary to the Congress. The *Social Security Bulletin* regularly contains useful analyses. The National Center for Health Statistics within HEW issues a large number of reports throughout each year. The Health Care Financing Administration has initiated a new publication, *Health Care Financing Review*, which will take over somewhat from the *Social Security Bulletin*, and a new series, *Health Care Financing Trends*.

HOSPITAL ORGANIZATION AND ADMINISTRATION

The governing board of a hospital not only establishes policies for the institution but also hires the administrator and other key personnel. The board also grants admitting privileges to physicians and dentists and others, usually on recom-mendation of the medical staff.

The administrator of a hospital may have been trained for that role with a baccalaureate degree in health administration or with a master's degree in that field from some graduate program. Some administrators have no formal academic training in the health field. Many hospitals, however, have as their administrator a nurse; some of these are small rural hospitals; many are Catholic hospitals run by the various nursing orders. The rationale for the nurse as administrator in the smaller hospitals is based on the fact that nurses constitute the largest body of specialized personnel in the institution. These hospitals, moreover, because of their relatively small size, have a limited range of services, and the complexities of management may not require specialized training. Many of the very large hospitals have physicians as the administrator, only some of whom have special training. Mental hospitals characteristically have a psychiatrist as administrator.

The organizational functioning of a hospital is not as clear-cut as it is in business and industry. The lines of authority are not precise. The board appoints the administrator and his or her chief deputies. The board also appoints the medical staff. While the medical staff is technically accountable to the board, it has a daily functional relationship with the administrator. Nursing service is administratively accountable to the administrator but professionally accountable to the medical staff. Other personnel, such as the pharmacists, lab and x-ray technicians, and dietitians, are also administratively accountable to the administrator but professionally accountable to the medical staff.

The hospital is really the physician's workshop, although some argue that it is now the center for meeting all community health needs. However, it is only the physician who can admit a patient (except in a few circumscribed areas in which admitting and treatment privileges are held by dentists), and all others must act on the physician's orders. But the physician typically does not hire or fire unless, as a member of the medical staff, the physician is an employee of the hospital. But even then the physician's authority is circumscribed by a certain administrative accountability to the administrator.

Thus, the physician asks that something be done for the patient or that certain supplies or equipment be purchased. It is up to the administrator and the nurses and others working with the administrator to cooperate to the greatest extent possible with the physician. As one might guess, blocks and conflicts occur: Personality clashes, misunderstandings, as well as insufficient funds create problems. The various parties try to work out the problems—to resolve differences, to figure out ways to get the needed funds, and to reach agreement on outstanding issues. When the medical staff and administrator cannot resolve differences, then the board must enter to decide.

A number of courses of action have been proposed over the years to make the hospital function more smoothly. One proposal is that physicians should be on the board; in some institutions, this has taken place. Some hospitals are shifting to the corporate model of organization, making the administrator president of the hospital with membership on the board and the medical staff reporting to the president. Some contend that this creates the form but not the substance of a good organization because in most hospitals the physicians are not employees and will talk and badger anyone they care to, and there is little the president can do about it whether the president is a trained administrator or a physician.

In practice, the hospital tends to function reasonably well; over the years, accepted patterns of functioning have been agreed to so that each group knows what its role is, what its responsibilities are, and what its authority is. The medical staff, in particular, has delegated to it by the board certain professional responsibilities, and these are typically described by the medical staff bylaws, which the board has approved. More importantly, however, the smooth functioning can be attributed to improved quality of administration, which came with the introduction of sound management practices and appropriately trained administrators.

MEDICAL STAFF PRIVILEGES

Physicians apply to a hospital for staff privileges. If the hospital is a closed group practice hospital, then the only way to become part of the hospital staff is to be accepted by the medical group. Hospital bylaws will define how a physician may secure admitting privileges. Typically, in community general hospitals, the physician who seeks privileges makes application to the board. The board typically seeks the advice of its medical staff. It judges the applicant's qualifications and character and makes a recommendation. The decision on appointment to the medical staff is based on a variety of factors and not just whether the physician is licensed and of good character. Specific items considered include such things as what kinds of admitting privileges are sought? Does the physician seek surgical privileges? If so, what kind? Is the applicant qualified for that kind of surgery? Do the qualifications warrant authority to read electrocardiograms? Is the applicant qualified to treat the kinds of patients for whom admitting privileges are sought? Does the hospital have the needed support services for this physician? Are there enough beds to accomodate his or her patients?

The larger and more complex the hospital, the more precisely defined the admitting privileges are. In some remote rural hospitals, a family practitioner may be doing general medical care, reading electrocardiograms, handling obstetrics, and performing a variety of surgical operations. The same physician moving to a large urban teaching hospital might be restricted to carefully circumscribed family practice privileges—no reading of ECGs, no obstetrics, no surgery.

Staff privileges also fall into several categories. The *active medical staff* consists of those physicians accorded all rights and privileges and responsibilities; they provide most of the care, leadership in various committees, and may hold a variety of medical staff offices.

Associate medical staff is for the more junior physicians or for those who wish to become active staff when vacancies occur. Their access to beds for their patients may be limited.

The *courtesy medical staff* is the category for those physicians who seek the privilege of admitting only occasional patients and who do not wish to become part of the active staff either because the bulk of their admissions are to other hospitals or because the physicians do not seek or have practices that necessitate frequent admission of patients.

The *consulting medical staff* consists of those who serve primarily as specialty consultants to members of the active staff. In some types of cases, for example, the law or hospital or medical-staff bylaws may require the attending physician to secure consultation, and this staff is available in the event an appropriate consultant is not on the active or associate staffs.

The *honorary medical staff* is reserved for distinguished physicians whom the hospital may wish to honor as well as those members of the active staff who have retired.

The medical staff organization—its bylaws, rules and regulations, and its offices—will vary from hospital to hospital. Typically, however, each staff has what is usually called a chief of staff. This physician is usually elected by the medical staff for a fixed term and represents the staff's interests to the board and to the hospital administration. This is the formal line for communication, particularly on major issues, but hospitals also have a wide informal mechanism that functions as the rule. In some hospitals, the chief of staff is called the medical director. Usually, this signifies that the physician is full time and salaried and appointed by the board. Full-time salaried physicians, other than radiologists, pathologists, anesthesiologists, and emergency-room physicians, are usually found in the larger teaching hospitals. When a hospital has divided its staff into clinical departments or services, there is typically a chief of service for each clinical area, and each chief reports to the chief of staff.

CLINICAL AND SUPPORTING DEPARTMENTS

The clinical organization of the general hospital will vary depending on its size (typically indicated by the number of beds), the pattern of patient mix among the various specialties, and the extent of specialization of the medical staff. Except in the very small hospitals, obstetrics tend to be segregated in a separate wing or on a separate floor of the hospital along with the newborn nursery. This is principally done to minimize the risks of infection to the newborn and mother. Pediatric cases also tend to be segregated. The assignment of other patients to clinical services or departments will vary considerably. If there is any departmental breakdown in the smaller hospitals, it will tend to be into medicine and surgery, with patient assignment as appropriate. As specialization increases in a hospital and an increased volume of patients within each specialty, there is a tendency for departments to be established with beds assigned to that specialty. Where the volume of patients is sufficient to justify it, the specialty beds may be located in a separate wing or on a separate floor. The establishment of specialty services with assigned beds permits a more effective and efficient concentration of support services that are peculiar to that specialty—equipment, specially trained nurses and other personnel—and contributes to the development of the specialty and its scientific work. In very large hospitals, one may find not only separate pediatric and obstetric units but also separate units or floors or wings for most of the medical specialties, and in some cases even for some of the subspecialties.

While assignment of beds to a given specialty has clinical advantages, it decreases institutional flexibility in terms of bed use. There may be more patients needing admission in medicine, for example, then there are beds to accomodate them, yet there may be empty beds on one of the surgical floors that normally cannot be used for those medical patients. Why not? Because the surgical floor may not be staffed or supplied to handle medical cases, and the surgical specialists would be very upset to find the beds assigned to them used to service medical cases. The surgeons may find, if the beds were used to service medical cases, that they cannot admit their patients, and the delays may well cut into the surgeons' incomes and interfere with efforts to strengthen the surgical service. If a hospital wants to build or strengthen a clinical service, it usually has to give assurances to the specialists that they will have an appropriate environment in which to do their work. Part of that is beds.

This is perhaps illustrated by a community that was seeking a urologist. One visited, was impressed, and then asked, "How many beds will I have?" He was told that he would have to queue up like the other physicians; he gets a bed if one is available. The urologist replied, "I have five beds assigned to me in the community where I am presently located; I see no reason why I should move to this community."

There are two additional units of the general hospital that need to be identified because of the increased importance they play. The first of these is the *emergency room*, and the second is the *outpatient* or *ambulatory services* (or *care*) department.

Historically, the smaller hospitals handled emergencies by calling on a member of the medical staff who happened to be in the hospital at the time. Night coverage was frequently handled by members of the active staff taking turns sleeping in the hospital to handle any emergencies that arose. In teaching hospitals, the interns and residents handled the emergency rooms. In recent years, there has developed a trend whereby emergency rooms are staffed by full-time physicians 24 hours a day; more recently, these physicians have undergone special training in trauma medicine. The emergency room is not only for emergencies. It has become also the family physician at night and on weekends. One even hears of patients calling up at night to find out which of the emergency room physicians is on duty in hopes of getting to see the one they prefer. Emergency room physicians are typically paid a salary and receive, in many hospitals, a percentage of the business over a certain amount.

The *outpatient* or *ambulatory-care department* was a feature common to many of the larger general hospitals, particularly teaching hospitals. Generally speaking, it provided a wide range of specialty consultation services for physicians in the community and, in particular, for those patients who could not afford private consultation. Because these departments often duplicated the services available from private specialists in the community, the departments were largely for care of the poor except in those areas in which community-based specialists were not readily available. Recent surgical practice developments, whereby an increased amount of surgery is performed on an ambulatory basis (in and out on the same day), surgery that had previously required two- and three-day admissions, have prompted more general hospitals to develop ambulatory care or outpatient departments. Further encouragement for this was the tendency for an increased number of other specialists to enter salaried

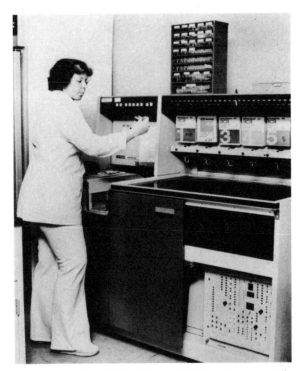

Figure 6–1. Automated chemical analyzer. This unit can perform 30 discrete chemistry tests on blood and other fluids. Approximate 1978 cost, $125,000. (Courtesy, Hamot Medical Center, Erie, Pennsylvania.)

hospital practice. In some instances, these ambulatory services may be provided in the emergency room. This is likely to occur in smaller hospitals in which space is at a premium. Ambulatory surgery is, of course, less costly than the surgery done on an inpatient basis, and it frees inpatient beds for other cases. In some hospitals, it may even cause the institution to be overbedded, that is, to have more beds than it needs. We might note here that whether or not a hospital has too many beds is normally determined by its occupancy rate, the average percentage of beds occupied over a fixed period of time. Most authorities suggest that the occupancy rate should be between 80% and 90%, which allows for room renovations, emergencies, and weekend and holiday drops in occupancy.

Some of the larger teaching hospitals are developing departments of *family medicine*. These departments serve as family physician to a community or to an enrolled group.

Supporting these patient-care services are three medically supervised departments: *anesthesiology, radiology,* and *pathology*. In smaller hospitals, these

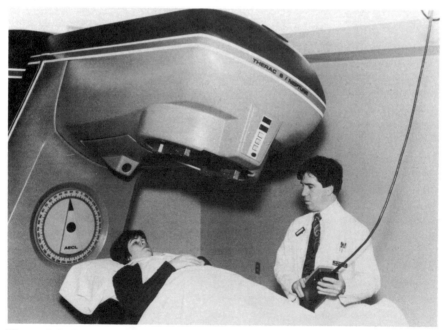

Figure 6–2. Linear accelerator. This radiation therapy machine is a major instrument in the treatment of cancer patients. Approximate 1978 cost, $210,000. (Courtesy, Hamot Medical Center, Erie, Pennsylvania.)

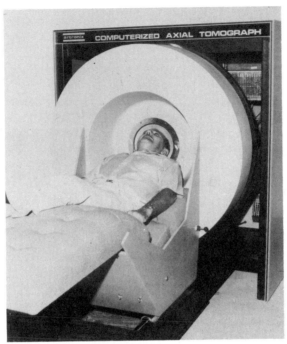

Figure 6–3. CAT scanner. Computerized axial tomography (CAT) is a highly sensitive radiological device that produces detailed pictures of any portion of the head or body, including areas that could not be visualized with previous radiological equipment. This head scanner cost in 1978 about $150,000. (Courtesy, Hamot Medical Center, Erie, Pennsylvania.)

may be supervised by part-time specialists; in larger hospitals, however, the specialists are full time, paid by salary, salary plus a percentage of the business, or sometimes on a fee for service basis. Both radiology and pathology are rapidly expanding departments due to rapidly developing technology (Figs. 6-1—6-5)

All hospitals have, of course, a number of other support services. Whether they have departmental status or not depends on the size of the institution and the rationale of those responsible for establishing the organizational arrangements. Some of these services are nursing, pharmacy, medical records, dietary. Larger hospitals will also have such services as inhalation therapy, physical therapy, occupational therapy, and medical social work.

Increasingly, hospitals are seeking new ways to cope with rising costs. *Shared services*—services shared with other hospitals—such as laundry, purchasing, and computers is one such mechanism. Whether a hospital participates in a

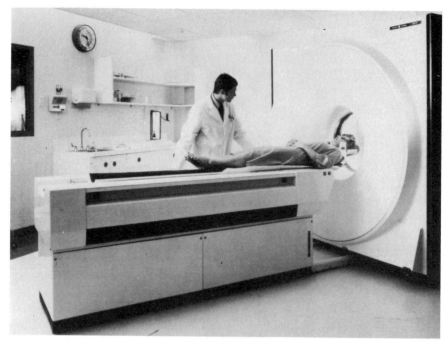

Figure 6–4. Whole-body CAT scanner. This advanced unit cost in 1979 between $615,000 and $735,000. (Courtesy of General Electric Co.)

given shared service depends on whether its needs can be adequately met in this way and whether it is economically advantageous.

PRIVATE, SEMIPRIVATE, AND WARD BEDS

Most general-hospital beds fall in one of these categories. *Private-room* beds are for only one patient and provide for a maximum amount of privacy. They cost more than *semiprivate rooms*, which have two or more beds in them. Most health insurance coverage is for care in a semiprivate room, with the patient paying an additional amount if he or she elects a private room. (Some health insurance policies will pay for private room care if the private room is medically necessary.) *Ward beds* were historically for charity cases, and they were usually in a large room with beds (sometimes as many as 100 or more) lined up on each side, some of which were placed in the middle of the ward. While some wards such as this still exist, there is a tendency for these beds to be in smaller rooms of from five to eight beds. The use of the word *ward* is

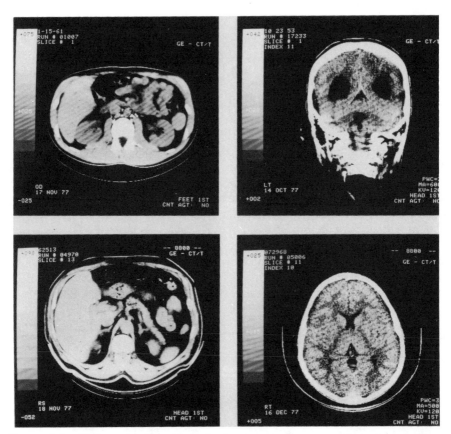

Figure 6–5. CAT scans. The whole body scanner is a versatile unit permitting patient scans feet first or head first. The two scans on the left are abdominal scans, and the scans on the right are head scans. (Courtesy of General Electric Co.)

perhaps becoming obsolete in the charity sense because most patients are now covered by some form of insurance.

The distribution in the number of beds between private, semiprivate and ward will vary from hospital to hospital.

HOSPITAL LICENSURE AND ACCREDITATION

Hospitals are licensed to operate by state governments, and each state has its own requirements. Generally, the various states have focused their attention for licensure on hospital physical plants—fire safety, heating, space allocations, sanitation, and so on. Very few states have moved beyond this to tie licensure to professional standards. In 1978, Pennsylvania sought to move in this direction and found itself sued by the hospital association and a number of its member hospitals. They argued that the state, in seeking to set optimal standards, was exceeding its authority, that state standards, as in all state regulatory matters, must be minimal standards, the floor below which the hospital may not go. Among the concerns was that by state-mandated optimal standards, the state could conceivably bankrupt every hospital in the state. The concern was more than just "We don't want regulation"; the state's track record in support of health services was not one that would make any person believe the state could do a better job if it did bankrupt the hospitals. More to the point, however, is that government has rarely been a leader in raising standards; it has almost always come from the nongovernmental sectors. So, too, in matters relating to hospitals.

We noted in an earlier chapter that the ACS suppressed its 1919 hospital inspection report because the conditions it found were so poor. The ACS and the AMA, however, worked consistently for reform of hospitals. While they were concerned, as were the states, with physical plants, these professional bodies were also concerned with matters relating to quality of care.

Their efforts at reform culminated in 1952 with the initiation of a hospital-accreditation program by the JCAH.

JOINT COMMISSION ON ACCREDITATION OF HOSPITALS (JCAH)

The history, philosophy, and activities of the JCAH are described in the *JCAH Corporate Brochure*, from which the following excerpts are taken (6, pp.2-3, 5, 8-9):

THE HISTORY OF THE JOINT COMMISSION

The history of the Joint Commission on Accreditation of Hospitals began, essentially, in 1913 when the American College of Surgeons was formed. The College's charter included an expression of intent to improve the care of the American hospital patient. Its Articles of Incorporation stated that:

> . . .some system of standardization of hospitals and hospital work should be developed. In this way patients and the public will have some means of recognizing those institutions devoted to the highest ideals of medicine.

The College soon saw how imperative the need was for such a "system of standardization." A surgeon's application for admission to the College required the submission of 100 medical records of patients upon whom he had operated. Sixty percent of otherwise approvable candidates were rejected because of the miserably poor records kept in hospitals. It was also discovered that a large number of hospitals lacked organized medical staffs and services essential to the surgeon, such as laboratory, X-ray, and other diagnostic facilities.

In 1915, in an effort to improve these conditions, the College allocated $500 to establish standards for hospitals. By 1917, with the financial assistance of the Carnegie Foundation, a list of standards was compiled. It was one page long and was called the "Minimum Standard for Hospitals."

In 1918, the College began on-site inspections of hospitals of over 100 beds. Of nearly 700 hospitals inspected, only 89 could meet the minimum standard. In the basement of the Waldorf Astoria Hotel in New York, the list of approved hospitals was burned. To the embarrassment of the profession, some of the country's most prestigious hospitals were omitted from the list. The College decided to release the statistics, but not the names. The mere publication of the figures, however, so shocked physicians, administrators, and trustees that widespread support of a hospital standardization program was obtained. With this support, the program grew over the next 33 years until more than 3,000 hospitals were able to meet the minimum standards.

As the success of the standardization program increased, so did the costs. By 1950, more than two million dollars had been spent on the program, and the College began to feel the financial strain. Membership dues, the College's only source of income, were not enough. So reiterating its belief in the broad, general approach, but unable to continue sole support of the growing program, the College solicited the participation of other national professional organizations.

Subsequently, the American College of Physicians, the American Hospital Association, the American Medical Association, the Canadian Medical Association (which withdrew in 1959 to participate in its own national hospital accrediation program) joined with the American College of Surgeons to form the Joint Commission on Accreditation of Hospitals. In 1951, the JCAH was incorporated in Illinois as a not-for-profit corporation. In June of 1952, the Joint Commission's Hospital Accreditation Program began surveying hospitals.

The Program was successful, and by 1966 the Joint Commission was well aware that the type of accreditation services it provided for hospitals was desperately needed in other specialized areas of health care and human services. That year, the Joint Commission began surveying long term care facilities in conjunction with its hospital program, which led, in 1971, to the formation of the Accreditation Council for Long Term Care Facilities. By that time, however, other accreditation programs had come under the purview of the JCAH. The Accreditation Council for Services for Mentally Retarded and Other Developmentally Disabled Persons had been formed in 1969, and the Accreditation Council for Psychiatric Facilities in 1970. In 1975, the Accreditation Council for Ambulatory Health Care was organized. The JCAH is governed by a Board of Commissioners, 20 individuals appointed by four parent Member Organizations. Three Commissioners are selected by the American College of Physicians, three by the American College of Surgeons, seven by the American Hospital Association, and seven by the American Medical Association. Commissioners serve for three-year terms without compensation. While mindful of the objectives of the organizations by which they are appointed, the Commissioners act independently while sitting as the governing body of the JCAH.

Originally, the Joint Commission's operations were financed solely by contributions from its Member Organizations. But because the scope of JCAH activities and the increasing number of facilities, services, and programs requesting surveys imposed a growing financial burden on the Member Organizations, the practice of charging for accreditation surveys was introduced in 1964. The survey fee schedule is established on the basis of cost and is subject to change from time to time in accordance with cost experience.

Today, the accreditation programs of the Joint Commission survey over 4,500 facilities, services, and programs in the course of a year, and approximately 7,300 facilities, services, and programs currently hold JCAH accreditation. The Quality Resource Center of the Joint Commission provides educational programs annually to more than 10,000 individuals directly concerned with the quality of care and services. In a quarter of a century of operation, the Joint Commission has made a widespread and positive impact on the delivery of health care and related human services in America. . . .

THE MEANING OF ACCREDITATION

Accreditation by the Joint Commission means that a facility has voluntarily sought to be measured against optimal achievable standards for quality of care and services, standards that apply to the performance of each function in the overall operation of a facility. It means that a facility has been found to be in substantial compliance with the standards, and is making an effort to provide even better care and services. Accreditation can thus document accountability of a facility to those who support it and to those it serves.

Accreditation is much more than an evaluation, however. Elements of consultation and education are found throughout the accreditation process. The presurvey activities such as self-evaluation are distinctly educational. The summation conference in which surveyors meet with representatives of the facility to discuss on-site survey findings and to make suggestions for improvement provides valuable consultation. The complete report of survey findings that accompanies each accreditation decision is also a consultative service that details the facility's strengths and weaknesses and makes recommendations for correcting deficiencies and raising the level of performance. Even after the accreditation decision has been made, the Joint Commission stresses that the facility maintain programs of continuing education and self-evaluation that will lead to improvement.

The meaning of accreditation is sometimes misunderstood. A common misconception is that the Joint Commission is a regulatory agency of the government. This is not so. The Joint Commission is a private, not-for-profit corporation. Accreditation by the JCAH is a voluntary process that uses optimal and yet achievable criteria as a basis for evaluating quality of performance. It encompasses more than, and should be distinguished from, certification or licensure, which are regulatory governmental determinations of a facility's ability to operate, most often based on minimum requirements.

However, JCAH accreditation is often used as a benchmark of quality by some regulatory agencies in granting certification and licensure. It is also used by some insurance agencies as a condition for honoring reimbursement claims, and as a criterion by some educational accrediting committees of professional organizations. Accreditation may also be used in decisions on funding or for purchasing services. Additionally, it can provide qualified professionals seeking employment and members of the public seeking health care with a guide to facilities that are known to strive to offer services of recognized quality. Use of accreditation in this manner is welcomed as a reinforcement of the objectives of the JACH. . . .

THE ACCREDITATION PROCESS

Because the Joint Commission is involved in promoting quality in many areas of health care and related human services, the evaluation processes employed by its accreditation programs must vary according to the nature of the facilities, programs, and services they survey. To gain a basic understanding of the accreditation process, however, a general model of the elements likely to be found in one or more of the JCAH programs may be helpful. This model reflects no one particular program's accreditation procedures, but is composed of elements that may appear commonly among them.

The accreditation process begins when a facility voluntarily applies to the Joint Commission for an on-site survey. Generally, upon receipt of the completed application, a document for self-evaluation is mailed to the facility to aid in comprehending JCAH standards and their interpretations, and to provide an inventory of the facility's compliance with the appropriate standards.

The next step in the process is the on-site visit by Joint Commission surveyors. During the visit, the surveyors, often using the completed self-evaluation as a guide, check every aspect of the facility's operation covered by the relevant Joint Commission standards.

Surveyors are recruited by the JCAH and are thoroughly trained in the standards and survey procedures of the accreditation program in which they serve. A typical hospital survey team consists of a physician, a registered nurse, and a hospital administrator. A psychiatric facility survey team must include a psychiatrist and frequently includes an administrator, a psychiatric nurse, or a social worker. In all accreditation programs, surveyors are drawn from the ranks of practicing professionals, individuals skilled and knowledgeable in their particular fields. The reliability of surveyors' assessments is monitored regularly.

An initial conference may be held on arrival by the surveyors with representatives from the governing body and the administration, major department heads, and members of the medical staff (if applicable). At this conference, the nature and purpose of the survey are explained and discussed.

A summation conference is always conducted by the surveyors at the end of the on-site visit. At this conference, attended by representatives of the facility's administration and staff, the surveyors report their findings, discussing deficiencies that they have observed and suggesting measures that may be taken to correct them.

After the on-site visit, the surveyors send a report of their findings to the appropriate accreditation program. The facility's file, including additional information submitted by the public or by federal or state agencies or associations, is assembled for review and analysis. After all pertinent information concerning a facility has been considered, a report of the survey is submitted to the accreditation committee of the relevant accreditation council or, in the case of hospital surveys, to the Accreditation Committee of the JCAH Board of Commissioners.

An accreditation decision is made on the basis of each survey report. Decisions made by the accreditation council are ratified by the Accreditation Committee of the Board of Commissioners, which meets once a month. Accreditation decisions are based on an evaluation of all available information and, although the survey necessarily addresses a sampling of conditions obtained at a point in time, an effort is made to assure that these conditions are typical. Major factors in the accreditation decision include evidence of overall compliance with standards, progressive advancement toward more complete compliance, and the absence of any serious impediment to patient safety or the quality of care.

The JCAH may grant two-year or one-year accreditation or it may deny accreditation. In the event that a facility receives a nonaccreditation decision or its accreditation is revoked, the JCAH provides an impartial process by which the facility may appeal the decision. The appeals process includes the right to an interview, a hearing, and formal reconsideration by the Board of

Commissioners. While the Joint Commission will release to the public the accreditation status of a facility it has surveyed, the criticisms and recommendations it makes to the facility are held in confidence, except as otherwise required by law. The Board of Commissioners has not deviated from this policy, as it believes that criticisms, including self-criticisms, of surveyed facilities, when kept confidential, are more likely to be uninhibited and to promote needed improvements. . . .

JCAH PERFORMANCE

The JCAH has, over the years, contributed much to the improved quality of care in hospitals. Its standards, which cover the gamut of hospital activities from fire safety to sanitation to bed-space allocation to professional services are designed to assure an optimal environment within which quality professional services can be provided. It does not seek to second guess the appropriateness or quality of care in given cases, but it wants to make certain that an appropriate professional body within the institution is looking at such questions. To do that adequately, for example, the JCAH argues, and its standards require, that the hospital must see to it that doctors keep their medical records on patients up to date, that there is a regular review of pathology reports on all tissues removed in surgery as a check on unnecessary surgery, that medical audits of patient medical records are made as a check on the quality and appropriateness of medical care, and that there is a regular review of utilization as a check on the necessity or appropriateness for admission and length of stay.

Over the years, the commission has sought to raise standards and has moved from what was minimally essential to the optimum achievable. As part of this move, it has reduced its accreditation period from three to two years. During the first 11 months of 1977, it surveyed 2,988 hospitals: while most (59 percent) were granted full two-year accreditation, 40 percent received only one-year provisional accreditation, and one percent were not accredited. The work entailed by a hospital in preparing JCAH review is considerable, and the AMA in mid-1979 decided to ask JCAH to grant three year accreditation for those hospitals which have repeatedly demonstrated excellence of patient care and conformance to JCAH standards.

Perhaps the most important part of the accreditation process is the self-evaluation survey that the hospital must go through in preparation for the JCAH visit. As it looks at itself and at JCAH standards, it can determine whether or not, in its judgment, the hospital meets those standards, and if it does not, what it can do to meet them. There lies the power of the JCAH standards, for if, on visitation, the hospital does not adequately measure up, it risks loss of accreditation. The hospital staff can, therefore, use the JCAH standards as leverage to bring about needed change even before the JCAH team visits. If the hospital staff recognizes deficiencies and cannot secure their correction, then criticism by the JCAH can be the needed ingredient of the outside voice. With serious deficiencies, loss of accreditation or provisional one-year accreditation may be the needed shock treatment that leads to the correction of deficiencies. Many will acknowledge that in some cases the best thing that can happen to a hospital is for it to lose its accreditation, for that short-term loss can be the vehicle for securing a long-term solution to its problems.

Failure to receive accreditation can have serious effects on a hospital. It loses its automatic Medicare certification; it must, in this event, be specially inspected and approved by state-government officials in order to be eligible for Medicare reimbursement. Most health insurance contracts, moreover, will only pay for care in an accredited hospital. Failure to win accreditation also makes it more difficult for a hospital to recruit medical staff, as well as residents if it is a teaching hospital: After all, failure to be accredited tells everyone that the hospital does not have the environment that it should have to provide the optimal conditions for quality care. Who would want to practice or be trained in that kind of institution? And so far as patients are concerned, what informed patient would want major surgery or intensive care in a nonaccredited hospital?

The JCAH is not without critics. Some administrators are critical of its concentration on housekeeping matters, contending that it places too much emphasis on these and not enough on the end product, that is, quality of patient care. Others contend that its standards are not high enough. Some critics are unhappy over the fact that the JCAH sponsors (AHA, AMA, ACP, and ACS) have too much of a stake in the hospitals and are therefore not as critical or as demanding of the health system. Some support for the latter seemed to come in 1975 when HEW conducted a series of validation surveys on JCAH accredited hospitals. "The government sent in five-man teams for five days . . . and made a painstaking search for fire and safety hazards. They found them: fully two-thirds of the 105 hospitals surveyed failed to meet the government's standards" (7, p.13). The director of the JCAH described HEW's validation surveys as "a search and destroy mission. Government set out to prove the voluntary process was sub-par" (7, p.13). The surveyors, in his judgment, focused on relatively minor issues. Fires, he noted, were extremely rare in hospitals (8, p.43). Significantly, the validation teams all had fire safety professionals, whereas the JCAH teams do not. The JCAH's principal complaint was that the validation surveys should have been just that, but to do so would require similar type teams rather than differently constituted teams.

As one views these charges and counter-charges, one should bear in mind that they represent a form of partisan or political debate, the kind of dialogue that has historically always been carried out between parties who have different views of the universe or different roles to play. The charges are challenges that typically cause adjustments on the part of those on whom they are levied, and so, too, the countercharges. At the end of the dialogue, the world and each of the partisans have usually changed somewhat. That is, of course, how progress is made.

The JCAH is under constant challenge. New groups want to join as sponsors of the organization; the ANA is one (JCAH declined), and the AAFP is another (JCAH declined and AAFP planning to sue). In addition, federal-sponsored programs such as the PSROs have potential widespread implications for JCAH long-term survival because of the potential for duplication of effort.

COMMISSION ON PROFESSIONAL AND HOSPITAL ACTIVITIES (CPHA)

The CPHA was established in 1955, sponsored by the the ACP, ACS, AHA, and the Southwestern Michigan Hospital Council. The presence of this substate regional council among national organizations stems from the council's pioneering work beginning in 1950 under a Kellogg Foundation grant for the study of professional activities in hospitals through interhospital comparisons of hospital statistical reports. The 1950 project was known as the Professional Activity Study (PAS), and it continues as the largest program under CPHA.

At the heart of PAS and of other studies carried out by CPHA are the medical abstracts of all hospitalized patients in participating hospitals. Kuehn, of the ACS described CPHA activities this way (9):

In the participating hospital, medical record personnel work with the usual clinical records, condensing the record of every patient discharged on a one-page PAS abstract. The abstracts are mailed to CPHA, where they are checked, rechecked, and then processed by computer systems. When the hospital completes submission of data for a period, the commission prepares a variety of standard reports and mails them immediately to the hospital.

PAS reports are prepared monthly, semiannually, and annually. Their most important function lies in providing a display of all aspects of hospital practice. For example, monthly reports analyze discharges for all patients grouped by hospital service, and for all patients grouped by final diagnosis explaining admission. Other monthly reports list all patients in sequence by patient number; all patients in sequence by final diagnosis explaining admission; all patients who were operated on, in sequence by most important operation; and all deaths in sequence by final diagnosis explaining admission. Semi-annual reports include indexes of all patients in sequence by diagnosis; all patients who were operated on, in sequence by operation; all patients for each physician in sequence by diagnoses; and of all patients who were operated on, for each surgeon in sequence by operation. Annual reports furnish discharge analyses of all patients grouped by hospital service, and of all patients grouped by final diagnosis explaining admission. . . .

By furnishing basic statistics of patients and medical record indexes, PAS reports form an integral system of accounting for professional service. They offer to the hospital a practical time-saving approach to the medical audit, and provide profiles of care for utilization review. As useful by-products, they also simplify the work of the medical record department, and increase a hospital's capability for research.

THE MEDICAL AUDIT PROGRAM

Among the several extensions of the PAS system, the Medical Audit Program (MAP) is the most important one. MAP is defined by the commission as a tool for evaluating the quality of care reflected in medical records. MAP is principally designed to help the hospital's medical staff match the care actually given to patients against standards of care agreed upon by all members of the staff. Using most of the statistics furnished through PAS abstracts, the PAS-MAP reports display clinical departmental practice in detail. The reports are prepared quarterly to allow the accumulation of enough records so that trends in medical practice can be detected. This three-month interval also permits thorough review without placing an unreasonable burden on the medical staff.

PAS-MAP reports consist of separate reports for each of the four major clinical services, and one report for newborn infants. Additionally, they include three reports, categorized by operation, for adult, pediatric, and obstetrical patients, as well as a summary comparing the reports of the four services, making a total of nine sets of reports each quarter.

The CPHA reports can clearly help a hospital in its self-assessment work, for it enables it to strengthen its JCAH required peer review activities by introducing to that process objective data from other institutions. A hospital no longer relies solely on the judgments of its own staff but now has available a standard against which its performance can be measured. The PAS program in early 1978 had approximately 2,200 participating hospitals with some 17 million discharges per year. This represented approximately 42 percent of the short-term discharges in the United States and about 28 percent in Canada.

HOSPITAL UTILIZATION PROJECT (HUP)

HUP is a program similar to and competitive with CPHA and serves over 600 facilities throughout the country with some three million annual discharges.

The development of HUP is worth describing because it illustrates a point made at the end of the discussion on JCAH, that is, the challenge made to an organization, the response to which typically represents some kind of changed behavior and is the stuff of which progress is made.

During the late 1950s, Blue Cross and Blue Shield plans in many parts of the country were experiencing high utilization and increased costs, and they made applications to the various state insurance commissioners, which regulated them, for rate increases. Generally, insurance commissioners had little data to work with other than that provided by the applicants. There was concern, however, because of frequent charges about unnecessary surgery, unnecessary admissions, and unnecessary lengths of stay. For example, one hospital administrator in upstate New York had put a notice on the doctor's bulletin board urging the physicians to admit patients and keep them in a little longer in order to maintain the hospital's occupancy rate. Most Blue Cross plans were, moreover, well aware of those two-day admissions for acute medical problems, many of which turned out to be admissions for costly diagnostic examinations that the plans did not cover.

In some states, the insurance commissioners commissioned studies to ascertain the extent of need for rate increases and the extent and nature of the problems. The studies were informative, but, in many instances, the data were inconclusive. This was often the case, for example, with regard to necessity for surgery, which is frequently a highly judgmental matter on which doctors may disagree. In Pennsylvania, in 1958, the insurance commissioner leveled his charge against the physicians in the Pittsburgh area, stating that they used hospital services unnecessarily and that patient stays were prolonged beyond the point of need. The physicians were taken aback and had no data with which to refute the charges. But they began to collect the data by reviewing the medical records. The process was slow and difficult, so they turned for help to the Allegheny County Medical Society and the Hospital Council of Western Pennsylvania. Over 30 local corporations contributed start-up money, and in 1963 HUP was operational.

While the physicians reacted defensively to the insurance commissioner's charges, his charges led to the creation of a new process for strengthening the peer-review processes in hospitals.

PROFESSIONAL STANDARDS REVIEW ORGANIZATIONS (PSROs)

Since the advent of Medicare and Medicaid, government has been assuming an increasing share of the costs of medical care, and the costs have been rising rapidly.

The initial legislation for Medicare in 1965 required utilization review; in 1967, this was extended to Medicaid. The 1971 amendments to the Social Security Act mandated the development of PSROs throughout the nation to give assurance that services paid for under Medicare, Medicaid, and under the Maternal and Child Health and Crippled Children's Programs are medically necessary, of high quality, and delivered at the lowest possible cost.

PSROs carry out their responsibilities by reviewing admissions to a health care facility, certifying the necessity for continuing treatment in an in-patient facility, reviewing other extended or costly treatment, conducting medical evaluation studies, regularly reviewing facility, practitioner, and health care service profiles of care, and reviewing facility and practitioner records as applicable to a particular review process. (10, pp.2-3)

Each PSRO must be a nonprofit, professional organization of licensed physicians. To be legitimate in the government's eyes, it must have as members at least 25% of the physicians in the area covered by the PSRO. But the legislation provides, however, that in the event that a medical PSRO cannot be organized to carry out the mandated activities, then the secretary of HEW may turn to some other qualified group to do the job. In other words, Congress said, Doctors, you do it, but if you don't do it in a satisfactory manner, then HEW can turn to nonmedical controlled groups to monitor quality and efficiency of care.

It is still too early to determine the extent to which PSROs are effectively carrying out their mandate. HEW reports some successes, particularly in terms of reduced average lengths of stay. Whether these are due to the sensitivities resulting from the presence of PSRO review activities or more basic changes in the practice of medicine, one cannot say with certainty. In one study,

HEW found that a few PSROs were effective in cutting admissions and lengths of stay. But these results were negated because, astoundingly, hospital use in other active PSRO areas actually increased . . . The study doesn't consider the quality of care, only the cost. It is possible, therefore, that PSROs are upgrading hospital care even though they're not curbing expenses. (11, pp. 15-16)

HEW concluded that the data strongly suggested that PSROs alone were not likely significantly to change hospital utilization rates or the level of government expenditures.

The work of a PSRO and some of its accomplishments were described by Bussman (12, pp.163-164)

The early experience of conditional PSROs has been to demonstrate a decrease in length of stay when review is begun in acute care institutions. The degree of reduction of length of stay has, of course, varied from one area to another largely depending on preexisting regional utilization patterns with reductions much less dramatic in those areas previously characterized by the shorter lengths of stay.

The effect on utilization of hospital days of care will inevitably reach a plateau as lengths of stay approach an irreducible minimum. Further impact on cost containment will thereafter be dependent on reduction in utilization of ancillary services and changing practice patterns to encourage care in ambulatory settings and increased use of outpatient surgical facilities wherever feasible.

Participation and support of physicians in PSRO functions has largely been enlisted through appeal to concerns for quality of care. While the principal avenue for improving quality in all settings has been structured around medical care evaluation studies, several PSRO's have demonstrated an impact on quality of care in acute care institutions through the concurrent review process. Identification of potential areas of less than adequate quality while the patient is still hospitalized allows an opportunity for intervention to correct the care of that particular patient rather than focusing only on patterns of care developed over a period of time. Physician education related to demonstrated deficiencies in quality of care has been shown to be significantly more effective if applied when the problem is first identified.

I would like to provide several examples of PSRO actions which have had an impact on utilization and quality of care.

One of our review coordinators identified in two hospitals that she was supervising that it was not a common practice to obtain the sputums and cultures in the case of low viral pneumonia. This was brought to the attention of the medical staff and was made a matter of a change in policy.

We have had a significant impact on mortality from myocardial infarction in one of our hospitals where the number of physicians qualified to deal with problems of myocardial infarction has increased dramatically since we pointed out their difference of results as compared to the rest of the community.

We have in several instances identified the use of saline in patients with congestive heart failure and myocardial infarction and intervened immediately to protect that patient's welfare.

Chest pain had, in one hospital, been treated in the emergency room without immediate referral to the coronary care unit. We have changed hospital policies in that area to lead to much more expedient management of the patient arriving in the emergency room with chest pain.

One of the hospitals discovered that there were unusual delays in their hospital days of care related to failure to request and expedite consultations. This has been changed through administrative action of the hospital.

In another hospital, we found that the resident house staff had been responsible for unusual lengths of stay prior to surgery. This has been changed through administrative action.

In another hospital, we identified rather inefficient programs of investigation of acute abdominal pain. This was made a matter of a medical care evaluation study which has increased the efficiency of the investigation process.

Improved documentation in almost all the hospitals has been a result of the advent of PSRO review.

In our community we have had a rather uncoordinated attitude toward discharge planning. In many hospitals, this is considered an ancillary service and is not initiated until the physician requests it. This has been coordinated through the PSRO to result in much more efficacious discharge planning procedures.

Despite the theoretical superiority of concurrent quality assurance, opportunities for this type of intervention will have of necessity [to] be limited, and most of the influence of PSRO in improving quality of care will occur through analysis of profiles of care delivered by various institutions and practitioners, with alteration of these patterns through intervention by education, or failing in this, by sanctions provided by the statute.

But PSRO survival as presently structured is in doubt. In early 1978, the President's Office of Management and Budget (OMB) proposed that PSRO funding be deleted from the budget request to the Congress because of an

HEW study that showed that PSROs did not have any significant effect on reducing costs and did not contribute significantly to increased quality of care. OMB's view did not prevail, but congressional dissatisfaction was also evident in that the appropriation for fiscal 1979 provided funds for hospital review activities but not enough for the reviews Congress had earlier directed for ambulatory and long-term care. In October 1978, the PSROs came under criticism from GAO. GAO criticized the salary schedules for PSRO executive directors that HEW had issued. GAO also felt that there was room for PSRO efficiency in terms of combining some administrative staffs and functions given the fact that in 21 states there was more than a single PSRO; there were in those 21 states a total of 164 PSROs. A month later, HEW's PSRO supervising office, the Health Care Financing Administration (HCFA) released a new evaluation that demonstrated PSRO effectiveness in both cost containment and cost control. Time and the Congress will tell about the future of the PSRO.

HOSPITAL COSTS

We hear a great deal of rhetoric about rising health costs, and in particular about rising hospital costs. And not without cause.

In 1950, for example, the average cost of hospital care was about $15.62 per day. In 1975, it was $151.42. In 1950, the average hospital stay totaled $127.23; in 1975, it was $1,166.80 (13, p.381). By 1977 it had risen to $1,318.31 (See Table 6-4). The bulk of these increased costs have been borne by industry and government, the former through the phenomenal growth of private (voluntary) health insurance that industry has increasingly paid for as an employee fringe benefit, the latter since the introduction of Medicare and Medicaid. Both industry and government have fretted over these rises, the former because it forces price increases in industrial products, the latter because it forces politically unpopular tax increases.

Three factors account for the rise in hospital costs and in health costs generally.

The first factor is population. We simply have more people today than we did in 1950 (216 million versus 153 million). This population is, moreover, an aging population, requiring more, longer, and costly types of care.

The second factor is inflation. Everything costs more — drugs, linens, food, fuel, and personnel. More than half of a hospital's budget is consumed by its payroll, and as a heavy employer of unskilled labor when the federally mandated minimum wage goes up (as it did in 1978 by 12%), hospital labor costs jump accordingly. So, too, with food and fuel and other items.

The third factor in hospital and health care cost increases is new technology

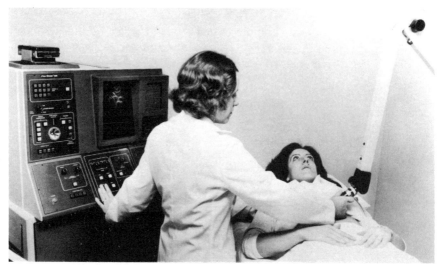

Figure 6–6. Ultrasound unit. This unit is a particularly useful diagnostic device in obstetrics when radiation is not desirable. This unit cost in 1978 about $90,000. (Courtesy, Hamot Medical Center, Erie, Pennsylvania.)

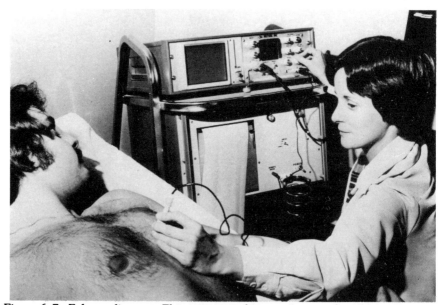

Figure 6–7. Echocardiogram. This unit uses ultrasound to test for abnormalities in the valves, muscles, and chambers of the heart. Unit cost in 1978 approximately $60,000. (Courtesy, Hamot Medical Center, Erie, Pennsylvania.)

and new services. As a result of scientific advances, we are able to do more things to help people than heretofore. But the price of new technology is high. Not only is the equipment expensive, but the personnel needed to operate it is also costly. Figures 6-1 to 6-10 show some of the latest technology and its approximate cost.

This will be discussed more thoroughly in the chapter on health care costs.

AN ANALYSIS OF HOSPITAL COSTS IN PENNSYLVANIA *

First, A Caution

A significant problem in analyzing hospital costs is finding an appropriate unit of statistical measurement. The hospital industry continues to report cost data on the basis of "cost per day" for consistency, and for the lack of a better alternative. However, we wish to caution that these figures can be misleading because they only measure costs on the basis of days spent in a hospital. If an institution has exactly the same expenses and admissions this year as last year, but because of new surgical procedures some patients were able to reduce their stays in the hospital, the same costs would be spread over fewer days of care, and the result would be an increase in the "cost per day" figure. Admittedly, this is an oversimplification since the hospital product is constantly changing as a result of new technology, new medicines, new procedures, and different methods of treating patients, to cite a few reasons.

If an item costs $1.00 this year and $1.10 next year, it is reasonable and accurate to say that the price of the item increased 10%. However, if the item has been changed in some manner — size, or material, or design, or quality for example — can we still say the price increased 10%, or are we not talking about a totally different item, thus precluding this type of comparison? A "patient day" is a day of care in a health care institution. However, it should be apparent that a day of maternity care differs significantly from a day of care for a patient who has had open heart surgery; yet the "cost per patient day" unit of measure does not reflect the shifting nature of patient days and associated costs.

As the subject of rising costs assumes increasing national importance, it is essential that the data upon which future public policy decisions are to be based be as authoritative and as detailed as possible. To that end, our Association is cooperating with the American Hospital Association in the

---

*This analysis was prepared by the Hospital Association of Pennsylvania in February 1977 and is printed with permission. Tables 6-1 and 6-2 have been updated, and Tables 6-4 and 6-6 have been added to the HAP analysis.

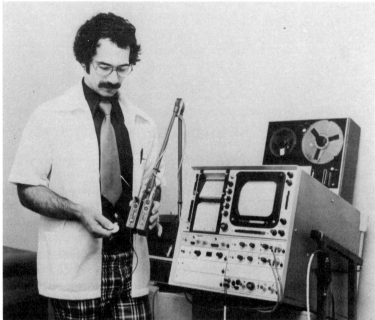

Figure 6–8. Electromyograph. This machine is used to detect nerve disorders by picking up and amplifying electrical potentials in the muscles and by measuring the velocity of electrical conduction along the nerves. Cost of this unit in 1978 was approximately $12,000. (Courtesy, Hamot Medical Center, Erie, Pennsylvania.)

development of two statistical indices, the hospital input price index, and the hospital intensity index which we believe improve upon existing statistical indices used to demonstrate the reasons for increases in hospital expenditures. These indices will be published monthly by the American Hospital Association and we will also be able to provide specific data for Pennsylvania. We think this will prove to be a useful tool in assisting all of us in achieving a better understanding and, therefore, developing a better explanation as to why hospital costs are increasing.

The data appearing in this analysis were developed from monthly reports generated for Pennsylvania hospitals by the American Hospital Association and covering the 12-month period ending June 30, 1976.

During that period, the average cost per day in Pennsylvania hospitals rose 15.7%, just slightly ahead of the national average of 15.2%. The average cost per case in Pennsylvania hospitals increased 14.9%, percentage of hospital bed occupancy rose 1.3%, and the average length of stay decreased 0.6%, or one-tenth of a day.

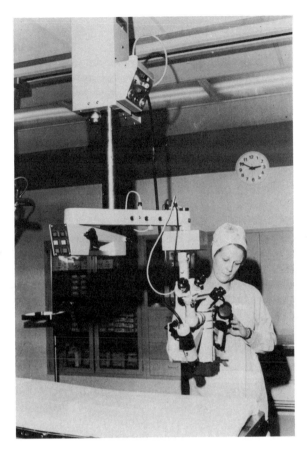

Figure 6–9. Ceiling-mounted microscope used in eye, neuro, and reconstructive surgery. Unit cost in 1978 about $45,000. (Courtesy, Hamot Medical Center, Erie, Pennsylvania.)

Personnel Costs

Of the 15.7% cost per day increase in Pennsylvania, more than half - 8.7% - is directly attributable to increased personnel costs. These increases can be further broken down into salary increases of 5.1%, added fringe benefit costs of 1.0% and an increase in the number of employees, reflecting 2.6% of the increased costs.

Hospitals spend approximately 51% of their budget on employee wages, while other industries spend a considerably smaller proportion of total budget. The nature of hospital service — care of the ill and injured — necessitates a person-to-person relationship; therefore, the hospital industry must employ large numbers of people (an average of 3.26 employees per patient,) as

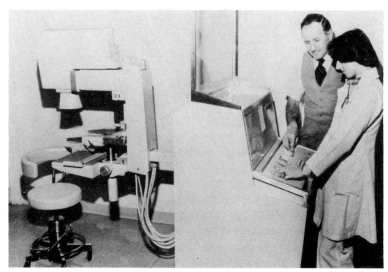

Figure 6–10. Mammograph. A diagnostic unit for breast cancer. Unit cost in 1978 about $35,000. (Courtesy, Hamot Medical Center, Erie, Pennsylvania.)

opposed to private industry which relies heavily on automation. Because of the number of persons employed by hospitals, and the degree of specialized training they require, wage increases have a much greater impact on hospitals than on other industries. These factors, coupled with a significant increase in union activity and the necessity of keeping wages of hospital workers competitive with other industries in the community have contributed to increased payroll costs.

Hospital wages, which for years were notoriously low, had begun to catch up with the rest of the economy until the economic stabilization program was begun in 1971, and wages were frozen at an average 5.5% increase annually for the next three years. Indeed, for about a year after controls were lifted from most of the rest of the economy, they remained in place for the health care industry. So, while the cost of living was increasing at record rates, hospital workers' wages were being depressed. Since wage and price controls were lifted for hospitals in April of 1974, there has been a moderate "catching up" period for employees, in an attempt to regain some degree of equity with workers in other fields. Recent data suggest that more pressure will be felt in this area. For example, medical or supportive service employees of the Pennsylvania government have average salaries of $11,101 and a significantly better fringe benefit package which places them over 20% higher than hospital employees with similar training.

Higher wages also bring attendant increases in fringe benefits through payment of higher Social Security taxes, increased workmen's compensation taxes, increased premiums for health care insurance, and increased retirement contributions (due in part to the Pension Reform Act.) New fringe benefits also have been added to attract and retain qualified personnel.

Other increases in personnel cost have been due largely to the hiring of additional employees (2.6% of the increase) in both patient and non-patient care areas. Many of these additional employees are directly related to the changing role of the hospital and the type of patient being treated. There was a time when the function of a hospital was more one of care than of cure. This custodial function called for employing personnel with a minimum of training and skill and permitted hospitals to employ persons from lower levels of the labor market as the bulk of their work force.

The introduction of new patient care techniques, diagnostic equipment and other medical advances has required a constant upgrading of the quality and an increase in the number of hospital employees. The miracles of modern medicine, demanded by a sophisticated public, have added heavily to the payroll costs for hospitals.

Today's modern hospital may have more than 200 different job classifications. Many of the employees have special skills that command relatively high salaries. On the average, one of every three hospital employees has specialized training, and most employees require special orientation and training on a continuous basis.

In the past ten years alone, dozens of new job titles have been created. These include respiratory therapist, surgical technician, cardiopulmonary technician, catheterization technician, nuclear medical technologist, electromedical equipment repairman, heart-lung machine operator and numerous other technicians and technologists. Nursing, too, has become more specialized because hospitals are offering more intensive care for the heart attack patient, for the critically ill medical-surgical patient, and for infants born with life-threatening problems.

The patient who is admitted to an inpatient service requires more intensive treatment than did his counterpart of several years ago. The number of x-rays, laboratory tests, physical therapy treatments and other ancillary services has increased by up to 25% during the past year alone. To adequately meet the increasing demand for these services, additional persons have been employed. While some of these treatments may be the result of "defensive medicine" practices, the majority have been used to maximize the certainty of diagnosis or the effectiveness of treatment, thereby minimizing danger to the patient.

The addition of some employees is a direct result of the increased record-keeping and data-generating requirements mandated by both governmental and voluntary agencies. Development of utilization review, quality assurance and Professional Standards Review Organizations has led to personnel increases in both medical records and social services. The large amount of information and data which must be provided to third party payers for the purposes of reimbursement, accreditation, and licensure has necessitated additional personnel in data processing and financial management. Finally, the deterioration of many urban areas has required hospitals in those areas to increase security personnel to protect both employees and patients.

Unlike most industries, hospitals must be staffed to provide services 24 hours a day, 365 days a year; and they must always be staffed at a specified level, with trained personnel available when needed. There is no such thing as a seasonal layoff should the patient census dip temporarily.

In addition, increases in personnel costs can be directly attributed to government law or regulation. For example, hospitals are now covered by the Fair Labor Standards Act, National Labor Relations Act, Equal Employment Opportunity Laws, Federal Unemployment Compensation Amendments, and the Employees Retirement Security Act. While most other industries are similarly covered, significantly more impact is shown in the health care industry because of its higher labor intensity. Some examples of this impact include:

THE FAIR LABOR STANDARDS ACT

The health care industry's exemption under this act was repealed by Congress in 1967. The act establishes a minimum hourly wage which the health care industry must pay covered employees. For health care employees, the minimum rose from $1.90 per hour in May, 1974, to $2.30 per hour in January, 1977. The act also requires that certain categories of employees be paid at the rate of time and one-half for all hours worked in excess of 40 hours in a single work week. The statute has had a dramatic effect on increasing direct personnel costs in health care institutions.

NATIONAL LABOR RELATIONS ACT

In July, 1974, Congress repealed the hospital exemption of the Taft-Hartley Act, making the law's terms and jurisdiction of the National Labor Relations Board applicable to non-profit hospitals. The law directs the National Labor Relations Board to perform two principal functions: to investigate and adjudicate unfair labor practices committed by employers and unions, and to conduct secret ballot elections for union representation where requested by employees. Inclusion of hospital employees under this statute has increased union activity considerably in the hospital industry. This has been a direct factor leading to increased employee wage and benefit packages in both unionized and non-unionized hospitals.

EQUAL EMPLOYMENT OPPORTUNITY LAWS

These laws, which include Title VII of the Civil Rights Act of 1964, the Equal Pay Act of 1963, the Age Discrimination and Employment Act, Section 304 (a) of the Consumer Credit Protection Act, the Vietnam Era Veterans' Readjustment Assistance Act, Executive Order 11246, Executive Order 11375, Executive Order 11141, and Section 503 and 504 of the Vocational Rehabilitation Act of 1973, forbid employment discrimination. The effects of these statutes and the regulations and rulings of the Equal Employment Opportunity Commission have necessitated the implementation of vastly expanded employee record and information systems and employee training programs to assure statutory compliance and to generate the statistical data necessary to prove compliance, should the institution be investigated by an enforcement agency. The cost of modifying existing record-keeping systems and hiring personnel to implement and maintain the additional paperwork generated also has had a significant impact on hospital costs.

FEDERAL UNEMPLOYMENT COMPENSATION AMENDMENTS OF 1970

These amendments required states to change their employment compensation statutes to provide for coverage of hospital employees. Although hospitals were given the option of paying for employee benefits on a reimbursement of cost basis, hospital unemployment compensation costs have soared because of the escalating expansion of benefit payments and the extension of benefit periods. Increased costs are incurred also in preparing adequately to contest and dispute claims and in pursuing appropriate hearing and appeals procedures.

EMPLOYMENT RETIREMENT INCOME SECURITY ACT OF 1974

This statute, more commonly referred to as the Pension Reform Act, mandates many pension plan requirements—including increased participation and vesting—which can have a significant impact on the cost to the employer of maintaining pension plans currently in effect. These increased requirements will undoubtedly result in more pressure by employees for establishment of pension plans where they do not exist. Finally, the new act provides for expanded reporting and funding requirements with stiff penalties to both employers and fiduciaries for failure to operate within its provisions. The results of these provisions have contributed to the increased cost of benefits for hospital personnel. With the labor-intensiveness of the hospital industry, the requirements of this statute will be inordinately expensive to implement.

Operating Costs

With about 8.7% of the 15% increase in hospital costs from 1975 to 1976 going for personnel-related items (salaries, fringe benefits, etc.), the other 7.0% can be accounted for in increased operating costs - principally in the areas of supplies and services (2.9%), capital expenditures for equipment (1.8%), capital expenditures for physical plant (2.0%) and interest expense (about 0.3%).

Increases in fuel and electricity costs continue to occur despite aggressive fuel energy conservation programs instituted by many hospitals which have resulted in less energy consumed. Likewise, where inpatient days have decreased, the actual number of meals served obviously has decreased; yet overall food costs have increased. Drug cost increases have resulted largely from both a greater use of medications and the higher purchase prices most hospitals have had to pay. These increased purchase prices are in part attributable to the increase of all petroleum-derivative pharmaceuticals. Telephone charges also have increased since hospitals lost their "charitable discount" status in 1974. Finally, despite the efforts of most hospitals throughout the state to hold costs down through effective loss control programs, and through the establishment of their own captive insurance company, malpractice insurance rates nevertheless have skyrocketed.

Capital expenditure for equipment is another major cost of providing hospital care. The constantly changing technological environment, intensity of illness, and public demand have prompted increased capital outlays. The total cost of equipping an average operating room is $20,000 or more. A television monitoring system, for instance, allowing the x-ray department to view and diagnose from x-ray pictures originating in surgery, costs $3,000. The ultrasonic cleaner used to clean various surgical utensils, costs over $4,500; an autoclave, also used in sterilizing equipment, costs over $5,700; an operating room table, over $4,400; surgical lights for the operating room cost over $5,800.

The total cost for buying intensive care unit equipment and installing the equipment can easily exceed $12,000 (Figs. 6-11 and 6-12). This figure includes a $2,300 defibrillator and oscilloscope, a $200 suction machine, a $1,300 electrocardiograph, a $100 portable oxygen machine, a $4,300 automatic respirator, and a $3,700 "crash cart" complete with synchronized direct current defibrillator, oscilloscope, internal-external pacemaker, and ECG machine. Equipment costs become much more pronounced in highly

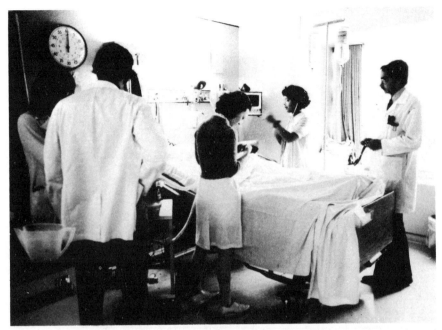

Figure 6–11. Respiratory intensive care unit specializing in care of patients with such conditions as tuberculosis, lung cancer, emphysema, pneumonia, and bronchitis. (Courtesy, Thomas Jefferson University Hospital, Philadelphia, Pennsylvania.)

specialized areas. For example, the initial cost for facilities and all equipment in a ten-bed kidney dialysis center has been estimated at over $300,000 (Fig. 6-13); a cardiac catheterization lab can cost over $250,000; and a highly sophisticated radiology department can cost well over $1,000,000.

However, not all equipment is purchased to provide a more sophisticated level of care. Some machines, particularly in the laboratory areas, are designed to increase efficiency. For example, the coulter counter blood machine automatically counts white and red blood cells, measures hematocrit and hemoglobin, calculates three other items about red blood cells, and prints the results on a computer card - all in forty seconds. The same procedure by hand would take twenty to thirty minutes. The machine costs over $35,000.

The prime goal of medical care is to save lives and ease suffering, and to that end science has developed and is developing amazing new methods of treatment. Of necessity, this rapid progress has been directed towards increasing the sophistication of care. To that end, technology continues to strive (Fig. 6-14).

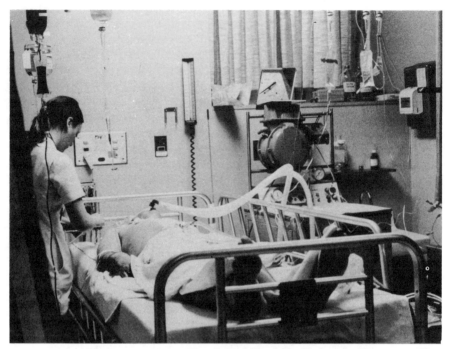

Figure 6–12. Intensive-care-unit, The Johns Hopkins Hospital. (Courtesy, The Johns Hopkins Hospital, Baltimore, Maryland.)

Legislation, too, has created additional operating cost burdens for health care institutions. Examples include:

OCCUPATIONAL SAFETY AND HEALTH ACT OF 1970

This law was enacted to assure " . . . every working man and woman in the nation, safe and healthful working conditions . . .". All employers are required to provide employment conditions that are free from hazards which might cause death or serious physical harm and to comply with the safety and health standards promulgated under the act. The OSHA standards presently include hundreds of pages of printed material encompassing thousands of detailed matters. These standards include, but are not limited to, the following areas: housekeeping; aisles and passageways; floorloading protection; means of egress; fire protection; sanitation; electrical requirements; protective equipment for personnel; accident prevention signs and tags; and laundry machinery and operations. The cost of complying with these standards and maintaining the proper records and documentation to monitor compliance imposes an additional expenditure of limited health care resources.

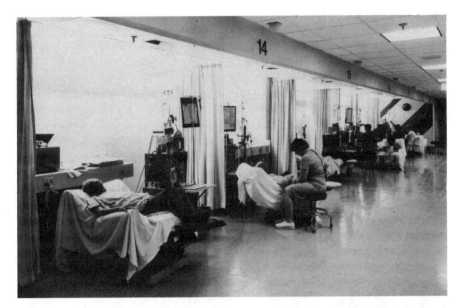

Figure 6–13. Renal (kidney) dialysis center. The lives of some kidney disease patients can be extended by many years with dialysis therapy on a regular basis. (Courtesy, Hamot Medical Center, Erie, Pennsylvania.)

LIFE SAFETY CODE REQUIREMENTS

Titles XVIII and XIX of the Social Security Act require all hospitals to be in compliance with the 1967 Life Safety Code as a condition for participation in these federal programs. However, hospitals receiving grants or loans under the Hill-Burton Act must comply with the 1973 Life Safety Code. If a hospital has a skilled nursing facility, the skilled nursing facility must be in compliance with the 1973 Life Safety Code to be approved for participation in the Medicare program while the rest of the hospital must still comply with the 1967 Life Safety Code. Finally, hospitals also must comply with a wide variety of differing state and local fire and safety codes. As a result of conflicting and differing standards/procedures of these codes, some hospitals have spent thousands of dollars to maintain compliance under one code only to have been found out of compliance when a new code or amended standard has been adopted.

The enormous outlay required to keep pace with technology and maintain existing facilities has required that hospitals borrow significant sums of money in recent years. Interest costs on these loans have also contributed to the rising costs per patient day in Pennsylvania.

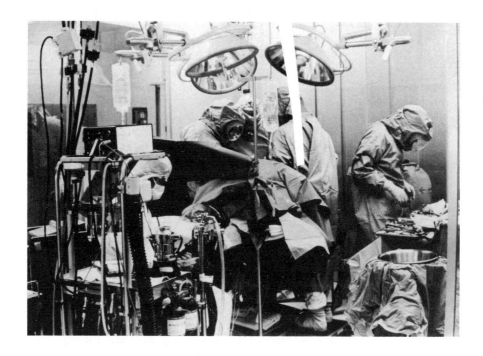

Figure 6–14. Laminar air flow operating room. This operating room (OR) is specially designed for total joint replacements (hip, knee, ankle, shoulder) by orthopedic surgeons.

Laminar flow is a method of air purification whereby the body of air moves through the work chamber along parallel flow lines in a constant direction and at uniform velocity.

This means the same air is recycled about 200 times per hour through high-efficiency hepafilters to remove contaminated particles. The cleanest air flows over the operative field, around partitions, and then returns to the filters.

Even the physicians are plugged into the system. The bubble-type face shields and helmets they wear prevent exhaled air from flowing downward to the patient by returning it via hoses for filtration.

Also, to minimize contamination, each of the team wears a paper scrub suit, reducing the amount of lint in the room that potentially can clog the filters.

This space-age concept was developed in the early 1960s to meet aerospace program needs. Modifications for medical purposes put laminar air flow into hospital operating rooms a decade later. (Courtesy, Hamot Medical Center, Erie, Pennsylvania.)

Cost Containment Activities

Although many cost areas are out of an institution's control, hospitals are doing their best to economize in areas which are under their control, without sacrificing the quality of the care they provide.

One area includes intensified programs of ongoing utilization review activities to assure that unnecessary admissions are not being made, and that hospital stays last no longer than necessary. The system also takes into consideration whether or not the treatment being provided is proper and consistent with the diagnosis, and whether any unnecessary treatment or tests are being ordered.

Hospitals continue to pursue their emphasis on outpatient or "vertical" care, through same-day surgical services, expanded outpatient departments, coordinated home care programs, and testing of elective surgery patients on an outpatient basis prior to admission for surgery. These programs - and others like them-are designed for more appropriate and effective delivery of care, with resulting reductions in the overall cost to the public. The increasing trend toward coverage of such outpatient services by insurance companies is encouraging, but there is potential for even more significant savings in this area.

Another area of cost saving by hospitals comes through participation in regional efforts such as group purchasing cooperatives for food, medical supplies and the like; and in the development of shared laundry services at strategic geographic locations. Still another facet of cost saving involves statewide efforts coordinated by The Hospital Association of Pennsylvania through its shared services corporation, the Pennsylvania Hospital Services Association (PHSA). Four areas of PHSA involvement are insurance, computer services, management engineering and biomedical engineering.

In insurance, the Association offers nine programs ranging from workmen's compensation insurance to liability protection for hospital employees and trustees. Annual premiums for these nine programs exceed $15,000,000 - substantially less than participating hospitals would have to pay on an individual basis.

In addition, over fifty Pennsylvania hospitals participate in PHSA's shared computer services program. Services include patient billing, accounts receivable, payroll, cost allocation, medical records, and many others. Participation in such joint efforts eliminates duplication of facilities and services and reduces administrative costs.

Likewise, a number of hospitals are utilizing the services of PHSA's Management Engineering and Cost Control Service, sponsored jointly with the New Jersey Hospital Association. The program provides services in manpower utilization, work and systems analysis, quality control and statistical analysis and cost reduction control. Over 225 engineering projects were completed in Pennsylvania through 1975, with verified savings to the hospitals of over $15,000,000. PHSA's recently established biomedical engineering program offers to institutions scheduled inspections of clinical equipment for safety and performance, training of clinical personnel to use medical devices safely and effectively, and assurance for both hospitals and their patients that the technology on which they both rely is safe, cost-effective, and reliable.

Participation in all of these programs represents good management practice, as do cooperative efforts in education, training, manpower recruitment and regional planning, among others; but they lack the visibility and the dramatic impact on the cost of health care of some of the areas previously mentioned. Nevertheless, the hospitals of the Commonwealth—on their own, as well as through their state and regional associations—are continuing to strive toward maintaining and improving the quality of care they provide to their communities, while trying to keep the cost within the ability of the public to pay for that care.

Summary

Increasing hospital costs have been, and will continue to be, significantly related to the inflationary economy of recent years. The industry's highly-trained professional personnel and wide range of services and supplies sharply reduce its ability to control costs without curtailing necessary community services and/or reducing the quality of patient care. Although hospitals must buy, build and hire in the same market place, they cannot offset costs by increasing production - as can industry, or by levying additional taxes - as can government.

In most cases, the additional costs have been offset by improvements in medical technology and the addition of new services. These have directly contributed to the decreasing average length of stay for hospital patients in the Commonwealth.

In addition, hospitals have taken considerable steps toward minimizing costs in areas under their control. Economies of scale have been obtained largely through the cooperative efforts of many institutions by participation in numerous shared service programs. Also increased efficiency and better management techniques have been produced through management engineering studies and elaborate management reporting systems.

These cost containment activities will continue and new ones will be developed. However, the industry cannot begin to solve the problems beyond the realm of its own control.

Statistical information at the national and state levels is attached.

Table 6-1. A Statistical Look At Community Hospitals in Pennsylvania

	1972	1973	1974	1975	1976	1977
Total hospitals reporting	232	232	239	240	246	246
Total beds	54,092	53,633	55,087	54,907	55,696	55,488
Total admissions	1,702,615	1,721,811	1,810,733	1,820,715	1,896,130	1,881,993
Total inpatient days	15,452,735	15,260,286	15,694,182	15,462,326	15,924,015	15,733,983
Total emergency visits	3,501,170	3,771,359	4,241,973	4,268,824	4,545,559	4,544,960
Total outpatient visits	13,655,547	14,011,261	15,897,416	16,028,180	16,779,071	15,745,490
Total equivalent full-time personnel	125,551	126,768	134,180	138,461	145,732	151,591
Total payroll expense	$894,431,000	$952,855,000	$1,060,481,000	$1,215,094,000	$1,401,767,000	$1,544,536,000
Total annual expense	$1,519,708,000	$1,654,256,000	$1,882,072,000	$2,210,611,000	$2,619,574,000	$2,970,334,000
Average daily census	42,222	41,882	42,996	42,409	43,512	43,152
Average length of stay (days)	9.10	8.86	8.67	8.49	8.40	8.36
Adjusted expenses per inpatient day	$87.48	$95.39	$104.36	$124.28	$142.26	$162.91
Adjusted expenses per admission	$796.07	$848.97	$907.93	$1,056.38	$1,197.50	$1,367.97
Average no. of employees per patient	2.97	3.03	3.12	3.26	3.35	3.51
Average salary per employee	$7,124.05	$7,516.53	$7,903.42	$8,775.71	$9,618.80	$10,188.84
Occupancy rate (percent)	78.1	78.1	78.1	77.2	78.1	77.8
Outpatient visits to admissions (ratio)	8.0 to 1	8.1 to 1	8.8 to 1	8.8 to 1	8.8 to 1	8.4 to 1

Source: Hospital Statistics, American Hospital Association, 1973_78.

301

Table 6-2. Community Hospitals Comparisons With Nearby States

Adjusted Expenses Per Inpatient Day

State	1972	1973	1974	1975	1976	1977
New York	$118.20	$128.32	$140.02	$164.41	$169.00	$193.66
Maryland	109.50	120.85	130.44	153.78	171.46	187.36
Delaware	103.03	109.83	113.15	139.19	157.22	175.59
New Jersey	88.83	98.97	109.58	125.88	142.51	159.69
PENNSYLVANIA	**87.48**	**95.39**	**104.36**	**124.28**	**142.26**	**162.91**

Adjusted Expenses Per Admission

State	1972	1973	1974	1975	1976	1977
New York	$1,134.72	$1,257.54	$1,372.20	$1,627.66	$1,673.10	$1,887.59
Maryland	919.80	1,003.06	1,095.70	1,276.37	1,457.41	1,587.83
Delaware	834.54	900.61	950.46	1,155.28	1,320.65	1,479.65
New Jersey	781.70	870.94	964.30	1,095.16	1,254.09	1,381.05
PENNSYLVANIA	**796.07**	**848.97**	**907.93**	**1,056.38**	**1,197.50**	**1,367.97**

Source: Hospital Statistics, American Hospital Association, 1973-1978.

Table 6-3. Community Short-Term General Hospitals Average Cost per Inpatient Day Equivalent 1974 and 1975

Rank	State	Cost per Inpatient Day Equivalent			Increase 1974 to 1975
		1975	1974	(Rank)	
1	California	$185.61	$155.78	(2)	$29.83
2	Alaska	183.65	163.04	(1)	20.61
3	District of Columbia	180.31	146.38	(4)	33.93
4	Massachusetts	176.02	152.33	(3)	23.69
5	New York	164.41	140.02	(7)	24.39
6	Connecticut	163.31	141.56	(6)	21.75
7	Rhode Island	161.52	133.41	(8)	27.91
8	Nevada	159.41	142.41	(5)	17.00
9	Maryland	153.78	130.44	(9)	23.34
10	Washington	151.54	125.83	(11)	25.51
11	Arizona	149.99	129.45	(10)	20.54
12	Michigan	144.08	122.46	(12)	21.62
13	Illinois	143.44	121.01	(13)	22.43
14	Oregon	140.68	116.82	(15)	23.86
15	Delaware	139.19	113.15	(17)	26.04
16	Florida	136.85	113.13	(18)	23.72
—	U.S. AVERAGE	133.81	113.55	(16)	20.26
17	Colorado	131.24	111.74	(19)	19.50
18	Hawaii	130.21	118.19	(14)	12.02
19	Utah	126.99	110.27	(20)	16.72
20	New Jersey	125.88	109.58	(21)	16.30
21	New Mexico	124.86	103.23	(24)	21.63
22	Ohio	124.81	107.36	(22)	17.45
23	Louisiana	124.68	103.03	(25)	21.65
24	PENNSYLVANIA	124.28	104.36	(23)	19.92
25	Georgia	121.82	102.57	(26)	19.25
26	Oklahoma	117.80	98.22	(28)	19.58
27	Maine	117.10	96.54	(33)	20.56
28	Texas	116.82	97.17	(32)	19.65
29	Missouri	116.74	97.90	(30)	18.84
30	Vermont	115.32	99.49	(27)	15.83
31	Wisconsin	114.42	98.20	(29)	16.22
32	Indiana	112.19	95.43	(34)	16.76
33	New Hampshire	111.62	95.12	(35)	16.50
34	Minnesota	111.62	97.60	(31)	14.02
35	Virginia	109.25	91.81	(36)	17.44
36	Nebraska	108.16	90.93	(38)	17.23
37	Alabama	105.92	91.58	(37)	14.34

Table 6-3.   (continued)

Rank	State	Cost per Inpatient Day Equivalent			Increase 1974 to 1975
		1975	1974	(Rank)	
38	Tennessee	104.15	88.88	(39)	15.27
39	Wyoming	103.82	84.55	(46)	19.27
40	Idaho	102.89	88.40	(40)	14.49
41	Kansas	102.49	87.02	(42)	15.47
42	South Carolina	101.75	86.45	(43)	15.30
43	North Carolina	100.97	88.18	(41)	12.79
44	Iowa	99.36	85.52	(44)	13.84
45	Montana	99.28	82.56	(47)	16.72
46	Kentucky	98.33	85.26	(45)	13.07
47	West Virginia	97.06	82.08	(49)	14.98
48	Arkansas	94.57	82.27	(48)	12.30
49	Mississippi	93.62	80.36	(50)	13.26
50	North Dakota	92.88	78.40	(51)	14.48
51	South Dakota	92.01	77.86	(52)	14.15

Source: Hospital Statistics, American Hospital Association, August, 1976

HOSPITAL COST CONTAINMENT EFFORTS: "THE VOLUNTARY EFFORT"

During 1977 and 1978, the Carter administration moved to get from Congress mandatory controls on hospital costs. The chairman of the House Ways and Means Subcommittee on Health challenged the hospitals and others in the health sector to take steps to control, voluntarily, rising costs. His challenge led to concerted action by the AMA, AHA, and the FAH to develop a program designed to reduce the rate of increase in hospital expenditures to 2% a year for 1978 and 1979 (for a total of 4%), to allow no net increase in the number of beds for 1978, and to secure a reduction in 1978 of new capital investment by hospitals. The national effort led to the development of committees in all states to work toward attainment of these objectives.

The voluntary effort, according to its supporters, is working. The hospitals cite the fact that while the rate of hospital expenditure increase for 1977 was 15.6%, for 1978 (for the first 10 months), it was down to 12.9%. The Carter administration is, however, not satisfied. It wants the rate of increase cut to 9.7% by 1980, and it wants new equipment and services spending drastically cut as well. To secure this, the administration has asked Congress for mandatory standby controls that would be triggered if expenditure increases exceed 9.7%. This is well below the industry's pledged reduction of 4% over a two-year period, and the industry is clearly unhappy with the HEW secretary's targets. Whether Congress will grant the administration standby controls and, if so, at what triggering percentage cannot be forecast with certainty at this writing.

The Blue Cross-Blue Shield Associations took a major step to affect hospital expenditures in early February 1979 when they called on their member plans not to pay for the routine diagnostic tests that patients normally get on admission to the hospital, such as a complete blood count, chest x-ray film, urinalysis, blood chemistry, and so on. Instead, the associations called on their member plans to pay for these only when specifically ordered by the attending physician. This, when fully implemented, will, it is believed, slow the pressure for raising Blue Cross and Blue Shield rates as well as contribute to the voluntary effort.

What is occurring, of course, is a form of jawboning, a challenging of the industry by threatening drastic action, which, in turn, prompts an industry response designed to defuse the federal threat.

EXCESS GENERAL HOSPITAL BED SUPPLY

Government and others have been claiming that there are too many general hospital beds in the country. To some extent, the alleged excess bed capacity in the United States may be due to the assignment of beds to given specialties. Another area in which excess bed capacity appears is in obstetrics. It is generally acknowledged that as a result of a declining birth rate, we have more obstetric beds than we need. Closing the beds in many communities is, however, a very sticky problem, particularly when part of the excess capacity is in a Catholic hospital and part in a non-Catholic hospital. Can one force the Catholic hospital to close its beds, thus denying the right of a Catholic mother to have her child in a Catholic hospital? Can one force the other hospital to close its beds, thus denying some pregnant women the right to have an abortion? Pediatric units also typically have low occupancy: Children simply no longer are afflicted with conditions requiring hospitalization to the extent they did when the hospitals were built. Conversion of pediatric and obstetric beds for other uses sometimes poses problems due to structural features of the units and due to the desire to maintain segregated units: Is it advisable, for example, to place adult medical and surgical cases within pediatric or obstetric units? What would be the costs of conversion in such a way as to maintain separate sections? Are the costs so great as to make construction of new beds elsewhere more desirable particularly

Table 6-4. A Look At Community Hospitals' Expenses in Fiscal Year 1977

State	No. of Hospitals	Total Expenses Percent Change 1976 to 1977	Adjusted Expenses Per Inpatient Day		Adjusted Expenses Per Admission	
			Fiscal 1977	Percent Change 1976 to 1977	Fiscal 1977	Percent Change 1976 to 1977
UNITED STATES	**5,881**	**14.16%**	**$173.98**	**13.89%**	**$1,318.31**	**12.95%**
Alabama	131	19.05	141.65	14.66	1,009.27	14.09
Alaska	16	43.87	303.59	31.43	1,562.78	32.17
Arizona	58	14.54	197.19	16.10	1,424.48	14.12
Arkansas	91	17.55	129.46	16.00	833.21	17.29
California	527	16.67	245.57	14.79	1,607.55	14.89
Colorado*	84	15.16	172.79	11.93	1,172.09	13.64
Connecticut*	36	11.38	205.53	11.45	1,547.94	11.21
Delaware	8	14.04	175.59	11.68	1,479.65	12.44
District of Columbia	13	17.14	252.80	22.98	2,016.88	22.16
Florida	209	17.72	176.73	13.37	1,305.21	13.00
Georgia	157	13.36	153.89	11.89	991.91	12.60
Hawaii	20	22.92	176.22	12.14	1,276.26	17.30
Idaho	46	19.63	142.85	13.88	882.16	17.06
Illinois*	241	13.96	189.63	14.27	1,509.31	13.25
Indiana	114	16.38	149.66	16.17	1,170.73	15.34
Iowa	131	13.78	137.80	16.60	1,026.47	14.97
Kansas	143	18.98	140.26	18.34	1,064.66	17.02
Kentucky	107	13.83	128.63	13.34	907.58	12.45
Louisiana	141	19.16	159.34	15.94	1,014.61	14.10
Maine	49	18.31	155.89	17.48	1,170.78	17.59
Maryland*	51	11.78	187.36	9.27	1,587.83	9.08
Massachusetts*	119	13.66	227.59	13.76	1,931.44	13.42
Michigan	212	12.09	189.04	13.20	1,483.36	10.47

Minnesota	171	16.66	149.79	17.00	1,302.43	18.21
Mississippi	103	17.95	122.68	13.21	852.54	15.38
Missouri	148	17.16	154.97	14.83	1,279.08	15.89
Montana	57	14.74	134.88	15.44	865.35	16.95
Nebraska	96	10.17	138.38	13.04	1,100.74	12.26
Nevada	19	17.46	208.22	15.23	1,362.14	12.27
New Jersey*	103	11.84	159.69	12.06	1,381.05	10.74
New Mexico	37	11.36	177.50	19.09	989.90	13.93
New Hampshire	27	16.72	143.85	14.35	1,024.03	14.45
New York*	300	6.21	193.66	8.59	1,887.59	6.93
North Carolina	129	15.48	130.79	14.33	980.68	14.62
North Dakota	53	19.20	131.75	15.52	1,100.55	17.71
Ohio	208	14.03	166.08	15.19	1,333.05	13.61
Oklahoma	120	17.44	164.49	16.74	1,070.45	16.32
Oregon	78	15.56	188.92	13.26	1,180,81	12.91
PENNSYLVANIA	**246**	**13.39**	**162.91**	**14.52**	**1,367.97**	**14.06**
Rhode Island*	14	11.08	201.11	10.88	1,640.74	9.68
South Carolina	72	20.15	135.26	16.94	953.57	15.66
South Dakota	57	13.30	120.47	12.00	862.34	14.91
Tennessee	142	20.83	141.09	16.15	1,018.08	14.06
Texas	500	16.47	158.31	16.44	1,047.49	14.69
Utah	34	20.14	178.47	20.49	938.63	14.99
Vermont	16	10.25	137.54	9.40	1,154.23	10.25
Virginia	102	17.80	147.20	14.81	1,179.76	16.81
Washington*	108	15.17	200.01	13.96	1,104.27	12.74
West Virginia	67	13.71	132.12	16.36	986.43	16.81
Wisconsin*	144	12.30	157.11	18.34	1,251.57	12.57
Wyoming	26	14.14	144.04	21.45	754.15	8.80

*States with mandatory review and approval of hospitals' rates.
Source: *Hospital Statistics*, American Hospital Association, 1978.

**Table 6-5. Cost per Inpatient Day Equivalent of
the 25 Largest Cities (Community Short-Term
General Hospitals)**

		1975 C/IDE	Population Rank
1.	Boston	$271	(16)
2.	Los Angeles	247	(3)
3.	San Francisco	211	(13)
4.	New York, NY	196	(1)
5.	Seattle	180	(22)
6.	Washington, D.C.	180	(9)
7.	San Diego	178	(14)
8.	Chicago	178	(2)
9.	Detroit	171	(5)
10.	Baltimore	171	(7)
11.	Philadelphia	164	(4)
12.	Milwaukee	163	(12)
13.	Phoenix	163	(20)
14.	Cleveland	154	(10)
15.	New Orleans	153	(19)
16.	Denver	153	(25)
17.	Indianapolis	152	(11)
18.	Jacksonville	151	(23)
19.	Pittsburgh	141	(24)
20.	Houston	140	(6)
21.	Dallas	132	(8)
22.	Columbus, Ohio	131	(21)
23.	St. Louis	127	(18)
24.	Memphis	125	(17)
25.	San Antonio	123	(15)

Source: Hospital Statistics, American Hospital Association,
August, 1973, 1974, 1975, 1976.

Note: Amounts rounded to nearest dollar. Entire Standard
Metropolitan Statistical Area (SMSA) figures included for
each city.

since the pediatric and obstetric bed needs could change should the population
served by the community change or should the birth rate change?

A high percentage of the unused bed capacity is in the smaller hospitals. In
1974, for example, hospitals in the 6-24 bed capacity had an occupancy rate
of 48.4%. Hospitals in the 25-49 bed size averaged a 56.5% occupancy, and
those hospitals with a capacity in the 50-99 bed range had an average

Table 6-6. 1977 Adjusted Expenses Per Inpatient Day 25 Largest U.S. Cities

		City Only		Metropolitan Area	
		Hospitals	Expenses	Hospitals	Expenses
1.	Boston	20	$367.09	58	$274.69
2.	Los Angeles	49	313.74	172	261.48
3.	San Francisco	18	275.77	64	248.61
4.	Chicago	57	253.38	103	212.20
5.	Washington, D.C.	13	252.80	34	217.52
6.	Detroit	30	238.27	68	216.92
7.	Seattle	19	230.19	29	224.48
8.	New York	93	228.35	112	224.34
9.	Milwaukee	17	225.62	27	210.39
10.	San Diego	14	223.31	28	219.77
11.	Phoenix	11	214.36	22	209.37
12.	Baltimore	21	212.77	28	201.57
13.	PHILADELPHIA	40	211.24	73	192.28
14.	Houston	39	201.38	60	194.78
15.	Cleveland	20	200.99	37	187.90
16.	Denver	16	200.84	23	195.60
17.	Indianapolis	7	191.08	16	180.53
18.	PITTSBURGH	21	189.38	39	168.64
19.	Jacksonville	9	186.45	16	183.63
20.	New Orleans	15	185.74	25	178.88
21.	Memphis	11	170.97	12	170.64
22.	Dallas	25	170.71	75	165.92
23.	Columbus	11	167.06	15	164.73
24.	St. Louis	28	165.00	34	163.42
25.	San Antonio	13	155.21	15	153.79

Source: Hospital Statistics, American Hospital Association, 1978

occupancy of 65.4%. Larger hospitals averaged higher occupancy rates, with the national average of all hospitals being 75.3%. The smaller hospitals, of course, tend to be lower cost institutions because they do not maintain the costly specialty and support services. Many of them are in rural areas.

It is argued that we cannot afford to maintain such excess capacity. Typically, proponents of this view cite the cost of maintaining an empty hospital bed. But figures are terribly misleading. If the costs they cite are based on the average cost per patient day when the hospital is operating at optimal capacity, it does not follow that it costs the hospital the same if beds are not occupied, yet this is frequently what is implied.

The average cost per patient day is determined by dividing the total cost of running the hospital by the number of patient days during a fixed time period. Let us assume that a 100-bed general hospital runs at 85% occupancy and has a total operating cost of $3,102,500 for the year. That would compute to $100 average cost per patient day. Does this mean, however, that if the hospital's occupancy drops to 75%, the ten extra unused beds per diem cost the hospital $1,000 a day to maintain? This is where the figures used are often misleading. If occupancy drops to 75%, the hospital may still incur some expenses for those empty beds with regard to heating, electricity, and cleaning, though even these items are not necessarily continuing expenses if the construction permits turning down the heat and closing off the rooms. But those 10 empty beds will not be drawing upon drugs, food, linens, laboratory and radiology services, nursing services, and so on. The total hospital costs would, therefore, drop because over time fewer items would be purchased, fewer nurses hired. What, then, would be the cost of an empty bed? Certainly not the average cost per patient day. Even the estimate of 50% of the cost of an occupied bed seems high, and the assumption that the initial costs of construction and finance expenses of what is now an unused bed should be considered is a debatable point (14, p.15). In late 1976, a committee of the Institute of Medicine of the National Academy of Sciences issued a report entitled *Controlling the Supply of Hospital Beds* (14). It concluded "that significant surpluses of short-term general hospital beds exist or are developing in many areas of the United States and that these are contributing significantly to rising hospital care costs . . ." (14, pp. vii, 16). In a sharp dissent, Shropshire (a committee member and administrator of the Tucson Medical Center) stated that this statement (14, p. 55).

---

appears to take some questionable research at face value and makes a critical assumption that there are substantial savings in bed reductions. Is this another example where we are looking for a scapegoat or a convenient 'red herring' in order to avoid addressing such other factors as costs from excess regulation, unrestrained hospital services generated by private practice, society's infinite demands and inability to cope with 'who shall live,' government's generous promises and arbitrary payment system, CAT scanners, open-heart surgery, and other significant clinical program developments? It avoids the whole question of the major impact that intensification of hospital services has had on the inflation rate in the hospital industry.

The committee, as a result of its calculations and analyses, calls for at least a 10% reduction in the ratio of short-term general hospital beds to population.

The 1976 ratio of about 4.4 nonfederal beds per 1,000 population should be reduced to about four beds per thousand by the end of 1981. The committee noted that "an effective control on hospital bed supply would lead to some waiting lists of patients for elective admissions to hospitals. We believe that manageable waiting lists for such patients are acceptable trade-offs for the economies to be realized by decreasing hospital beds to reasonable levels. (14, p. 41).

A careful reading of the report leaves one uneasy over the refined calculations with their apparent slavish obsession with ratios, ignoring some of the harder issues that Shropshire identified. The almost offhanded mention of waiting lists, as though they are minor considerations, displays a lack of awareness for the public irritation with such lists in both Great Britain and New Zealand, where they have prompted the rapid growth of the private, nonregulated health sector.

The real issue here is that government is now paying a heavy proportion of total hospital costs in the country, and it is searching for some quick way to control government outlays.

When Bunker et al., in their study of elective hysterectomies, conclude that "society, if it is to pay the costs, must decide whether to allocate public funds for a procedure if it appears to be more of a convenience or luxury than a necessity" (15, p.270), they open, of course, a Pandora's box, for the issue is not only payment of the physician's fee and hospital's bill but also whether or not we want to allow the health system even to have the capacity to handle such cases. Under current legislation, buttressed by reports such as the one just cited from the Institute of Medicine, we seem to be moving in the direction of a negative response. This raises some interesting questions regarding the rights of individuals in a free society, including the right to freely dispose of earned income. In Great Britain and New Zealand, nonregulated private sectors have at least provided a safety valve for calculation errors and for individual choices. But we do not in the United States. Schwartz, writing in *The New York Times* (16), notes how some of the advocates of cost control and of one standard of care for all change their attitudes when it hits home: then, either because of personal wealth or influence, "only the best is acceptable, regardless of cost." And there is, for them, no queuing, no waiting list. Yet Schwartz goes on to note:

The currently fashionable rhetoric, which has been heard from both major political parties, is that every American has a right to first-class medical care, but after 11 years of Medicare and Medicaid costs, politicians are seeking ways to reduce medical costs, not to provide for care of the quality received by Mrs. Carter, Senator Humphrey, or Edward M. Kennedy, Jr.

UTILIZATION REVIEW (UR) AND CERTIFICATE OF NEED (CON)

Government has sought to put a lid on rising costs through mandated utilization review and control of hospital expansion through CON legislation.

Utilization review was to focus on appropriateness for admission to hospital and on length of stay. Aspects of this will be considered in later sections of this chapter. Suffice it to say here that the aim was to assure government expenditures were necessary and not wasted.

CON legislation was directed toward the control of hospital expansion. Typically, any new service, beds, or equipment that cost more than $100,000 ($150,000 in early 1979) required a certificate of need from the state government. Without a CON, government reimbursement for care using those beds and services or equipment under Medicare, Medicaid, and other programs would be denied. As Blue Cross and other insurance programs faced cost pressures, many of them also sought shelter in CON legislation as a hoped-for way to control spiraling costs. Clearly, CON may slow down expansion; in slowing down, it serves to contain costs. Whether the health needs of the population are served by this is open to some question. Whether there is a real cost saving is also open to question: Denial of a CON to a hospital in one community because of unused capacity at a hospital in another community to some extent hides some costs, that is, the costs incurred by patients who are now forced to go to the other community. These consumer-borne costs may include transportation, food, hotel, lost time at work, as well as personal inconvenience. These costs are rarely, if ever, calculated. Whether CON laws, which Congress has now mandated for all states, can effectively contain direct costs for government programs remains to be seen. The history of regulatory agencies in the United States does not provide much encouragement. Even in states in which CON laws have been operational, ingenious hospitals have often found ways to get what they want overtly or covertly.

UNNECESSARY SURGERY

Surgeons are among the most highly paid physicians. Drama surrounds them, and the more dramatic the procedure, the more it costs, not only in terms of the surgeon's fee but also in terms of the hospital support system needed to back up whatever the surgeon does.

We are told often about unnecessary coronary bypass operations, unnecessary hysterectomies, unnecessary mastectomies, unnecessary tonsillectomies, and so on. And we know that in Britain the surgical rate for some procedures is half what it is here. The reports make good news, but, typically, the full story is much more complicated.

Take, for example, needless mastectomies. In 1977, a peer review subcommittee connected with the NIH reviewed 506 breast lesion cases that were discovered by mammography in breast screening centers. (It should be noted that there are disagreements within the profession as to the appropriateness of mammography screening.) The subcommittee found 66 questionable cases and concluded that 53 of those cases had undergone what appeared to be needless mastectomies. The findings made good copy in the nation's press, but the professional criticisms of the subcommittee findings caused the parent committee to reconvene, and it found that most of the cases in question were the result of the subcommittee's having reviewed the wrong slides (17, p.7)

For nearly all the 53 mastectomy patients . . . surgery was delayed anywhere from three days to several months—contrary to the impression that there was a rush to surgery. In 11 cases, biopsies were diagnosed as malignant by [breast screening center] pathologists but not by the hospital pathologists. Appropriately . . . there was no mastectomy in these cases. In two, though the diagnosis was questionable, mastectomies were performed on women at their own insistence because of personal and family histories of breast cancer.

The full committee found that the clinical management was appropriate in nearly every case. In what may be one of the understatements of the year, an NIH spokesman stated, "I think there's going to be a credibility problem . . . No matter what happens, doubt is going to be thrown on the other minimal [size] lesions the panel agreed on. People will wonder about the whole report's accuracy."

A favorite whipping post is the surgical removal of the uterus (hysterectomy). One of the best discussions of the clinical indications for elective hysterectomy appeared in *The New England Journal of Medicine* on July 29, 1976, under the heading of "Public Health Rounds at the Harvard School of Public Health." The discussants described what were in their judgment the clinical indications for elective hysterectomy, and the indications were extensive and extended far beyond benign and malignant lesions; and they included birth control and improvement of the quality of life. It is clear from that discussion the medical profession is not in agreement as to the indications for elective hysterectomy.

In an assessment of the costs, risks, and benefits to be derived from elective hysterectomy, Bunker et al. concluded (15, p.270):

The principal benefits of elective hysterectomy, it is assumed, are improvements in the quality of life. Menstrual discomfort and inconvenience will be relieved, but these benefits may be offset by a variety of unpleasant sequelae associated with hysterectomy and castration. There are no data on what proportion of women, on the balance, are benefited by elective hysterectomy. While the benefits are unmeasured and uncertain, the costs are large. These costs are rarely paid by the patient. Society, if it is to pay the costs, must decide whether to allocate public funds for a procedure if it appears to be more of a convenience or luxury than a necessity.

They also noted that "the individual patient may consider that the quality of life benefits of hysterectomy are sufficient to offset attendant risks; indeed, based on the extremely high hysterectomy rates reported for physician's wives, who should be reasonably well informed 'consumers', it seems likely that many women will make this choice." (15, p.269).

Quality of life may well account for some of the surgical rate differences between the United States and Britain. In Britain, surgical care is rationed by use of a surgical waiting list for elective surgery. The rationing is dictated by the inability of the government to provide sufficient beds and professional and support services to eliminate the backlog of cases and to deal with new cases as they come along. Depending on the condition, a patient may have to wait six months, a year, or longer unless the patient chooses to incur the cost of private care. By the time the hospital gets around to the elective surgical case, the patient may well have decided to live with it or may even have died from some other condition. Varicose veins won't kill a person, but they can be discomforting and downright painful. Many people with gallstones can keep them and bear with the occasional attack. So, too, with many inguinal hernias. The sociology of the society may also have a bearing on these cross-national differences and merits study. Is the American patient, for example, a more decisive-oriented person, more desirous of a quick, radical solution rather than living with whatever life or the authorities serve?

This is not to say that there is no unnecessary surgery, rather to suggest that the extent to which it exists is not easily determined, nor is the cause. Professional judgments and patient choices all play a role. Recent findings regarding coronary bypass surgery, for example, reflect current disagreement among professionals: There is a professional debate going on as to the appropriateness of this procedure. Moreover, when the debate is ended, we are probably going to find a time lag before all get the message, reflecting the slowness by which new knowledge and new technology are disseminated. One needs to bear in mind—and the coronary bypass operation may or may not fit here—that what may have been medically indicated yesterday may have become contraindicated today because of new knowledge. Whether the surgery is necessary or not may thus reflect on when it was done, whether or not there were any special clinical considerations, and whether the information on necessity had been disseminated.

Dyck et al., in a Canadian study of hysterectomies, illustrate the complexities in making determinations as to necessity for surgery (18, pp.1326-1328):

It should be emphasized that the difficulty in establishing rigid criteria for performing a hysterectomy is well known and was recognized by the Committee. The list of indications has already been criticized by some as being too liberal and by others as being too restrictive . . . The Committee realizes that some of the accepted indications might not, in everyone's opinion, justify hysterectomy.

Dyck et al. go on to cite two U.S. studies. In one study, the investigator found hysterectomies unnecessary in 30.8% of the cases, but he did not consider as an indication for surgery a condition that the Canadian group considered appropriate. In the second U.S. study, the investigator concluded that 39.3% of the hysterectomies in his sample were questionable. But Dyck et al. note that he did not include three conditions that the Canadians believed were appropriate indications for surgery. Such cross-national differences can also appear between regions within the United States, affecting not only necessity for surgery but also necessity for admission and length of hospital stay.

The extent to which unnecessary surgery stems from sloppy diagnosis and avarice is simply not known, though it is probably slight, for the various peer checks (JCAH review, residency training programs, tissue committees, PAS-MAP, HUP, PSRO review, family-physician referrals, second opinions before surgery) as well as the risks of malpractice suits serve as regulatory devices. Certainly unnecessary surgery resulting from sloppy diagnosis and avarice is much less frequent today than in years past and is becoming less of a problem as peer review mechanisms are strengthened. As a case in point, though not necessarily due to sloppy diagnosis or avarice, Dyck et al. noted that their review committee was appointed by the Saskatchawan College of Physicians and Surgeons as a result of Saskatchawan Health Department data that showed a sharp rise in the hysterectomy rate. Concurrent with the Committee's review was a sharp drop in the number of hysterectomies in the hospitals studied. The authors state that "there is indirect evidence that the work of the Committee has made doctors more critical in their judgment of when a hysterectomy is required, as evidenced by the drop in the percentage of unjustified hysterec-tomies." They conclude by observing that "it must also be said that there should never have been any need for the creation of the Committee, which resulted from a breakdown of adequate review at the hospital level."

If one were to hazard a guess as to where to look for unnecessary surgery resulting from sloppy diagnosis or avarice, it would be, as the Canadian study suggests, where the peer review mechanisms are weakest. Weaknesses can, of course, develop in any system, but the checks are weakest, if existent at all, in nonaccredited hospitals and physician's offices. This is not to say that surgery in nonaccredited hospitals and doctors offices is unnecessary surgery or that it may only be found there but that the peer review checks are weakest in those locales.

Organized medicine—that is, medical societies and associations—is under-standably sensitive to charges that reflect on the profession, and "unnecessary surgery" is one such area of sensitivity. The editor of JAMA dealt with this topic in an editorial in 1976. He wrote (19, pp.387-388):

Physicians have a responsibility to advise, prescribe, and perform only that which is in the best interest of their patients. To subject a patient to a procedure that the physician believed to be of no benefit and that might even result in harm would be reprehensible. Most physicians are highly ethical people and try to use their best judgment and their clinical skills for the benefit of and not harm to their patients.

Recently the Subcommittee on Oversight and Investigations of the Com-mittee on Interstate and Foreign Commerce of the US House of Representatives held hearings on the subject of "unnecessary surgery." The report of the Committee, entitled "Cost and Quality of Health Care: Unnecessary Surgery," alleges that 2.38 million unnecessary operations performed in the United States in 1974 resulted in 11,900 deaths and an expenditure of 3.92 billion dollars. These are serious charges and should not be made without incontro-vertible factual support.

However, the procedure followed, the definitions employed, and the data used call into serious question the conclusions at which the committee arrived. It began its study of a complex issue without first defining the nature of the problem being investigated. This approach has been taken by many people embarking on research who have subsequently realized that finding the correct answers depends on asking the right questions.

Definitions of what constitutes unnecessary surgery were developed during the hearings, and thus the problem was defined in terms of the answers that the committee wanted to hear. This backward approach was further distorted by anecdotal evidence from persons who had undergone surgery and by testimony only from physicians prejudiced to one side of the question. Finally, data developed from limited regional studies were extrapolated to encompass all surgical procedures performed in the United States.

The six categories accepted by the committee as defining unnecessary surgery are worth a critical examination by the profession and the public:

Category I.   Completely discretionary operations for asymptomatic, nonpathologic, nonthreatening disorders.

Category II. Operations where no pathologic tissue is removed.

Category III. Operations where indications are a matter of difference in judgment and opinion among experts.

Category IV. Operations to alleviate endurable or tolerable symptoms.

Category V.   Operations formerly performed in large numbers, now considered outdated, obsolete, or discredited.

Category VI. Operations done primarily for the personal gain of the surgeon, wherein the weight of informed opinion would deny any indication to the present.

Of these categories, only V and VI are acceptable definitions. Category I condemns some plastic and most cosmetic surgery as unnecessary. Under Category II, procedures such as hernia repair would have to be eliminated. Category III is indeed strange, for the assumption is made that if experts differ in their opinion about the advisability of surgery, then the procedure is unnecessary. Under Category IV, both surgeon and patient may wish to abolish symptoms, but a third party could judge that the symptoms could be endured, and therefore, the proposed surgery was unnecessary. It is unlikely that this category would find wide public acceptance.

Unfortunately, reports of congressional committees become part of a permanent public record regardless of whether or not the findings are factual. The report of this committee has libeled the medical profession, and some action should be taken to set the record straight.

The House Subcommittee on Oversight and Investigation was not to be cowed by the AMA counterattack. The subcommittee held additional hearings and issued another report (*Surgical Performance: Necessity and Quality*) in December 1978 and concluded that "unnecessary surgery remains a monumental problem for the American public." The subcommittee went on to conclude that it is "appalled at the amount of evidence of incompetent as well as unnecessary surgery. There appears to be a lack of desire or ability on the part of the states, organized medicine, or existing PSROs to take corrective action."

Whether the problem is "monumental" and merits the subcommittee's being "appalled" is difficult to judge. A lone subcommittee dissent by Congressman James M. Collins, Republican from Texas, noted:

The medical profession has a long and successful history of improving the quality of surgery. Unfortunately, recognition of these gains seems to have been submerged in the atmosphere of sensationalism that has surrounded this Subcommittee's work. All too often, what should be a search for an improved partnership between government and medicine has bogged down in acrimony and distrust . . . I believe that there is some surgery performed that should not be, just as any human endeavor includes the questionable acts of some; however, neither we, nor anyone else, knows how much. I recognize that the studies of Doctors McCarthy, Bluestone, John Morris, and others raise questions about the rationale for the performance of some surgery. However, other witnesses have questioned their findings.

Clearly, whatever questions are raised as to the amount of "unnecessary" surgery are still only questions. No final judgment has been reached. Further, I do not believe that those raising the questions have adequately solved the puzzle of how to prevent such unneeded procedures, regardless of the percentage.

PROLONGED HOSPITAL STAYS

The accepted practice in patient care changes as new knowledge and new technology are acquired. In recent decades, there has been a tendency to shorten the length of hospital stay. Since hospital care is so costly today, there is keen interest in making certain that patients stay only as long as is necessary.

But not everyone shares such a view. The patient, for example, may prefer to stay in the hospital a few extra days rather than go to an intermediate care facility if that facility, in the patient's judgment, is not adequate. Or the patient or physician may feel it appropriate to keep a patient in a few extra days if there is no one at home to assist the patient on discharge. The hospital administration may also be anxious to keep patients in longer, particularly if the hospital's occupancy is down: If the patient stays in when not really necessary, the level of service required does not cost as much as normal—no definitive nursing or laboratory services may be necessary, and the only cost may be the cost of meals and laundry. But the hospital collects its usual amount from Blue Cross, the government, or other insurers. What an easy way for a hospital to make money to offset losses or high charges in other areas! It might be noted that if such prolonged lengths of stay are reduced, it does not mean that the overall cost of care will be reduced accordingly; in the long run, it may simply be redistributed, driving the remaining costs up, or it may mean the hospital will not be able to finance whatever purchases it feels are necessary or desirable. Depending on one's viewpoint, the latter may be good or bad. If the purchase will increase utilization, the insurer may not like it, but the patient or physician may find it quite desirable. The increased use of utilization review is making prolonged stays less and less of a problem: not only are physicians and hospital personnel becoming more critical in their judgments regarding need to stay in the hospital, but also someone is watching to blow the whistle.

UNNECESSARY HOSPITAL ADMISSIONS

Utilization review is making this less and less of a problem. However, it is worth noting some of the factors that have gone into this alleged abuse of hospitals because allegations tend to persist long after the disappearance or lessening of a problem.

During the 1970s, there was a marked shift in how physicians provided hospital care. Increasingly, physicians began to utilize outpatient services. Outpatient or ambulatory surgery is perhaps the most noteworthy advance: instead of admitting a patient for two or three days for certain types of surgery, the patient would go to the ambulatory or outpatient department, have the surgery done, and be sent home a few hours later. One has to be careful, however, in judging current inpatient care for what is now typically done on an outpatient basis. The physician may feel that there are clinical or other considerations that may make admission desirable. Unnecessary admissions are a little like unnecessary surgery; clinicians may disagree over the appropriateness for admission, and the disagreements may be pronounced as quality-of-life considerations enter (such as there being no one at home to take care of the ambulatory patient).

Another type of "unnecessary" admission develops from the way health insurance policies are written. Health insurance typically, but not always, does not cover tests for diagnosis. The basis for this exclusion is historical: there was no way the health insurance firm could predict what its utilization would be, and without an ability to predict utilization, there was no way to calculate a rate. Therefore, diagnostic tests were excluded, as were admissions to the hospital primarily for diagnosis. Many policies, however, did cover these diagnostic tests in hospital *if* they were part of or incidental to an admission primarily for treatment. While this may seem like hairsplitting, it was very important for the solvency of the health insurance company, for the admission for treatment was calculated in the premium; therefore, all accompanying expenses were coverable. The "unnecessary" aspect of admission came when physicians admitted their patients for two or three days for purposes of diagnosis, claiming, however, that the admission was for treatment and the tests for diagnosis incidental or an integral part of the treatment process. They did this mostly to help the patient get covered for tests that were felt necessary and that the patient might not otherwise be able to afford.

There are considerable data now to calculate rates for diagnostic test coverage, but most insured people do not have the coverage. They don't have it because it is very expensive. Many employers who may be paying the premiums for the employees won't do it for the same reason or, if willing but a union shop, won't do it because it can be an important management concession in the next set of negotiations with the union. While the data to calculate a rate exist, we should note that their reliability may be open to question unless there are controls or limits to prevent new abuses, for example, extensive physical exams, routine GI series every couple of years for those over 40 or 50, and so on.

HOSPITAL COMPETITION

Every few years, there is a new controversy in the health field, a controversy that arises from new technology. The new technology permits the management of cases in new ways—lifesaving, more effective clinical management, better diagnosis. Each in its time—cobalt therapy, coronary care, renal dialysis, open-heart surgery, computerized axial tomography—occupied center stage because of the high cost and the alleged desire of all hospitals to develop the new services. Now that the computerized axial tomography (CAT) scanner price (originally costing as high as $600,000 plus $100,000 a year to operate) is beginning to drop, and the utility of the scanner demonstrated, we can anticipate its more widespread use and, in time, replacement of it by some new item of controversy.

There is some duplication of very costly services, and there is competition among some hospitals to acquire the latest in technology. But the documentation to support the free-wheeling rhetoric is often weak. The fact is that no one really knows the extent to which there is competition, whether it is bad when it does exist, and the extent to which it causes unnecessary expenses and contributes to less than adequate care. Relatively few studies are made; usually, studies that are done focus on large metropolitan areas and on selected issues; in some of these studies, documentation is made. For example, the *American Medical News* carried this item in 1976 (20):

A recent controversy over open-heart surgery in Boston has resulted in a hospital just outside of Boston moving to discontinue its program of cardiovascular surgery requiring extracorporeal support.

The decision to discontinue the program was arrived at after a six-month dispute that began when the assistant director for acute and ambulatory care of the state Dept. of Public Health received a complaint that the open-heart surgery program at Malden Hospital in Malden, Mass. showed an unusually high death rate—32 deaths representing 49% of the cases over a seven-year period.

The state then instructed the hospital to investigate the charges. The hospital's board of trustees asked the American Assn. for Thoracic Surgery to conduct a study of all aspects of the program. The association conducted its review April 16-17.

According to the hospital, the review team was provided with curriculums vitae of all pertinent staff members and pump technicians, a breakdown by procedure of the cases to be studied, a description of the hospital's anesthesia, radiology, respiratory departments, and all lab procedures associated with open-heart surgery.

Said the review committee after a two-day look at the program: " . . . the results of open-heart surgery in the Malden Hospital program from 1968 through 1975, do not compare favorably with average reported results of comparable cases in the United States for the same period."

The review committee presented a number of factors which it noted as contributing to the untoward results:

- Insufficient quantity of cardiovascular clinical material requiring extracorporeal support was available.
- Surgical teams had insufficient experience in cardiovascular surgery requiring extracorporeal support.
- Though anesthesia services were found to be acceptable as provided since September, 1975, an inability to evaluate the quality of anesthesia services prior to that time led the committee to conclude the anesthesia services might have been a contributing cause to the high mortality rate.
- A large number of the patients operated upon were critically ill.
- Autopsy reports were inadequate.

Said the hospital, in response to the committee's report, "The report reinforces our initial concerns that the relatively limited number of open heart surgical cases presented does not permit the development of the team coordination . . . which depends on frequent and repeated interaction of the team members in a pump assisted setting."

"The trustees accept the premise of the American Assn. for Thoracic Surgery that a viable open heart surgical program cannot be sponsored by the Malden Hospital at this time," said a report of the hospital's board.

It is more difficult to judge those instances in which there is duplication or unused capacity but no health indicators suggesting lessened quality of care. While some condemn hospitals that compete with others, others might well applaud such competition because it may serve to improve the overall quality of care in a given institution, indeed even in the community for the ripple effect it will create.

Let us assume, for example, that a large hospital decides to develop an open heart surgery unit. Physicians on the staff may want such a service available to their patients when necessary. Let us also assume that other open heart surgery units in the community are not operating at full capacity. For the sake of efficiency, should the new unit develop? If it does develop, the cost of care in the community may indeed be higher than need be because of the inefficiencies resulting from unused capacity. But what would be the salutary effect on the hospital that seeks to develop the service? Not only would the physicians have greater pride in their institution and a new resource, but the very presence of the open heart surgery unit would cause other associated units to be strengthened, which would have the effect of an overall strengthening of the hospital clinically. If the hospital is denied the opportunity to develop the service, one can safely say that the quality of care in that hospital may not be the best because of the weaker associated services; also, the hospital might lose some of its clinicians, who will feel frustrated over the inability to see developed an optimal professional environment. This would further weaken the hospital clinically. The same "rats leaving a sinking ship" syndrome could also develop if hospitals are forced to close some units because of low occupancy. This is no idle threat, for we have considerable evidence of physicians leaving Great Britain, Canada, and New Zealand because of what they felt were unsatisfactory professional environments.

The problem today is that because hospitals are reimbursed close to cost by most health insurance policies, and because it is relatively easy for them to borrow money because they are good risks, and because there is very little good community health planning, it has been too easy for a hospital to charge ahead and develop new services without thinking about the ability of the hospital to maintain a high quality service with necessary supporting services, and it has been too easy not to think about cost implications.

As we shall see in the chapter on health planning, the health systems agencies have been placed in the position of both planning and regulating despite the fact that there is ample evidence to suggest that when the two are combined, regulation holds sway and little hard planning is undertaken. Shropshire alludes to this in his dissent to the Institute of Medicine's report on *Controlling the*

Supply of Hospital Beds when he says that "focus on bed ratios will give the Health Systems Agencies a simple way to avoid doing any true planning for the community and probably will not have much impact on cost inflation (14, p. 55)." (The health systems agencies referred to are the officially designated area-wide health planning agencies that blanket the nation and whose recommendations go to the state health planning and resource development agencies.) It will be suggested in the later chapter that effective voluntary controls on development are possible and can come about through long-range community health planning in which the providers are full participants.

HOSPITAL RATES AND COST CONTROL

As hospital costs rise, the amount charged by the hospital for patient care also rises. Most of the increased charges are paid for by health insurance or by some government sponsored program—Medicare and Medicaid being the two most important. As suggested earlier, the hospitals contend that they have little control over most of the cost elements in their operations; they have to pay at least the minimum wage, they are now subject to malpractice suits, and they have to bear the increased costs of food, fuel, telephones, drugs, new equipment and the cost of meeting the ever-changing regulations set by various government agencies.

The pressures on government and on the insurance companies are somewhat different. While sometimes sympathetic to the plight of the hospitals, government can't afford a continued price rise without an eventual tax increase, nor can the insurance companies without rate increases. Both government and the health insurance industry have thus sought ways to contain costs. CON legislation, utilization review, and PSROs have been steps that, in part, seek the goal of cost control. Direct control over hospital costs is also being explored in an increasing number of states. In early 1978, at least 24 states had some type of rate review program, some of which were mandatory, some voluntary. In a survey of half of the states with rate-review programs by the *American Medical News* (21), it was found that in at least five states (New York, Maryland, Connecticut, Washington, and Indiana):

---

the rate of increase in either total hospital expenditures or expenses per in-patient day was held to approximately ten percent in the past year or two. The national average rise in total hospital expenditures is estimated at about 16 percent during that period, and per day in-patient costs have risen at 15.4 percent a year nationwide.

Most of the rate review programs rely on *prospective reimbursement* as the preferred method for setting a hospital's rate. Under prospective reimbursement, a hospital negotiates in advance the rate it will be paid by the government, health insurance companies, and/or paying patient. The laws vary as to whom and to what the negotiated rate applies. In New York, for example, it applies only to Medicaid (a state/federal-funded program) and Blue Cross reimbursement. The hospitals negotiate separate rates with the federal government for Medicare (a federal/consumer funded program) reimbursement, and they do whatever they can with commercial insurance companies and self-paying patients, negotiating whatever rate the traffic will bear. The Maryland rate review body, on the other hand, regulates all hospital rates, and its power is even believed to encompass the regulation of rates charged by hospital based radiologists, pathologists, and cardiologists, although this point is in litigation. In Connecticut, a trial referee held that the existing law there did not apply to regulation of physician charges. There is, of course, some historical precedent for routine control of physician fees, but one has to go back to colonial America in which some colonial legislative bodies did just that. Because some hospitals and physicians are seeking to avoid the constraints set by CON laws by physicians purchasing the expensive equipment for their private offices, states are looking at ways to apply CON or rate review laws to physicians' offices.

Under *prospective reimbursement*, the negotiated rate applies for a fixed time period. If the hospital is able to keep its costs or charges below the negotiated rate, it still collects the negotiated rate and makes a profit that it can use for other purposes. If, on the other hand, its costs exceed its reimbursement, it has to bear the loss. How it makes up the loss is up to the hospital: It can dip into reserves held for upcoming renovation or construction, or it can appeal to its constituency for donations. But the sums involved can be substantial. In Maryland during 1976, three hospitals had operating deficits of more than $500,000. In New York, only 12 out of 225 hospitals avoided operating deficits over the past four years; 77 of the voluntary hospitals sustained operating losses in 1976 alone, totaling $116 million, and the public hospitals (not counting those in New York City) sustained an operating loss in 1976 totaling $54 million (22, p.20). What is not clear is the extent to which efficient hospitals will be penalized for the profit they show at the next rate review go around. One can't help but feel that rate regulation is aimed not only at cost control but also at keeping the hospitals threadbare. This is indeed one of the very complaints of the New York Hospital Association in its suit contesting that state's decision to set the same rate for both Blue Cross subscribers and Medicaid recipients; while it assures the same level of reimbursement for all people, the rate is set so low (the amount the state is willing to pay for Medicaid recipients) that the hospitals are being denied reasonable costs for a level of care desired or demanded by Blue Cross subscribers.

New York hospitals also complain about the administration of the New York law. The state regulatory agencies are supposed to notify the hospitals by November 1 of the rate at which each will be reimbursed during the following year, but they usually are not told what the rate will be until the middle of the operating year (20). This obviously makes efficient management of hospitals most difficult.

While the rate review statutes and CON laws seem to have slowed the rate of hospital expenditures and charges, it is really too early to proclaim success for these legislative ventures. First of all, it is not altogether clear as to the extent to which hospitals made their big investments in advance of the new legislations, getting in under the wire. Second, we do not know the extent to which subterfuge also hides current or later price rises, such as physicians buying the equipment and charging for its use rather than the hospital or hospitals building large entranceways (because the planning agencies don't look at that, only at beds, and space allocations for the various services) where the inexpensive movement of a wall later on will permit the expansion of a revenue producing hospital department. Third, the success stories mostly depend on data supplied by the regulatory agencies. Their data tend to minimize or clothe the adverse effects on the hospitals. Indeed, if hospitals continue to sustain losses, as in New York and Maryland, bankruptcy is inevitable for some. This is not necessarily bad if the hospitals are poorly managed, nor is it a matter of great concern if the hospitals are few in number. But if the bankruptcy is widespread, or if it hits some of the tertiary care facilities (the large referral hospitals), then there is legitimate concern that the ultimate effect would be the expropriation of the voluntary sector by the state. But the risks of this occurring are relatively slight, given the fact that the power structure of communities still dominate hospital boards. Of greater concern, perhaps, is that state prospective reimbursement regulatory bodies have been endorsed by the AHA, which is certainly a representative body of at least the acute general hospitals.

Commenting on the regulatory trend, Fuchs states (23, p.103):

Although some deviation from a purely competitive solution seems inevitable, regulation of hospitals by state public utility commissions would, in my opinion, be a disaster. In the first place, our experience with other industries has taught us that regulation is frequently introduced at the behest of the regulated as a device for achieving legal cartelization and restricting competition. Hospitals would certainly be no exception to this rule. The leading proponent of state public utility regulation approach is the American Hospital Association. Second, experience has shown that regulation rarely works to lower prices and frequently results in inefficiency and undesirable costs. Finally, regulation would tend to inhibit technological and organizational innovation.

CONCLUSION

The hospital, and particularly the general hospital, is a complex institution buffeted today by conflicting forces and winds of change. On the one hand, hospital leadership and the public want higher standards of care, and so does Congress. On the other hand, government and business want costs controlled. But, even without new technology and without improvements in the quality of care, the hospital today is under an enormous cost squeeze, and most of the causative factors are beyond the institution's control. It is remarkable that the hospital has been able to do as well as it does, given the difficult circumstances under which it operates. But the hospital is still a vibrant institution: It is moving in many ways to strengthen its ability to meet the challenges of the day through support of strengthened accreditation procedures, improved peer review mechanisms, strengthened monitoring of hospital efficiency, and positive cost containment efforts. Some of the steps taken by hospitals are conceived and initiated by the hospitals, and some are responses to challenges from Blue Cross, state insurance commissioners, Congress, HEW, and the courts. Whatever the source, the hospital is demonstrating daily its resiliency. While critics are many, the fact remains that we need hospitals, and with new knowledge and new technology and an aging population, we shall need them more and more as each day passes. The bottom line is: What kind of hospitals do we want, how much are we willing to pay, and to what extent are we willing to let the hospitals do the job without negative interference?

REFERENCES

1. MacEachern, M. T.: *Hospital Organization and Management,* 3rd ed., Beowyn Physicians' Record Company, 1969.
2. Wing, K. T.: *The Law and the Public's Health,* St. Louis, Mosby, 1976.
3. Quoted by Stewart, D. A.: *The History and Status of Proprietary Hospitals.* Research Series #9, Blue Cross Association, Chicago 1973.
4. American Hospital Association: *Hospital Statistics,* Chicago 1977 edition, Table 1.
5. American Hospital Association: *Guide to the Health Care Field,* Chicago 1977 edition.
6. *Joint Commission on Accreditation of Hospitals,* Chicago JCAH, 1976.
7. *American Medical News,* April 4, 1977.
8. *New York Times,* March 23, 1975.
9. Kuehn, H. R.: The commission on professional and hospital activities, *Bulletin,* American College of Surgeons, Chicago, October 1973.
10. *PSRO Factbook,* U.S. Department of Health, Education, and Welfare, May 1977.
11. *Medical World News,* November 28, 1977, p. 15f.

12. Bussman, J. W.: *Professional Standards Review Organizations.* Hearings before the Subcommittee on Oversight of the Committee on Ways and Means. U.S. House of Representatives, 95th Congress, first session, Serial 95-25.

13. *Health * United States * 1976-1977,* U.S. Department of Health, Education, and Welfare, DHEW Publication No. (HRA) 77-1232.

14. *Controlling the Supply of Hospital Beds,* Institute of Medicine, Washington National Academy of Sciences, October 1976.

15. Bunker et al.: *Costs, Risks, and Benefits of Surgery,* New York, Oxford University Press, 1977.

16. Schwartz, H.: "Paying for Health Care," *New York Times,* August 14, 1977.

17. *Medical World News,* November 28, 1977.

18. Dyck, F. J.: Effect of surveillance on the number of hysterectomies in the province of Saskatchewan, *New Engl. J. Med.,* 296: 1977.

19. Barclay, W. R.: Unnecessary surgery. JAMA, 236: July 26, 1976.

20. *American Medical News,* May 31, 1976.

21. "State Review Programs Effective in Slowing Hospital Cost Spiral," *American Medical News,* March 6, 1978.

22. *Hospitals,* JAHA, December 1, 1978.

23. Fuchs, V. R.: *Who Shall Live?* New York, Basic Books, Inc., 1974.

7

Nursing Homes and Community Health Agencies

NURSING HOMES

The nursing home, which is one type of long-term-care facility*, represents one of our more difficult problems. With fair regularity scandals erupt in homes that cheat patients, physically abuse and neglect patients, provide inadequate medical and nursing care, and that are fire traps. To make matters worse, we have an insufficient number of good nursing home beds to deal with the growing number of aged persons who need such care.

The roots of this problem lie in history. Nursing homes have their origins in the county poorhouses (or almshouses) of the eighteenth and nineteenth centuries. Local governments established these institutions to care for the poor, to provide them with shelter, food, clothing, and with work to help pay the costs of their care. As might be expected, many, if not most, of these people were older folks who had no families to care for them; being older, many were also invalids. Over time, these almshouses became the community dumps for all of their castoffs, not only the poor and the physically ill but also the mentally ill, the mentally retarded, and the alcoholics because there were often no places for them to go except the local poorhouses. Generally, conditions in these homes were not good, for they had to get along on meager public appropriations and on charity. The appropriations were meager because the public had little sense of identity with these institutions or for the people in them; the inmates were poor and noncontributing to the general welfare, and many were transients without a previous history of community contributions. Why reward

---

*Long-term care facilities are facilities that provide inpatient care for patients who need care over a longer period of time than care needed in an acute general hospital. Long term care facilities include nursing homes, psychiatric and mental-retardation hospitals, TB hospitals, chronic-disease hospitals, and rehabilitation hospitals.

them with ideal facilities? Why tax the hard working, thrifty citizenry to support those who were not that way? The politicians gave the almshouses the levels of support the electorates wanted: bare minimum.

But a society gets what it pays for; periodically, scandals erupted, as they do today, and public consciences were pricked. Over time, the mentally ill and retarded were pulled out and sent to more appropriate institutions—mostly state, rather than local, administered. In Maryland, the conditions in county almshouses were so bad that the state set up state run chronic disease hospitals to care for the infirm in return for closing of the county almshouses. In other states, improvements were made from time to time, and these county homes, as patients were reassigned, were left mainly with the aged poor and the physically disabled who did not need hospital care but who were unable to subsist without some form of health service support.

In recent decades, the state governments began to regulate these homes along with all other nursing homes—church, fraternal, proprietary—inspecting them and setting standards for performance. But the hands of state regulation were generally lightly applied, for few states were prepared to close many of the county, the voluntary, and the proprietary homes, for that would force the state to assume full responsibility.

As noted above, there developed nursing homes under other sponsorships. Church groups and fraternal organizations started homes for care of their members. These were mainly homes for the aged, but they had to develop over time supporting health services to meet the needs of their residents. These homes received strong support from their sponsoring bodies, not only direct financial aid but also much "in kind" support in terms of gifts of equipment, volunteer maintenance, and—where there were farms—harvesting services, as well as a variety of volunteer, direct, patient care services such as help in feeding patients, occupational and play therapy, and social visiting. It is widely acknowledged that the quality of service in church and fraternal sponsored homes is high, and one rarely finds in them the shortcomings often found today in local government nursing homes and in some of the proprietary nursing homes.

The private (for profit or proprietary) nursing homes emerged as a force during the 1930s as a result of the Social Security Act of 1935, which provided welfare benefits for patients in nongovernmental institutions. The original exclusion of benefits for patients in public institutions (since repealed) apparently stemmed from congressional concern over conditions in county poorhouses and a desire to get them closed.

But many health professionals and civic leaders were concerned over the resulting rapid growth in the private nursing home sector, believing that high quality care could not be developed and maintained if the homes depended on income derived primarily from welfare recipients, for these homes not only had to provide the needed care but also leave enough profit to make the owner's investment of money worthwhile. Resulting scandals in the proprietary sector have borne out the fears of these people. Not only were the payments insufficient to maintain both quality care and assure a reasonable return on the owner's investment, but also the very availability of large sums of money to pay for care in facilities that were in short supply proved to be an open invitation for the unscrupulous to enter the business.

Foreseeing these kinds of circumstances developing, there were attempts by health professionals and civic leaders to encourage the development of non-profit nursing homes. Congress responded by amending the Hill-Burton Act to make construction grants available for public and nonprofit nursing homes, and some states also developed grant programs. The resistance of the proprietary sector to such grant programs was vigorous and highly political. One of the successful efforts of the proprietary sector was to get Congress to approve its eligibility for FHA (Federal Housing Authority) guaranteed contruction loans. The distribution of nursing homes and beds between the public, proprietary, church and fraternal, and other nonprofit sponsorships shifts constantly but the proprietary sector is clearly dominant, with over 70% of the beds and over 75% of the homes. Growth in the public and nonprofit sectors is slow, and many factors affect this slow growth. Local governments, for one, are financially hard pressed and may be reluctant to extend their commitments in the nursing home area, for the population is aging, costs are rising, and insurance and government programs do not pay all of the costs, and their length of benefit periods are also limited, and sometimes there are retroactive denials of payment. The fear is that local government will not only be saddled with the initial investment, but also the unmet costs and the costs forced by changing federal requirements for Medicare and Medicaid and changing state requirements for state licensure. Add to this the bureaucratic hassles and paper work that a nursing home has to put up with, and the motivation to launch an expanded effort often dissipates. Similar considerations affect the nonprofit sector. This, then, leaves the field open to the proprietary sector in which one finds some very good homes as well as many which are very bad.

The unmet need for nursing home beds has persisted for some years and is, in fact, becoming more critical. Our population is aging, and with it comes an increased amount of chronic disease. As family units become smaller and all able persons working, no one is at home to care for the older folks, thus further increasing the demand for facilities for care of the aged. The demand accelerated enormously with the implementation of Medicare and Medicaid, which paid for some of this care, and also with the rapid growth of catastrophic health insurance coverage, which also paid for some (typically 80%) of this care. The demand also increased as government and health insurance companies sought to reduce the lengths of stay in acute hospitals by moving patients to a lesser level of care.

With the advent of Medicare and Medicaid and the accompanying large sums of money that would become available for nursing home care, the federal government had to establish definitions as to the types of institutions that would fall within the framework of those eligible for reimbursement, as well as standards to govern and assure quality of care in those homes eligible to participate. No longer could a "home for the aged" be synonymous with "nursing home". If a home for the aged wanted to be paid under Medicare or Medicaid for care to eliigible patients, the home had to meet certain standards. The federal government now recognizes two types of homes as being eligible. The first is a *skilled nursing facility* (SNF) and the second is an *intermediate care facility* (IFC). HEW provides these definitions (1, pp.4-5):

A *skilled nursing facility (SNF)* is a nursing home that has been certified as meeting Federal standards within the meaning of the Social Security Act. It provides the level of care that comes closest to hospital care with 24-hour nursing services. Regular medical supervision and rehabilitation therapy are also provided. Generally, a skilled nursing facility cares for convalescent patients and those with long-term illnesses.

An *intermediate care facility* (ICF) is also certified and meets Federal standards and provides less extensive health related care and services. It has regular nursing service, but not around the clock. Most intermediate care facilities carry on rehabilitation programs, but the emphasis is on personal care and social services. Mainly, these homes serve people who are not fully capable of living by themselves, yet are not necessarily ill enough to need 24-hour nursing care.

Medicare provides coverage in SNFs (but not in ICFs) for up to 100 days of care for each illness, provided the patient has spent first at least three days in a hospital. But the 100 days is not fully paid for: after the first 20 days, the patient must pay a portion of each day's care. Medicaid pays for care in both SNFs and ICFs, but the exact benefits will vary from state to state. There are, of course, other kinds of homes, homes for the aged and the like. Some of these will have sections that are approved as an SNF or ICF for which they can receive payment.

Many general hospitals will also have skilled nursing facilities under their management, developed in part to provide a more efficient use of their acute beds and sometimes as a justification for building or retention of acute beds. On this last point, some hospitals are experimenting with "swing beds," which can handle acute cases one day and SNF cases the next. This allows a hospital some flexibility and is a particularly inviting approach to a hospital that has low occupancy and doubly inviting if there is a shortage of SNF beds in its area.

Rather than close beds or keep them unoccupied, they can be used and be income producing, but for a level of care less than acute general hospital care. If the hospital is pressed for acute beds at any time, it then has the option of converting the long term care beds back to acute beds.

While federal standards were meant to raise the quality of nursing homes, at the time of Medicare and Medicaid implementation, the standards were applied liberally, that is to say, homes were approved even though they did not fully meet the standards. The decision by HEW to do this was, of course, political: The homes were already in business, and not to certify them and thus deny benefits to the population who thought they were getting benefits would be a political liability for the president and for the legislators who passed the legislation. But another consideration undoubtedly operated: Getting marginal homes in would, over time, provide an opportunity to force them to raise the quality of their services, which would be easier to bring about the more dependent the homes were on Medicare and Medicaid payments. Frank (2, pp.538-545) notes in this connection that the federal regulations:

... represented the first attempt by government to impose comprehensive national quality controls over nursing homes. This attempt was particularly important because the states had failed to provide adequate and uniform standards through their own licensure laws; furthermore, the Joint Commission on Accreditation of Hospitals, which attempted to accredit nursing homes meeting relatively high standards, never accredited more than a minute fraction of the nation's nursing homes. The federal standards are designed not only to improve care, but also to reorient it.

The process for elevating the quality of nursing homes, and of the care they provide, continues. Apart from the notorious homes that provide substandard care and which abuse both the patients and the agencies that pay the bills, the process of reform and upgrading is still uphill because of the rising number of people needing care, the increased recognition as to the new types of care needed, and the rising costs of care in an economy that is experiencing difficulty.

AMBULATORY CARE: NEIGHBORHOOD AND PRIMARY CARE CENTERS

Neighborhood health centers (NHCs) began to develop in the late 1960s, initially with funding from the Office of Economic Opportunity (OEO) and, later, HEW. These centers were to provide, primarily, comprehensive ambulatory services for a defined population of poor people. The poor had, of course, always received large amounts of care from health departments, indigent hospitals, and on charitable or government-financed bases in nongovernmental general hospitals. The larger hospitals, and particularly medical school hospitals, had long histories in care of the poor on both inpatient and outpatient bases. But the outpatient care was often demeaning: impersonal, crowded surroundings, and long waits on hard benches. The neighborhood health center was designed to overcome these demeaning features not only by providing a broad range of primary and secondary ambulatory care services by salaried physicians and other health professionals but also by emphasizing prevention, having available a wide range of supporting nonmedical services, and providing these services in the neighborhoods in which the people lived. Importantly, too, was the concept that the people served, the consumers, should be involved in the control of their centers.

Where possible, the centers were financed on a fee for services basis from Medicare and Medicaid and other vendor payments and from government grants. But the future of these centers is clouded. As with so many government programs, there comes a time when priorities shift and funding tapers off. Bowers notes (3, p.177):

By 1972, start-up funds for NHCs were shrinking as the future of OEO became uncertain. (It was soon merged with HEW.) A significant stricture was the limitation on coverage for ambulatory care services under most State medical programs. Further, as we have noted, States were tightening the belts of their medicaid programs, thereby eroding the financial base of NHCs.

In the fall of 1973, Yohalem and Brecher reported serious problems faced by NHCs. "The chief problem in the operation of these centers," they noted, "is one of finances. Because not all services are necessarily covered by Government programs, and because eligibility is based on income levels, the neighborhood center and its sponsor are dependent on an unstable flow of funds." Deficient eligibility criteria, variations in benefits covered, and the diversity of fiscal administrative controls are other shortcomings of NHCs.

In 1975, there were 123 neighborhood health centers.

Primary health care centers are like neighborhood health centers except that they provide a more limited range of services and focus on primary care. The number of primary care centers is increasing rapidly, particularly in underserved rural areas. Like the NHC, the primary care centers have major financial problems, and the rural centers also have difficulty attracting and retaining professional staffs. Many of these centers have developed with support from one of several federal programs: National Health Service Corps (NHSC), Rural

Health Initiative (RHI), Health Underserved Rural Areas (HURA), and the Appalachian Regional Commission (ARC), support that augmented local organizational efforts and local building of the facilities. The typical federally supported center will have two family practitioners and one dentist. The supporting services beyond nursing will vary from center to center. Some will have visiting consultant services, some pharmacy services, some nutrition services, and some other services. The financial problems are varied. Some result from community overbuilding of the facility, incurring a debt that is difficult to pay off from center earnings. Some centers overextend themselves in terms of the supporting services they provide. A steady flow of patients who pay a fee for service is also a problem: being rural, there is a frequent turnover of the professional staffs, and with each turnover, the centers lose patients— people seeking older practitioners who are likely to stay around—even though the patients may have to travel greater distances. Some centers also report a drop in patients due to the unaccustomed high cost of care; the newer and younger doctors who practice in these centers typically practice a type of care that employs more tests than the old-time practitioners used. The patients sometimes reject this more advanced type of care, preferring to find an older practitioner who won't be as fancy, substituting clinical judgment for tests and consequently delivering care that will not be as costly. The long term survival of these centers will depend not only on attaining financial stability but also on finding a way to attract and retain professional personnel.

COMMUNITY MENTAL HEALTH CENTERS

Following the Second World War, psychiatric theory began to shift more and more to notions of community care. The community psychiatry theories were greatly abetted by the advent of tranquilizing pills in the 1950s, for with tranquilizers, the need to keep many patients in mental hospitals was obviated. The tranquilizers suppressed symptoms sufficiently that patients could be treated in the community. In many of the states during the 1950s, general hospitals, mental hospitals, health departments, and others began to experiment with new types of community based ambulatory therapeutic programs, and success stories began to be heard with increased frequency. Some local health departments had a wide range of services for psychiatric emergencies and both individual and group psychotherapy. Some hospitals and health departments established day hospitals in which patients who lived at home could go during the day for psychiatric treatment, and also established night hospitals in which patients who lived and worked in the community could go after work for needed psychiatric care. New York State, in 1954, enacted its Community

Mental Health Services Act. By 1963, sufficient experience was at hand for Congress to pass the Mental Retardation Facilities and Community Mental Health Center Construction Act of 1963.

The aim of the federal legislation with subsequent amendments was to stimulate, via grants of money, the development of comprehensive mental-health services through community mental-health centers. Grants included monies for construction and operations.

Purpose: To provide comprehensive mental health services through a community mental health center via six grant programs: (1) staffing grants, (2) planning grants, (3) grants for initial operations, (4) consultation and education services, (5) conversion grants, and (6) distress grants. The comprehensive services which centers must provide are: inpatient, outpatient, day care, and other partial hospitalization services and emergency services; specialized services for the mental health of children; specialized services for the elderly; consultation and education services, assistance to courts and other public agencies in screening catchment area residents considered for referral for inpatient treatment in a State mental health facility; follow-up care for catchment area residents discharged from a mental facility; transitional half-way house services for catchment area residents discharged from mental health facilities or who would require inpatient care without such halfway house services; unless there is insufficient need, or the need is otherwise being met, specialized programs for the prevention, treatment, rehabilitation of alcohol and drug abusers, alcoholics, and drug addicts. (4, p.13)

The centers were to be the focal point for development and coordination of services in their areas. Some services the centers provided, other services were developed by appropriate agencies, often at the proddings of the centers, and still other services, which had been operational long before the advent of the centers, were tied into the centers by formal and informal working agreements.

By the mid-1970s, federal grant support began to taper off. By 1978, only continuation staffing grants were available. At the end of fiscal 1975, there were 603 centers supported by federal grants, serving about 87 million people. More than half of the centers were in poverty areas (3, p.179). The decline in federal monies and the concentration of centers in poverty areas highlight the major problem facing these centers: Despite all the good they may do, financial problems are major and inevitably must affect the comprehensiveness of service, let alone the survival of the centers.

HOME HEALTH AGENCIES

These agencies operate under various names, with varying organizational ties and differing services. Generally, these agencies, whether they are independent, hospital operated, or health department managed, provide a variety of health and health supporting services in patient homes. Some agencies, however, are single purpose, offering only one type of service, for example, Meals-on-Wheels. Financial support for these agencies vary. Medicare, Medicaid, and insurance companies pay for some services. Government grants pay for some; patients also pay; charity contributes.

A *visiting nurse association* (VNA) is one type of home health service in which a nurse, usually a nurse with public health training, visits a patient's home to provide some type of nursing service, for example to change a dressing or give an injection. Many of these VNAs will also provide physical therapy and speech therapy services by qualified personnel.

Some home health agencies will provide needed health aids for the home, such as crutches, walkers, wheelchairs, and other equipment and appliances.

Some agencies will provide *homemaker* services: housecleaning, maintenance and repairs, cooking.

Meals-on-Wheels are common in most cities today when an agency supplies usually one hot meal a day to those confined to their homes. This is typically the noon meal, the assumption being that someone is at home in the morning and evening to provide the other meals. Many of these agencies use volunteers to deliver the meals. The meals are secured from various agencies, the hospital or the school kitchen being two common suppliers.

AMBULANCE SERVICE

Ambulance services are provided by a variety of agencies. Funeral homes are frequently the source for this service, but it is also available, depending on the community, from the police or fire departments, hospitals, volunteer groups, private ambulance companies. Considerable effort has been made in recent years to train ambulance crews in dealing with the kinds of emergencies they are likely to encounter.

SHELTERED WORKSHOP

Sheltered workshops exist for the physically and mentally handicapped. They are places of work where the worker is sheltered from the normal pressures of the work world. The work and production schedules are geared not to commercial demands but to the capabilities of the worker.

HEALTH AND WELFARE COUNCILS

Health and welfare councils are voluntary agencies usually representative of the smaller health and welfare agencies in a community, though the larger agencies may sometimes belong. The councils serve a very useful service not only in terms of representing the small agencies but also in providing a research and planning capability that the agencies individually, because of their size, could not afford.

CLINICAL LABORATORIES

The physician may require a variety of laboratory analyses to facilitate his or her diagnosis and treatment. Some physicians have their own lab technicians to carry out whatever tests are desired. Some tests are, however, very complicated and require rather costly equipment. For these tests, as well as some of the simpler tests if the physician has no lab technician or does not do the tests himself or herself, the physician may have an arrangement with the nearby hospital. Very often, however, the physician may use a free-standing clinical laboratory run by a pathologist or by a registered medical technologist. Sometimes the physician sends the patient to the lab; sometimes the physician sends the specimen to the lab. In rural settings, the doctors may have to mail the specimen to a lab, or the lab may arrange for periodic pickups of the specimens.

Although there is state licensing of clinical laboratories and federal monitoring of those labs that work across state lines, there has been concern over the years as to the quality of laboratory analyses. Periodically, studies are completed that call into question the accuracy of clinical lab results. This is, of course, a serious matter because a physician treats a patient on the basis of lab reports.

AMBULATORY SURGICAL CENTERS

In recent years, there has been an upsurge in the amount of surgery performed on an ambulatory basis. Hospitals all over the country are experiencing a rise in the number of surgical cases on patients who come into the hospital and go home the same day, surgical care for cases that previously had required at least an overnight stay in the hospital if not a two or three day stay. One can appreciate how this can affect a hospital's need for beds and its overall organization.

Many surgeons, however, have been accustomed to performing ambulatory surgery in their offices, the limit on what they did depending on the surgeon's facilities, support services, and self imposed limits. One of the major limits was anesthesia. The surgeon typically would employ a local anesthetic, not a general anesthetic, since the latter should be administered by board certified anesthesiologists.

During the 1970s, a number of free-standing—that is to say, not hospital based—surgical centers began to develop in several parts of the country, the surgical center having more complete facilities, support services, anesthesia services, and, significantly, an augmented system (over the surgeon's office) for monitoring the quality of surgical practice. The number of centers is apparently quite small but growing. It already appears, however, that a professional conflict is emerging over the desirability of independent centers over hospital based centers (5).

FAMILY PLANNING CENTERS

Family planning services are provided by local health departments, some hospitals, and by free standing family planning centers or clinics. The latter are supported primarily by government grants and charity.

VOLUNTARY HEALTH AGENCIES

There are a large number of national health agencies that operate state and sometimes local chapters. These agencies are typically special disease oriented and are financed largely by charitable contributions. Some of the more prominent agencies include: The American Heart Association, National Society for the Prevention of Blindness, National Tuberculosis and Respiratory Disease Association, American Association on Mental Deficiency, American Red Cross, and the National Association for Mental Health. Some of these agencies will provide some direct service (e.g., diagnostic services, clinic consultation), some will support research, some will help finance needed services, most will conduct some health education activities to educate the population about the health problem of their concern.

PHARMACEUTICAL COMPANIES

The pharmaceutical industry is large and profitable. Major pharmaceutical (drug) companies carry out research, develop, manufacture, and market a large number of drugs. *Ethical* drugs are sold only by prescription and are not advertised to the public, only to the health professions, which can legally prescribe them. *Proprietary* drugs are sold over the counter without prescription, and the companies advertise in the general public media.

Physicians learn about prescription drugs—what they can do and cannot do—principally from advertisements in professional journals, from exhibits at medical conventions, and from literature mailed or delivered in person. The delivery of literature, and often samples of the drugs, is done by specially trained persons who visit physicians' offices, physicians' cloakrooms at the hospitals, and who staff exhibits at conventions. These pharmaceutical people are called *detailers.* While some physicians learn about new drugs from scientific articles and a number of other scientific publications, such as *The Physician's Desk Reference, The Merck Manual,* and so on, the detailers, backed by their companies, are the principal vehicle for new information.

Physicians get to know the representatives of the various companies, for they are visited regularly by them. As a physician learns from a detailer about a particular product, the physician tends to prescribe that company's product rather than the same drug produced by some other company. Price variations exist between companies making the same scientific formula due to advertising and marketing costs, developmental costs, and desired profit levels. In the nonprescription area, one can cite acetylsalicylic acid, better known as aspirin. Five grains of acetylsalicylic acid are identical whether marketed by Bayer or under the label of a discount drug store. So, too, with many prescription drugs, though, not infrequently, the major companies have new drugs that their competition has not duplicated.

Since drugs constitute a major cost item in health care costs, governments have sought to get physicians to prescribe by scientific (generic) name rather than brand name so that the drug used can be that of the manufacturer whose price is the lowest. In some states, the pharmacist is able to make substitutions, provided the substitute is scientifically identical. The large pharmaceutical companies are not happy with this trend, arguing that when they have higher costs, it is due to several factors: higher developmental costs, higher production costs due to quality control, and the need to cover losses from research that does not produce a drug that is marketable on a profitable basis in the United States. Over the years, the U.S. government has been unhappy over this situation, and Congress has many times conducted hearings looking into the drug industry. The fact remains, however, that the pharmaceutical companies are highly competitive businesses, providing products that are needed. The

FDA monitors the industry and must approve the marketing of new drugs in terms of their safety and effectiveness and assure that the literature used is accurate and not misleading.

REFERENCES

1. *How to Select a Nursing Home,* Office of Nursing Home Affairs, Washington, HEW.
2. Frank, Kenneth D., Government support of nursing home care. *New Eng. J. Med.* 287: 1972.
3. Bowers, John Z. *An Introduction to American Medicine-1975.* Washington, HEW, 1977.
4. *Profiles of Financial Assistance Programs.* Washington, HEW, 1978.
5. O'Donovan, Thomas R. *Ambulatory Surgical Centers.* Germantown, Aspen Systems Corporation, 1976.

8

Health Costs

If one were to place a current dollar value on all goods and services produced in a country during any one year, the resulting sum would constitute what is known as the Gross National Product (GNP). Economists have been able to use such a figure as a rough index of a nation's economy, as a measure from one year to the next of the increasing or decreasing wealth in a society as measured by its productive capacity, and as a comparative measure of the economic vitality and productive capacity of one country against another.

In the United States, the defense industry has long accounted for producing the greatest proportion of the GNP. The second largest industry, as measured by the percentage of the GNP credited to it, is the health industry: the physicians, nurses, optometrists, dentists, physiotherapists, and other health-sector workers, and the hospitals, nursing homes, health insurance companies,

---

Most of the data in this chapter are drawn from two articles in the *Social Security Bulletin*, both authored by Robert M. Gibson and Charles R. Fisher: "National Health Expenditures, Fiscal Year 1977" (*Social Security Bulletin* Vol. 41, July 1978) and "Age Differences in Health Care Spending, Fiscal Year 1977" (*Social Security Bulletin* Vol. 42, January 1979). These articles are updated annually and should be consulted for the most current figures, although significant annual changes do not usually occur. Beginning with 1979, the articles will appear in a new HEW publication, *Health Care Financing Review*.

As the galley proofs for this book were being checked in mid-September 1979 the author received the Summer 1979 issue (Vol. 1, No. 1) of the *Health Care Financing Review* with the 1978 figures on health expenditures. Since the data on health care costs by age groups were not reported it was decided to use the 1977 figures in this book. The 1978 data do not seem to change significantly except that HEW is now reporting the data on a calendar year basis rather than fiscal year, and it has recalculated all data back to 1965 (and some back to 1929) to reflect, as the author (Gibson, R.M.) puts it, "changes in some basic data sources as well as improvements in methodology." Some of the 1978 data are given by footnotes in this chapter but the reader is cautioned that the data may not always describe the same universe, and comparison of 1978 calendar data with 1977 fiscal year data may not be valid. This can be seen from Table 8-16 when the data there is compared with the data in Table 8-1.

medical equipment manufacturers, and pharmaceutical companies. The health sector has, over the years, captured a growing share of the GNP. In 1950, for example, national health expenditures constituted only 4.6% of the GNP. Since that time it has risen steadily to 8.7% in 1976 and 8.8% in 1977. (See Fig. 8-1 and Table 8-1.) All indicators point to a continued rise.

Another important point to note (Table 8-1) is that the public (government) sector has, over the years, accounted for an increased share of the health expenditures. In 1929, for example, only 13.3% of the total health expenditures were from tax sources. That 13.3% was for the health services provided by the armed forces, the VA hospitals, Public Health Service hospitals and services, and health services provided by state and local health departments, care in government mental and mental retardation hospitals, and comparatively limited monies provided by the federal government for medical research and for health services for mothers and children. Since that time, there has been a growth in

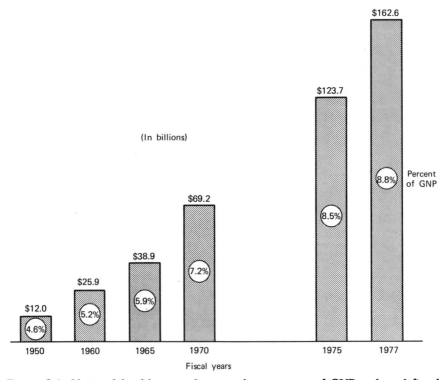

Figure 8-1. National health expenditure and percentage of GNP, selected fiscal years 1950-1977. (*Source:* Gibson R.M., and Fisher, C.R.: National health expenditures, fiscal year 1977. *Social Security Bulletin* 41:1978.)

Table 8-1. Aggregate and per Capita National Health Expenditures, by Source of Funds and Percent of Gross National Product, Selected Years, 1929-77

Year	Gross National Product (in billions)	Health Expenditures								
		Total			Private			Public		
		Amount (in millions)	Per Capita	Percent of GNP	Amount (in millions)	Per Capita	Percent of Total	Amount (in millions)	Per Capita	Percent of Total
Ending June—										
1929	$101.3	$3,589	$29.16	3.5	$3,112	$25.28	86.7	$477	$3.88	13.3
1935	68.9	2,846	22.04	4.1	2,303	17.84	80.9	543	4.21	19.1
1940	95.4	3,883	29.98	4.1	3,101	23.14	79.9	782	5.84	20.1
1950	264.8	12,027	78.35	4.5	8,962	58.38	74.5	3,065	19.97	25.5
1955	381.0	17,330	103.76	4.5	12,909	77.29	74.5	4,421	26.47	25.5
1960	498.3	25,856	141.63	5.2	19,461	106.60	75.3	6,395	35.03	24.7
1965	658.0	38,892	197.75	5.9	29,357	149.27	75.5	9,535	48.48	24.5
1966	722.4	42,109	211.56	5.8	31,279	157.15	74.3	10,830	54.41	25.7
1967	773.5	47,897	237.93	6.2	32,026	159.15	66.9	15,853	78.78	33.1
1968	830.2	53,765	264.37	6.5	33,725	165.83	62.7	20,040	98.54	37.3
1969	904.2	60,617	295.20	6.7	37,680	183.50	62.2	22,937	111.70	37.8
1970	960.2	69,201	333.57	7.2	43,810	211.18	63.3	25,391	122.39	36.7
1971	1,019.8	77,162	368.25	7.6	48,387	230.92	62.7	28,775	137.32	37.3
1972	1,111.8	86,687	409.71	7.8	53,214	251.50	61.4	33,473	158.20	38.6
1973	1,238.6	95,383	447.31	7.7	58,715	275.35	61.6	36,668	171.96	38.4
1974	1,361.2	106,321	495.01	7.8	64,809	301.74	61.0	41,512	193.27	39.0
1975[a]	1,454.5	123,716	571.21	8.5	71,348	329.42	57.7	52,368	241.79	42.3
1976[a]	1,625.4	141,013	645.76	8.7	80,831	370.16	57.3	60,182	275.60	42.7

Table 8-1. (continued)

		Health Expenditures								
		Total			Private			Public		
Year	Gross National Product (in billions)	Amount (in millions)	Per Capita	Percent of GNP	Amount (in millions)	Per Capita	Percent of Total	Amount (in millions)	Per Capita	Percent of Total
Ending September—										
1975	1,487.1	127,719	588.48	8.6	73,238	337.45	57.3	54,481	251.03	42.7
1976	1,667.4	145,102	663.06	8.7	83,560	381.84	57.6	61,542	281.22	42.4
1977[b]	1,838.0	162,627	736.92	8.8	94,185	426.78	57.9	68,442	310.13	42.1

[a]Revised estimates.

[b]New Federal fiscal year.

Source: Gibson, R. M., and Fisher, C. R. National health expenditures, fiscal year 1977. *Social Security Bulletin* Vol. 41, July 1978.

Note: The federal fiscal year was changed in 1977. Instead of July 1 through June 30, it is now October 1 through September 30. Yearly comparisons are likely to be complicated and confusing for a number of years not only because of the fiscal year change but also because in 1979 HEW decided to report this data initially on a calendar year basis and later on on a fiscal year basis. See footnote at the beginning of this chapter.

government expenditures to the point where government at all levels was responsible in 1976 for 42.4% of all health expenditures and in 1977 for 42.1%. (See *note* accompanying Table 8-1.)

The rise in terms of *government's share* of the GNP for health can be attributed to new or expanded government activities such as medical research, the Hill-Burton Construction Act, and such health services programs as crippled children's services, Kerr-Mills health insurance for the aged, mental health, Medicare, Medicaid, as well as a vast number of other programs that, in their own way, added to the total public share. In 1967, we note a sharp rise in government expenditures. This was due in large measure to the implementation of Medicare and Medicaid. The growth in the public sector in subsequent years can largely be attributed to growth in the expenditures for these two programs.

The factors that go into the overall rise in the health sector's share of the GNP (both public and private) can be attributed to technological advances and other changes in the health system, price rise (inflation), and population increases (more people demanding more services). We might examine these briefly.

Technological advances have been enormous: New drugs, which permit the more effective treatment of disease; new anesthetics, which are safer and often more effective; new instrumentation, permitting the electronic monitoring of patients requiring intensive care and high risk surgery; a variety of sophisticated diagnostic and therapeutic radiological devices (such as the CAT scanner, cobalt therapy units, as well as diagnostic units that do exactly what other units do except with much less radiation exposure to the patient); renal dialysis equipment; autoanalyzers and an array of other laboratory equipment, which permit faster and more accurate and more sophisticated analyses; heart-lung machines, which permit open heart surgery; new metals and materials, which permit the replacement of hip and knee joints; and our list could go on and on.

The developmental costs of new equipment are typically high; many require highly trained technicians to operate them, and they cost money. The very development of this new technology increases utilization and accompanying expenditures. New drugs and new anesthetics likewise frequently lead to expanded services and increased utilization and costs.

Increased concern over quality of care, accompanied by an increase in malpractice suits, has caused both hospitals and physicians to accelerate their technological capabilities and to utilize various tests and procedures more frequently. The substitution of tests for professional judgments may or may not improve the overall quality of care; it certainly increases costs.

There are some technological advances that cost money but could be considered by some as unnecessary frills. For example, therapeutically, we could probably provide as effective care using the hand cranked iron posted beds of old. Instead, we are shifting to more expensive, electronically controlled beds in which the patient is able, by the push of a button, to raise and lower the head, the foot, and the knees. This is a convenience for the patient—the extent to which the hospital personnel costs can be reduced by not employing aides to do this work is perhaps negligible.

Another change in the health system rather than technological advance is the availability of semiprivate and private rooms rather than use of the open wards, though the construction of open wards would be less expensive. The question here is really one of social choice—what a society wants in respect to the setting in which care is to be provided. Does it want a stripped down, bare essentials model, or does it want some of the comforts and conveniences that are possible? We have opted for the latter.

Inflation is another factor in rising health costs. Part of this is that the cost of everything is rising—food, electricity, telephones, fuel, supplies, equipment, construction materials, labor, and liability insurance rates. For some of these items, the health industry must simply pay the going rate. It can't do much about the cost of fuel, electricity, telephones, or food. It can't do much about the going wage rates: As a labor-intensive industry and as a traditional heavy employer of unskilled labor (as well as skilled labor), it is acutely sensitive to congressionally mandated rises in the minimum wage; hospitals, moreover, only recently came under the requirements of the minimum wage and work- man's compensation acts. This is not to decry these last developments but to note that they had a significant impact on hospitals, in particular, whose labor costs in 1976 represented 54.2% of total costs (1, p.xiii). Some economies can sometimes be achieved through group purchasing and by establishment of medical society and hospital association liability (malpractice) insurance com- panies. Critics of the health industry focus often on the elements of inefficiencies, but it is questionable if all of the inefficiencies in the overall amount to a significant component. Getting an effective handle, in terms of cost containment or control, on the major components still eludes the critics; the best they can do is advocate ceilings (often called *lids* or *caps*), which tend to suppress demand, decrease services, and lessen quality of care.

It is true, of course, that the way we pay for hospital care, reimbursement at cost or close to cost, does not inhibit expansion and does not encourage either provider or consumer economies. But this, in itself, is not to be construed as inefficiency, though critics of the health industry are inclined to do so. In fact, the goals of health insurance and of many pieces of legislation—Medicare, Medicaid, community mental health centers, and others—were to facilitate access to care by removing the cost barriers, by assuring the hospitals through proper reimbursement that they would be able to provide all of the services necessary. The enormous expansions of NIH further encouraged the develop- ment of new technology. And it was, after all, the Congress that passed, in 1966, Public Law 89-749, which declared that "fulfillment of our National purpose depends on promoting and assuring the highest level of health attainable for every person, in an environment which contributes positively to healthful individual and family living . . ." *Population increases,* therefore, were not only direct population growth but also the opening of access to needed care to the aged, the poor, the mentally ill, and to those who could now benefit from new technology.*

Table 8-2 provides a detailed breakdown of the expenditures for fiscal 1977. Hospitals account for 40.4% of all expenditures in 1977, followed by physicians, who accounted for 19.8% of the expenditures. Drugs and drug sundries accounted for 7.7%, and nursing home care for 7.8%. These four items thus account for nearly three-quarters or 75% of all health expenditures in 1977.** Small wonder that these are the areas of focus by Congress and by federal, state, and local governments since between them they spent $68.442 billion, 42.1% of the total $162.627 billion spent for health. (*Note:* Most tables show expenditures in the millions. The discussion in this text uses billions, which is achieved by moving a decimal point.)

It might be noted that included in the hospital total are the sums paid to hospital based salaried physicians. It should also be noted that the drug and drug-sundries figures do not include hospital-, clinic-, and physician-dispensed drugs. Finally, the cost of private physician office and laboratory facilities are not included in the medical facilities expenditure figure.

Table 8-3 shows an interesting breakdown of the $142.586 billion expenditures for *personal* health care (as distinct from health expenditures for public health activities, research and construction) in terms of who pays for it. An analysis of this table tells us a good deal about the state of health insurance today: 69.7 percent ($99.312 billion) of the $142.586 billion was covered by health insurance or government.† (Together, the insurance companies and government are *third party* payers, the health unit and patient being the other two parties.) The consumer paid directly for 30.3% ($43.274 billion). This might at first suggest how woefully inadequate our health insurance and government protections are. To understand this a bit more, however, one has to look at parts of the $142.586 billion. If we look, for example, at hospital care, we find that of the total $65.627 billion, a little more than 94.1% ($61.761 billion) was covered, leaving the consumer to pay only 5.9%. The 5.9%

---

*Gibson (*Health Care Financing Review,* Vol.1, No.1, Summer 1979) attributes the sources of increase from 1969 to 1978 as follows: 63% due to price rise, 30% due to technology and utilization resulting from technological changes, and 7% to population.

**For calender year 1978 the relationships remained fairly constant: hospitals accounted for 39.5%, physicians 18.3%, drugs and drug sundries 7.9%, nursing home care 8.2%; for a total of 73.9% of all expenditures.

†See footnote on page 349.

Table 8-2. National Health Expenditures, by Type of Expenditure and Source of Funds, Year Ending September 1977
in millions

Type of Expenditure	Total	Private			Public		
		Total	Consumers	Other^a	Total	Federal	State and local
				1977^b			
Total	$162,627	$94,185	$87,807	$6,378	$68,442	$46,563	$21,879
Health services and supplies	153,887	91,294	87,807	3,487	62,594	42,542	20,051
Personal health care	142,586	85,465	82,574	2,891	57,121	39,823	17,299
Hospital care	65,627	29,427	27,887	1,540	36,199	25,715	10,484
Physicians' services	32,184	24,360	24,318	42	7,824	5,808	2,016
Dentists' services	10,020	9,520	9,520	0	500	310	190
Other professional services	3,212	2,288	2,175	113	924	683	241
Drugs and drug sundries	12,516	11,373	11,373	0	1,143	614	529
Eyeglasses and appliances	2,086	1,956	1,956	0	130	66	64
Nursing-home care	12,618	5,434	5,343	91	7,184	4,204	2,980
Other health services	4,322	1,105	0	1,105	3,217	2,424	793
Expenses for prepayment and administration	7,572	5,829	5,233	596	1,743	1,430	313
Government public health activities	3,729				3,729	1,289	2,440
Research and medical-facilities construction	8,739	2,891		2,891	5,848	4,020	1,828
Research^c	3,684	284		284	3,400	3,139	261
Construction	5,055	2,607		2,607	2,448	881	1,567

^aIncludes spending by philanthropic organizations and for industrial in-plant health services.

^bPreliminary estimates.

^cResearch and development expenditures of drug companies and other manufacturers and providers of medical equipment and supplies excluded from "research expenditures" but included in the expenditure class in which the product falls.

Source: Gibson, R. M. and Fisher, C. R.; National health expenditures, fiscal year 1977. Social Security Bulletin Vol. 41; July 1978.

($3.886 billion) represents expenditures by people not covered in any form by health insurance (one recent estimate placing this at only 6% of the population [2]) and expenditures not covered by a patient's policy (such as care of newborns and excluded services—preexisting conditions, excluded procedures, extra charges for private rooms). The unprotected people represent the poor who cannot afford private insurance but are not poor enough to be eligible for Medicaid, some self-employed who elect not to purchase policies or who are in small employee groups that have not bought it, and some who are uncovered because they are between jobs. The high-percentage payment of hospital care and the high percentage of those covered by insurance for hospital bills suggest that close to 100% coverage of hospital care by at least some combination of government and private insurance is within our grasp. It is worth comparing the improvements in coverage from 1975 through 1977, by comparing Table 8-3 with Tables 8-4 and 8-5.

If we look (Table 8-3) at physician services, we find a picture not quite as rosy. Of $32.184 billion, only 61.2% ($19.682 billion) is covered by insurance or government programs. The remaining $12.502 billion is paid directly by the consumer. While some of the $12.502 billion is for physician charges above what the insurance company or government pays, the bulk of this sum is for physician care in the office and home, services typically not covered by insurance. There is, of course, serious question as to the advisability of covering routine home and office visits because of the high administrative costs involved, the increased utilization such coverage would stimulate, and the potential for physician abuse.

Perhaps a more accurate picture of health insurance adequacy comes from a survey conducted by the Health Insurance Association of America of the 1977 expenses for *group* insured persons. This is reported in Table 8-6. Table 8-7 tells us how *all government* health expenditures (not just personal health expenditures) were allocated by program, by level of government, 1976.

AGE DIFFERENCES IN HEALTH-CARE SPENDING

The preceding section looked briefly at *what* the key elements are in health costs and *what* causes these costs to rise. In Chapters 3 and 6, we examined

---

†Comparison with 1978 data would be difficult because of the different methodologies employed including the use of the calendar year rather than the fiscal year. On a *calendar* basis, for example, for 1976 and 1977, HEW reports that 68.3% and 67.4% of the total personal health care costs were covered by government or health insurance. *Fiscal* year data for the same years are reported to be 68.8% and 69.7%. Thus on a calendar year basis third parties covered in 1977 a lesser percentage of the personal health care costs but on a fiscal year basis covered a greater percentage.

Table 8-3. Aggregate and per Capita Amount and Percentage Distribution of Personal Health Care Expenditures Met by Third Parties by Type of Expenditure, Year Ending September 1977.

Source of Payment	Total	Hospital Care	Physicians' Services	Dentists' Services	Other Professional Services	Drugs and Drug Sundries	Eyeglasses and Appliances	Nursing-Home Care	Other Health Services
					1977[a]				
Aggregate amount (in millions)									
Total	$142,586	$65,627	$32,184	$10,020	$3,212	$12,516	$2,086	$12,618	$4,322
Direct payments	43,274	3,866	12,502	7,965	1,398	10,401	1,918	5,226	
Third-party payments	99,312	61,761	19,682	2,055	1,814	2,115	169	7,393	4,322
Private health insurance	39,299	24,021	11,817	1,554	777	973	39	118	
Philanthropy and industrial inplant	2,891	1,540	42		113			91	1,105
Government	57,121	36,199	7,823	501	924	1,142	130	7,184	3,217
Federal	39,823	25,715	5,807	311	683	613	66	4,204	2,424
Medicare	20,770	15,520	4,431		457			362	
Medicaid	9,181	3,368	1,032	225	184	573	66	3,603	195
Other	9,872	6,827	344	85	42	40		238	2,229
State and local	17,299	10,484	2,016	190	241	529	64	2,980	793
Medicaid	7,076	2,596	795	173	142	442	64	2,777	150
Other	10,223	7,888	1,220	17	99	87		203	642
Per capita amount									
Total	$646.11	$297.38	$145.84	$45.41	$14.56	$56.72	$9.45	$57.18	$19.59
Direct payments	196.09	17.52	56.64	36.10	6.34	47.13	8.69	23.68	
Third-party payments	450.02	279.86	89.19	9.31	8.22	9.59	.77	33.49	19.59
Private health insurance	178.08	108.85	53.55	7.04	3.52	4.41	.18	.53	
Philanthropy and industrial inplant	13.10	6.98	.19		.51			.41	5.01
Government	258.84	164.03	35.45	2.27	4.19	5.18	.59	32.55	14.58
Federal	180.45	116.52	26.32	1.40	3.09	2.78	.30	19.05	10.99
Medicare	94.12	70.33	20.08		2.07			1.64	

350

Medicaid	41.60	15.26	4.68	1.02	.83	2.60		16.33	.88
Other	44.73	30.93	1.56	.38	.19	.18	.30	1.08	10.10
State and local	78.39	47.51	9.13	.86	1.09	2.40	.29	13.50	3.59
Medicaid	32.06	11.76	3.60	.78	.64	2.01		12.58	.68
Other	46.33	35.75	5.53	.08	.45	.39	.29	.92	2.91
Percentage distribution									
Total	100.0	100.0	100.0	100.0	100.0	100.0	100.0	100.0	100.0
Direct payments	30.3	5.9	38.8	79.5	43.5	83.1	91.9	41.4	
Third-party payments	69.7	94.1	61.2	20.5	56.5	16.9	8.1	58.6	100.0
Private health insurance	27.6	36.6	36.7	15.5	24.2	7.8	1.9	.9	
Philanthropy and industrial inplant	2.0	2.3	.1		3.5			.7	25.6
Government	40.1	55.2	24.3	5.0	28.8	9.1	6.2	56.9	74.4
Federal	27.9	39.2	18.0	3.1	21.3	4.9	3.2	33.3	56.1
Medicare	14.6	23.6	13.8		14.2			2.9	
Medicaid	6.4	5.1	3.2	2.2	5.7	4.6		28.6	4.5
Other	6.9	10.4	1.1	.8	1.3	.3	3.2	1.9	51.6
State and local	12.1	16.0	6.3	1.9	7.5	4.2	3.1	23.6	18.3
Medicaid	5.0	4.0	2.5	1.7	4.4	3.5		22.0	3.5
Other	7.2	12.0	3.8	.2	3.1	.7	3.1	1.6	14.9

*Preliminary estimates.

Source: Gibson R. M., and Fisher, C. R.; National health expenditures, fiscal year 1977. Social Security Bulletin Vol. 41: July 1978

Table 8-4. Aggregate and per Capita Amount and Percentage Distribution of Personal Health-Care Expenditures Met by Third Parties, by Type of Expenditure, Year Ending September 1976

Source of Payment	Total	Hospital Care	Physicians' Services	Dentists' Services	Other Professional Services	Drug and Drug Sundries	Eyeglasses and Appliances	Nursing-Home Care	Other Health Services
					1976				
Aggregate amount (in millions)									
Total	$126,217	$57,497	$28,504	$8,987	$2,849	$11,472	$1,986	$10,834	$4,088
Direct payments	39,425	3,423	11,394	7,250	1,398	9,597	1,831	4,532	
Third-party payments	86,792	54,074	17,110	1,737	1,451	1,875	155	6,302	4,088
Private health insurance	33,618	20,589	10,194	1,270	631	799	34	101	
Philanthropy and industrial inplant	2,698	1,457	40		107			86	1,007
Government	50,477	32,028	6,876	468	713	1,076	121	6,115	3,081
Federal	34,990	22,538	5,059	290	508	585	65	3,615	2,329
Medicare	17,643	13,274	3,734		309			326	
Medicaid	8,142	2,926	1,011	213	159	549	65	3,095	189
Other	9,206	6,338	314	77	40	36		194	2,140
State and local	15,488	9,490	1,817	177	204	491	56	2,500	752
Medicaid	5,859	2,100	732	154	114	395		2,228	136
Other	9,628	7,390	1,085	23	90	96	56	273	616
Per capita amount									
Total	$576.77	$262.74	$130.25	$41.07	$13.02	52.42	$9.07	$49.51	$18.68
Direct payments	180.16	15.64	52.07	33.13	6.39	43.85	8.37	20.71	
Third-party payments	396.61	247.10	78.19	7.94	6.63	8.57	.71	28.80	18.68
Private health insurance	153.62	94.09	46.58	5.80	2.88	3.65	.15	.46	
Philanthropy and industrial inplant	12.33	6.66	.18		.49			.39	4.60
Government	230.66	146.35	31.42	2.14	3.26	4.92	.56	27.94	14.08

Federal	159.89	102.99	23.12	1.33	2.32	2.68	.30	16.52	10.64
Medicare	80.62	60.66	17.06		1.41			1.49	
Medicaid	37.21	13.37	4.62	.97	.73	2.51		14.14	.86
Other	42.07	28.96	1.44	.35	.18	.17	.30	.89	9.78
State and local	70.77	43.37	8.31	.81	.93	2.24	.26	11.43	3.43
Medicaid	26.77	9.60	3.35	.70	.52	1.81		10.18	.62
Other	44.00	33.77	4.96	.11	.41	.43	.26	1.25	2.81
Percentage distribution									
Total	100.0	100.0	100.0	100.0	100.0	100.0	100.0	100.0	100.0
Direct payments	31.2	6.0	40.0	80.7	49.1	83.7	92.2	41.8	
Third-party payments	68.8	94.0	60.0	19.3	50.9	16.3	7.8	58.2	100.0
Private health insurance	26.6	35.8	35.8	14.1	22.2	7.0	1.7	.9	24.6
Philanthropy and industrial inplant	2.1	2.5	.1		3.8			.8	
Government	40.0	55.7	24.1	5.2	25.0	9.4	6.1	56.4	75.4
Federal	27.7	39.2	17.7	3.2	17.8	5.1	3.3	33.4	57.0
Medicare	14.0	23.1	13.1		10.8			3.0	
Medicaid	6.5	5.1	3.5	2.4	5.6	4.8	3.3	28.6	4.6
Other	7.3	11.0	1.1	.9	1.4	.3		1.8	52.3
State and local	12.3	16.5	6.4	2.0	7.2	4.3	2.8	23.1	18.4
Medicaid	4.6	3.7	2.6	1.7	4.0	3.4		20.6	3.3
Other	7.6	12.9	3.8	.3	3.2	.8	2.8	2.5	15.1

Source: Gibson R. M., and Fisher, C. R.; National health expenditures, fiscal year 1977. *Social Security Bulletin* Vol. 41: July 1978.

Table 8-5. Aggregate and per Capita Amount and Percentage Distribution of Personal Health Care Expenditures, Met by Third Parties by Type of Expenditure, Year ending September 1975

Source of Payment	Total	Hospital Care	Physicians' Services	Dentists' Services	Other Professional Services	Drug and Drug Sundries	Eyeglasses and Appliances	Nursing-Home Care	Other Health Services
					1975				
Aggregate amount (in millions)									
Total	$110,665	$49,973	$24,553	$8,034	$2,463	$10,582	$1,822	$9,620	$3,616
Direct payments	34,697	2,589	9,622	6,573	1,248	8,953	1,682	4,029	
Third-party payments	75,968	47,385	14,931	1,461	1,215	1,628	140	5,592	3,616
Private health insurance	28,514	17,446	8,723	1,014	568	656	29	79	
Philanthropy and industrial inplant	2,419	1,313	36		97			77	896
Government	45,035	28,626	6,171	447	550	973	112	5,436	2,720
Federal	30,290	19,534	4,427	270	378	510	63	3,100	2,009
Medicare	14,880	11,233	3,140		222			285	
Medicaid	7,084	2,461	998	197	119	478	63	2,647	184
Other	8,326	5,841	289	73	36	32		168	1,825
State and local	14,745	9,092	1,745	177	172	463	49	2,336	711
Medicaid	5,579	1,938	786	155	94	377	49	2,085	145
Other	9,166	7,154	959	22	78	86		251	566
Per capita amount									
Total	$509.90	$230.25	$113.13	$37.02	$11.35	$48.76	$8.40	$44.33	$16.66
Direct payments	159.87	11.93	44.34	30.29	5.75	41.25	7.75	18.57	
Third-party payments	350.03	218.33	68.79	6.73	5.60	7.50	.65	25.76	16.66
Private health insurance	131.38	80.39	40.19	4.67	2.62	3.02	.13	.36	
Philanthropy and industrial inplant	11.14	6.05	.17		.44			.36	4.13

Government	207.50	131.90	28.43	2.06	2.54	4.48	.52	25.05	12.53
Federal	139.57	90.01	20.40	1.24	1.74	2.35	.29	14.28	9.26
Medicare	68.56	51.76	14.47		1.02			1.31	.85
Medicaid	32.64	11.34	4.60	.91	.55	2.20	.29	12.20	8.41
Other	38.36	26.91	1.33	.34	.17	.15		.77	
State and local	67.94	41.89	8.04	.82	.79	2.13	.23	10.76	3.28
Medicaid	25.71	8.93	3.62	.71	.43	1.74		9.61	2.61
Other	42.23	32.96	4.42	.10	.36	.40	.23	1.16	.67
Percentage distribution									
Total	100.0	100.0	100.0	100.0	100.0	100.0	100.0	100.0	100.0
Direct payments	31.4	5.2	39.2	81.8	50.7	84.5	92.3	41.9	
Third-party payments	68.6	94.8	60.8	18.2	49.3	15.4	7.7	58.1	100.0
Private health insurance	25.8	34.9	35.5	12.6	23.1	6.2	1.6	.8	24.8
Philanthropy and industrial inplant	2.2	2.6	.1		3.9			.8	
Government	40.7	57.3	25.1	5.6	22.3	9.2	6.1	56.5	75.2
Federal	27.4	39.1	18.0	3.4	15.4	4.8	3.4	32.2	55.6
Medicare	13.4	22.5	12.8		9.0			3.0	5.1
Medicaid	6.4	4.9	4.1	2.5	4.8	4.5	3.4	27.5	50.5
Other	7.5	11.7	1.2	.9	1.5	.3		1.7	
State and local	13.3	18.2	7.1	2.2	7.0	4.4	2.7	24.3	19.7
Medicaid	5.0	3.9	3.2	1.9	3.8	3.6		21.7	15.7
Other	8.3	14.3	3.9	.3	3.2	.8	2.7	2.6	4.0

Source: Gibson, R. M. and Fisher, C. R.: National health expenditures, fiscal year 1977. Social Security Bulletin, Vol. 41: July 1978.

Table 8-6. Percentage of Expenses Covered by Group Health Insurance Plans

Type of Expense	Percentage of Covered Expenses Reimbursed 1977
Hospital	90.3
Surgery	83.8
Private duty nursing	82.7
Anesthetist	82.6
Diagnostic x-ray and lab	81.5
Doctor visits, in hospital	74.1
Prescribed drugs	63.6
Doctor visits, office and home	59.4

Source: Source Book of Health Insurance Data, 1977-78, Health Insurance Institute.

some of these elements also as we reviewed the service units that were the principal sources of these costs, that is, the physician and the general hospital. Another important factor to consider is *who* creates those costs by demand for the services of those service units. The *who* is obviously patients. But it is useful to examine those patients in terms of who they are, for we find significant differences if they are grouped by ages. These age differences have a bearing on any plan to phase in a national health insurance system by age groups (which some advocate) as well as indicate what the long term cost prospects are as our population grows and ages.

The principal breakdown of the population for health care is: under 19, 19-64, 65 and over. Table 8-8 shows the distribution of the population within these categories and the percentage distribution of personal health care expenditures. We can quickly see that the younger group accounts for a very low share of the expenditures: While they represent 31.6% of the population, they incur only 12.6% of the costs. By contrast, the elderly represent only 10.8% of the population but incur 28.9% of the costs. This is reflected in the average medical care bill (Table 8-9): the under-19 group averaged only $252.96, the middle-age group averaged $660.78, whereas the 65-and-over group had an average bill of $1,745.17. The average for people of all ages was $646.11.

These figures simply reflect the state of the nation's health: The young are relatively healthy, the costs incurred tend to be for acute and ambulatory care, and the costs are much less than for the other groups; the elderly suffer from a variety of chronic disabling conditions, have longer lengths of institutional stay, and call on the services of the health industry more frequently—and the resulting costs are the highest.

In terms of national health insurance, if we were to phase in a comprehensive

Table 8-7. Expenditures for Health Services and Supplies Under Public Program, Type of Expenditure, and Source of Funds, Year Ending September 1977.

(In Millions)

Program and Source of Funds	Total	Hospital Services	Physicians' Services	Dentists' Services	Other Professional Services	Drugs and Drug Sundries	Eyeglasses and Appliances	Nursing-Home Care	Government Public Health Activities	Administration	Other Health Services
						1977[a]					
Total	$62,594	$36,199	$7,824	$500	$924	$1,143	$130	$7,184	$3,729	$1,743	$3,217
Medicare (health insurance for the aged and disabled)[b]	21,591	15,520	4,431		457			362		821	
Temporary disability insurance (medical benefits)[c]	103	74	25		2	1	1				
Workers' compensation (medical benefits)[c]	2,609	1,315	1,109		80	52	52				
Medicaid[d]	17,103	5,964	1,827	398	325	1,016		6,380		846	346
Other public assistance medical-vendor payments	517	190	58	13	10	32		203			11
General hospital and medical care	8,296	6,877	21	4		3					1,391
Defense Department hospital and medical care[e]	3,392	2,459	91	8		12				31	791
Maternal and child health services	637	97	60	15	49	14	19			5	378
Government public health activities[f]	3,729	3,729							3,729		
Veterans' hospital and medical care	4,334	3,589	58	63		13	31	238		40	302

357

Table 8-7. (continued)

Program and Source of Funds	Hospital Services	Physicians' Services	Dentists' Services	Other Professional Services	Drugs and Drug Sundries	Eyeglasses and Appliances	Nursing-Home Care	Government Public Health Activities	Administration	Other Health Services
Medical vocational rehabilitation										
Federal	283	115								
	42,542	25,715	310	683	614	27	4,204	1,289	1,430	2,424
Medicare (health insurance for the aged and disabled)[b]		142				66				
	21,591	15,520		457			362		821	
Workers' compensation (medical benefits)[3]		4,431								
	69	45	225	4	1	1				195
Medicaid[d]	9,713	17		184	573		3,603		533	984
		3,368								
General hospital and medical care	1,605	1,032	4		3					
		592								
Defense Department hospital ard medical care[e]	3,392	21	8		12				31	791
		2,459								
Maternal and child health services	322	91	10	38	11	12			5	152
		50								
Government public health activities[f]	1,289	44						1,289		
Veterans' hospital and medical care	4,334	3,589	63		13	31	238		40	302
		58								
Medical vocational rehabilitation										
State and local	227	92				22				
	20,051	113	190	241	529	64	2,980	2,440	313	793
		2,016								
Temporary disability insurance (medical benefits)[c]	103	74	2	2	1	1				
		25								

Workers' compensation (medical benefits)[c]	2,540	1,270	1,092		76	51	51				
Medicaid[d]	7,389	2,596	795	173	142	442		2,777		313	150
Other public assistance medical-vendor payments	517	190	58	13	10	32		203			11
General hospital and medical care	6,691	6,284									406
Maternal and child health services	315	47	17	4	11	3	7				225
Government public health activities[f]	2,440								2,440		
Medical vocational rehabilitation	57	23	28				5				

[a]Preliminary estimates.

[b]Represents total expenditures from trust funds for benefits and administrative costs. Trust fund income includes premium payments paid by or on behalf of enrollees.

[c]Includes medical benefits paid under public law by private insurance carriers and self-insurers.

[d]Includes funds paid into Medicare trust funds by States under "buy-in" agreements to cover premiums for public assistance recipients and for persons who are medically indigent.

[e]Includes care for retirees and military dependents. Payments for services other than hospital care and other health services represent only those made under contract medical programs.

[f]Includes expenditures before 1974 reported under the Office of Economic Opportunity.

Source: Gibson, R. M., and Fisher, C. R.: National health expenditures, fiscal year 1977, *Social Security Bulletin* Vol. 41: July 1978.

Table 8-8. Personal Health Care Expenditures by Age Distribution for Year Ending September, 1977

	Population		Personal Health Care Expenditures	
Age	Number (in millions)	Percentage distribution	Amount (in billions)	Percentage distribution
All ages	220.7	100.0	$142.6	100.0
Under 19	70.8	31.6	17.9	12.6
19-64	126.2	57.6	83.4	58.5
65 and over	23.6	10.8	41.3	28.9

Source: Gibson, R. M., and Fisher, R. S.: Age differences in health care spending, fiscal year 1977. Social Security Bulletin, Vol. 42: January 1979.

plan with the younger age group, initial costs would clearly be minimized. On the other hand, if we began a national scheme with the older age group, the group already covered by Medicare (and some also by Medicaid), a different and slightly greater cost would be incurred even if we discount the amounts already paid by government. If national health insurance covered both groups initially (the under 19 and the over 65), it would be less initial additional government cost than if the middle-age group were covered. But any calculation should be done with caution: Medicare, part B premiums paid by the aged are reported not as private expenditures but as federal expenditures. Hence, it could be reasonably argued that the federal government's data mislead us as to the extent to which Medicare removes the financial burden from the aged. Of concern to national health planners, however, is that the percentage of the population that is 65 and over is increasing, which means that not only will overall costs rise but also that the costs will probably have to be borne under any public program by the dwindling percentage of younger people. The problem this poses is demonstrated by Table 8-10, which shows the percentage of people hospitalized by sex and age, as well as the number of hospital stays and the average length of stay for each age group. It should be noted that as the population ages, the percentage hospitalized increases, as does the average length of stay. The one exception is that percentage of women hospitalized in the 20-34 age group. This can be accounted for by the fact that this is the main childbearing age range, and most babies are born in hospitals.

The third column of Table 8-9 states the public or government expenditures by age group. Table 8-11 breaks this down into level of government, federal and state/local. Figure 8-12 shows the relationship between age groups and the payors. Some of the state/local monies include federal revenue sharing funds given to the states. In 1976, for example, the total state/local expenditure

Table 8-9. Personal Health Care Expenditures for Three Age Groups: Aggregate and per Capita Amount and Percentage Distribution, by Type of Expenditure and Source of Funds, Years Ending September 1975-77

Table 8-9a.

1977ᵃ

	All ages			Under 19		
Type of expenditure	Total	Private	Public	Total	Private	Public
Aggregate amount (in millions)						
Total	$142,586	$85,465	$57,121	$17,909	$12,392	$5,517
Hospital care	65,637	29,427	36,199	6,333	3,448	2,885
Physicians' services	32,184	24,360	7,824	4,924	4,180	744
Dentists' services	10,020	9,520	500	2,144	1,925	220
Other professional services	3,212	2,288	924	305	169	136
Drugs and drug sundries	12,516	11,373	1,143	2,319	2,161	158
Eyeglasses and appliances	2,086	1,956	130	270	248	21
Nursing-home care	12,618	5,434	7,184	341	162	178
Other health services	4,322	1,105	3,217	1,272	98	1,174
Per capita amount						
Total	$646.11	$387.27	$258.84	$252.96	$175.03	$77.92
Hospital care	297.38	133.35	164.03	89.45	48.70	40.76
Physicians' services	145.84	110.39	35.45	69.55	59.05	10.51
Dentists' services	45.41	43.14	2.27	30.29	27.19	3.10
Other professional services	14.56	10.37	4.19	4.31	2.39	1.92
Drugs and drug sundries	56.72	51.54	5.18	32.76	30.52	2.23
Eyeglasses and appliances	9.45	8.86	.59	3.81	3.51	.30
Nursing-home care	57.18	24.62	32.55	4.81	2.29	2.52
Other health services	19.59	5.01	14.58	17.97	1.39	16.58

361

Table 8-9. (continued)

Table 8-9a.

	All ages			Under 19		
Type of expenditure	Total	Private	Public	Total	Private	Public
Percentage distribution						
Total	100.0	100.0	100.0	100.0	100.0	100.0
Hospital care	46.0	34.4	63.4	35.4	27.8	52.3
Physicians' services	22.6	28.5	13.7	27.5	33.7	13.5
Dentists' services	7.0	11.1	.9	12.0	15.5	4.0
Other professional services	2.3	2.7	1.6	1.7	1.4	2.5
Drugs and drug sundries	8.8	13.3	2.0	12.9	17.4	2.9
Eyeglasses and appliances	1.5	2.3	.2	1.5	2.0	.4
Nursing-home care	8.8	6.4	12.6	1.9	1.3	3.2
Other health services	3.0	1.3	5.6	7.1	.8	21.3
			1976[b]			
Aggregate amount (in millions)						
Total	$126,217	$75,740	$50,477	$16,104	$10,987	$5,117
Hospital care	57,497	25,470	32,028	5,646	3,067	2,580
Physicians' services	28,504	21,628	6,876	4,460	3,741	719
Dentists' services	8,987	8,519	468	1,956	1,749	207
Other professional services	2,849	2,136	713	278	158	120
Drugs and drug sundries	11,472	10,396	1,076	1,964	1,814	150
Eyeglasses and appliances	1,986	1,864	121	269	249	21
Nursing-home care	10,834	4,718	6,115	252	120	132
Other health services	4,088	1,007	3,081	1,279	90	1,190

Per capita amount

Total	$576.77	$346.10	$230.66	$225.01	$153.52	$71.50
Hospital care	262.74	116.39	146.35	78.89	42.85	36.05
Physicians' services	130.25	98.83	31.42	62.32	52.27	10.05
Dentists' services	41.07	38.93	2.14	27.33	24.44	2.89
Other professional services	13.02	9.76	3.26	3.88	2.21	1.68
Drugs and drug sundries	52.42	47.51	4.92	27.44	25.35	2.10
Eyeglasses and appliances	9.07	8.52	.56	3.76	3.48	.29
Nursing-home care	49.51	21.56	27.94	3.52	1.68	1.84
Other health services	18.68	4.60	14.08	17.87	1.26	16.63

Percentage distribution

Total	100.0	100.0	100.0	100.0	100.0	100.0
Hospital care	45.6	33.6	63.4	35.1	27.9	50.4
Physicians' services	22.6	28.6	13.6	27.7	34.0	14.1
Dentists' services	7.1	11.2	.9	12.1	15.9	4.0
Other professional services	2.3	2.8	1.4	1.7	1.4	2.3
Drugs and drug sundries	9.1	13.7	2.1	12.2	16.5	2.9
Eyeglasses and appliances	1.6	2.5	.2	1.7	2.3	.4
Nursing-home care	8.6	6.2	12.1	1.6	1.1	2.6
Other health services	3.2	1.3	6.1	7.9	.8	23.2

Table 8-9. (continued)

Table 8-9a.

1975

Type of expenditure	All ages			Under 19		
	Total	Private	Public	Total	Private	Public
Aggregate amount (in millions)						
Total	$110,665	$65,630	$45,035	$14,393	$9,681	$4,711
Hospital care	49,973	21,348	28,626	5,007	2,635	2,372
Physicians' services	24,553	18,382	6,171	3,928	3,201	727
Dentists' services	8,034	7,587	447	1,788	1,590	198
Other professional services	2,463	1,913	550	248	149	100
Drugs and drug sundries	10,582	9,609	973	1,843	1,708	136
Eyeglasses and appliances	1,822	1,710	112	247	228	19
Nursing-home care	9,620	4,185	5,436	190	91	99
Other health services	3,616	896	2,720	1,141	80	1,061
Per capita amount						
Total	$509.90	$302.40	$207.50	$196.10	$131.90	$64.18
Hospital care	230.25	98,36	131.90	68.22	35.90	32.32
Physicians' services	113.13	84.70	28.43	53.52	43.61	9.90
Dentists' services	37.02	34.95	2.06	24.36	21.66	2.70
Other professional services	11.35	8.81	2.54	3.38	2.03	1.36
Drugs and drug sundries	48.76	44.28	4.48	25.11	23.27	1.85
Eyeglasses and appliances	8.40	7.88	.52	3.37	3.11	.26
Nursing-home care	44.33	19.28	25.05	2.59	1.24	1.35
Other health services	16.66	4.13	12.53	15.55	1.09	14.46

Percentage distribution

Total	100.0	100.0	100.0	100.0	100.0	100.0
Hospital care	45.2	32.5	63.6	34.8	27.2	50.3
Physicians' services	22.2	28.0	13.7	27.3	33.1	15.4
Dentists' services	7.3	11.6	1.0	12.4	16.4	4.2
Other professional services	2.2	2.9	1.2	1.7	1.5	2.1
Drugs and drug sundries	9.6	14.6	2.2	12.8	17.6	2.9
Eyeglasses and appliances	1.6	2.6	.2	1.7	2.4	.4
Nursing-home care	8.7	6.4	12.1	1.3	.9	2.1
Other health services	3.3	1.4	6.0	7.9	.8	22.5

[a]Preliminary estimates.

[b]Revised estimates.

Source: Gibson, R. M., and Fisher, R. S.: Age differences in health care spending, fiscal year 1977. *Social Security Bulletin* Vol. 42: January 1979.

Table 8-9. (continued)

Table 8-9b.

1977[a]

Type of Expenditure	19-64			65 and over		
	Total	Private	Public	Total	Private	Public
Aggregate amount (in millions)						
Total	$83,422	$59,449	$23,973	$41,256	$13,624	$27,631
Hospital care	41,109	23,840	17,269	18,185	2,140	16,045
Physicians' services	20,115	17,291	2,824	7,145	2,889	4,255
Dentists' services	6,854	6,620	234	1,022	976	46
Other professional services	2,091	1,794	298	816	325	490
Drugs and drug sundries	7,338	6,790	549	2,859	2,423	436
Eyeglasses and appliances	1,505	1,405	100	312	303	9
Nursing-home care	1,741	737	1,004	10,536	4,535	6,001
Other health services	2,669	973	1,695	381	33	348
Per capita amount						
Total	$660.78	$470.89	$189.89	$1,745.17	$576.33	$1,168.84
Hospital care	325.62	188.83	136.78	769.25	90.52	678.73
Physicians' services	159.33	136.96	22.37	302.23	122.23	180.01
Dentists' services	54.29	52.43	1.86	43.24	41.28	1.96
Other professional services	16.56	14.21	2.36	34.51	13.77	20.75
Drugs and drug sundries	58.13	53.78	4.35	120.94	102.48	18.46
Eyeglasses and appliances	11.92	11.13	.79	13.20	12.83	.37
Nursing-home care	13.79	5.84	7.95	445.68	191.82	253.86
Other health services	21.14	7.71	13.43	16.12	1.41	14.71

Percentage distribution

Total	100.0	100.0	100.0	100.0	100.0	100.0
Hospital care	58.1	15.7	44.1	72.0	40.1	49.3
Physicians' services	15.4	21.2	17.3	11.8	29.1	24.1
Dentists' services	.2	7.2	2.5	1.0	11.1	8.2
Other professional services	1.8	2.4	2.0	1.2	3.0	2.5
Drugs and drug sundries	1.6	17.8	6.9	2.3	11.4	8.8
Eyeglasses and appliances	0.	2.2	.8	.4	2.4	1.8
Nursing home care	21.7	33.3	25.5	4.2	1.2	2.1
Other health services	1.3	.2	.9	7.1	1.6	3.2

1976^b

Aggregate amount (in millions)

Total	$23,868	$11,802	$35,670	$21,492	$52,951	$74,443
Hospital care	13,900	1,877	15,777	15,548	20,526	36,074
Physicians' services	3,640	2,469	6,108	2,517	15,418	17,935
Dentists' services	43	859	902	218	5,911	6,129
Other professional services	344	377	722	248	1,601	1,850
Drugs and drug sundries	413	1,912	2,325	513	6,670	7,184
Eyeglasses and appliances	9	2.56	265	92	1,360	1,452
Nursing home care	5,190	4,022	9,212	794	577	1,370
Other health services	330	30	360	1,561	887	2,448

Per capita amount

Total	$1,035.31	$511.93	$1,547.24	$173.03	$426.29	$599.32
Hospital care	602.93	81.42	684.35	125.17	165.25	290.42
Physicians' services	157.89	107.10	264.94	20.26	124.13	144.39
Dentists services	1.87	37.26	39.13	1.76	47.59	49.34

367

Table 8-9. (continued)

Table 8-9b.

Type of Expenditure	19-64			65 and over		
	Total	Private	Public	Total	Private	Public
Other professional services	14.89	12.89	2.00	31.32	16.35	14.92
Drugs and drug sundries	57.84	53.70	4.13	100.85	82.94	17.91
Eyeglasses and appliances	11.69	10.95	.74	11.49	11.10	.39
Nursing-home care	11.03	4.65	6.39	399.58	174.46	225.12
Other health services	19.71	7.14	12.57	15.62	1.30	14.31
Percentage distribution						
Total	100.0	100.0	100.0	100.0	100.0	100.0
Hospital care	48.5	38.8	72.3	44.2	15.9	58.2
Physicians' services	24.1	29.1	11.7	17.1	20.9	15.2
Dentists' services	8.2	11.2	1.0	2.5	7.3	.2
Other professional services	2.5	3.0	1.2	2.0	3.2	1.4
Drugs and drug sundries	9.6	12.6	2.4	6.5	16.2	1.7
Eyeglasses and appliances	2.0	2.6	.4	.7	2.2	0
Nursing-home care	1.8	1.1	3.7	25.8	34.1	21.7
Other health services	3.3	1.7	7.3	1.0	.3	1.4

1975^b

Type of Expenditure	19-64			65 and over		
	Total	Private	Public	Total	Private	Public
Aggregate amount (in millions)						
Total	$65,006	$45,617	$19,389	$31,266	$10,331	$20,935
Hospital care	31,238	17,091	14,147	13,728	1,621	12,107
Physicians' services	15,523	13,237	2,286	5,103	1,944	3,159
Dentists' services	5,455	5,246	209	792	751	41
Other professional services	1,595	1,394	201	621	371	250
Drugs and drug sundries	6,619	6,156	463	2,119	1,745	374
Eyeglasses and appliances	1,308	1,224	85	267	259	8
Nursing-home care	1,131	479	652	8,299	3,614	4,685
Other health services	2,136	789	1,347	339	27	312

Per capita amount

Total	$536.54	$376.51	$160.03	$1,391.08	$459.65	$931.44
Hospital care	257.83	141.06	116.77	610.78	72.12	538.65
Physicians' services	128.12	109.25	18.87	227.02	86.47	140.55
Dentists' services	45.02	43.30	1.73	35.23	33.41	1.82
Other professional services	13.16	11.51	1.66	27.61	16.49	11.11
Drugs and drug sundries	54.63	50.81	3.82	94.28	77.64	16.65
Eyeglasses and appliances	10.80	10.10	.70	11.88	11.52	.37
Nursing-home care	9.33	3.95	5.38	369.23	160.79	208.43
Other health services	17.63	6.51	11.12	15.06	1.20	13.86

Percentage distribution

Total	100.0	100.0	100.0	100.0	100.0	100.0
Hospital care	48.1	37.5	73.0	43.9	15.7	57.8
Physicians' services	23.9	29.0	11.8	16.3	18.8	15.1
Dentists' services	8.4	11.5	1.1	2.5	7.3	.2
Other professional services	2.5	3.1	1.0	2.0	3.6	1.2
Drugs and drug sundries	10.2	13.5	2.4	6.8	16.9	1.8
Eyeglasses and appliances	2.0	2.7	.4	.9	2.5	0
Nursing-home care	1.7	1.1	3.4	26.5	35.0	22.4
Other health services	3.3	1.7	6.9	1.1	.3	1.5

aPreliminary estimates.

bRevised estimates.

Source: Gibson, R. M., and Fisher, R. S.: Age differences in health care spending, fiscal year 1977. *Social Security Bulletin* Vol. 42: January 1979.

Table 8-10. Hospitalization by Age Group

Age	Total Number Hospitalized (in thousands)	Percent Hospitalized			Mean Rate per Hospital User per Year		Average Length of Stay[a]
		Total	Men	Women	Inpatient Days of Care	Hospital Stays	
20-64	13,637	12.8	10.1	15.3	10	1.20	8.3
20-34	6,181	14.8	8.1	20.7	7	1.14	6.1
35-44	2,377	10.8	10.6	11.1	9	1.16	7.8
45-54	2,698	11.4	10.9	12.0	12	1.29	9.3
55-64	2,381	12.5	13.1	12.0	15	1.31	11.5
65 and over	4,245	20.5	21.8	19.5	18	1.41	12.8

[a]Computed by author.
Data for aged 20-64 group from Social Security Administration 1972 Survey of the Disabled. Data for age 65 and over from health insurance program statistics, Health Care Financing Administration.
Source: Gibson, R. M., and Fisher, R. S.: Age differences in health care spending, fiscal year 1977. Social Security Bulletin Vol. 42: January 1979.

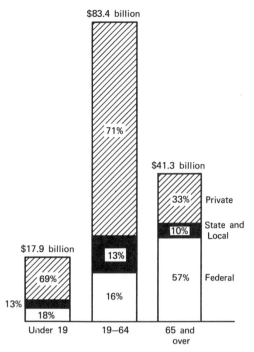

Figure 8–2. Percentage distribution of expenditures for personal health care, by source of funds and age group, fiscal year 1977. (*Source*: Gibson, R.M., and Fisher, C.R.: Age differences in health care spending, fiscal year 1977. *Social Security Bulletin* 42:1979.)

for health came to $17.299 billion; the federal revenue sharing contribution for the first half of that year (the only figures reported) came only to $.232 billion. For 1977, of the total public expenditures, the state/local share was 30%, but the federal share is really inflated because it includes all of the premium contributions from the aged and disabled under part B of Medicare. If these citizen contributions are deducted ($2.193 billion in 1977)*, then the public expenditure drops from $57.121 billion to $54.928 billion, and the state/local share of that ($17.299 billion) represents 31.5% of the total public expenditures for personal health care. It might be noted at this juncture that personal health care expenditures represent "that portion of the total national health care expense representing health services and supplies received directly by individuals. They make up total national expenditures for health, together with spending for research and medical facilities construction, identifiable adminis-

_____

*Per telephone inquiry to HEW, Medicare Bureau.

Table 8-11. Estimated Personal Health Care Expenditures Under Public Programs, by Type of Expenditure and Source of Funds, for Three Age Groups, Years Ending September 1975-77 (In Millions)

Table 8-11a.

Type of Expenditure	All Ages			Under 19		
	Total	Federal	State and Local	Total	Federal	State and Local
			1977[a]			
Total	$57,121	$39,823	$17,299	$5,517	$3,186	$2,331
Hospital care	36,199	25,715	10,484	2,885	1,777	1,108
Physicians' services	7,824	5,808	2,016	744	440	304
Dentists' services	500	310	190	220	124	96
Other professional services	924	683	241	136	84	52
Drugs and drug sundries	1,143	614	529	158	91	67
Eyeglasses and appliances	130	66	64	21	15	7
Nursing-home care	7,184	4,204	2,980	178	98	81
Other health services	3,217	2,424	793	1,174	558	616
			1976[b]			
Total	$50,477	$34,990	$15,488	$5,117	$3,008	$2,109
Hospital care	32,028	22,538	9,490	2,580	1,608	972
Physicians' services	6,876	5,059	1,817	719	428	292
Dentists' services	468	290	177	207	118	89
Other professional services	713	508	204	120	75	45
Drugs and drug sundries	1,076	585	491	150	87	62
Eyeglasses and appliances	121	65	56	21	14	6

Nursing-home care	6,115	3,615	2,500	132	73	58
Other health services	3,081	2,329	752	1,190	605	585

1975[b]

Total	$45,035	$30,290	$14,745	$4,711	$2,708	$2,003
Hospital care	28,626	19,534	9,092	2,372	1,456	916
Physicians' services	6,171	4,427	1,745	727	416	310
Dentists' services	447	270	177	198	109	89
Other professional services	550	378	172	100	62	38
Drugs and drug sundries	973	510	463	136	76	59
Eyeglasses and appliances	112	63	49	19	13	6
Nursing-home care	5,436	3,100	2,336	99	53	46
Other health services	2,720	2,009	711	1,061	523	538

[a]Preliminary estimates.

[b]Revised estimates.

Source: Gibson, R. M., and Fisher, R. S.: Age differences in health care spending, fiscal year 1977. *Social Security Bulletin* Vol. 42: January 1979.

Table 8-11. (continued)

Table 8-11b.

Type of Expenditure	19-64			65 and Over		
	Total	Federal	State and Local	Total	Federal	State and Local
			1977[a]			
Total	$23,973	$13,244	$10,729	$27,631	$23,393	$4,239
Hospital care	17,269	9,172	8,096	16,045	14,766	1,280
Physicians' services	2,824	1,249	1,575	4,255	4,119	137
Dentists' services	234	154	80	46	32	15
Other professional services	298	139	158	490	460	31
Drugs and drug sundries	549	283	266	436	240	197
Eyeglasses and appliances	100	44	56	9	7	2
Nursing-home care	1,004	592	412	6,001	3,514	2,487
Other health services	1,695	1,610	85	348	256	91

Total	$21,492	$11,849	$9,643	$23,868	$20,133	$3,735
Hospital care	15,548	8,203	7,345	13,900	12,727	1,173
Physicians' services	2,517	1,119	1,398	3,640	3,512	128
Dentists' services	218	143	75	43	29	14
Other professional services	248	115	134	344	318	26
Drugs and drug sundries	513	269	244	413	229	184
Eyeglasses and appliances	92	44	48	9	7	1
Nursing-home care	794	474	319	5,190	3,068	2,122
Other health services	1,561	1,481	80	330	243	87

1975[b]

Total	$19,389	$10,238	$9,151	$20,935	$17,345	$3,590
Hospital care	14,147	7,113	7,034	12,107	10,965	1,141
Physicians' services	2,286	983	1,303	3,159	3,028	131
Dentists' services	209	134	75	41	27	14
Other professional services	201	88	113	250	228	21
Drugs and drug sundries	463	234	229	374	199	175
Eyeglasses and appliances	85	43	42	8	7	1
Nursing-home care	652	377	275	4,685	2,670	2,015
Other health services	1,347	1,266	81	312	220	92

[a]Preliminary estimates
[b]Revised estimates.
Source: Gibson, R. M., and Fisher, R. S.: Age differences in health care spending, fiscal year 1977. *Social Security Bulletin* Vol. 42: January 1979.

trative costs of government programs, government public health activities, expenses incurred by philanthropic organizations in raising funds for health care, and the net cost of private health insurance (the difference between premiums and benefit payments)" (3, p. 3-4).

Table 8-12 analyzes the public program expenditures by program and whether the money comes from federal or state/local funds. The overall impact of Medicare and Medicaid is clearly evident: Together, they represent 64.8% of all government expenditures *for personal health programs.* In terms of federal government expenditures, these two programs represent 75.2% of the federal effort. If one totals the federal figures for Medicare, Medicaid, Defense Department programs, and VA programs, the resulting sum represents 94.4% of the total *federal* expenditures for personal health care.

Gibson and Fisher note that one of the most significant changes in recent years has been the rise in government expenditures for the midage group (19-64), reflected in Medicare and Medicaid as a result of legislation:

In July 1973, certain disabled workers (and their dependents) eligible for OASDI benefits and persons suffering from end-stage renal disease became eligible for Medicare benefits. In January 1974, the public assistance program for the permanently disabled was abolished and the new Federal supplemental security income (SSI) program for the aged, blind, and disabled began operation. In 35 states, these persons are also eligible for Medicaid; the remaining states make separate determinations on their eligibility for Medicaid. (3, p.9)

From fiscal 1974 to fiscal 1977, reflecting these changes, Medicare and Medicaid expenditures rose from $5.3 billion to $9 billion.

Table 8-13 shows a detailed analysis of the expenditures for persons 65 and over. Noteworthy are the shortcomings of Medicare and Medicaid: Overall, these programs covered only 44.3% and 16.7% of the expenditures for personal health care of the aged, who must pay, through health insurance or their own funds, 33% of the cost. Actually, the aged pay more than that percentage, since their part B Medicare premiums are counted as a public expenditure. If that consumer contribution is taken into account, the 44.3% is reduced to 41%. (3, p.13)

Of the 22.9 million persons 65 and over in 1976 (*note:* not 1977), an estimated 15.7% (3.6 million) were also covered by Medicaid either because

Table 8-12. Estimated Personal Health Care Expenditures Under Public Programs, by Program and Source of Funds, for Three Age Groups, Years Ending September 1975-77 (In Millions)

Table 8-12a.

Program	All Ages			Under 19		
	Total	Federal	State and Local	Total	Federal	State and Local
		1977[a]				
Total	$57,121	$39,823	$17,299	$5,517	$3,186	$2,331
Medicare (health insurance for the aged and disabled);[b]	20,770	20,770		29	29	
Temporary disability insurance (medical benefits)[c]	103		103			
Workers' compensation (medical benefits)[c]	2,609	69	2,540			
Medicaid;[d]	16,257	9,181	7,076	2,852	1,610	1,241
Other public assistance medical vendor payments	517		517	91		91
General hospital and medical care	8,296	1,605	6,691	1,108	388	721
Defense Department hospital and medical care[e]	3,361	3,361		845	845	
Maternal and child health services	632	317	315	535	269	267
Veterans' hospital and medical care	4,293	4,293		57	45	11
Medical vocational rehabilitation	283	227	57			

Table 8-12. (continued)

Table 8-12a.

	All Ages			Under 19		
Program	Total	Federal	State and Local	Total	Federal	State and Local
				1976[b]		
Total	$50,477	$34,990	$15,488	$5,117	$3,008	$2,109
Medicare (health insurance for the aged and disabled)[b]	17,643	17,643		24	24	
Temporary disability insurance (medical benefits)[c]	90		90			
Workers' compensation (medical benefits)[c]	2,233	68	2,165			
Medicaid[d]	14,000	8,142	5,859	2,481	1,443	1,038
Other public assistance medical vendor payments	717		717	127		127
General hospital and medical care	7,845	1,536	6,309	1,123	437	686
Defense Department hospital and medical care[e]	3,178	3,178		799	799	
Maternal and child health services	599	307	292	507	260	247
Veterans' hospital and medical care	3,894	3,894				
Medical vocational rehabilitation	278	222	56	56	44	11

Total	$45,035	$30,290	$14,745	$4,711	$2,708	$2,003
Medicare (health insurance for the aged and disabled)[b]	14,880	14,880		18	18	
Temporary disability insurance (medical benefits)[c]	75		75			
Workers' compensation (medical benefits)[c]	1,926	54	1,872			
Medicaid[d]	12,663	7,084	5,580	2,259	1,264	995
Other public assistance medical vendor payments	670		670	119		119
General hospital and medical care	7,503	1,281	6,222	1,011	364	647
Defense Department hospital and medical care[e]	3,110	3,110		782	782	
Maternal and child health services	554	281	273	469	238	231
Veterans' hospital and medical care	3,389	3,389				
Medical vocational rehabilitation	265	212	53	53	42	11

[a]Preliminary estimates.

[b]Represents total expenditures from trust funds for benefits and administrative costs. Trust fund income includes premium payments paid by or on behalf of enrollees.

[c]Includes medical benefits paid under public law by private insurance carriers and self-insurers.

[d]Includes funds paid into Medicare trust funds by States under "buy-in" agreements to cover premiums for public assistance recipients and medically indigent persons.

[e]Includes care for retirees and military dependents. Payments for services other than hospital care and other health services represent only those made under contract medical programs.

[f]Revised estimates.

Source: Gibson, R. M., and Fisher, R. S.: Age differences in health care spending, fiscal year 1977. *Social Security Bulletin* Vol. 42: January 1979.

Table 8-12. (continued)

Table 8-12b.

Program	19-64			65 and over		
	Total	Federal	State and Local	Total	Federal	State and Local
	1977[a]					
Total	$23,973	$13,244	$10,729	$27,631	$23,393	$4,239
Medicare (health insurance for the aged and disabled)[b]	2,459	2,459		18,282	18,282	
Temporary disability insurance (medical benefits)[c]	103		103			
Workers' compensation (medical benefits)[c]	2,530	67	2,463	79	2	77
Medicaid[d]	6,515	3,679	2,836	6,890	3,891	2,999
Other public assistance medical vendor payments	207	207		219		219
General hospital and medical care	6,150	1,122	5,028	1,038	95	943
Defense Department hospital and medical care[e]	2,421	2,421		95	95	
Maternal and child health services	97	49	48			
Veterans' hospital and medical care	3,271	3,271		1,022	1,022	
Medical vocational rehabilitation	221	177	44	6	5	1
	1976[f]					

Total	$21,492	$11,849	$9,643	$23,868	$20,133	$3,735

Category						
Total	$21,492	$11,849	$9,643	$23,868	$20,133	$3,735
Medicare (health insurance for the aged and disabled)[b]		2,027	2,027	15,591	15,591	15,591
Temporary disability insurance (medical benefits)[c]	90		90			
Workers' compensation (medical benefits)[c]	2,166	68	2,100	67	2	65
Medicaid[d]	5,602	3,259	2,343	5,917	3,439	2,478
Other public assistance medical vendor payments	287		287	303		303
General hospital and medical care	5,745	1,010	4,735	977	89	888
Defense Department hospital and medical care[e]	2,289	2,289		90	90	
Maternal and child health services	92	47	45			
Veterans' hospital and medical care	2,977	2,977		917	917	
Medical vocational rehabilitation	217	174	43	6	4	1

1975[f]

Category						
Total	$19,389	$10,238	$9,151	$20,935	$17,345	$3,590
Medicare (health insurance for the aged and disabled)[b]	1,489	1,489		13,373	13,373	13,373
Temporary disability insurance (medical benefits)[c]	75		75			
Workers' compensation (medical benefits)[c]	1,868	52	1,815	58	2	57
Medicaid[d]	5,031	2,815	2,217	5,373	3,005	2,368
Other public assistance medical vendor payments	266		266	285		285

Table 8-12. (continued)

Table 8-12b.

Program	19-64			65 and over		
	Total	Federal	State and Local	Total	Federal	State and Local
General hospital and medical care	5,537	842	4,695	954	74	880
Defense Department hospital and medical care[e]	2,240	2,240		88	88	
Maternal and health services	85	43	42			
Veterans' hospital and medical care	2,591	2,591		798	798	
Medical vocational rehabilitation	207	166	41	5	4	1

[a]Preliminary estimates.

[b]Represents total expenditures from trust funds for benefits and administrative costs. Trust fund income includes premium payments paid by or on behalf of enrollees.

[c]Includes medical benefits paid under public law by private insurance carriers and self-insurers.

[d]Includes funds paid into Medicare trust funds by States under "buy-in" agreements to cover premiums for public assistance recipients and medically indigent persons.

[e]Includes care for retirees and military dependents. Payments for services other than hospital care and other health services represent only those made under contract medical programs.

[f]Revised estimates.

Source: Gibson, R. M., and Fisher, R. S.: Age differences in health care spending, fiscal year 1977. *Social Security Bulletin* Vol. 42: January 1979.

Table 8-13. Estimated Amount and Percentage Distribution of Personal Health Care Expenditures for Persons Aged 65 and Over, by Type of Expenditure and Source of Funds, Years Ending September 1975-77

Table 8-13a.

Amount (in millions)

Type of Expenditure	Total	Private	Public			
			Total	Medicare	Medicaid	Other
1977[a]						
Total	$41,256	$13,624	$27,631	$18,282	$6,890	$2,459
Hospital care	18,185	2,140	16,045	13,533	638	1,874
Physicians' services	7,145	2,889	4,255	3,975	221	60
Dentists' services	1,022	976	46		31	15
Other professional services	816	325	490	425	61	4
Drugs and drug sundries	2,859	2,423	436		418	18
Eyeglasses and appliances	312	303	9			9
Nursing-home care	10,536	4,535	6,001	349	5,325	328
Other health services	381	33	348		196	152
1976[b]						
Total	$35,670	$11,802	$23,868	$15,591	$5,917	$2,360
Hospital care	15,777	1,877	13,900	11,614	538	1,748
Physicians' services	6,108	2,469	3,640	3,374	211	55
Dentists' services	902	859	43		29	14
Other professional services	722	377	344	288	51	5
Drugs and drug sundries	2,325	1,912	413		389	24
Eyeglasses and appliances	265	256	9			9
Nursing-home care	9,212	4,022	5,190	315	4,515	360
Other health services	360	30	330		184	146

Table 8-13. (continued)

Table 8-13a.

Amount (in millions)

Type of Expenditure	Total	Private	Public			
			Total	Medicare	Medicaid	Other
		1975[a]				
Total	$31,266	$10,331	$20,935	$13,373	$5,373	$2,189
Hospital care	13,728	1,621	12,107	9,998	471	1,638
Physicians' services	5,103	1,944	3,159	2,894	216	50
Dentists' services	792	751	41		28	13
Other professional services	621	371	250	206	40	4
Drugs and drug sundries	2,119	1,745	374		352	22
Eyeglasses and appliances	267	259	8			8
Nursing-home care	8,299	3,614	4,685	276	4,080	329
Other health services	339	27	312		186	125

[a]Preliminary estimates.
[b]Revised estimates.

Source: Gibson, R. M., and Fisher, R. S.; Age difference in health care spending, fiscal year 1977. Social Security Bulletin Vol. 42: January 1979.

Table 8-13b.

<table>
<tr><th rowspan="3">Type of Expenditure</th><th colspan="7">Percentage Distribution</th></tr>
<tr><th rowspan="2">Total</th><th rowspan="2">Private</th><th colspan="5">Public</th></tr>
<tr><th>Total</th><th>Medicare</th><th>Medicaid</th><th>Other</th></tr>
<tr><td colspan="7" align="center">1977[a]</td></tr>
<tr><td>Total</td><td>100.0</td><td>33.0</td><td>67.0</td><td>44.3</td><td>16.7</td><td>6.0</td></tr>
<tr><td>Hospital care</td><td>100.0</td><td>11.8</td><td>88.2</td><td>74.4</td><td>3.5</td><td>10.3</td></tr>
<tr><td>Physicians' services</td><td>100.0</td><td>40.4</td><td>59.6</td><td>55.6</td><td>3.1</td><td>.8</td></tr>
<tr><td>Dentists' services</td><td>100.0</td><td>95.5</td><td>4.5</td><td></td><td>3.1</td><td>1.4</td></tr>
<tr><td>Other professional services</td><td>100.0</td><td>39.9</td><td>60.1</td><td>52.1</td><td>7.5</td><td>.5</td></tr>
<tr><td>Drugs and drug sundries</td><td>100.0</td><td>84.7</td><td>15.3</td><td></td><td>14.6</td><td>.6</td></tr>
<tr><td>Eyeglasses and appliances</td><td>100.0</td><td>97.2</td><td>2.8</td><td></td><td></td><td>2.8</td></tr>
<tr><td>Nursing-home care</td><td>100.0</td><td>43.0</td><td>57.0</td><td>3.3</td><td>50.5</td><td>3.1</td></tr>
<tr><td>Other health services</td><td>100.0</td><td>8.8</td><td>91.2</td><td></td><td>51.3</td><td>39.9</td></tr>
<tr><td colspan="7" align="center">1976[b]</td></tr>
<tr><td>Total</td><td>100.0</td><td>33.1</td><td>66.9</td><td>43.7</td><td>16.6</td><td>6.6</td></tr>
<tr><td>Hospital care</td><td>100.0</td><td>11.9</td><td>88.1</td><td>73.6</td><td>3.4</td><td>11.1</td></tr>
<tr><td>Physicians' services</td><td>100.0</td><td>40.4</td><td>59.6</td><td>55.2</td><td>3.4</td><td>.9</td></tr>
<tr><td>Dentists' services</td><td>100.0</td><td>95.2</td><td>4.8</td><td></td><td>3.2</td><td>1.5</td></tr>
<tr><td>Other professional services</td><td>100.0</td><td>52.3</td><td>47.7</td><td>39.9</td><td>7.1</td><td>.7</td></tr>
<tr><td>Drugs and drug sundries</td><td>100.0</td><td>82.2</td><td>17.8</td><td></td><td>16.7</td><td>1.0</td></tr>
<tr><td>Eyeglasses and appliances</td><td>100.0</td><td>96.8</td><td>3.2</td><td></td><td></td><td>3.2</td></tr>
<tr><td>Nursing-home care</td><td>100.0</td><td>43.7</td><td>56.3</td><td>3.4</td><td>49.0</td><td>3.9</td></tr>
<tr><td>Other health services</td><td>100.0</td><td>8.4</td><td>91.6</td><td></td><td>51.1</td><td>40.5</td></tr>
</table>

Table 8-13. (continued)

Table 8-13b.

				Percentage Distribution			
					Public		
Type of Expenditure	Total	Private	Total	Medicare	Medicaid	Other
				1975[2]			
Total	100.0	33.0	67.0	42.8	17.2	7.0
Hospital care	100.0	11.8	88.2	72.8	3.4	11.9
Physicians' services	100.0	38.1	61.9	56.7	4.2	1.0
Dentists' services	100.0	94.8	5.2		3.5	1.7
Other professional services	100.0	59.7	40.3	33.2	6.4	.6
Drugs and drug sundries	100.0	82.3	17.7		16.6	1.0
Eyeglasses and appliances	100.0	96.9	3.1			3.1
Nursing-home care	100.0	43.5	56.5	3.3	49.2	4.0
Other health services	100.0	8.0	92.0		55.0	37.0

[a]Preliminary estimates.

[b]Revised estimates.

Source: Gibson, R. M., and Fisher, R. S.; Age difference in health care spending, fiscal year 1977. *Social Security Bulletin* Vol. 42: January 1979.

Table 8-14. Personal Health Care Expenditures for Two Age Groups: Total and Per Capita Amount and Percentage Distribution of Expenditures met by Third Parties, Fiscal Years 1966 and 1977

Source of Payment	Total Amount (in millions)		Per Capita Amount		Percentage Distribution	
	1966	1977	1966	1977	1966	1977
			All Ages			
Total	$36,216	$142,586	$181.96	$646.11	100.0	100.0
Direct payments	18,668	43,274	93.79	196.09	51.5	30.3
Third-party payments	17,548	99,312	88.17	450.02	48.5	69.7
Private health insurance	8,936	39,299	44.90	178.08	24.7	27.6
Government	7,892	57,121	39.65	258.84	21.8	40.1
Other	720	2,891	3.62	13.10	2.0	2.0
			Under 65			
Total	$27,974	$101,330	$154.96	$514.25	100.0	100.0
Direct payments	14,286	32,332	79.13	164.08	51.1	31.9
Third-party payments	13,688	68,999	75.82	350.17	48.9	68.1
Private health insurance	7,627	36,919	42.25	187.36	27.3	36.4
Government	5,432	29,490	30.09	149.66	19.4	29.1
Other	629	2,590	3.48	13.14	2.2	2.6
			65 and Over			
Total	$8,242	$41,256	$445.25	$1,745.17	100.0	100.0
Direct payments	4,382	10,943	236.72	462.89	52.5	26.5
Third-party payments	3,860	30,313	208.52	1,282.28	46.8	73.5
Private health insurance	1,309	2,380	70.71	100.70	15.9	5.8
Government	2,460	27,631	132.89	1,168.84	29.8	67.0
Other	91	301	4.92	12.75	1.1	.7

Source: Gibson, R. M., and Fisher, R. S.: Age differences in health care spending, fiscal year 1977. Social Security Bulletin Vol. 42: January 1979

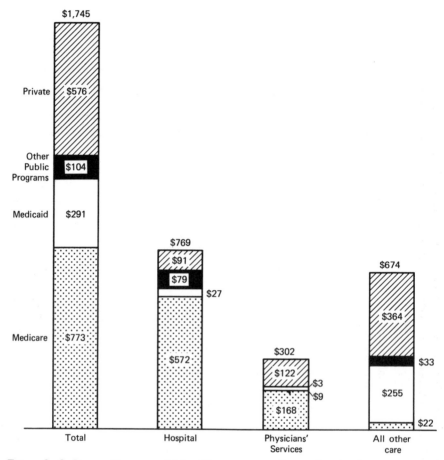

Figure 8–3. Per capita personal health-care expenditures for the Aged, by source of funds and type of care , fiscal year 1977. (*Source*: Gibson, R.M., and Fisher, R.S.: Age differences in health care spending, fiscal year 1977. *Social Security Bulletin* 42:1979.)

they qualified because of extremely low incomes or because they had incurred such large medical bills that they qualified as medical indigents (3, p. 13). In 1977, these persons accounted for 16.7% of the expenditures (Table 8-13). The remaining public expenditures were provided by the VA, Defense Department (for retired military persons and their dependents), and state mental hospitals.

Of the expenditures for personal health care, Table 8-14 breaks the figures down, showing who pays. For the average $1,745 bill for those 65 and over, 67% is paid by Medicare, Medicaid, and/or other government programs. Approximately 5.8 percent is paid by private health insurance taken out by the elderly to protect themselves against noncovered Medicare expenses; 26.5% of the average $1,745 bill is paid directly by the patient from his or her own resources. When one adds to these percentages (26.5% and 5.8%) miscellaneous private funding (.7%), the sum reaches the 33% figure found in Table 8-13 and Figure 8-3. But the 26.5% (which equals $463) should have added to it the sums paid out by the elderly for part B Medicare coverage. For a person enrolled in part B for fiscal 1977, the premiums would total $75. In addition, those elderly who took out private health insurance to supplement Medicare also incurred the cost of that insurance coverage, an estimated $75. Table 8-15 illustrates this: out-of-pocket expenses are closer to $613 than $463. Gibson and Fisher note, however, that during the 1966-1977 time frame shown in Table 8-15, the per-capita income of the aged rose at a rate of 10% per year, whereas the rise in out-of-pocket expenses rose at only 6.6% annually, and that out-of-pocket spending as a percentage of average income declined from 15% to 11% (3, p.15).

Table 8-15. Out-of-Pocket Expenses

Out-of-pocket Expense	Amount, Fiscal Year	
	1966	1977
Total	$300	$613
Direct payments	237	463
Premiums		
Private health insurance	63	75
Medicare SMI	(a)	75

[a]Data not available.

Source: Gibson, R. M., and Fisher, R. S.: Age differences in health care spending, fiscal year 1977. Social Security Bulletin Vol. 42: January 1979.

Table 8-16. Aggregate and per Capita National Health Expenditures, By Source of Funds and Percent of Gross National Product, Selected Calendar Years*

Calendar Year	Gross National Product (in billions)	Total — Amount (in billions)	Total — Per Capita	Total — Percent of GNP	Private — Amount (in billions)	Private — Per Capita	Private — Percent of Total	Public — Amount (in billions)	Public — Per Capita	Public — Per Percent of Total
1929	$103.1	$3.6	$29.49	3.5	$3.2	$25.49	86.4	$.5	$4.00	13.6
1935	72.2	2.9	22.65	4.0	2.4	18.30	80.8	.6	4.34	19.2
1940	99.7	4.0	29.62	4.0	3.2	23.61	79.7	.8	6.03	20.3
1950	284.8	12.7	81.86	4.5	9.2	59.62	72.8	3.4	22.24	27.2
1955	398.0	17.7	105.38	4.4	13.2	78.33	74.3	4.6	27.05	25.7
1960	503.7	26.9	146.30	5.3	20.3	110.20	75.3	6.6	36.10	24.7
1965	688.1	43.0	217.42	6.2	32.3	163.29	75.1	10.7	54.13	24.9
1966	753.0	47.3	236.51	6.3	34.0	169.81	71.8	13.3	66.71	28.2
1967	796.3	52.7	260.35	6.6	33.9	167.61	64.4	18.8	92.74	35.6
1968	868.5	58.9	288.17	6.8	37.1	181.40	63.0	21.8	106.76	37.0
1969	935.5	66.2	320.70	7.1	41.6	201.83	62.9	24.5	118.87	37.1
1970	982.4	74.7	358.63	7.6	47.5	227.71	63.5	27.3	130.93	36.5
1971	1,063.4	82.8	393.09	7.8	51.4	244.12	62.1	31.4	148.97	37.9
1972	1,171.1	92.7	436.47	7.9	57.7	271.78	62.3	35.0	164.69	37.7
1973	1,306.6	102.3	478.38	7.8	63.6	297.17	62.1	38.8	181.22	37.9
1974	1,412.9	115.6	535.99	8.2	69.0	319.99	59.7	46.6	216.00	40.3
1975	1,528.8	131.5	604.57	8.6	75.8	348.61	57.7	55.7	255.96	42.3
1976	1,700.1	148.9	678.79	8.8	86.6	394.73	58.2	62.3	284.06	41.8
1977	1,887.2	170.0	768.77	9.0	100.7	455.27	59.2	69.3	313.50	40.8
1978[a]	2,107.6	192.4	863.01	9.1	114.3	512.62	59.4	78.1	350.40	40.6

[a]Preliminary estimates.

Source: Gibson, R. M., "National Health Expenditures, 1978," *Health Care Financing Review*, Vol. 1, Summer 1979, Washington, HEW.

*Cautionary Note: This table contains data on a *calendar* year basis. Other tables are on a *fiscal* year basis. In addition, a different methodology was employed for structuring this table. See footnote at the beginning of this chapter and Table 8-1.

REFERENCES

1. *Hospital Statistics,* 1977 ed., Chicago, American Hospital Association.
2. Sudovar, S. G., and Sullivan, K.: *National Health Insurance Issues: The Unprotected Population.* Roche Laboratories, 1977.
3. Gibson, R. M., and Fisher, R. S.: Age differences in health care spending, fiscal year 1977. *Social Security Bulletin* Vol.42; January 1979.

9

Health Insurance

Health insurance is a hot issue when it comes to discussions of the health field. The cost of policies are rising enormously, reflecting the rises in the health industry costs against which the insurance is designed to protect. The range of benefits—what is covered and what is not—is uneven. Mueller notes (1, pp.3-4):

That the insured person cannot expect to receive truly comprehensive health care services in return for his premium payments is just one of the deficiencies in the private health insurance system. Individual buyers frequently encounter age-limit restrictions or the termination of insurance benefits after stated ceilings are reached. They often are subject to waiting periods and sometimes are even excluded from coverage because of preexisting conditions. Hospital coverage under group policies may be of limited duration, and some kinds of illness may not be covered for treatment and care.

Almost 60 percent of the persons with group insurance policies that covered basic hospital expense (first-dollar coverage) had to make up the difference out of pocket between the semiprivate room-and-board charge and the room-and-board allowance paid by their insurance policies. Only one-third of the newly covered had full dollar protection under their basic plans when an intensive-care unit was required. Only 36 percent were covered for hospital stays of 120 days and over. About 16 percent had maximum surgical benefits of less than $500. About 69 percent received less than $8 for each physician in-hospital visit. Major-medical benefits helped to meet these deficiencies, but almost 30 percent of those covered in 1975 under major-medical policies were subject to maximum benefit limits of $100,000 or less.

Such shortcomings, along with the fact that many are not covered by health insurance, have provided some of the fuel for advocacy of a single, comprehensive national health-insurance system. But Fuchs reminds us (2, pp.17-19):

392

The most basic level of choice is between health and other goals. While social reformers tell us that 'health is a right,' the realization of that 'right' is always less than complete because some of the resources that could be used for health are allocated to other purposes. This is true in all countries regardless of economic system, regardless of the way medical care is organized, and regardless of the level of affluence. It is true in the communist Soviet Union and in welfare-state Sweden, as well as in our own capitalist society. No country is as healthy as it could be; no country does as much for the sick as it is technically capable of doing.

The constraints imposed by resource limitations are manifest not only in the absence of amenities, delays in receipt of care, and minor inconveniences; they also result in loss of life. The grim fact is that no nation is wealthy enough to avoid all avoidable deaths . . .

. . . Within limits set by genetic factors, climate, and other natural forces, every nation chooses its own death rate by its evaluation of health compared with other goals.

. . . If better health is our goal, we can achieve it, but only at some cost.

Yet, though as a people Americans are very lightly taxed compared with persons in other industrialized nations, our attempts to date at a national system for a limited population group (Medicare) have evidenced an unwillingness to provide even there comprehensive coverage. What Mueller noted above applies even to federal programs, as we noted in the preceding chapter on the amount of money Medicare recipients had to pay themselves.

Why? Why can't we have a truly comprehensive benefit structure for all peoples? The answer lies in large part in the history of health insurance in America.

HISTORICAL DEVELOPMENTS: BLUE CROSS AND BLUE SHIELD

The year 1929 is generally credited as marking the birth of modern health insurance. It was in that year that Justin Ford Kimball established a hospital insurance plan at the Baylor University Hospital for the schoolteachers of Dallas, Texas. As a one-time superintendant of the Dallas public schools, he was sensitive to the plight of schoolteachers, particularly so when he found many of them had unpaid bills at the hospital. Working from hospital records, he calculated that the schoolteachers as a group "incurred an average of 15 cents a month in hospital bills. To assure a safe margin, he established a rate of 50 cents a month . . . " (3, p.19). In return, the schoolteachers were assured of 21 days hospitalization in a semiprivate room.

Kimball's success spread, and over the years, his approach became the model for what became the Blue Cross plans around the country—the concept of assuring the benefit not of cash but of *service*, the emphasis on semiprivate accommodations, and even the time frame of 21 days of benefits.

But though 1929 is cited as the beginning, there were antecedents. Anderson notes, for example (3, p.17):

Between 1916 and 1918, attempts were made by 16 state legislatures from New York to California to establish some form of compulsory health insurance, essentially a mechanism to help families pay for health services, which were already being felt as costly and unpredictable episodes. The necessary mass political support in the states was not present, however, and the solid opposition of the American Medical Association, insurance companies, and the pharmaceutical industry, not to mention business and industry opposed to unaccustomed payroll taxes, stopped the movement.

The Health Insurance Institute also cites antecedants (4, p.7):

When health insurance began some 130 years ago, it met a far simpler need—coverage against rail and steamboat accidents.

The nation's first health insurance company came into being in 1847. Three years later another company was organized specifically to write accident insurance. By 1864, coverages were available for virtually every type of accident. At the turn of the century, 47 companies were issuing accident insurance.

In addition, the mutual aid society concept, which originated in Europe, was adopted in the United States in the latter half of the 1800s. Small contributions were collected from members of workers' groups in return for the promise to pay a cash benefit for disability through accident or sickness. Fraternal benefit societies also were important early providers of health insurance in the U.S.

Mutual benefit associations, or "establishment funds," began in 1875 in the United States. These funds—sometimes financed partially by employers—provided small payments for death or disability of workers in a single organization.

Both accident insurance companies and life insurance companies entered the health insurance field in the early 1900s. At the beginning, the insurance largely covered the policyholders' loss of earned income due to a limited number of diseases, among them typhus, typhoid, scarlet fever, smallpox, diphtheria and diabetes. . . .

This was the birth of modern health insurance. The demand for the new product grew as the Depression of the 1930s deepened. Out of this emerged the Blue Cross service concept, which foreshadowed insurance company reimbursement policies for hospital and surgical care. Also during the 1930s, insurance companies began to emphasize the availability of cash benefit plans for hospital, surgical and medical expenses. The first Blue Shield type of plan for surgical and medical expenses was formed in 1939.

And there was the single hospital benefit plan organized in 1912 at Rockford, Illinois; the Grinnell, Iowa, hospital plan in 1921; the Brattleboro, Vermont, plan in 1927. Each offered payment for limited hospital services. But the idea as developed at Baylor by Kimball was the model that spread. The AHA requested Kimball to describe the Baylor plan at its annual meeting in 1931. Other hospital people also developed interest, and by 1935 there were 15 hospital insurance plans in 11 states and six additional plans developed during 1936. "Concurrently, there was a move to create a coordinating agency of some sort to give the now rapidly growing movement a national focus and a broad base" (3, p.36). And this was done within the framework of the AHA, evolving over the years to a semiautonomous body and eventually to a completely independent Blue Cross Commission and, later, Blue Cross Association.

Anderson notes that the early leadership came not from the hospitals but from early pioneers, far-sighted individuals, some of whom were hospital accountants. The hospitals, says Anderson, were "timid in their backing of prepayment."(3, p.42) It was, after all, a new idea, an experiment. "Originally, the plans covered only employees and not their dependents; the dependents were an unknown and feared quantity actuarially. But common sense and equity would shortly have it that dependents should be covered too, and so they were" (3, p.43).

Anderson goes on to note that the Blue Cross movement surged ahead in the 1940s, with a nationwide enrollment of 6 million subscribers in 1940 spread through 56 independent Blue Cross plans. "By 1945, the enrollment was up to 19 million in 80 plans, and by the early 1950's it was 40 million. By that time, private insurance companies were also coming up from behind after an early lack of interest in insuring against hospital costs" (4, p.45).

The Health Insurance Institute states (3, p.8):

During World War II, as a result of the freezing of wages, group health insurance became an important component of collective bargaining.

Even greater impetus came in the postwar era when the U.S. Supreme Court ruled that enployee benefits, including health insurance, were a legitimate part of the labor-management bargaining process.

After that, health insurance protection expanded rapidly. For instance, in 1950 some 77 million people had hospital expense insurance. By 1976, some 177 million Americans were protected, or more than 8 out of 10 of the civilian noninstitutional population.

Traditionally, the greatest emphasis has been on hospital coverage because health services revolve around the hospital as the center of medical technology.

The dramatic progress of surgery and its increasing cost also spurred the demand for insurance for these expenses. In 1950, 54 million people had surgical expense insurance. By 1976, this coverage had tripled, with 167 million having such protection.

In 1950, more than 21 million people had coverage for physicians' fees other than surgery. In 1976, 163 million persons were covered.

In general, coverage for the cost of hospital care, surgery and physicians' services is called "Basic Protection."

As Blue Cross began to demonstrate the feasibility of covering hospital expenses via the insurance mechanism, pressures to do likewise for physician services also developed. The pressures accelerated following the report of the Committee on Costs of Medical Care with its challenge to organized medicine. In 1939, the California Medical Association established the California Physicians Service, which was the first of what became known as the Blue Shield plans for payment of doctors' bills. Like Blue Cross, Blue Shield operated on a *service benefits* principle: the California plan provided complete physician's service at a rate of $1.70 per month.

Enrollment was limited to employed persons earning less than $3,000 per year. Physicians were reimbursed on a 'unit' basis, the unit having a par value of $2.50 (the fee for an office visit), with other services being valued at multiples of this unit. Experience in the early years, however, was unfavorable, as demand for services far exceeded expectations, and the effect was to devalue the unit. So, beginning in 1941, all contracts were modified. This resulted in much more favorable experience, and the unit value now approximates par. (5, p.36)

We might digress for a moment to note two things. First, California developed the unit-value scale, more recently known as the relative-value scale, the legality of which is in dispute. Most Blue Shield plans did not, however, use this method for establishing their schedules of allowances. Second, the need to devalue the unit was acceptable to the medical profession because the plan was medical society sponsored: The physicians were obligated to deliver the service regardless of what the plan could pay. This is acceptable if one has a say in the management, as the physicians did. Throughout the Blue Shield movement, physicians have dominated the boards of directors not only because they underwrote the plan but also because the plans were truly *their* plans as a response to the challenge for insurance coverage, and they were in keeping with AMA principles of keeping medical matters in the hands of physicians. A similar situation existed with Blue Cross: The hospitals agreed to accept the Blue Cross payment as full payment for care in a semiprivate room. If the Blue Cross plan could not pay the agreed-to cost, then the hospital would accept whatever Blue Cross could pay and *not* bill the patient for any additional monies. Thus, Blue Cross offered its subscribers *service benefits* rather than lump-sum or *indemnity benefits*. In the early days of Blue Cross, quite a few plans had to pay hospitals less than 100 cents on the dollar, and hospitals tend to dominate Blue Cross boards, though both Blue Cross and Blue Shield are under pressures to change their board structures since the underwriting of the plans by the providers of service is now less a fact of life. We might note here that even when Blue Cross paid a hospital full cost, it was frequently discounted and acceptable to the hospital since it was assured payment.

Medical society sponsorship of Blue Shield plans had its origins as early as 1917 in the state of Washington, in which county medical societies established "county medical service bureaus" that contracted with employers to provide medical care for employees. According to Hawley, these bureaus developed as a result of some competitive abuses that arose among some of the medical-care plans in the state (5, pp.35-36).

Both Blue Cross and Blue Shield were service-benefit plans, the former relying mainly on type of accommodation (semiprivate room) as the determinant of service-benefit eligibility. Blue Shield relied on income of the patient or patient's family. Both Blue Cross and Blue Shield provided benefits for subscribers who used private rooms or were above income, the patient paying the additional charges, if any.

Blue Cross worked quite well. The Blue Shield service-benefit principle did not work well. The reasons for this failure were historical and developmental. When Blue Shield first began, physicians commonly charged patients on a sliding-fee scale—soak the wealthy to pay for care of the poor, and so on, in between. The early Blue Shield schedules for various services were pitched to the going rate in the service-benefit income category. As the economy developed, and along with it inflation, the Blue Shield schedule of payments was service-benefit payments for fewer and fewer subscribers since they were increasingly above income. This led some Blue Shield plans to develop different types of contracts with different service-benefit income levels, allowance schedules geared to each level, and, of course, premiums geared to the allowances. In time, some Blue Shield plans developed contracts with *usual, customary,* and *reasonable* (UCR) allowances. But the point is that the Blue Shield service benefits, when geared to subscriber income, did not work well because of inflation and the difficulties in determining subscriber income. It was left to the patient to discuss with the physician, and both parties were reluctant to talk about money when the patient was sick. Resulting misunderstandings were common.

Another problem faced by Blue Shield with regard to service benefits developed as a result of the changing health system. Initially, radiology, pathology, and anesthesiology were hospital services covered by Blue Cross. During the 1950s and 1960s, many of the hospital based physicians in those specialties moved out from under the hospital umbrella to do their own billing while still housed in the hospital, and many also established their own offices. Blue Cross generally was not allowed by law to pay for physician services as such, only for hospital services. Blue Shield rate structures were not geared to pay these professional services since they had never been calculated or anticipated in structuring the rates. For a while, the subscribers were caught in a bind and had to pay the bills until such time as Blue Shield was able to adjust its rates to incorporate these benefits. But then Blue Shield had to get the groups, mainly the employers, to go along with the increased rates. As one can imagine, not all were willing to do so unless they had to, and others wouldn't do so until the next round of collective bargaining sessions began when these new benefits could become a management concession.

Both Blue Cross and Blue Shield also faced similar situations in later years as new technology developed, often horrendously expensive. If paid for under existing rates because payments were close to or at cost, it would encourage hospitals, particularly, to expand and write off the increased costs on Blue Cross: The new equipment would be averaged with all other costs and be built into what all admissions would cost. If Blue Cross covered such items, it would eventually force a rate increase, and if there was a rate increase, then competitors would gain an advantage. The pressures on both Blue Cross and Blue Shield became even more acute as they acted as fiscal intermediaries (the agency handling the payments) for Medicare: The federal government, bitten by rising costs, sought to pressure the Blues (a frequently used word for the Blue Cross/Blue Shield movement) and others, and pressure also came from state governments, which were bitten by the rising costs of Medicaid—if only the Blues can hold the line, the federal/state Medicaid program will benefit.

The shortcomings in private health insurance are set in the main by the leadership roles of Blue Cross and Blue Shield; their shortcomings, however, are not always of their doing but are affected by the attitudes and willingnesses of employers and of federal and state governments.

According to the national Blue Shield Association, in 1977, there were 70 Blue Shield plans covering 70.9 million persons. About 38 million of these people were covered by policies that provide UCR allowances—in effect, service benefits. The remaining subscribers were covered by indemnity contracts. In addition to these 70.9 million subscribers, 32 Blue Shield plans administered part B of Medicare, and 14 plans were the fiscal intermediaries for Medicaid. In all, Blue Shield plans served 20.1 million Medicare and Medicaid persons, close to half of the total population served by these programs.

The count of Blue Cross plans by the end of 1977 was also 70. There were, in addition, five affiliated plans in Canada and one in Jamaica.

The number of Blue Shield and Blue Cross plans in recent years varies slightly due to mergers. Each plan, as member of a national movement, has an exclusive territory so far as the national association is concerned.

Sensitive to criticism of hospital domination, the national Blue Cross Association, in its *Fact Book* 1978, reports:

As of December 31, 1977, there were 70 Blue Cross Plans in the United States and Puerto Rico, 5 affiliated Plans in Canada and 1 in Jamaica. All are nonprofit, community oriented, voluntary health care pre-payment Plans. On December 31, 1977, the 70 member Blue Cross Plans reported having 1,790 board members. Of this amount, 67 per cent represented the public (8 per cent were hospital trustees) and 33 per cent represented the providers of health care (16 per cent were hospital administrators and 17 per cent were M.D.s and other providers). Counting the hospital trustees as a public representative, 58 Plans enrolling 90 per cent of the Blue Cross Plan membership have a majority of public representatives on their governing boards.

The *Fact Book 1978* goes on to summarize the kinds of benefits currently available:

In their basic contracts, Blue Cross Plans generally offer service benefits rather than cash indemnities regardless of the hospital's charges. Payment for care is made by the Plan to the hospital or other provider rather than to the subscriber. Preadmission testing is covered by more than 45 Plans. Outpatient services (usually for accidental injury and minor surgery, although some Plans cover medical emergencies, diagnostic testing, physical therapy, kidney dialysis and chemotherapy treatments) are also covered in Blue Cross Plans' basic certificates. Under family contracts, 58 Plans cover handicapped dependent children regardless of age as long as the physical or mental condition exists.

In addition, most Blue Cross Plans offer supplementary variable front-end deductibles and 80 per cent coinsurance. Maximums vary from $5,000 to an unlimited amount of extended benefits beyond the basic certificate which may include the services of a physician, surgeon and physiotherapist, nursing home care, care in the home after hospitalization, ambulance services, prosthetic appliances, blood transfusions, prescription drugs, rental or payment for durable equipment, therapy treatments, diagnostic x-rays and laboratory services, catastrophic illness coverage as well as coverage for private duty and licensed practical nursing care in the hospital; treatment of nervous or mental conditions, drug addiction or alcoholism usually is at 50 per cent coinsurance.

Blue Cross Plan subscribers receive benefits anywhere in the country. They can transfer from one Plan area to another and may change their coverage from single to family, family to single, family member to individual, group to nongroup, or from regular to complementary, without losing continuity or fulfilling any waiting periods.

The 76 Blue Cross Plans, 70 Blue Shield Plans, and all offices of the national Blue Cross and Blue Shield organizations are linked with a 40,000-mile network of electronic communications through the computerized Telecommunications Center located at the Blue Cross Association headquarters in Chicago.

Each of the Blue Cross plans, like each of the Blue Shield plans, is an independent corporation with its own benefit packages, and as the above account suggests, benefits vary from plan to plan—how many days covered in hospital at full benefit (from 14, 21, 30, 90, to 365 days) as well as out-of-hospital, diagnostic, and highly specialized services. Each of the plans has its own corporate title and organization, and each is permitted to use a national symbol (Blue Cross or Blue Shield), having met the stipulated national requirements, which include, among other things, being nonprofit and agreeing to work cooperatively with other plans for the benefit of subscribers.

Generally, the Blue Cross plans provided great support and assistance to the developing Blue Shield plans. Typically, they used the same salaried sales forces, the same personnel systems, the same offices, and sometimes the same executive staffs, although the governing boards were generally different and the corporations generally separate, from a legal standpoint. In nearly all states, there was special enabling legislation for both plans that made them legally different from ordinary insurance companies. In some states, there were bitter conflicts between the Blue Cross plan and local medical societies that sponsored Blue Shield, and these conflicts even reached the national level in 1948, for example, when the AMA opposed a proposed merger of Blue Cross and Blue Shield at the national level for purposes of enrolling national accounts. Why the conflict? The AMA's position was based on fear that it would again be accused of restraint of trade, and well it might have been, and also because it feared that Blue Cross, representing the hospitals, would dominate the national joint venture and the the views of medicine would not be adequately represented (3, pp.53-67). This, like the conflicts within the states, reflected an age-old fear on the part of physicians that this would lead to nonmedical people telling doctors how to practice medicine. Hospitals, by the same token, were wary of physicians telling them how to run the hospital. These conflicts became more pronounced as one moved up the hierarchies: In the small town, the physicians and hospital people may get along fine (but not always) in their small hospital, but as organizations become larger, the need for a bureaucracy develops and, with it, the insensitivities and misunderstandings and resulting fears that pervade all large social institutions and organizational arrangements. While a mechanism for enrolling national accounts was eventually successful, it was not until 1978 that there was a successful merger of the national Blue Shield and Blue Cross organizations. Part of the reason for successful merger was that by 1978, under pressures from state insurance departments and the federal government, the Blue Cross and Blue Shield plans had become less than surrogates for the providers; they were becoming true third parties.

The efficiency of Blue Cross and Blue Shield is truly remarkable. Enrolling 38.5% (83.9 million) of the U.S. population in 1976, Blue Cross had a total national subscription income of $13.597 billion. It paid out in benefits (the claims expense) 95.5% of the earned subscription. Its operating expenses were 5.9%. Since operating and claims expenses exceeded earned subscription income, the Blue Cross plans overall had to decrease their reserves, though this, naturally, varied from plan to plan. Blue Shield claimed coverage of 40.6% (86.3 million) of the U.S. population and had an earned subscription income of $9 billion, a claims expense of 91.9% and an operating or administrative expense of 8.3%.

Generally, Blue Shield administrative expenses are higher than those of Blue Cross, primarily because Blue Shield deals with a larger number of providers (physicians rather than hospitals) and its claims payments are in smaller amounts. It might be noted, however, that the lingering conflict between physicians and hospitals persists in those Blue Shield people who argue that their administrative costs are higher than those of Blue Cross in part because Blue Cross charges to Blue Shield for sales and other services are not equitably distributed.

SOME ELEMENTS OF HEALTH INSURANCE RATE STRUCTURING

Blue Cross was initially underwritten by the hospitals. They agreed to accept less than 100 cents on the dollar (apart from the discounts) if Blue Cross was in a financial bind and this reduction in payments to hospitals did occur in some areas, forced largely by errors in calculating and setting the premiums and errors in enrollment procedures. We might look at these because of the understandings they should yield about health insurance costs and benefits in general.

Premium errors in the early days of Blue Cross came about because the plans did not have available a reliable statistical base for predicting what their utilization would be. No one else had the data, either. Thus, for a given premium, should Blue Cross provide 14 days of in-hospital care or 21 days or 30 days; should it cover maternity; what about pre-existing conditions, conditions that existed at the time a person joined Blue Cross; if a pre-existing condition exists when a person joins Blue Cross, should that person have to wait a period of time before Blue Cross covers it, or can it be covered immediately? Blue Cross, and Blue Shield, also, had to weigh such questions and to build the answers into the equation for calculating what the premium should be.

To illustrate this in simple form, let us suppose that a community of 100 people is debating whether or not to join Blue Cross and be covered for only one kind of hospitalization: removal of gallbladder. Let us further assume that the cost of care in the hospital is $200 a day and that, on the average, a gallbladder removal case stays in the hospital for five days. Let us further assume that, on the average, one can predict five cases a year for every 100 people.

Given these assumptions, Blue Cross could antitipcate for that community a cost of $200/day × 5 days × 5 cases, or $5,000. But the laws governing Blue Cross as a nonprofit company generally require Blue Cross to set aside an additional sum of money for the unforeseen. This would be a *contingency fund,* or *reserves.* In this instance, the law might require Blue Cross to provide for a possible sixth case, thus another $1,000 needed by Blue Cross. But the people at Blue Cross have to live; they need income and, therefore, must be paid for their services: the selling of the policy, negotiating with the hospital, and administering the claims. They also need an office in which to work, and that means rent, electricity, fuel bills, and so on. Typically, this will come, for Blue Cross, to about 6% of its income. Thus, add about $360 for administration. Total cost to Blue Cross would thus come to $6,360.

Blue Cross can thus say to the community: We calculated a rate; it's a *community rate* to cover all of you for gallbladder removal. Since there are

100 people, it will cost each of you $63.60 a year for coverage, about 17 cents a day. That will cover you only for hospital care relating to gallbladder removal. It will not cover the doctor's bill or other conditions or admission for gallbladder when surgery is not performed. You get what you pay for, and all you are paying for is gallbladder surgery. If all of you join *now,* you'll be covered immediately—no waiting periods—and all of you are covered even if you have gallbladder problems before joining. We can do this because you represent the average, and we have calculated our premium rate on that basis.

It is this kind of exercise that Blue Cross went through originally in deciding what to charge and for what. In real life, however, it was much more complicated because Blue Cross covered most acute conditions. Moreover, since Blue Cross worked with the community rate idea, in the beginning, it enrolled not communities but representative bodies or groups of the community—typically, groups of employees. But let us carry our hypothetical model a step further.

Let us suppose that not everyone in the community or group of 100 wants to join. Let us suppose that only 20 choose to do so. Blue Cross would probably refuse to let only 20 join because the group of 20 is not a community average and, thus, does not meet the requirements of a community rate. In all probability, more than one gallbladder case will occur in the 20. Blue Cross will probably not allow a group such as this to be organized even at a higher rate. But let us suppose that instead of only 20, 60 want to join. Now Blue Cross has a problem. Is 60 average enough? Probably not. But can't the rate be tinkered with to make the group financially acceptable? While each Blue Cross plan has its own enrollment requirements, in this hypothetical case, Blue Cross might well say that it could enroll the 60 but that the rate would have to be tinkered with. It would tinker not by setting a different rate but by imposing an 11-month waiting period for pre-existing conditions, in this case, for any gallbladder surgery if the subscriber had any reason to believe he or she had abdominal problems.

Let us assume now that in the next isolated community or employee group there are four people. They hear about the Blue Cross coverage and seek to join. But here Blue Cross would probably say that a community or group of four is not typical for its rate. However, Blue Cross might say that if any member of that group of four wants to join, it will write an individual contract or policy, but it will not cover any gallbladder operation if the subscriber had reason to believe something was amiss. Moreover, Blue Cross will charge more for the policy because of higher risks and higher administrative costs. Thus, Blue Cross (and Blue Shield) typically offers *nongroup* enrollment for those who are not eligible for *group* enrollment. But what about that group of 20? Can they get nongroup enrollment? No, because Blue Cross must rely on group enrollment if it is to succeed in its mission of covering everyone at a community rate. By denying the 20, the 20 will become a pressure group within the larger group, agitating for more to seek Blue Cross enrollment.

We can appreciate the need for enrollment minimums if we make another assumption. Let us suppose that two more groups of 100 each want to join, and let us assume that all 100 join in each group. The two groups contribute $2,000 to the contingency fund. The first group (60 subscribers) will also probably be contributing to that fund; we don't know for sure, but the waiting period (the Blue Cross equalizer) has probably assured us that instead of five cases, there will only be three. Proportionally, $600 from the 60-person group will go into the contingency fund. Thus, there is $2,600 in the fund.

But let us further suppose that a fourth group of 100 joins. As the year progresses, Blue Cross may find that this group has many more than five gallbladder operations. Let us say it has eight. Well, the group's premiums cover five of those operations; the group's contingency fund contribution covers a sixth. That would leave Blue Cross $2,000 short if it did not have the contributions from the other groups that it uses to cover the high utilization group. If there were no other groups, only this group with eight operations, Blue Cross would have to seek a rate increase, and it might have to say to the hospital that for this year the hospital will be asked to underwrite the Blue Cross policy by accepting $6,000 as though $8,000 were paid. If, moreover, Blue Cross had not adhered to its enrollment minimum, it might not have enough reserves and would have to pay less to the hospital. One can say, in fact, that enrollment minimums not only protect the hospital but also protect the subscribers against rate increases.

This is how Blue Cross and Blue Shield developed. They gambled, they made mistakes, but they won more than they lost.

Enter now another complication. Let us suppose that one of our groups of 100 is a community of young people in their twenties, working for the same company. The employer provides them with Blue Cross coverage as well as a life insurance policy and a good retirement plan. The complication is that some other large insurance company would love to get the insurance policy and the retirement plan away from a competitor. It has a handle on this business by way of health insurance. It could offer a health insurance policy with about the same benefits as Blue Cross at a lower cost because the group is low risk. It would base its rate on the group's experience (or performance). Alternatively, the insurance company could charge the same as Blue Cross but provide greater benefits. The commercial company doesn't need the unused premium money from the low-risk group to carry the losses incurred with a high-risk group, as does Blue Cross. If the commercial company enrolls a high-risk group, its rate would bear a relationship to its experience or anticipated claims performance. With an experience rated policy, the commercial insurance company is thus not likely to lose even if it doesn't get the life policy and retirement plan business. At worst, it takes a loss for one year only and then adjusts its premiums accordingly the next year. But what is the effect on Blue Cross? Blue Cross won't have as much money in the contingency fund. If, moreover, the competition takes away too many low-risk groups, Blue Cross will be forced to seek a rate increase that, in turn, may make it noncompetitive.

Blue Cross has thus had to engage in experience rating, also, simply to remain competitive and keep, if nothing else, a few pennies of contribution to the contingency fund. But the process has undermined the concept of the community rate and has had the effect of driving up health insurance costs and of charging those who are more sick higher premiums.

In practice, the group commerical insurance companies do not provide quite as high a ratio of benefits on the income dollar as Blue Cross (See Table 9-4.) Their indemnity benefit packages are, however, typically very good. The competition has, in many cases, stimulated Blue Cross to do better, but it has also had, in some cases, adverse costs effects on some groups because of the undermining of the community rate concept.

In recent years, the underwriting by hospitals and physicians has been inconsequential because the economic pressures that exist today militate against any subsidization; hospitals, at least, are not able to afford subsidization, which can, in these days, be considered a luxury. And rates rise rather than hospitals or doctors subsidizing the inability of Blue Cross or Blue Shield to pay 100 cents on the dollar. And, as noted earlier, even in the best of times, in many areas, the Blue Cross plan never paid hospitals 100 cents on the dollar but negotiated a discounted rate since Blue Cross was assuring payment. In today's environment, hospitals have been rebelling against this cost squeeze practice.

Nongroup commercial policies are available, and many are sold via mail and magazine and newspaper advertising. But while the Blue Cross and Blue Shield policies pay out generally in excess of 90 cents on the income dollar and the group commercials in excess of 80 cents on the income dollar, the nongroup commercial policies tend to be highly selective and pay out mostly less than 60 cents on the income dollar, some as low as 30 cents. These policies, like group commercial policies, are nearly all indemnity policies.

NUMBER OF PEOPLE COVERED AND EXTENT OF COVERAGE

Estimates vary as to the number of people covered by health insurance, the two principal estimates being from HEW and the Health Insurance Association of America (HIAA). The counting process is complicated by duplication of coverage (e.g., husband and wife each covered through places of employment), by Medicare beneficiaries who also elect to take out health insurance because of shortcomings in Medicare, by the unknown number of dependents (estimates run from 5 to 7 million) covered under the Civilian Health and Medical Care Program for the Uniformed Services (CHAMPUS), by VA patients who are without health insurance because they are totally dependent on the VA system for care (also an unknown number) and by long-term residents of state and local mental hospitals and prisons, many of whom are without insurance.

Great care needs to be taken in looking at HEW and HIAA data, for one can very easily misinterpret or misread the maze of charts and tables.

Working with HEW figures (Table 9-1), we note that the U.S. Bureau of the Census estimated the U.S. *civilian* population to be 213,863,000 as of January 1, 1977. Of this population, 190,628,000 were estimated to be under 65 years of age, and 23,235,000 aged 65 or over.

Of the 190 million under age 65, 78.5% (149,643,000) were estimated to be covered for hospital insurance. If we add to this 150 million those covered by Medicare (25.2 million—22.8 million 65 and over, 2.4 million under 65) and Medicaid (20.8 million), we arrive at a hospitalization covered figure of 195.6 million people out of a total estimated population of 213.9 million. (*Note:* in Table 9-1, the 65-and-over population covered should not be misunderstood; this 14 million represents the Medicare covered people who elected to take out hospitilization insurance to supplement Medicare coverage and some over-65 people who were not originally eligible for Medicare but who could, following the 1972 Social Security amendments, buy Medicare coverage at full cost—for this latter group private health insurance may have been more advantageous.) Does this mean that 18.3 million people (the difference between 213.9 and 195.6) have no coverage? Some, but not all, for in this 18.3 million are the CHAMPUS beneficiaries (perhaps as many as 5 or 7 million, nearly 1 million American Indians, and over 1 million veterans under VA care.* This would leave an unprotected civilian population of somewhere around 9 or 11 million. But these figures have to be treated with caution: The base figure is that 149.6 million people under 65 who have hospital insurance coverage, but the estimate for the preceding year was 154.2 million. The unprotected may be 9-11 million, but it may also be several million less.

Who are the uncovered? Some have, by choice, chosen not to secure coverage. Some are in small groups that have not been able to meet the group enrollment minimums. Some are between jobs or are not eligible on their new job until they have been employed a certain period of time. Some are the poor, who are too well off to be eligible for Medicaid but not well off enough to be able to afford the cost of health insurance. Some are probably the

---

*Developed from data presented by Sudovar, S. G. and Sullivan, K.: *National Health Insurance Issues: The Unprotected Population*. Roche Laboratories, 1977, pp. 2 and 17.

Table 9-1. Estimates of Net Number of Different Persons Under Private Health Insurance Plans and Percent of Population Covered, by Age and Specified Type of Care, as of December 31, 1976

	All Ages		Under Age 65		Aged 65 and Over	
Type of Service	Number (in thousands)	Percentage of Civilian Population[a]	Number (in thousands)	Percentage of Civilian Population[b]	Number (in thousands)	Percentage of Civilian Population[c]
Hospital care	164,235	76.8	149,643	78.5	14,592	62.8
Physicians' services:						
Surgical services	162,179	75.8	149,262	78.3	12,917	55.6
In-hospital visits	155,548	72.7	145,470	76.3	10,078	43.4
X-ray and laboratory examinations	150,897	70.6	142,942	75.0	7,955	34.2
Office and home visits	124,124	58.0	118,522	62.2	5,602	24.1
Dental care	46,578	21.8	45,808	24.0	770	3.3
Prescribed drugs (out-of-hospital)	150,222	70.2	145,440	76.3	4,782	20.6
Private-duty nursing	147,311	68.9	142,668	74.8	4,643	20.0
Visiting-nurse service	145,863	68.2	140,841	73.9	5,022	21.6
Nursing-home care	70,422	32.9	65,560	34.4	4,862	20.9

[a]Based on Bureau of Census estimate of 213,863,000 as of Jan. 1, 1977.
[b]Based on Bureau of Census estimate of 190,628,000 as of Jan. 1, 1977.
[c]Based on Bureau of Census estimate of 23,235,000 as of Jan. 1, 1977.

Source: Carroll, M. S.: Private health insurance plans in 1976: an evaluation. Social Security Bulletin Vol. 41: September 1978.

custodial patients and inmates in state, local, and federal hospitals and prisons.

The distribution of health insurance enrollees by type of coverage and type of insurance company is shown in Table 9-2. Table 9-3 breaks this down in terms of percentages. Again, a cautionary note: The aged 65-and-over categories in both tables represent not all Medicare eligibles but only those who chose to supplement Medicare coverage or, in some fewer cases, those who opted for private insurance rather than bear the full cost of Medicare because they were not eligible to belong to it as were most aged 65-and-over persons.

Hospital cost coverage is had by most of the people, followed by surgical fee payments and then in-hospital medical visits. This follows the pattern of development in health insurance—first Blue Cross, then Blue Shield surgical coverage, and later medical coverage as experience was gained. Some of the x-ray and laboratory examination coverage for physician services is for out-of-hospital coverage, some for in-hospital service, where the physician does the billing. Much coverage for these services is not shown, for they are included in the hospital care category.

As health insurance statistical experience developed, Blue Cross and Blue Shield and the group commercial companies were able to develop their benefit packages, offering new and expanded coverages. The companies could, at times, gamble because of the lessened insurance company risk that accompanied the growth of experience rated contracts. Pressures for expanded coverage also came because of the rapidly rising in-hospital costs: If outpatient or ambulatory services could be used, or if people could be encouraged to see physicians at the first sign of symptoms by paying for the visits, or if preventive services could be covered, then the cost of expensive in-hospital services could be eliminated or lessened.

These arguments are attractive, but whether they are sound remains to be seen. There is a view that holds that the more you look for disease and disability, the more you will find, and this will lead to increased utilization, which must be added to the cost of case finding. There is also the view that medical preventive services won't really pay off in terms of improved health.

Major medical expense or *catastrophic insurance* has experienced the most rapid growth. Initiated in 1951 by the commercial companies, it is now available also through some Blue Cross and Blue Shield plans. The number covered is estimated to be from 92 million to 146 million persons, the former estimate by HIAA and the latter by HEW.

Major medical expense policies help protect against large, unpredictable costs. There are two basic types: one supplements hospital-surgical-medical insurance programs, the other provides comprehensive protection where both basic protection and extended health care benefits are a unit.

Table 9-2. Gross Enrollment Under Private Health Insurance Plans, by Age, Type of Plan and Specified Type of Care, as of December 31, 1976* (In Thousands)

Type of Plan	Hospital Care	Physicians' Services				Dental Care	Prescribed Drugs (Out-of-Hospital)	Private-Duty Nursing
		Surgical Services	In-Hospital Visits	X-ray and Laboratory Examinations	Office and Home Visits			
All Ages								
Total	208,575	192,813	190,723	184,768	151,844	47,036	157,491	153,817
Blue Cross-Blue Shield	85,528	76,952	74,684	68,438	35,958	4,363	46,253	41,620
Blue Cross	83,054	4,629	4,121	(1)	1,369	(1)	(1)	(1)
Blue Shield	2,474	72,323	70,563	(1)	34,589	(1)	(1)	(1)
Insurance companies	113,820	104,399	105,027	105,027	105,027	26,662	105,027	105,027
Group policies	86,824	88,327	98,355	99,355	98,355	26,562	98,355	98,355
Individual policies	26,996	16,072	6,672	6,672	6,672	100	6,672	6,672
Independent plans	9,227	11,462	11,012	11,303	10,859	16,011	6,311	7,170
Community	4,070	6,205	6,204	6,137	6,044	1,802	2,034	4,857
Employer-employee-union	5,005	5,095	4,646	5,004	4,653	2,137	4,240	2,299
Private group clinic	152	162	162	162	162	72	37	14
Dental service corporation						12,000		
Under Age 65								
Total	191,989	180,381	180,353	175,819	145,460	46,266	152,713	149,081
Blue Cross-Blue Shield	76,956	69,100	67,288	62,423	32,479	4,358	44,001	39,480
Blue Cross	74,756	4,120	3,757	(1)	1,277	(1)	(1)	(1)
Blue Shield	2,200	64,980	63,531	(1)	31,202	(1)	(1)	(1)

[1]Data not available.

[2]Includes disabled persons under age 65 who are eligible for Medicare.

Source: Carroll, M. S.; Private health insurance plans in 1976: an evaluation. *Social Security Bulletin*, Vol 41: September 1978.

*Table continued on following page.

Table 9-2. (continued)

Type of Plan	Hospital Care	Physicians' Services				Dental Care	Prescribed Drugs (Out-of-Hospital)	Private-Duty Nursing
		Surgical Serives	In-Hospital Visits	X-ray and Laboratory Examinations	Office and Home Visits			
Insurance companies	106,613	100,626	102,869	102,869	102,869	26,240	102,869	102,869
Group policies	84,876	86,390	96,344	96,344	96,344	26,140	96,344	96,344
Individual policies	21,737	14,236	6,525	6,525	6,525	100	6,525	6,525
Independent plans	8,420	10,655	10,196	10,527	10,122	15,688	5,843	6,732
Community	3,835	5,893	5,891	5,824	5,733	1,770	1,926	4,627
Employer-employee-union	4,446	4,613	4,156	4,554	4,230	2,021	3,882	2,091
Private group clinic	139	149	149	149	149	70	35	14
Dental service corporation						11,807		
				Aged 65 and Over				
Total	16,586	12,432	10,370	8,949	6,384	770	4,878	4,736
Blue Cross-Blue Shield	[2]8,572	[2]7,852	[2]7,396	[2]6,015	[2]3,479	5	2,252	2,140
Blue Cross	[2]8,298	[2]509	[2]364	(1)	[2]92	(1)	(1)	(1)
Blue Shield	[2]274	[2]7,343	[2]7,032	(1)	[2]3,387	(1)	(1)	(1)
Insurance companies	7,207	3,773	2,158	2,158	2,158	422	2,158	2,158
Group policies	1,948	1,937	2,011	2,011	2,011	422	2,011	2,011
Individual policies	5,259	1,836	147	147	147		147	147
Independent plans	807	807	816	776	747	343	468	438
Community	235	312	313	313	311	32	108	230
Employer-employee-union	559	482	490	450	423	116	358	208
Private group clinic	13	13	13	13	13	2	2	0
Dental service corporation						193		

Type of Plan	All Ages			Under Age 65			Age 65 and Over		
	Visiting Nurse Service	Nursing-Home Care	Vision Care	Visiting Nurse Service	Nursing Home Care	Vision Care	Visiting Nurse Service	Nursing Home Care	Vision Care
Total	152,566	71,782	(1)	147,443	66,871	(1)	5,123	4,911	(1)
Blue Cross-Blue Shield	37,420	37,023	763	34,898	33,221	742	[2]2,522	[2]3,802	21
Blue Cross	(1)	(1)	(1)	(1)	(1)	(1)	(1)	(1)	(1)
Blue Shield	(1)	(1)	(1)	(1)	(1)	(1)	(1)	(1)	(1)
Insurance companies	105,027	28,852	(1)	102,869	28,207	(1)	2,158	645	(1)
Group policies	98,355	23,189	(1)	96,344	22,721	(1)	2,011	468	(1)
Individual policies	6,672	5,663	(1)	6,525	5,486	(1)	147	177	(1)
Independent plans	1,119	5,907	7,127	9,676	5,443	6,624	443	464	503
Community	7,379	3,347	4,558	7,099	3,163	4,285	280	184	273
Employer-employee-union	2,740	2,410	2,415	2,577	2,143	2,198	163	267	217
Private group clinic	0	150	154	0	137	141	0	13	13

[1]Data not available.

[2]Includes disabled persons under age 65 who are eligible for Medicare.

411

Table 9-3. Percentage Distribution of Total Gross Enrollment Under Private Health Insurance Plans, by Age, Type of Plan, and Specified Type of Care, as of December 31, 1976

Type of Plan	Hospital Care	Physicians' Services			
		Surgical Services	In-Hospital Visits	X-Ray and Laboratory Examinations	Office and Home Visits
All Ages					
Total	100.0	100.0	100.0	100.0	100.0
Blue Cross-Blue Shield	41.0	39.9	39.1	36.8	23.6
Insurance companies	54.6	54.1	55.2	57.0	69.3
Group policies	41.6	45.8	51.5	53.4	64.8
Individual policies	12.9	8.3	3.6	3.6	4.4
Independent plans	4.4	6.0	5.8	6.2	7.1
Under Age 65					
Total	100.0	100.0	100.0	100.0	100.0
Blue Cross-Blue Shield	40.1	38.3	37.3	35.5	22.3
Insurance companies	55.5	55.8	57.0	58.5	70.7
Group policies	44.2	47.9	53.4	54.8	66.2
Individual policies	11.3	7.9	3.6	3.7	4.5
Independent plans	4.4	5.9	5.7	6.0	7.0
Aged 65 and over					
Total	100.0	100.0	100.0	100.0	100.0
Blue Cross-Blue Shield	51.7	63.2	68.6	67.2	54.5
Insurance companies	43.4	30.3	23.8	24.1	33.8
Group policies	11.7	15.6	19.9	22.5	31.5
Individual policies	31.7	14.7	3.9	1.6	2.3
Independent plans	4.9	6.5	7.6	8.7	11.7

Type of Plan	Dental Care	Prescribed Drugs (Out-of-Hospital)	Private-Duty Nursing	Visiting-Nurse Service	Nursing-Home Care
All Ages					
Total	100.0	100.0	100.0	100.0	100.0
Blue Cross-Blue Shield	9.3	29.4	27.1	24.5	51.6
Insurance companies	56.7	66.6	68.3	68.8	40.2
Group policies	56.5	62.4	63.9	64.4	32.3
Individual policies	.2	4.2	4.3	4.4	7.9
Independent plans	34.0	4.0	4.6	6.7	8.2
Under Age 65					
Total	100.0	100.0	100.0	100.0	100.0
Blue Cross-Blue Shield	9.4	28.8	26.5	23.7	49.7
Insurance companies	56.7	67.4	69.0	69.8	42.2
Group policies	56.5	63.1	64.6	65.3	34.0
Individual policies	.2	4.3	4.4	4.4	8.2
Independent plans	33.9	3.8	4.5	6.5	8.1
Aged 65 and Over					
Total	100.0	100.0	100.0	100.0	100.0
Blue Cross-Blue Shield	.6	46.2	45.2	49.2	77.4
Insurance companies	54.8	44.2	45.6	42.1	13.1
Group policies	54.8	41.2	42.5	39.2	9.5
Individual policies	0	3.0	3.1	2.9	3.6
Independent plans	44.6	9.6	9.2	8.7	9.5

Source: Carroll, M. S.: Private health insurance plans in 1976: an evaluation. Social Security Bulletin Vol. 41: September 1978.

Major medical benefits are paid toward all kinds of health care prescribed by a physician, including treatment performed in and out of a hospital, special nursing care, X-rays, prescriptions, medical appliances, nursing home care, ambulatory psychiatric care and many other health care needs. Maximum benefits range from $10,000 to $25,000 per person or higher, and in some cases they are unlimited. All are subject to deductibles and coinsurance payments by the person insured. (4, p.24)

The deductible typically runs from $50 to $150, that is, the patient pays that amount initially. After the deductible, all expenses are covered, but the patient coinsures. Typically, this means that a patient pays, depending on the policy, from 20% to 30% of the remaining expenses.

Both deductibles and coinsurance are mechanisms designed to limit costs and to give greater assurance that the use of services is appropriate, that there is no unnecessary expense or use. To the extent they are successful in this, all can be appreciative; but for the person who really needs the added services, the costs can be significant, and, in some cases in which deterrence is effective, it may not be in the best interest of the patient.(6)

How well the various kinds of insurance companies do in terms of payments (claims expense—how much they pay out on the income dollar) and how efficient they are in terms of operating expenses is revealed by Table 9-4. Clearly, other things being equal, that is, benefits covered under the policies, the companies with the highest claims expense best serve the subscribers' interests, and the higher the operating expenses, the less there is for payment of claims.

Where a plan operates at a loss, it must draw on its reserves. In time, if the loss persists, there must be a rate increase. Blue Cross plans in 1976, for example, had reserves drop to an average of 1.13 months of claims, that is, they could pay claims for that length of time without income. The Blue Cross Association recommends three months of claims reserve. If the plans continue to experience losses, we can anticipate a round of rate increases, depending on each plan's reserve situation. Again, each plan is independent, with its own benefit packages and rate structures. To get a rate increase, each has to secure the approval of its state insurance regulatory agency.

INDEPENDENT PLANS—HIP AND KAISER-PERMANENTE

The Blues (Blue Cross and Blue Shield) and the group commercial companies so dominate the health insurance field that it is all too easy to forget the important role played by some of the independents. Two, in particular, merit examination at this junction: the Health Insurance Plan of New York (HIP) and Kaiser-Permanente.

HIP

The Health Insurance Plan of New York stands as one of the most successful health insurance programs, providing comprehensive medical services through organized medical groups of family physicians and specialists. Each medical group has specialists in 13 basic specialities: dermatology, general surgery, internal medicine, neurology, obstetrics and gynecology, ophthalmology, orthopedics, otolaryngology, pathology, pediatrics, psychiatry, radiology, and urology. When necessary to secure the services of physicians skilled in highly specialized fields that are beyond the capabilities of the medical group, they can be drawn from an approved list and paid out of a special fund.

HIP is the organizing force that handles enrollments (726,445 persons at the end of 1976), sets standards, monitors performance. It requires that all enrolled subscriber groups have hospital insurance for its members. This is usually Blue Cross. HIP then contracts with independent medical group partnerships—28 at present—spelling out the conditions for their participation in the HIP program and paying each group an annual sum for the complete care of each enrolled subscriber in the group. How each group divides the sum of capitation payments is up to the group. At present, only one hospital is operated by HIP; most HIP subscribers who need hospital care go to the hospital in which the attending HIP physician has privileges. New subscribers are encouraged to select a family physician within the group as soon as possible. They may change physicians and groups.

The following services are available without charge to each enrolled subscriber (7):

- General medical, specialist, surgical and obstetrical care;
- Laboratory and diagnostic procedures;
- Periodic health examinations, immunizations, and other measures for the prevention and detection of diseases;
- Physical therapy, radiotherapy, and other therapeutic measures;
- Professional services for the administration of blood or plasma.
- Eye refractions;
- Visiting nurse service at the insured person's residence as prescribed by a physician of the Group;
- Ambulance service from the insured person's residence or, in an emergency, from other locations within the area served by the Group, to a hospital, when ordered by a physician or the administrator of the Group.

Table 9-4. Financial Experience of Private Health Insurance Organizations, 1976
(Amounts in Millions)

Type of Plan	Total Income	Subscription or Premium Income	Claims Expense	
			Amount	Percent of Premium Income
Total	(1)	$39,422.3	$34,985.1	88.7
Blue-Cross-Blue Shield	$17,560.1	17,268.1	16,226.5	94.0
Blue Cross	12,242.9	12,037.4	11,624.9	96.6
Blue Shield	5,317.2	5,230.7	4,601.6	88.0
Insurance companies	(1)	19,504.0	16,280.2	83.5
Group policies	(1)	16,222.0	14,549.0	89.7
Individual policies	(1)	3,282.0	1,731.2	52.7
Independent plans	2,698.0	2,650.2	2,478.4	93.5
Community	1,175.8	,162.1	1,069.3	92.0
Employer-employee-union	1,177.2	1,147.8	1,090.1	95.0
Private group clinic	45.0	40.3	34.0	84.4
Dental service corporation	300.0	300.0	285.0	95.0

Type of Plan	Operating expense		Net underwriting gain		Net income	
	Amount	Percent of Premium Income	Amount	Percent of Premium Income	Amount	Percent of Total Income
Total	$5,048.1	12.8	-$611.0	-1.5	(1)	(1)
Blue-Cross-Blue Shield	1,192.8	6.9	-151.2	-.9	$140.8	.8
Blue Cross	623.3	5.2	-210.8	-1.8	-5.3	-.04
Blue Shield	569.5	10.9	59.6	1.1	146.1	2.7
Insurance companies	3,689.0	18.9	-465.2	-2.4	(1)	(1)
Group policies	2,154.0	13.3	-481.0	-3.0	(1)	(1)
Individual policies	1,535.0	46.8	15.8	.5	(1)	(1)
Independent plans	166.3	6.3	5.5	.2	53.3	2.0
Community	76.2	6.6	16.6	1.4	30.3	2.6
Employer-employee-union	69.7	6.1	-12.0	-1.1	17.4	1.5
Private group clinic	5.4	13.4	.9	2.2	5.6	12.4
Dental service corporation	15.0	5.0	0	0	0	0

1Data not available.

Source: Carroll, M. S.: Private health insurance plans in 1976: an evaluation. Social Security Bulletin Vol. 41: September 1978.

While HIP makes every effort to persuade physicians to work fulltime with the organization, it has allowed part-time affiliations.

Mechanic notes that "HIP is a less attractive national prototype than Kaiser because it does not control the hospitals it depends on, and it is believed that the incentives for economy that can be developed under such circumstances are considerably weaker than those at Kaiser, where doctors can allegedly be penalized for excessive use of hospital facilities" (8, p.107). Whether the recently acquired hospital in Queens, New York, will alter this remains to be seen. Mechanic is, however, correct. On the other hand, the HIP model in some ways may offer a more realistic (though not an ideal or as attractive) approach in that the spread of the HIP model can more easily adapt to existing hospital arrangements. A new HIP group does not need to buy or build a hospital; all it needs are admitting privileges at an existing hospital.

Kaiser-Permanente

Mechanic noted that "HIP is a less attractive national prototype than Kaiser," and so it is. Kaiser has captured the imagination of many. Like HIP, it provides for comprehensive care and places considerable emphasis on prevention. The prevention component of Kaiser-Permanente has been especially enticing because of its modern profile: regular checkups employing a battery of diagnostic tests (this process is known as multiphasic screening) with medical assessment at the end of the process. With over 2 million members, the plan operates in six states: California, Colorado, Hawaii, Ohio, Oregon, and Washington. Its West Coast base stems from its beginning in the late 1930s when the Kaiser Industries had to develop a mechanism for hospital and medical care for its employees at remote construction sites. The experience led Kaiser to extend the effort to its shipyards and steel plants during World War II, a necessity in part because it was felt that community facilities could not handle the influx of workers and their families. Following the war, the program was opened to the public.

In mid-1976, it had about 3,000 full-time physicians, providing care to its more than 2 million members, and it owned and operated 25 community hospitals with some 5,400 beds. It had, in addition, 66 medical-office facilities throughout the system. Weissman describes the principle operating units as follows (9):

Kaiser Foundation Health Plan, Inc.—a nonprofit organization which enrolls members and arranges for their health care services. Membership in the health plan is voluntary. The health plan contracts with six *Permanente Medical*

Groups, one in each region, which are organized as partnerships (or, in one instance, a professional corporation). These medical groups, functioning on a group practice basis, undertake to provide all professional services to health plan members. The health plan also contracts with *Kaiser Foundation Hospitals*—a nonprofit chaitable organization which assumes the responsibility for providing hospital services to the members enrolled in the health plan and to persons in other segments of the communities in which they operate.

While studies have shown lower hospital utilization rates, Kaiser-Permanente has acknowledged that its clientele are *not* representative of the population: It is a younger group and "relatively under represented in certain population groups . . . the unemployed, the indigent, the wealthy, the self-employed, and people living in rural and other metropolitan areas (10, p.165).

COMPARATIVE COSTS OF HEALTH INSURANCE

The cost of health insurance policies will vary considerably depending on the items of service covered, the amounts paid for the services, utilization, and administrative costs. The costs of policies will, moreover, change from year to year. But to give some idea of what policies cost per month, the following figures are given. Compared is HIP and Blue Shield in New York City for individual and family *group* enrollment as of August 1978. The Blue Shield policy is its most common policy with a maximum surgical indemnity of $1,500. Also shown is the cost of New York (City) Blue Cross, which both HIP and Blue Shield use for hospital coverage.

	HIP	Blue Cross	Total Monthly Costs
Individual	$12.25	$14.70	$26.75
Family	36.75	39.50	76.25
	Blue Shield	Blue Cross	Total Monthly Costs
Individual	$ 5.05	$14.70	$19.75
Family	14.84	39.50	54.34

For comprehensive HIP/BC coverage for a family, the cost is $76.25 per month, $915 per year. For limited BS/BC without routine office medical visits, the cost is $54.34 per month, $652 per year.

MEDICARE AND MEDICAID

Congress amended the Social Security Act in 1965, adding to it Title XVIII and Title XIX. Title XVIII was Medicare; Title XIX was Medicaid.

Medicare

Medicare is a health insurance program for the aged 65 and above regardless of income or wealth, and it also covers disabled persons under 65 who have been entitled to Social Security or Railroad Retirement disability benefits for at least two consecutive years or who suffer from chronic renal (kidney) disease that requires a kidney transplant or routine dialysis treatment. The "under 65" provisions were added to Medicare by the Social Security Amendments of 1972.

The program consists of two parts: parts A and B. Part A is the hospital insurance portion of Medicare, providing coverage for in-hospital care, needed skilled nursing facility care, and home health care. The last two benefits require that the patient first be in the hospital for three consecutive days. Financed by Social Security taxes, part A benefits provide:

1. Up to 90 days inpatient care for each benefit period; a new benefit period begins after the patient has been out of hospital and/or skilled nursing facility for 60 consecutive days. But this coverage does not cover all of the charges. The patient must pay, in 1979, the first $160 of the hospital bill and, after 60 days, the patient must pay $40 a day up to the ninetieth day. If a patient must stay in hospital beyond 90 days, Medicare permits the patient to draw upon a lifetime reserve of 60 extra days, with the patient paying $80 for each day used out of this reserve.
2. Up to 100 days in a skilled nursing facility, with Medicare paying the full cost for the first 20 days and the patient, in 1979, paying $20 a day for each day thereafter.
3. Up to 100 home health visits for the further treatment of the condition for which the patient was in hospital or skilled nursing facility. The visits must include part-time nursing care, physical therapy, or speech therapy.

As costs go up, Medicare payments go up, as do the amounts the patient must pay.

Part B of Medicare is Supplementary Medical Insurance (SMI); it is optional, and part A-eligible persons must pay for it if they elect to take it out; most people do take it out. Part B provides some important insurance benefits:

1. Payment of reasonable physician charges (after the patient pays the initial $60 annual deductible). But the payment is not full payment, only 80%,

with the patient paying the balance. Exceptions are pathology and radiology service charges when the patient is in hospital, and then the SMI pays 100%. Psychiatric service payments are limited to $250 each year. If the physician is unhappy with the amount Medicare determines as "reasonable," he or she may elect to have the 80% paid to the patient and is then free to bill the patient for whatever amount the physician feels is appropriate.

2. Hospital outpatient and emergency room services.

3. Up to 100 home health visits that do not require prior hospitalization or skilled nursing facility care and that are in addition to the 100 visits for posthospital and skilled nursing facility care under Part A.

4. A number of other services and supplies such as outpatient physical and speech therapy, diagnostic x-ray examinations, wheelchairs, artificial limbs, limited chiropractic services, and so on.

As of July 1978, the SMI cost the insured person $8.20 per month. Additional costs come out of federal general revenue. As health care costs go up, so do the premium charges, but the law requires that the premium increase be limited to the percentage rise in the Social Security income. In July 1979, the part B premium had risen to $8.70 per month, a little less than the 6.5% rise in 1978 Social Security payments.

HEW's Health Care Financing Administration (HCFA) oversees the Medicare program. While it handles some payments directly, most payments for care are made by fiscal intermediaries for part A and carriers for part B with whom HCFA contracts. The contractors are mainly Blue Cross, Blue Shield, and commercial insurance companies.

Medicare has clearly helped the aged and other eligibles pay for needed health services. But these people are generally on fixed incomes, and not high incomes at that. Yet they have to pay considerable sums when hospitalization and skilled nursing facility care are necessary, and there are some expensive items not covered that many elderly people require—specifically, hearing aids and eyeglasses. The medical insurance payments, while significant, may still not cover all a physician's fee: Physicians may charge what they believe their services are worth; Medicare pays what its insurance carriers have calculated as reasonable charges, which are based on the customary charges in that medical practice area.

While the direct costs of care borne by Medicare recipients are considerable, the cost of benefits paid by the government has been frighteningly high, far exceeding the early calculations when the legislation was being considered. Benefit costs for example, more than tripled from fiscal 1967 to fiscal 1975. The reasons for increased costs will be considered following a description of the Medicaid program.

Medicaid

Medicaid, authorized by Title XIX of the Social Security Act, is a federal-state financed program to pay for health services for the *categorically needy* and the *medically needy*. The *categorically needy* are those receiving public assistance from the Aid for Dependent Children (AFDC) program and those who receive Supplementary Security Income (SSI) because they are aged, blind, or disabled. (Some people are eligible for both Medicare and Medicaid.) The *medically needy* may be covered under Medicaid if their state has opted to provide coverage for their care; 28 states plus Puerto Rico, the Virgin Islands, Guam, and the District of Columbia have chosen to provide benefits for these low-income people; 21 states have not. Arizona does not have a Medicaid program. It is up to each state to define income eligibility for classification as medically needy, and this, as might be expected, varies from state to state.

The benefit structure under Medicaid varies from state to state. If the state has a Medicaid program, and all but Arizona do, it must at least provide for inpatient and outpatient hospital services, skilled nursing facility services, physician services, home health care, family planning services, and early and periodic screening, diagnosis, and treatment (EPSDT) of children under 21 who are eligible. A state, at its option, may elect to pay for dental services, prescribed drugs, eyeglasses, intermediate care facility services, and some other services.

Medicaid is financed out of general revenues. The federal government share ranges from 50% in the most wealthy states to 78% in those states with the lowest per capita income. In some states, local governments share a portion of the state costs. The program is administered by each state under federal regulations and guidelines.

Like Medicare, Medicaid costs have risen rapidly. These costs have been of growing concern to both state and federal governments.

Reasons for Increased Costs of Medicare and Medicaid (11)

The primary cause for the increase in Medicare costs since the inception of the program has been inflation. Increased numbers of beneficiaries, and an increase in the utilization of services by beneficiaries have also contributed to the growth in Medicare costs.

Medicaid cost increases can be attributed to a number of reasons. The two main reasons are an increase in the number of people eligible for benefits and inflation. Another contributing factor was the election by some States to include additional optional services under their program.

Cost Increases in Medicare

The cost of the Medicare program has more than tripled since its first year of operation. During fiscal year 1967, part A benefits cost about $2.9 billion for its 19 million eligibles and part B benefits approximately $1.2 billion for the 18 million people enrolled.

By fiscal year 1975, Medicare costs had increased to $10.5 billion for the 23.7 million part A eligibles and $4 billion for the 23.2 million part B enrollees. Thus, while the number of part A eligibles increased only 25 percent, part A costs increased 263 percent, (an average annual rate of 17.5 percent). Also, part B costs increased 243 percent, (an average annual rate of 16.7 percent) while part B enrollees increased only 30 percent.

The cost of providing benefits, the number of people eligible for benefits, the cost per eligible enrollee and the percent change in this cost for fiscal years 1967 through 1975 are presented in Table 9-5 for part A and Table 9-6 for part B.

EFFECT ON COSTS OF INCLUDING THE DISABLED AND THOSE WITH CHRONIC KIDNEY DISEASE UNDER MEDICARE

The Social Security Amendments of 1972 added provisions to the Social Security Act which included coverage under Medicare of individuals under

Table 9-5. Medicare Hospital Insurance Experience:
Fiscal Years 1967-75 (Part A)

Fiscal Year	Total Cost (millions)	Total Number of Eligibles (millions)	Cost per Eligible	Percent Change in Cost per Eligible
1967	$ 2,886	19.0	$151.70	—
1968	3,841	19.4	198.35	30.8
1969	4,641	19.6	236.21	19.1
1970	4,992	19.9	250.30	6.0
1971	5,602	20.3	276.44	10.4
1972	6,161	20.6	299.28	8.3
1973	6,743	20.9	322.26	7.7
1974[a]	8,201	23.1	354.96	10.1
1975[a]	10,471	23.7	442.34	24.6

[a]Includes data for the disabled and those with chronic kidney disease. These individuals accounted for part A costs of $657 million in fiscal year 1974 and $945 million in fiscal year 1975.

Table 9-6. Medicare Supplementary Medical Insurance Experience: Fiscal Years 1967-75 (Part B)

Fiscal Year	Total Cost (millions)	Total Number of Enrollees (millions)	Cost per Enrollee	Percent Change in Cost per Enrollee
1967[a]	$1,163	17.8	$65.52	—
1968	1,490	18.0	82.60	26.1
1969	1,748	18.8	92.82	12.4
1970	1,896	19.3	98.18	5.8
1971	2,072	19.7	105.37	7.3
1972	2,299	20.0	114.70	8.8
1973	2,454	20.4	120.13	4.7
1974[b]	3,256	22.6	143.82	19.7
1975[b]	3,993	23.2	171.84	19.5

[a]Enrollees had only 6 months in which to meet the calendar year 1966 deductible which could effect the total costs of the part B program for fiscal year 1967. Also, since this was the first year of the program, utilization may have differed from subsequent years and this could have effected total part B costs.

[b]Includes data for the disabled and those with chronic kidney disease. These individuals accounted for part B costs of $487 million in fiscal year 1974 and $651 million in fiscal year 1975.

age 65 who had been entitled to social security or railroad retirement disability benefits for 24 months or more, and the coverage of individuals suffering from chronic renal disease if they require regular dialysis treatment or kidney transplantation. The primary effect of this legislative change was to increase the number of people eligible for Medicare.

The disabled and those with chronic kidney disease use part A benefits which cost about the same per person as those used by Medicare eligibles 65 years of age or older. However, part B benefits cost substantially more per person for the disabled and those with chronic kidney disease than they do for Medicare eligibles 65 years of age or older. The cost of covering the disabled and those with chronic kidney disease amounted to about $1.1 billion in fiscal year 1974 and about $1.6 billion in fiscal year 1975.

COST OF INPATIENT GENERAL HOSPITAL CARE

To determine the factors which have resulted in the large increases in Medicare costs per beneficiary we analyzed the costs of providing care in general hospitals and in nursing homes. General hospital costs accounted for about 70 percent of total Medicare benefit costs and about 96 percent of total part A benefit costs during fiscal year 1975.

The cost of providing inpatient general hospital care for Medicare beneficiaries increased from $2.7 billion in fiscal year 1967 to $10.1 billion in fiscal year 1975. Table 9-7 gives the cost of providing inpatient hospital care, the number of days of care provided, the cost per day of care, the percent change in this cost, and the economic inflation rate for the fiscal years 1967 through 1975.

The total cost of providing inpatient hospital care increased about 270 percent from fiscal year 1967 to fiscal year 1975 and the cost per day of care increased about 173 percent. The increased cost per day of care was due primarily to inflation with some of the increase probably due to more extensive types of care being provided in the hospitals. The increase in the cost per day of care accounts for about $6.2 billion of the increase in hospital costs of fiscal year 1975 over those in fiscal year 1967.

The remainder of the increased costs not attributable to inflation is the result of increased utilization of the hospital benefit by Medicare part A eligibles and the increase in the number of eligibles. We analyzed Medicare hospital utilization data to determine the increase in utlization.

Table 9-8 gives the number of hospital admissions, the admissions per

Table 9-7. Cost of Inpatient General Hospital Care Under Medicare Part A

Fiscal Year	Total Cost (millions)	Total Days of Care (thousands)	Cost per Day of Care	Percent Change in Cost per Day of Care	Economic Inflation Rate (note a)
1967	$2,729	71,245	$38.30	—	18.6
1968	3,465	77,712	44.59	16.4	15.1
1969	4,200	81,716	51.40	15.3	14.7
1970	4,662	80,554	57.87	12.6	10.6
1971	5,354	80,553	66.47	14.9	13.2
1972	5,945	80,038	74.28	11.7	9.4
1973	6,505	81,081	80.23	8.0	5.0
1974[b]	7,911	89,361	88.53	10.3	6.0
1975[b]	10,090	96,441	104.62	18.2	16.4

[a]Consumer Price Index for semi-private hospital room charge.

[b]Includes data for the disabled and those with chronic kidney disease.

Table 9-8. General Hospital Utilization Under Medicare

Fiscal Year	Admissions (millions)	Admissions per 1,000 Eligibles per Year	Average length of Stay (days)	Days of Care per 1,000 Eligibles per Year
1967	5.13	269	13.9	3,475
1968	5.47	283	14.2	4,013
1969	5.75	293	14.2	4,159
1970	5.92	297	13.6	4,039
1971	6.24	308	12.9	3,975
1972	6.45	314	12.4	3,888
1973	6.81	326	11.9	3,875
1974[a]	7.68	332	11.6	3,868
1975[a]	8.29	350	11.6	4,074

[a]Includes data for the disabled and those with chronic kidney disease.

1,000 eligibles per year, the average length of stay, and the days of care per 1,000 eligibles per year.

Table 9-8 shows that there has been a 62 percent increase in the number of admissions and a 30 percent increase in the admissions per 1,000 eligibles. However, because of the 16 percent decrease in the average length of stay, there has been an increase of only about 9 percent in the days of care per 1,000 eligibles provided by Medicare, which is the increase in the utilization of the hospital benefit by Medicare eligibles. In other words, the average Medicare eligible used 9 percent more hospital days in fiscal year 1975 than was used in fiscal year 1967. This increased utilization rate accounted for about $315 million of the increases in hospitalization costs between fiscal years 1967 and 1975.

The last major factor explaining the increase in Medicare hospital costs is the increase in the number of eligibles. There were about 4.7 million eligibles more in fiscal year 1975 than in fiscal year 1967. These people accounted for about $870 million in increased costs.

In summary, our analysis of the Medicare hospital data indicates that, of the $7.4 billion increase in the cost of providing hospital benefits, $6.2 billion was due to inflation (and possibly the provision of more extensive services in the hospital), $870 million was due to more people being eligible for Medicare hospital benefits, and $315 million was due to an increase in the use of the hospital benefit by eligibles.

If data for the disabled and those with chronic kidney disease is excluded, the total increase in the costs of providing hospital care to those 65 years of age or older was $6.4 billion. Of this $6.4 billion increase, $5.7 billion was due to inflation, $460 million was due to increased numbers of eligibles and $260 million was due to increased utilization.

COST OF NURSING HOME CARE

In fiscal year 1968, about 21 million days of nursing home care were provided to Medicare beneficiaries at a cost of more than $341 million. By fiscal year 1975, both the cost and the total days of nursing home care had decreased to about $243 million and 8.6 million days, respectively. Table 9-9 presents the cost of providing nursing home care, the total days of care provided, the cost per day of care, the percent change in this cost, and the economic inflation rate.

The reason for the decrease in utilization of nursing home services under Medicare was a stricter enforcement of the requirement included in the Social Security Act that nursing home services be necessary medically. However, even though total utilization and costs are now lower than they were in fiscal year 1968, the cost per day of care in nursing homes has increased about 99 percent between fiscal years 1967 and 1975. Inflation was primarily responsible for this increase.

We analyzed nursing home utlization data to determine the costs avoided by Medicare because of the decreased utilization. Table 9-10 gives the number of admissions, admissions per 1,000 eligibles per year, the average length of

Table 9-9. Cost of Nursing Home Care Under Medicare

Fiscal Year	Total Cost (millions)	Total Days of Care	Cost per Day of Care	Percent Change in Cost per Day of Care	Economic Inflation Rate[a]
1967[b]	$139	9,797,000	$14.19	—	8.0
1968	341	21,050,000	16.20	14.2	7.9
1969	392	20,454,000	19.16	18.3	7.6
1970	277	13,223,000	20.95	9.3	7.3
1971	204	8,592,000	23.74	13.3	7.8
1972	167	6,588,000	25.35	6.8	5.3
1973	180	6,989,000	25.75	1.6	3.6
1974[b]	213	8,162,000	26.10	1.4	6.4
1975[c]	243	8,617,000	28.20	8.0	13.3

[a]Consumer Price Index for all medical services.

[b]Benefit only available for 6 months.

[c]Includes data for the disabled and those with chronic kidney disease.

Table 9-10. Nursing Home Utilization Under Medicare

Fiscal Year	Admissions (millions)	Admissions per 1,000 Eligibles per Year	Average Length of Stay (days)	Days of Care per 1,000 Eligibles per Year
1968	.45	23	47	1,087
1969	.45	23	45	1,041
1970	.33	16	40	663
1971	.27	13	32	424
1972	.25	12	26	320
1973	.28	13	25	334
1974[a]	.30	13	27	353
1975[a]	.31	13	28	364

[a]Includes data for the disabled and those with chronic kidney disease.

stay, and the days of care per 1,000 eligibles per year for nursing homes for fiscal year 1968 through 1975.

Between fiscal years 1968 and 1975 the number of nursing home admissions decreased 31 percent, the admissions per 1,000 eligibles per year decreased 43 percent, the average length of stay decreased 40 percent, and the days of care provided per 1,000 eligibles per year decreased 66 percent. Thus, the average eligible used 66 percent fewer nursing home days per year in fiscal year 1975 than he did in fiscal year 1968. This decrease in utilization enabled the Medicare program to avoid paying for about 17 million days of nursing home care during fiscal year 1975. This represents, at 1975 prices, about a $479 million cost avoidance. However, because of inflation, Medicare paid $121 million more for the care provided in fiscal year 1975 than this care would have cost in fiscal year 1967.

Cost Increases in Medicaid

Since its inception, the Medicaid program, like Medicare, has experienced a large increase in the cost of providing health care. In fiscal year 1967 the cost of providing Medicaid services was about $2.3 billion. By fiscal year 1975, the cost had risen to approximately $12.1 billion. Table 9-11 lists the total cost of Medicaid services, the number of people who received Medicaid services, the cost per recipient, and the percent change in cost per recipient for fiscal year 1967 through fiscal year 1975.

Table 9-11 shows that there has been a 433 percent growth in total

Table 9-11. Medicaid Experience: Fiscal Years 1967-75

Fiscal Year	Total Cost (millions)	Total number of Recipients (millions)[a]	Cost per Recipient	Percent Change in Cost per Recipient
1967	$2,269	5.2	$436	—
1968	3,538	8.6	411	−5.7
1969	3,988	9.5	420	2.2
1970	4,634	15.0	309	−26.4
1971	5,895	18.2	324	4.8
1972	8,138	20.6	395	21.9
1973	8,714	23.5	371	−6.1
1974	9,756	24.3	401	8.1
1975	12,086	22.5	537	33.9

[a]The number of recipients is the number of people who received Medicaid services at some time during the year. Since some people eligible for Medicaid never receive services, the figures given do not represent the number of eligibles.

Medicaid costs, a 333 percent increase in the number of people who received Medicaid services, and that the cost per recipient has increased 23 percent. However, the cost per recipient figures given in the table can be misleading. The number of recipients represents the number of people who, at some time during the year, actually had at least one medical service paid for by Medicaid. These recipients may have been eligible for Medicaid for the entire year or only for 1 month during the year. Also, the number of recipients figure does not give the total number of people eligible for Medicaid because some eligibles never receive a medical service during a particular year. Because of these factors, the cost per recipient is not equal to the cost per year of eligibility, and therefore, is not strictly comparable from year to year. Data to determine cost per year of eligiblity is not available in HEW.

The large increase in the number of persons receiving Medicaid services was caused by (1) additional States starting Medicaid programs (in January 1967, 25 States and 3 jurisdictions representing about 75 percent of the Nation's population had Medicaid programs in operation, but by August 1972, 49 States and 4 jurisdictions representing 99 percent of the Nation's population offered Medicaid services); (2) an increase in the number of States covering the medically needy (in July 1970, 27 States and jurisdictions had Medicaid programs covering the medically needy, but as of July 1975, 32 States and jurisdictions with about 65 percent of the Nation's population covered the medically needy), and (3) an increase in the welfare rolls (about 7.5 million persons were receiving some form of public assistance in 1967 compared to 15.5 million in June 1975).

Because of this increase in Medicaid eligibles, the total number of services used and the total cost of providing those services have increased significantly. For example, Table 9-12 shows that from calendar year 1968 to fiscal year 1974 the total days of care provided to Medicaid recipients in general hospitals has more than doubled and the cost of providing this care rose about 260 percent.

Because of the difficulty in obtaining comparable data for specific types of services for Medicaid from one year to another, we believe that analysis of the available data would not be meaningful. Therefore, we selected 3 States that had reported data for calendar years 1968 and 1969 and fiscal years 1972 through 1974. We selected California, Michigan, and New Mexico because they represent a large, medium and small State. Using these 3 States' data, we compiled cost data for inpatient general hospital services and nursing home services.

Table 9-13 presents the experience the 3 States reported having in providing inpatient hospital services to Medicaid recipients and table 9-14 does the same for nursing home services. California's cost per day of general hospital care increased by 40 percent from calendar year 1968 to fiscal year 1974.

Table 9-12. Cost of Inpatient General Hospital Care Under Medicaid[a]

Year	Total Cost (thousands)[b]	Total Days of Care[b]	Cost per Day of Care[b]	Percent Change[b]	Economic Inflation Rate[c]
CY 1968	$445,406	7,554,432	$59	—	13.6
CY 1969	946,554	11,908,554	79	33.9	13.4
CY 1970	1,412,827	[d]	[d]	—	12.9
FY 1972	2,220,662	22,841,411	97	—	9.4
FY 1973	1,558,137	16,732,238	93	−4.1	5.0
FY 1974	1,605,201	16,556,175	97	4.3	6.0

[a]Figures include data for persons under 65 years of age. Most Medicaid eligibles over 65 are also covered by Medicare and Medicaid only pays for the Medicare deductible until Medicare benefits are exhausted. Thus, data for those over 65 was deleted to prevent distortion of the cost data.

[b]Because not all States having programs reported data for each year, the figures cannot be accurately compared from year to year. For example, the fiscal year 1972 data includes the information for New York while the fiscal year 1974 data does not.

[c]Consumer Price Index for semi-private hospital room charge.

[d]Not available.

Table 9-13. General Hospital Costs for the Medicaid Program in Three Selected States (Recipients Under 65 Years of Age)

	California			Michigan			New Mexico			
Year	Total Cost (millions)	Cost per Day of Care	Percent Change	Total Cost (millions)	Cost per Day of Care	Percent Change	Total Cost (millions)	Cost per Day of Care	Percent Change	Economic Inflation Rate[a]
CY 1968	$185.8	$100	—	$ 41.1	$53	—	$3.7	$ 52	—	13.6
CY 1969	230.6	111	11.0	44.8	69	30.2	3.6	58	11.5	13.4
FY 1972	314.3	102	([b])	101.7	91	([b])	5.2	80	([b])	9.4
FY 1973	316.7	114	11.8	135.4	84	-7.7	6.8	99	23.8	5.0
FY 1974	369.5	140	22.8	147.0	94	11.9	7.8	105	6.1	6.0

[a]Consumer Price Index for semi-private hospital room charges.

[b]Percent changes were not calculated because of the change from calendar year to fiscal year data.

Table 9-14. Nursing Home Costs for the Medicaid Program in Three Selected States

	California			Michigan		
Year	Total Cost (millions)	Cost per Day of Care	Percent Change	Total Cost (millions)	Cost per Day of Care	Percent Change
CY 1968	$165.4	$10.83	—	$ 89.7	$11.67	—
CY 1969	194.3	11.14	2.9	80.9	15.29	31.0
FY 1972	227.7	11.14	b	116.6	14.99	b
FY 1973	258.5	11.99	7.6	159.8	14.76	−1.5
FY 1974	305.1	14.26	18.9	130.1	17.22	16.7

aThe inflation rate is for all medical care services not just services provided in nursing homes. The inflation rate is taken from the Consumer Price Index.

bPercent changes were not calculated because of the change from calendar year to fiscal year data.

During the same period, this cost rose by 77 percent in Michigan and 102 percent in New Mexico. Similarly, California's cost per day of nursing home care increased 32 percent, Michigan's by 48 percent, and New Mexico's by 36 percent. Most of the increases in hospital and nursing home costs per day of care are attributable to inflation.

Cost Control Efforts

States and the federal government have taken steps to control the increased costs of these programs. Some of these steps were described in Chapter 6 and included cutting back on allowable hospital costs, paying less than full hospital costs for what is covered, creating deterrents by charging Medicare-eligible people more for part B premiums as costs go up, and increasing the amount of the deductible and coinsurance payments they must make. HEW has also altered its calculations of reasonable charges for medical care, which has prompted more physicians to refuse Medicare assignments—the physician billing the patient what the physician feels is a reasonable charge rather than what HEW and the insurance carrier have determined. In addition, many people lose their Medicaid eligibility as wages rise in line with the overall cost of living: when the Medicaid eligibility income levels for the medically needy remain fixed in face of rising wages and cost of living, some people begin to earn more than the income eligibility level, yet their ability to pay the costs of health care have not, in reality, improved.

Table 9-14. (continued)

Year	New Mexico			Economic Inflation Rate[a]
	Total Cost (millions)	Cost per Day of Care	Percent Change	
CY 1968	$3.5	$10.63	–	7.3
CY 1969	2.2	12.22	15.0	8.1
FY 1972	1.7	13.97	[b]	5.3
FY 1973	.8	13.93	–0.3	3.6
FY 1974	.1	14.48	3.9	6.4

Determined efforts have been made to tackle inefficiencies in claims payment. In New York, for example, double billing and claims for services not covered were, in fact, paid by Medicaid to the tune of $60 million over a two-year period from 1975 to 1977. Of this, $15 million was paid to one public hospital in New York City for nonreimbursable services (12). Other abuses of Medicaid include "Ping-Ponging" of patients back and forth between physicians in a clinic to justify additional visits, ordering unnecessary lab tests and medications (with some kickbacks), "gang" visits in which a physician visits all members of a family, or patients in a nursing home, when visit only to one is necessary.

Hospitals, nursing facilities, pharmacies, physicians, ambulance services, and other health professions have yielded their share of cheaters. While the number of cheaters to the total number of participants may be small, the sums involved have been considerable, newsworthy, and embarrassing to the groups from which the cheaters sprang. The abuses should also have been embarrassing to the governments, fiscal intermediaries, and insurance carriers who failed to set up more sound practices and controls at the outset. They failed to realize that whatever the enterprise or endeavor, when a large sum of money becomes available, it will draw out the worst in some people, who will do whatever they can to get more than they are entitled to.

NATIONAL HEALTH INSURANCE (NHI)

The idea of a universal NHI scheme is very appealing and also very much misunderstood. NHI would provide a uniform range of benefits for all citizens and most other permanent residents of the United States. Its aim would be to enable all people to secure care without being deterred over cost considerations and assure all that they will not be bankrupted by the bills that come in following illness.

But NHI would not be free, nor would it pay for everything. NHI would cost money—through increased taxes and through increased cost of manufactured goods (since employers are likely to be called upon to pay a major portion). Nearly all NHI proposals, moreover, have limited benefit structures, particularly as regards care in skilled nursing facilities.

NHI is, nonetheless, a politically popular issue despite the fact that the vast majority of people already have fairly good coverage for surgical and in-hospital medical care. In the 94th Congress, as of February 1976, there were 18 different NHI bills introduced. The Ullman Bill (H.R. 1) was supported by the AHA. The Corman-Kennedy Bill (H.R. 21 and S.3) was supported by the AFL-CIO. The Burleson-McIntyre Bill (H.R. 5990 and S.1438) was supported by the Health Insurance Association of America. The Fulton Bill (H.R. 6222) was endorsed by the AMA. The Waggonner and Long-Ribicoff Bill (H.R. 10028 and S.2470), while not endorsed by any national organization, received considerable attention. Of the 18 bills, most had been introduced in similar or identical versons in the previous Congress. No congressional consensus developed on any of these bills, and no formal action was taken by either branch of the Congress. Whether the bills introduced into the 96th Congress will all be the same or modified and whether they will receive the same endorsements cannot be gauged as of this writing (September 1979), although it appears that the AMA, at least, will not endorse any bill at this time and that the Kennedy bill is somewhat altered.

Of the various bills and of proposals not yet in bill form, it is clear that there is no agreement as to the scope of benefits to be provided, nor is there agreement on how any NHI scheme should be financed. Many political and health leaders are becoming increasingly concerned over the cost projections with regard to NHI. Writing in *The New York Times,* Richard D. Lyons stated, (13),

"Missing from the last week's rhetorical skirmish between President Carter and Senator Edward M. Kennedy over national health insurance was mention of its cost. That is probably because Mr. Carter wishes the issue would go away, while Mr. Kennedy knows that the estimates would stagger even his own supporters."

At a period when there is increasing public resistance to tax increases, the prospects for NHI in the near future are not bright. Reports from overseas regarding the allegedly progressive systems in England, Sweden, and Australia further frighten health and political leaders. Australia, for example, which introduced its national program some years ago, dismantled it in 1978 and decided to rely instead on health insurance and a supplementary program similar to Medicare and Medicaid. In England and Sweden, access to some types of needed care is being denied some people, particularly the elderly, and long waiting lists exist for non-emergency surgery. Further frightening political leaders are the rapidly rising costs in the United States of Medicare and Medicaid and the inability to control those costs.

The issue of NHI, despite these frightening cost signs, will probably stay with us nonetheless. President Carter is committed to some type of NHI and has made a first step, a modest proposal for catastrophic coverage. In May 1979, Senator Kennedy introduced his latest proposal, the *Health Care for All Americans Act of 1979.*

The benefits, costs, and issues raised by a number of national health insurance proposals will be topics for public debate for quite some time. Should a NHI proposal reach the floor of either the House or Senate it is likely to be the descendant of one of the bills which has received support from some large interest group—the AHA, HIAA, Chamber of Commerce, AFL-CIO, AMA, some leading member of Congress, or the President. Figures 9-1 to 9-6 are summaries of some of the major bills introduced in the 94th Congress as of February 1976.*

Figure 9-7 is a summary of the Kennedy, *Health Care for All Americans Act of 1979.* This summary was released May 14, 1979 by the senator's office. It does not show the benefit limitations that are contained in the full proposal as regards home health servcices (100 visits per year), skilled nursing facility services (100 days after a hospitalization of three days or more), and a variety of limited benefits for psychiatric inpatient and outpatient care. Nor does the summary list some of the exclusions such as services not reasonable or necessary for diagnosis or treatment, personal comfort items, and custodial care. All NHI schemes, including the most comprehensive ones, thus have benefit limitations and exclusions, and clearly indicate that in addition to the increased costs borne by the public through increased taxes and cost of goods and services, which reflect increased operating costs due to health insurance premium costs to employers, some of the very ill at least will still have to pay for some health care. Commenting on the Kennedy proposal, *TIME* magazine (May 28, 1979) wrote: "Employers would be liable for the premium payments, estimated at $11.4 billion a year more than they pay now, but they could require workers to provide up to 35% of that amount. . . . The Federal Government, as it does now, would pay the bills for most elderly and poor patients, but at a cost estimated at $28.6 billion a year more than it now pays. . . . Opponents claim that the Kennedy plan would cost closer to $45 billion."

---

*Figures 9-1 through 9-6 are reprinted from *National Health Insurance Proposals,* Provisions of Bills Introduced in the 94th Congress as of February, 1976, compiled by Saul Waldman, HEW.

Figure 9-1. Mixed Public and Private—Ullman Bill

Subject	Provisions
General concept and approach	A 3-part program including: (1) a plan requiring employers to provide private coverage for employees, (2) a plan for individuals, and (3) federally contracted coverage for the poor and aged. State establishes a health care plan, supervises carriers and insurers, and promotes a system of health care corporations (HCC). Supported by American Hospital Association.

	Private plans	Plan for low income and aged
Coverage of the population	Employees of employers under social security and of State and local governments. Also, individuals who elect coverage.	Low-income and medically indigent families, and aged persons.

Benefit structure	Benefits phased in over 5-year period. Final benefits: Institutional services: Hospital: 90 days, $5 copayment per day. Skilled nursing facility: 30 days, $2.50 copayment per day. Nursing home: 90 days, $2.50 copayment per day. Personal services: Physicians: 10 visits per year, $2 copayment per visit. Laboratory and X-ray: 20 percent coinsurance. Home health services: 200 visits per year, $2 copayment per visit. Dental services: Children age 7-12: 1 exam per year, other services, 20 percent coinsurance.

436

Other services and supplies:

Prescription drugs: Limited to specified conditions, $1 per prescription.

Medical equipment and appliances and ambulance service: 20 percent coinsurance.

Eyeglasses: Children to age 12, 1 set per year, 20 percent coinsurance.

Catastrophic coverage: Payable when certain noncovered expenses reach a specified limit, which varies by family income and age; would remove the cost sharing on all benefits and the limitation on number of hospital days and physicians' visits.

Administration	Administered by private insurance carriers under State supervision, according to Federal guidelines.	Federal Government would contract with private insurance carriers who issue policies to eligible persons.
Relationship to other Government programs	Medicare: Abolished. Medicaid and other assistance programs: Would not pay for covered services. Other programs: Mostly not affected.	Would not pay for covered services.
Financing	Employee-employer premium payments, with employer paying at least 75 percent. Federal subsidy of premium for low-income workers and certain small employers, and 10 percent subsidy for HCC enrollees. Individuals pay own premium.	Financed in part by premium payments by medically indigent, but with no premium for lowest income group. Balance of cost financed by Federal general revenues and the payroll taxes of the present Medicare program.

Figure 9-1. (continued)

Subject	Provisions
Standards for providers of services	All institutions and HCC's must meet Medicare standards. Skilled nursing facilities must be under supervision of a hospital medical staff or have its own organized staff. Use of paramedical personnel must meet Federal standards. All providers and HCC's must establish systems of peer review, medical audit and other procedures to meet Federal-State requirements on quality and utilization of services.
Reimbursement of providers of services	Institutions and HCC's: State commission would establish prospective payment methods and review proposed charges. Physicians and other professionals: Reasonable fee, salaries, or other compensation, as approved by State commission.
Delivery and resources	State health commission: Establishes a State health plan, including provisions for regulation of providers and insurance carriers. Takes responsibility for health planning and must approve, in advance, proposed capital expenditures of providers. Health care corporations: State commissions would incorporate system of HCC's, approved to operate in designated geographical areas. HCC must furnish all covered services through its own facilities or affiliated providers (and permit all qualified practitioners to furnish services for it). Would be required to hold open enrollment for public and eventually offer services on a capitation basis. Federal grants provided for HCC's for planning, development, outpatient centers, medical and data equipment, and to cover initial operating deficits.

Source: National Health Insurance Proposals, Provisions of Bills Introduced in the 94th Congress as of February 1976, HEW.

Figure 9-2. Mixed Public and Private—BURLESON-McINTYRE BILL

Subject	Provisions	

Subject	Provisions
General concept and approach	A 3-part plan including a voluntary employee-employer plan and a plan for individuals, under which contributors would receive tax advantages, and a State plan for the poor. All plans administered through private insurance carriers and provide same benefits. Supported by the Health Insurance Association of America.

	Private plans	State plan
Coverage of the population	Employee-employer plan includes employees (and their families) of employers who voluntarily elect a qualified plan. Individual plan includes persons who voluntarily elect.	Low-income families.

Benefit structure	Benefits phased-in over a 8-year period, final benefits as follows: Deductible of $100 per person and 20% coinsurance, except where noted. Institutional services: Hospital. Skilled nursing facility: 180 days. Personal services: Physicians. Dentists. Home health services: 270 days. Laboratory and X-ray: No cost sharing. Health exams and family planning. Well-child care with no cost sharing.

Source:*National Health Insurance Proposals.* Provisions of Bills Introduced in the 94th Congress as of February 1976, HEW.

Figure 9-2. (continued)

Subject	Provisions	
	Private plans	State plan
	Other services and supplies: Medical appliances. Eyeglasses. Prescription drugs.	Reduced cost sharing and family maximum according to family income.
	Annual limit for all cost sharing of $1,000 per family.	
Administration	Insurance administered by private carriers under State supervision. Treasury Department determines tax status of plan.	Insurance administered by private carriers under agreement with the State. Regulations for program established by DHEW.
Relationship to other Government programs	Medicare: Continues to operate. Medicaid and other assistance programs: Would not pay for services under programs. Other programs: Most not affected.	
Financing	For employee-employer plan, premium paid by employers and employees, as arranged between them, but contributions of low-income workers limited according to their wage level. For individual plan, policyholder pays entire premium.	No premium required for lowest income group; for others, premium paid by enrollees, varying according to family income. Federal and State governments pay balance of costs from their general revenues, with Federal share 70 to 90 percent, depending on State per capita income.

440

	Employees and individuals who itemize deductions can take entire premium as deduction on income tax return.[1] Employers can take their entire premium as normal business deduction as under present law (but contributions to nonqualified plans would not be deductible).
Standards for providers of services	Same as Medicare.
Reimbursement of providers of services	Hospitals and other institutions: Prospectively approved rates for various categories of institutions. Hospitals prepare budgets and schedule of charges which are reviewed by a State commission which approves or disapproves charges, subject to DHEW review of rate levels. Physicians and dentists: Reasonable charges, based on customary and prevailing rates.
Delivery and resources	Health planning: Planning agency approval required for capital expenditures to be recognized for reimbursement. Health maintenance organizations: Must be made available as an option to persons enrolled in State plan. Ambulatory health centers: Grants, loans, and loan guarantees for construction and operation of centers. Health manpower: Increases loans and grants for students, with special provisions for shortage areas.

[1]Under present law, deduction of premium is limited to one-half the premium cost up to a maximum of $150.

Source: National Health Insurance Proposals. Provisions of Bills Introduced in the 94th Congress as of February 1976, HEW.

441

Figure 9-3. Mixed Public and Private—FANNIN BILL

Subject	Provisions	
General concept and approach	A 2-part program including (1) a plan requiring employers to offer health insurance coverage to their employees and (2) a State plan for low-income families. Supported by U.S. Chamber of Commerce.	
	Employer-employee plan	*Low-income plan*
Coverage of the population	Full-time employees, including employees of Federal, State, and local governments.	Low-income families.
Benefit structure	No limit on amount of benefits, except where indicated: Institutional services: Hospital. Skilled nursing facility: By regulation. Personal services: Physicians. Laboratory and X-ray. Other services and supplies: Prescription drugs. Medical supplies and appliances. Deductible of $100 per person and 25 percent coinsurance, but total limit to $2,600 annually per family. Actuarially equivalent benefits may be substituted for specified ones.	10-percent coinsurance, but limited to 5 percent of annual family income.

442

Administration	Private health insurance carriers (or self-insured arrangements) supervised by the States, under Federal regulations.	Administered by States through private carriers.
Relationship to other Government programs	Medicare: Continues. Medicaid: Abolished. Other programs: Most not affected.	
Financing	Employee-employer premium payments, with employer required to pay at least 50 percent of cost. Special pools for small employers and self-employed.	Premium payments from enrollees according to family income, with none for lowest income group. Balance of cost from Federal general revenues.
Standards for providers of services	Same as under Medicare.	
Reimbursement of providers of services	Institutions: Prospective budgets with uniform payment rates per specified period of time (e.g. per day) for all patients. Physicians: Usual and customary charges.	
Delivery and resources	Health maintenance organizations: Under both plans, option available to enroll in approved HMO's. Professional Standards Review Organization (PSRO): Would apply to all services under program. Regulation of providers: Proposed and existing capital facilities and services must be approved by local planning agency.	

Source: *National Health Insurance Proposals. Provisions of Bills Introduced in the 94th Congress as of February 1976*, HEW.

Figure 9-4. Mixed Public and Private—CARTER BILL [Rep. Tim Carter, R-Ky]

Subject	Provisions		
General concept and approach	A 3-part program including: (1) a plan requiring employers to provide private health insurance for employees, (2) an assisted plan for the low-income and high medical-risk populations, and (3) an improved Federal Medicare program for the aged. The States would supervise providers of health service and insurance carriers, under Federal guidelines. Supported by the Administration in the 93rd Congress.		
	Employee plan	*Assisted plan*	*Plan for aged*
Coverage of the population	Full-time employees, including employees of State and local governments.	Low-income families, employed or nonemployed. Also, families and employment groups who are high medical risks.	Aged persons insured under social security.

Benefit structure	No limits on amount of benefits listed below, except where indicated:
	Institutional services:
	  Hospital inpatient and outpatient.
	  Skilled nursing facility: 100 days per year.
	Personal services:
	  Physicians.
	  Dentists: For children under age 13.
	  Laboratory and X-ray.
	  Home health services: 100 visits per year.
	  Family planning, maternity care, and health examinations; by regulation.
	Other services and supplies:
	  Prescription drugs.
	  Medical supplies and appliances.
	  Eyeglasses and hearing aids (and eye and ear exams): For children under age 13.		

444

	Deductible of $150 per person and 25 percent coinsurance, but total cost sharing limited to $1,500 annually per family ($1,050 for individuals).	Maximum cost sharing provisions are same as employee plan, but reduced according to individual or family income.	Deductible of $100 per person and 20 percent coinsurance, but total cost sharing limited to $750 per person annually. Reduced cost sharing according to individual income for low-income aged.
Administration	Insurance through private carriers (or self-insured arrangements) supervised by States, under Federal regulations.	Administration by States, using private carriers to administer benefits, under Federal regulations.	Administered by Federal Government in way similar to present Medicare program.
Relationship to other Government programs	Medicare: Program continues as the Federal plan for the aged. Medicaid: No Federal matching funds for covered benefits (or for premiums or cost sharing) under new program, but continues for specified noncovered services (such as intermediate-care facilities).		
Financing	Employer-employee premium payments, with employer paying 75 percent of premiums (65% for first 3 years). Temporary Federal subsidies for employers with usually high increases in payroll costs. Special provisions to assure coverage for small employers.	Premium payments from enrollees according to family income (none for lowest income groups). Balance of costs from Federal and State general revenues, with State share varied according to State per capita income.	Continuation of present Medicare payroll taxes and premium payments by aged (but no premiums for low-income aged). Federal and State general revenues used to finance reduced cost sharing and premiums for low-income aged.

Figure 9-4. (continued)

Subject	Provisions
Standards for providers of services	Similar to Medicare, with additional standards for participation of physicians' extenders.
Reimbursement of providers of services	Reimbursement rates established by States, according to Federal procedures and criteria. Providers of service who elect as "full participating" would be paid the State-established rates, including the cost sharing, as full payment of their charges. Providers who elect as "associate participating" could charge more than the State rate for employee plan patients, but must collect the extra charges and cost sharing from the patients. However, all hospitals and SNF's must be full participating providers.
Delivery and resources	Prepaid practice plans: Under all plans, option available to enroll in approved prepaid group or individual practice plans (which meet special standards). Regulation of insurance carriers: By State, including approval of premium rates, enforcement of disclosure requirements, annual CPA audit, and protection against insolvency of carriers. Regulation of providers: By State, including standards for participation in program approval of proposed capital expenditures, and enforcement of disclosure requirements. Professional Standard Review Organization (PSRO): Applies to all services under program.

Source: National Health Insurance Proposals. Provisions of Bills Introduced in the 94th Congress as of February 1976, HEW.

Figure 9-5. Mainly Public—CORMAN-KENNEDY BILL-94th Congress

Subject	Provisions
General concept and approach	A program administered by Federal Government and financed by special taxes on earned and unearned income and by Federal general revenues. Supported by Committee for National Health Insurance and AFL-CIO.
Coverage of the population	All U.S. residents.
Benefit structure	Benefits with no limitations, except as noted. No cost sharing by patient. Institutional services: Hospital Skilled nursing facility: 120 days. Personal services: Physicians. Dentists: For children under age 15; scheduled extension to age 25; eventually to entire population. Home health services. Other health professionals. Laboratory and X-ray. Other services and supplies: Medical appliances and ambulance services. Eyeglasses and hearing aids. Prescription drugs needed for chronic illness and other specified diseases.
Administration	Federal Government: Special board in DHEW, with regional and local offices to operate program.
Relationship to other Government programs	Medicare: Abolished. Medicaid and other assistance programs: Would not pay for covered services. Other programs: Most not affected.

Figure 9-5. (continued)

Subject	Provisions
Financing	Special taxes: On payroll (1.0% for employees and 2.5% for employers), self-employment income (2.5%) and unearned income (2.5%). Income subject to tax: Amount equal to 150% of earning base under social security (i.e., $22,950 in 1976). Employment subject to tax: Workers under social security and Federal, State, and local government employment. Federal general revenues: Equal to amount received from special taxes.
Standards for providers of services	Same as Medicare, but with additional requirements: Hospitals cannot refuse staff privileges to qualified physicians. Skilled nursing facilities must be affiliated with hospital which would take responsibility for quality of medical services in home. Physicians must meet national standards; major surgery performed only by qualified specialists. All providers: Records subject to review by regional office. Can be directed to add or reduce services and to provide services in a new location.
Reimbursement of providers of services	National health budget established and funds allocated, by type of medical services, to regions and local areas. Hospitals and nursing homes: Annual predetermined budget, based on reasonable cost. Physicians, dentists, and other professionals: Methods available are fee-for-service based on fee schedule, per capita payment for persons enrolled, and (by agreement) full- or part-time salary. Payments for fee-for-service may be reduced if payments exceed allocation. Health maintenance organization: Per capita payment for all services (or budget for institutional services). Can retain all or part of savings.

448

Delivery and resources	Health planning: DHEW responsible for health planning, in cooperation with State planning agencies. Priority to be given to development of comprehensive care on ambulatory basis.
	Health resources development fund: Will receive, ultimately, 5 percent of total income of program, to be used for improving delivery of health care and increasing health resources.
	Health maintenance organizations: Grants for development, loans for construction, and payments to offset operating deficits.
	Manpower training: Grants to schools and allowances to students for training of physicians for general practice and shortage specialties, other health occupations, and development of new kinds of health personnel.
	Personal care services: Demonstration projects to provide personal care in the home, including homemaker, laundry, meals-on-wheels, transportation, and shopping services.

Source: National Health Insurance Proposals. Provisions of Bills Introduced in the 94th Congress as of February 1976, HEW.

Figure 9-6. Tax Credits—FULTON BILL

Subject	Provisions
General concept and approach	A 2-part plan including (1) a plan requiring employers to offer private health insurance to employees and (2) a plan making available private insurance for the nonemployed and self-employed, with Federal subsidies of the premium provided through tax credits or subsidy certificates. Supported by American Medical Association.

	Employee plan	Plan for nonemployed and self-employed
Coverage of the population	Full-time employees of private employers and of Federal, State, and local governments (including persons under Medicare) and workers receiving unemployment insurance.	Low-income families, self-employed, and all others not under an employee plan (including persons under Medicare).

Benefit structure	No limits on benefits, except where indicated:

Institutional services:
  Hospital inpatient and outpatient.
  Skilled nursing facilities: 100 days.
Personal services:
  Physicians services.
  Dental care: Initially for children age 2-6, later extended to age 17.
  Home health services.
  Laboratory and X-ray.
  Health exams, maternity care, and well-child care.
Other services and supplies:
  Medical supplies and equipment.
  Cost sharing: 20% coinsurance, with maximum limit of $1,500 for individuals and $2,000 for families; cost sharing reduced or eliminated for low-income and unemployed families.

	Medicare beneficiaries: Same benefit coverage, but policy excludes the benefits provided by Medicare.
Administration	Insurance provided through private carriers, supervised by the States under regulations issued by a new Federal board. Employers purchase insurance from carriers.　Family purchases insurance from carriers.
Relationship to other Government programs	Medicare: Continues to operate. Medicaid: Would not pay for covered services.
Financing	Employee-employer premium payments, with employer paying at least 65% of cost. Special maximum limit on amount of premium costs for small employers. Federal subsidies for all employers with large increases in payroll costs. Premium for unemployed persons paid by Federal Government.	Federal subsidy of premium ranging from 100% to 10% of premium costs, varied according to annual tax payment of family; this subsidy is taken as income tax credit or by obtaining a subsidy certificate from DHEW. State insurance pools established to assure coverage.
Standards for providers of services	Standards could be issued by a new Federal board.
Reimbursement of providers of services	Hospitals: Reimbursement determined by State governments, based on prospective payment or other methods. Physicians: Payment on basis of usual and customary or reasonable charges.
Delivery and resources	Studies to be conducted by new Federal board.

Source: National Health Insurance Proposals. Provisions of Bills Introduced in the 94th Congress as of February 1976, HEW.

Universal Coverage—Every resident of the United States will be covered for mandated health insurance plans, with federal financing of coverage for the poor and the aged.

Comprehensive Benefits—There will be full coverage of inpatient hospital services, physicians' services in and out of hospital, home health services, x-rays, and lab tests. Costs of catastrophic illness will be covered since there will be no arbitrary non-medical limits on number of hospital days or physician visits. Medicare will be upgraded for the elderly and will also cover prescription drugs.

Cost Controls—Prospective budgeting of hospital and negotiated physician fee schedules will become the principal method of cost control.

Budgeting Costs—Hospitals and doctors will be paid on the basis of prenegotiated amounts. They will not be permitted to charge patients more than the insurance plan pays. National, area-wide and state budgets for health services will be set and any increases will be tightly controlled.

Administration—The program will be administered by a National Health Insurance Board whose members will be appointed by the President, subject to Senate confirmation. A majority will be consumer representatives.

State Role—The Board will contract with each state and territory to help administer the national health insurance program.

Insurance Plans and HMO Consortia—Most Americans will be insured by an insurer of health maintenance organizations which is certified and regulated by the federal government. The insurer must be a member of a consortium of (1) insurance companies, (2) Blue Cross/Blue Shield plans, (3) federally qualified health maintenance organizations, or (4) Independent Practice Associations. There will be a special consortium of plans such as those providing direct or those jointly administered by unions and employers.

Medicare—The elderly and eligible disabled people will continue to be covered by Medicare which will be upgraded. Physicians will no longer bill Medicare patients but will be paid directly by the insurance plan. Prescription drugs will be covered for the elderly.

Medicaid—The poor and near-poor will be covered by the national health insurance plan for all mandated benefits. Medicaid will cover only those services such as long-term nursing home care which are not incorporated in the national health insurance program. The states will contribute only what they are presently spending for Medicaid, and no more.

Health Insurance Card—Every resident of the United States will be issued a health insurance card. If a patient receives medical care without proof of insurance coverage, the provider will bill the state agency which will pay the bill and later determine the source of payment. With or without a card, every person will have a right to receive treatment.

Figure 9-7. (continued)

Federal Regulations—In order to be included in the program, an insurer will require federal certification and will be subject to ongoing federal regulation. The effect of certification and regulation will be to eliminate such long-standing practices as "risk selection" and discriminatory pricing, and to bring existing private insurance expenditures into conformity with public policy on cost controls and equity of benefits and financing.

Financing—Employers will pay a premium related to total wages. The premium will cover the full costs of the covered benefits. The wage-related amount will mean that employers paying high wages will pay more for health insurance than employers paying low wages, although the rate will be the same. Unless other arrangements are made, employees may pay up to 35 percent of premium costs. This means, for example, that unions may negotiate for employers to pay the entire costs.

Self-Employed—The self-employed will be guaranteed comprehensive coverage at income-related group rates not to exceed the value of the benefits covered. They will no longer have to purchase individual policies (if available) at high risk-related premium rates.

Costs—Total costs of health care will be less within a few years of the national health insurance program than they would be under current programs because of the immediate and long-range cost controls applied. New on-budget costs for coverage of the poor and for improving Medicare, would be $28 billion in 1980 dollars.

Quality Controls—Quality controls will be strengthened and the states will be required to implement these quality standards as a condition of participation in the program.

Health Maintenance Organizations—HMOs and other non-traditional forms of health care delivery, such as neighborhood health centers, will be fully supported and their development encouraged through incentives.

Competition—Insurers and HMO's will compete for enrollees, but not by selecting "risks." They will know what premium they will be entitled to receive for each person or family covered. They will compete on the basis of administrative efficiency and for supplemental coverages.

Equalization Program—To assure that no consortium member will be able to profit by selecting "risks," there will be an equalization fund to counterbalance member companies and consortia. The program will protect individual companies or plans against unforeseen costly events.

Existing Employer/Employee Arrangements—An employer will be obligated to maintain existing contractual or other arrangements for health benefits. If the employer's present costs exceed mandated premiums, the excess will be

Figure 9-7. (continued)

---

applied to other employee benefits, subject to negotiation with employee representatives.

Preventive Medicine and Health Promotion—Services for the prevention and early detection of disease will be covered, including immunization and health education.

Resource Distribution—A Resources Distribution Fund will be used to improve services for underserved populations and to develop new services for the full population's changing needs, in particular for home care of the elderly and chronically ill.

Consumer and Provider Advisory Councils—A National Health Insurance Advisory Council and State Councils with consumer majorities will advise Federal and State Public Authorities.

President Carter announced his plan in June 1979, and it was sufficiently close to the Long-Ribicoff proposal for catastrophic insurance that it received the endorsements of both Senator Long and Senator Ribicoff. The President's plan called for staged implementation, Phase I mandating that all employees and their families be covered by health insurance through place of employment by policies which may (but need not) have a co-insurance feature not to exceed $2,500 per year per family. Medicare and Medicaid covered individuals would be covered by a government plan but the co-insurance here would be limited to $1,250, and for very low income persons there would be no co-insurance. The co-insurance would not apply, however, to pre-natal care, delivery and infant care to age 1; full dollar coverage would apply for these services for all Americans. Coverage for skilled nursing home service would be limited to 100 days per year, home health visits would be limited to 100 visits per year, and mental health services would be limited to 20 days per year of inpatient care and $1,000 in ambulatory psychiatric care. For services beyond these limits the patient would be responsible. As with the Kennedy proposal there would be, however, unlimited acute inpatient hospital care and unlimited physician services. Hospital charges would be controlled, and physician fees would be fixed by negotiation and would constitute full payment for Healthcare clients (those formerly under Medicare and Medicaid). This means, of course, fixed maximum charges for physician services for those patients. For those covered by private health insurance plans, physician fees would not be fixed.

In a note of candor The White House, in announcing the President's plan stated: "The uncertainty as to the magnitude of savings brought about by these types of system reforms and cost constraints makes any projection of first year costs more problematic the further out in time the estimates are presented." The White House proceeded to forecast 1983 expenditures for covered services in terms of 1980 dollars. It predicted $4 billion less in individual expenditures and $2 billion less by state and local governments. But, employer expenditures would rise by $6 billion (and presumably be passed along to individuals through higher priced goods and services). Federal government expenditures would rise $18.2 billion. Phase II of this plan would come at some later, unspecified, date and constitute a broadening of the benefit structure.

In what may be the most accurate assessment as to the chances for the Carter, Kennedy and other national health insurance proposals, the chairman of the House Ways and Means Committee (Al Ullman) was reported to have said: "It is my judgment that Congress is in no mood to vote for a multi-billion dollar health package" (*Medical World News*, June 25, 1979).

REFERENCES

1. Mueller, M. S.: Private health insurance in 1975: Coverage, enrollment, and financial experience. *Social Security Bulletin*, Vol. 40; June 1977.

2. Fuchs, V. R.: *Who Shall Live?* New York, Basic Books, Inc., 1974.

3. Anderson, O. W.: *Blue Cross Since 1929: Accountability and the Public Trust.* Cambridge, Ballinger, 1975.

4. *Source Book of Health Insurance Data 1977-1978*, Washington, D.C., Health Insurance Institute.

5. Hawley, P. R.: *Non-Profit Health Service Plans*, Blue Cross Commission and Blue Shield Commission, Chicago, 1949.

6. Scitovsky, A. A., and McCall, N: Coinsurance and the Demand for Physician Services: Four Years Later. *Social Security Bulletin*, Vol. 40; May 1977.

7. *Thirty Years of Service to New York 1947-1977*, HIP, no date.

8. Mechanic, D: *Public Expectations and Health Care.* New York, John Wiley and Sons, 1972.

9. Weissman, A: *What One Group Practice Prepayment Plan Is Doing to Stem the Increase in Medical Care Costs.* Kaiser-Permanente, 1976; from public testimony before the Council on Wage and Price Stability.

10. Quoted in Bowers, J. Z.: *An Introduction to American Medicine—1975*, DHEW Publication No. (NIH) 77-1283, 1977.

11. *History of the Rising Costs of the Medicare and Medicaid Programs and Attempts to Control These Costs: 1966-1975*, General Accounting Office, February 11, 1976, pages 4-15; Footnotes have been deleted.

12. *New York Times*, December 18, 1977.

13. *New York Times*, December 17, 1978.

10
Public Health: State and Local

For analytic purposes, there are a number of ways for categorizing health services. One convenient way is to place the various services under two broad umbrellas: preventive and treatment. Thus far in the text, we have focused primarily on the organization of treatment services—how we train physicians, how we organize hospitals, how physicians practice, and how we pay for all of the treatment services that are provided by physicians and hospitals.

While physicians have always done some preventive work, including checkups and the education of their patients on matters relating to their health, the bulk of their activities has focused on crisis intervention, on dealing with the vast array of concerns and complaints registered by patients when they consult their physicians. This is not to suggest their lack of interest in, or concern for, prevention, rather, recognition of two fundamental facts:

First, the major preventive thrusts are beyond the organizational capacity of the individual physician. Required is a communal effort organized under the police powers of the state. The individual physician can do little, for example, to assure purity of water and air, the elimination from the environment of noxious weeds and substances, protection of people from a large number of communicable diseases and from the antisocial and self-destructive behavior of the mentally ill, from unsafe social and occupational environments, and to assure the safety of marketable products—drugs, foods, automobiles, and so on. The physician's authority is limited, but the physician can, as an expert in matters relating to health, advise those who have the authority to order and to otherwise take all necessary steps to protect society, that is, state government along with its agencies and subunits that exercise delegated authorities. This kind of advice individual physicians and medical societies have given throughout our history; indeed, if one looks at the leadership of government health departments in terms of their salaried directors and the boards of health that provide legislatively delegated policy or administrative direction to the departments, one finds medical practitioner domination. Health officers are mostly physicians, and boards of health that exercise policy or administrative authority tend to be controlled by physicians. In the extreme, Gossert and Miller report (1, p.488):

In 9 states professional societies or associations are mandated by law to provide a list of nominees from which the governor is obligated to make his selection. In two states, Alabama and South Carolina, the medical association is by statutory provision the state board of health; committees of the medical societies carry responsibility on behalf of the state for its public health functions.

They go on to note:

Boards with policy-making and administrative functions tend to have more professional representation than boards with only advisory functions. In every instance but one where physicians constitute a majority of the membership the board functions in policy-making and administrative capacities . . . In no instance do physicians constitute a majority where the board functions only in an advisory capacity . . .

Medical domination of health departments stems largely from the fact that, in the early days, legislatures and governors and mayors felt it necessary to delegate to "the doctors" all matters that related to health, for "the doctors" were recognized as the ones who were most knowledgeable in such matters. How deeply ingrained this notion is is perhaps illustrated by an experience the author had in Maryland in the early 1960s: A medically dominated planning committee was considering a recommendation to the governor for a reorganized state board of health; although the board was to be a policy board, the physicians on the committee were all agreed that in the 1960s there was no need for a board of health to have physicians on it so long as the board had medical advisory groups; a layman on the committee, a prominent and able legislator, objected and said that it was inconceivable to him to have a state board of health without physicians on it, and that if the committee stuck to its thinking and did not specify some physician membership, he could predict legislative bewilderment and subsequent legislative action—not sponsored or led by him—to create a board of health consisting of mostly physicians.

We'll return shortly to boards of health, but let us now note the second reason for physician concern for crisis intervention. Despite all that the theoreticians say about the primary importance of prevention, the fact remains that society demands, and will always demand, that the crises of life that call for physician intervention—the injured child, the complicated pregnancy, the victim of a heart attack, and so on—that these crises will be addressed, and prevention, if need be, will be deferred. First things first, and medical crises come first, and society demands physician intervention with whatever armamentarium is appropriate.

Having actively supported the creation of government health agencies, in various states, physicians have nonetheless, from time to time, been in conflict with these health departments, sometimes in disagreement as to how health department programs should develop professionally, sometimes in reaction to what the private physicians felt was government intrusion into their domain. The AMA, for example, while long supportive of many federal health initiatives, took issue with the Sheppard-Towner Act (1921) and unsuccessfully opposed that grant program for development in the states of child health programs. At the time, the AMA saw this as the opening wedge for the provision of all medical care by government. On the other hand, the AMA recognized and supported the need of government action to provide medical care for the poor but vigorously opposed, from 1933 until only recently, all proposals for compulsory National Health Insurance. Similar patterns appeared at the state level: The California Medical Association vigorously opposed, in 1949, a state legislative proposal for a compulsory health insurance program, a proposal that Hanlon maintains was almost identical to that which the association had proposed a decade earlier (2, pp.622-623). In some states, on the other hand, a happy and progressive relationship developed between the medical societies and the health departments: in Maryland, for example, for many years, leaders in the medical society and in private practice worked closely with the state health department to develop some of the most progressive public health programs in the nation. The qualities of leadership and political skill on the part of medical and government leaders often made the difference, along with some of the key issues of the times to which we all respond from time to time but over which we have little control. Miller et al., in a 1974 survey of local health departments, found that in only one of ten of the large city health departments and in only one in five of the small local health departments was the medical society viewed by the department as a constraint on the development of its services (3, p.935).

STATE HEALTH AGENCIES

Administrative Organization of State Health Agencies

How a state government organizes its public health functions will vary from state to state. History, personalities, federal grant programs, and chance all play a role. The traditional public health functions include *communicable disease control, maternal and child health services, environmental sanitation, health education, laboratory services,* and *vital statistics.* These were until recently placed administratively in state health or public health departments. In the last decade, there has been a tendency in some states to remove some of the environmental health activities and place them in new environmental protection agencies. But a state government's health responsibilities (and being government health activities, they are appropriately public health activities) go far beyond these basic six functions. Not only have the basic six functions spawned a large number of related program activities far beyond the original range of services, but the states have also been responsible for care of the mentally ill, mentally retarded, and professional and institutional licensure. Whether these latter functions are or are not located in the state's chief public health agency— the state health department—varies. Some states have all of these activities in a single agency. Some states break them out and place them in separate agencies. In any one state, the organizational pattern may from time to time change as new problems arise and as new opportunities are seized. As might be expected, reorganizations within bureaucracies are resisted by some and favored by others.

Within any one state, where health agency functions are split, there may be a variety of administrative forms. Gossert and Miller analyzed the state boards of health and published their results in 1973.

There are in the states three basic models. First is where the health agency is headed by a board of health with policy or administrative functions over the agency. The board is typically appointed by the governor and approved by the state senate, though the appointment and approval are not always this way. Board members are typically nonsalaried, and as we have noted, where the boards have policy or administrative roles to play, physicians tend to be in the majority. In addition to overall direction of the agency, boards of health (including boards that have only advisory functions) very frequently have authority to enforce public health laws by holding hearings on violations, hearing appeals on health officer actions, and by issuance of board orders for compliance with the laws. Board orders must be enforced by law enforcement agencies, although the recipient of a board of health order can, of course, appeal it in the state courts. Many boards either appoint key agency personnel or have a strong influence in their appointment. As one might expect, there have been good and bad boards of health, progressive as well as nonprogressive boards. Some boards have been highly politicized by the types of people appointed to them; other boards have been highly professional with no partisan politics or political hacks. Advocates of policy boards argue that they provide not only good professional advice to the agency (which they could get, of course, from advisory boards equally as well) but also a buffer when the chief health officer must take unpopular stands on public health issues or when the political leaders want something done or not done for political reasons, such as closing their eyes to a problem, not rendering advice that might prove costly and therefore politcally difficult for the elected official to deal with, or support for a budget cut. Critics of policy boards argue that they inhibit political accountability. How can a governor be held accountable if he or she must work through a board that the governor probably has mostly inherited? This criticism has not always been persuasive, given the frequently held belief that politicians, if at all possible, will avoid accountability when the going gets tough. Political escape acts have been common in the areas of mental health and mental retardation when poor conditions were publicized and are common today when government leaders complain about high costs; everyone is at fault except them.

A second pattern for health agency governance is to have a gubernatorial-appointed secretary or commissioner of health. Like boards, this type of leadership can be good or bad, depending on the quality of the appointed official and the quality of the governor. If a governor avoids tough issues, if a governor tends to appoint incompetents or political hacks, then the board system might be preferred. But here the *if* is *if* a good board is inherited or appointed. If, on the other hand, there is an unprogressive board, then a strong governor with a competent secretary of health would be preferred. The political style of a state often dictates how well each of the systems works. There is a tendency in recent years to move away from policy boards to the cabinet system of government in which the health agency head is the secretary of health. In at least one state in which this occurred, it has led to a marked deterioration in the quality of health programming. The cabinet approach allows for greater political management and fiscal control, which has clear political advantages but can also be professionally disadvantageous.

In recent years, a number of states have sought to create umbrella organizations, bringing together under one secretary several human service agencies of state government. Where these super agencies have been created (frequently called a *department of human resources*), no set pattern exists as to which agencies are included, though health, mental health and retardation, education, and welfare are most common. Other agencies may also be included, such as corrections. The rationale for these superagencies stems from the fact that many of the clientele of one agency are frequently the clientele of one or more of the other agencies, and by placing these agencies under one authority, improved coordination would take place, resulting in more effective and more efficient services. While success stories abound for this approach, the "successes" are usually reported by those who created these superagencies or who benefited job-wise by their creation. There are considerable anecdotal data to suggest that while the theory is true, the practice has, in fact, not been operationalized at the state levels due to the jealous guarding of prerogatives by the various bureaucracies: A health professional, for example, may be very supportive of new initiatives in education or corrections as long as it is not at the expense of the health budget.

Activities

Hanlon cites a 1961 unpublished survey of activities engaged in by 50 state health departments (2, pp.299-300). There were 103 different activities, some engaged in by all 50 departments (environmental health, health education, maternal and child health, nursing). Other activities reported by at least 40 departments included communicable diseases, dental health, engineering, hospital survey and planning and construction, licensure, laboratories, local health services, tuberculosis (TB) control, vital statistics. Other frequently reported activities (by more than 20 departments) included cancer control, chronic disease control, crippled children's services, food and drug control, heart disease control, industrial health, mental health, nutrition, personnel, venereal disease (VD) control, water and sewage.

The categorization of activities was based on the organization charts for 50 state health departments. What the summary indicates, therefore, are those activities in the various states that have been given organizational chart identity. The activity may well exist in other departments or in the health department but be submerged under another organizational unit. For example, 19 states had general sanitation units on their charts. The other 31 states probably had that activity but not on the organizational chart. General sanitation in the other 31 states might have been subsumed, at least in part, under engineering, environmental health, industrial health, water and sewage, and like categories. The listing is useful, however, in its identification of some of the major programmatic areas for health department programming.

Miller et al. conducted a similar analysis but used state laws instead of the organization charts (4, pp. 940-945). They identified 44 public-health areas specified in state laws:

Communicable Disease Control
Vital Statistics
Promulgate Rules and Regulations
Venereal Disease Control
Quarantines
Tuberculosis Control
Water/Stream Pollution Control
Facilities Inspection
Facilities Licensure

Qualifications of Local Health Officer
Chronic Disease Control
Crippled Children
Milk Inspection
Health Planning
Housing Inspection
PKU/Metabolic Screening
Alcohol and Addiction Control
Dental Health

Laboratory Services	Establish Local Hospitals
Refuse Disposal	Rabies Control
Air Pollution Control	Ambulance Service
Abate Nuisances/Filth	School Health
Health Education	Health Personnel Registration
Radiological Health	Home Health
Food Inspection	Needs and Resource Assessment
Mental Health	Nursing Care
Prevention of Blindness	Family Planning
Maternal/Child Health	Extermination Services
Immunizations	Compulsory Hospitalization
Occupational Health	Nutrition Program
Care of Indigent	Emergency Medical Service

Miller et al. discuss the problems that flow from the language of the statutes. For example, although only 60% of the states authorized immunizations by statutory language, 100% authorized communicable disease control activities. Miller et al. presume, and probably correctly, that immunizations in 40% of the remaining states are authorized under the broader mandate of communicable disease control.

Some public health programs are operated directly by a central department of state government (typically: state TB, MH, and MR hospitals; licensure of professional personnel, hospitals, nursing homes, and other health facilities). Some programs are decentralized to regional offices of the state agency if regional organization is employed. More frequently, programs have a shared responsibility between state and local government health agencies. Where this shared responsibility occurs, the state agency will typically set performance standards under which local programs will operate in return for which some state monies will be allocated to supplement local government resources. State standards also often govern the operation of nongovernmental agencies, sometimes standards that must be met in order to be eligible for a license or for payment under some state administered program.

Some programs for which there is shared responsibility will entail some state service along with complementary local services. Standards are typically minimal standards: If one proposes to provide a service, it must at least meet those standards. Standards are, in a sense, a floor below which a program is not considered acceptable. Standards have rarely been optimal standards because few, if any, could reach such levels without significant tax increases. Standards in public health, as in other areas, have been evolutionary in nature—initially, the bare essentials, which most could meet or which so clearly affected the public's health that no government could resist establishing them. As in medical education and with hospital accreditation standards, after initial establishment, public health standards become a mechanism for elevating the more marginal programs. Often, the standards by themselves were not enough; an added inducement was the offer of a grant of money for development and/or operation of a program that met the standards. Grant monies for local programs come from the state government and also from the federal government. As we shall note in the chapter on the federal government, the national government has been able to secure development of programs in the states and in communities by offering a bribe—a gift of money if the lower unit of government will develop the program to meet federal standards. Sometimes federal monies paid all of the costs of the program; sometimes federal monies paid only part of the cost. The federal strategy was to offer to pay a sufficient proportion of the costs to stimulate the desired state or local action.

The mix of programs, the sophistication of programs, the population served by programs, vary considerably from state to state and from unit to unit within a state. Most states serve all the people through environmental health programs, assuring the quality and safety of the environment through such program activities as were identified by Miller et al. and as reported by Hanlon. These activities involve health agency inspections, citations on deficiencies, and board of health or police action if deficiencies are not corrected. The variability from state to state in programs is illustrated by the rules and regulations governing restaurants in two large Eastern states. In one state, the local health ordinances require all restaurants to have two separate doors leading to the street to inhibit the flow of flies and animals into the restaurant. Also prohibited are the use of chemically treated fly-catching materials hung in the restaurant. In the nearby state, none of these requirements or prohibitions are present. The former state was practicing good public health, assuring the quality and safety of the environment. Whether it in fact prevented disease is not known. But it represented an attitude toward health matters that, along with other attitudes and measures, contributed to a pattern that militated against opportunities for disease causing agents to make inroads. An analogous situation occurs in surgical operating rooms. One break in sterile technique will not necessarily lead to infection, but a string of breaks may; if operating room people are finicky about technique, they are so organized as to inhibit opportunities for infectious agents to make inroads; where sterile technique is casual or sloppy, the chances of wound infection are greatly increased.

It is easy to demonstrate the value of immunizations as well as water quality control measures. It is more difficult to demonstrate and persuade people as to the value of many other public health measures. To do so often requires able professional and political leadership and an informed public.

Sometimes public health laws and ordinances serve not the public's health but the public's aesthetic tastes. The prohibition against swimming in reservoirs is an example: Since impounded water is almost always treated, there is really no reason why one can't swim in the reservoir.

Thus, while all states engage in environmental health activities, the degree and extent of activity varies.

Similarly, all states have some personal preventive service programs, particularly in areas relating to maternal and child health, school health, and immunizations. Most, moreover, have program activities relating to crippled children services with a variety of diagnostic and treatment services available. In some states, however, access can be a problem, particularly when the state may require referral from a private physician or makes access to the service difficult through lack of public information about the service, infrequency of services, and remoteness of service. Some of these barriers are intentional, some accidental.

In a great many states, public health agency services have moved far beyond the traditional areas of environmental, personal preventive, mental health, and mental retardation services, with the states, directly or through local public health agencies, providing many of the services that are provided by hospitals and private physicians in other states. Where this occurs, one often finds the public health agencies paying for care in general hospitals and hiring private physicians to provide special medical services, thus supplementing the more general services provided by the full time physician staff. While most of the personal preventive and the medical care services are provided to the poorer people of the state, some programs are available to all citizens regardless of income status. This, again, will vary considerably from state to state.

Mental Health and Mental Retardation in State Administrations

Mental health agencies were frequently spun off administratively. In the nineteenth century and for a great portion of this century, there was, in fact, little that could be done clinically for the mentally ill, and the mainstream of medical practice more or less washed its hands of the problem. The medical schools weren't very helpful either during the first half of this century; few had psychiatric departments, and the psychiatric components of the undergraduate medical education programs were thin at best. Since professional interest lagged due in large measure to the absence of knowledge as to how to treat these patients, the state, as in other countries, assumed responsibility for warehousing these patients in large, remote, custodial institutions. Typically, they were understaffed and poorly maintained, for what useful purpose would be served by pouring tax monies into them?

Efforts at reform were spotty at best and usually only temporary. But as the appalling conditions in most state institutions became known, as professional interest grew in the 1950s due to new knowledge and new insights on how to deal with the mentally ill, and as tranquilizers were developed that made possible, by suppression of symptoms, the treatment of many patients in out-of-hospital settings, and as the nation's economy improved and tax monies became more readily available, reformers began to be heard. Professionals argued that it was now time for psychiatry to re-enter the mainstream of medical practice, to subject its theories and its treatment modalities to the scrutiny of other medical people. Professionals and lay people also called for new monies for improved staffing as well as community programs. Moreover, in many states, inadequate and incompetent administration within the mental health units led to cries for administrative reform. Among the reforms suggested was to merge the health and mental health agencies where they were separate. In some states, this was accomplished. In other states, it was successfully resisted by the mental health bureaucracies. While I believe the clinical justification for merger is clear-cut, merger may at times be inadvisable for other reasons, particularly where the absorbing agency has a greater level of incompetence or is so highly politicized that merger would run the grave risk of inappropriate interference in the clinical programs.

The placement of mental retardation agencies in state bureaucracies also varies. They are sometimes separate, sometimes in the health department, very often in with mental health, and sometimes in other state agencies. These institutions have also suffered along similar lines and for similar reasons as the mental health institutions. In some respects, the controversy that flows from merger proposals has not been as spirited, for mental retardation has seemed to be more clearly physically based with behavioral manifestations, although some experts believe that some mental retardation is essentially the result of cultural deprivation. On the other hand, the controversy still exists between the psychiatrists and the pediatricians, the former having handled the mental retardation problem historically by default; no one else would deal with it, and so it fell to the psychiatrists. These two medical specialties often are engaged in a debate with the educators who argue that since mental retardation cannot be cured, it is the field of special education that must play the most prominent role in order to educate the mental retardation patients to as high a functioning level as possible. The controversy around mental retardation, while sometimes over merger, is more often over a question of professional responsibility for mental retardation program leadership.

Reformers also called for more modern residential facilities, improved staffing, and the development of a variety of nonresidential and community services—day hospitals, community mental health centers, emergency services, and so on. But state governments, faced with rising demands from many sectors of society along with rising costs, generally gave measured responses to the new demands. Major improvements were made in many states, but in many states progress was slow. The work environment of many state institutions left much to be desired; physically remote, old, and without adequate support services, they proved unattractive to many professionals. And with still low salaries, professional positions went vacant in many states; in others, they were filled by FMGs,many of whom had language problems and only temporary medical licenses. On the whole, the record of state governments was not good, even in the second half of the twentieth century.

The movement for community based care loomed as a solution to the state governments. If community care was the most appropriate locale for the mentally ill and retarded, why make heavy investments in state hospitals? Why not get the patients out to the communities in which they belong? Not only did this encourage states not to allocate large sums of new monies for hospitals and staff upgrading, but it also encouraged some states to accelerate the discharge of patients to the community. In California and New York, the dumping of patients reached scandalous dimensions, for the communities did not have the money to develop an adequate range of services, and the states released the patients without services in place. In New York City, which has been on the verge of bankruptcy for some time, the patients ended up in what are aptly called flophouses. In California, the Santa Clara County sheriff's department reported in 1974 that jail population there had more than tripled as a result of former mental hospital patients who were arrested for loitering and mischievous conduct. This, of course, prompts citizens to resist the release of patients to their communities and to the placement of community facilities near their homes. But it is not only California and New York: In a great many states, newspapers periodically report on community homes and nursing facilities that burn down or that drug, beat, or starve patients because the state governments have not enforced standards that, if they did, might only force the state to take back the patients. Becker and Schulberg concluded (5, pp.255-261):

The majority of patients currently cared for in state hospitals could be adequately treated in the community if a comprehensive spectrum of psychiatric services and residential alternatives were established. The failure to establish this network of community services before the discharge of thousands of patients has discredited the deinstitutionalization programs in many states, including California and New York, and forced California to abandon its plan to phase out all its state hospitals. Thus, although phase out of state hospitals is clinically feasible, it is unlikely at present since the fiscal and idealogical commitment to shift to community-based care is lacking.

LOCAL HEALTH ACTIVITIES

Miller et al., in their 1974 survey of local health departments, found that from 63% to 96% of the responding departments provided services in the following areas: immunization, environmental surveillance, TB control, maternal and child health (MCH), school health, VD control, chronic disease, home care, family planning, (4, p.934). They go on to note:

The majority of health departments are the sole sources in their localities for programs of environmental surveillance (70.4 percent), tuberculosis control (63.3 percent), and immunizations (57.7 percent). Other major obligations for which health departments are sole providers are maternal and child health (44.8 percent of reporting departments), school health (38.5 percent), family planning (38 percent), and chronic disease programs (25.7 percent) . . . Other functions, although less common, are of special interest: more than 7.5 percent of health departments are the sole source of ambulatory care in their area; and 20 health departments (1.4 percent) report themselves as the sole source of acute hospital services . . .

Respondents were asked to indicate their department's three most important functions; "disease prevention" and "environmental surveillance" head the list, each function being recorded as among the three most important functions for about three-fourths of the departments. Closely related functions are disease control (34 percent) and public education (23 percent). Slightly more than one-quarter of all departments list "direct delivery of medical care" as one of their most important functions.

They go on to report that about 60% of local health department funds come from local government, about 20% from the state, and at least 9% from the federal government. Medical doctors predominate: nearly two-thirds of local health department heads are physicians, but only about one-third of these have had special training leading to a public health or similar master's degree. Presumably the nonmedically qualified health officers head very small departments, although there was an uproar in New York City when for a short time the health department came under the supervision of a nonmedical administrator. It would be interesting to know the extent to which nonmedical health officers are in the departments that report the medical society as inhibiting or constraining the development of services.

Miller et al. conclude their survey of local health departments by noting that despite all of the recent federal efforts to influence health services in the United States, there has been "little acknowledgement that local health departments are part of that scene." They go on to note that "increasingly, when the nation's leaders speak of existing patterns of health service they refer to private professional practice, ignoring important resources and potentials in the public sector" (4, p.937). This lament is well taken. While critics, which Miller et al. note, cite inadequacies of local health departments to justify the diminished recognition given these public agencies, one can't resist observing that some of the diminished recognition stems from ignorance about what health departments do, some stems from irritation or frustration over the fact that an entrenched lower-level bureaucracy exists that has its own expertise and its own honestly held views on needs and on ways to do things, and some stems from individuals who are from those relatively few states in which the state health department is weak and the local scene and potential goes unrecognized and/or undeveloped.

It is important for us to appreciate more fully what a health department does, for it should go without saying that were it not for organized public health efforts, our nation would not be as stable, as successful, as livable as it is. It is the work of health officers and their collaborators that make our society a safe one in which to live and that is conducive to the healthy development of the individual.

The pattern of local health department organization varies from state to state. A few states have no local units; whatever services are provided are provided by the state. But most states have local departments; typically, some of their monies come from state and federal coffers. In New England, local departments tend to be on a city or town basis, county government being weak or nonexistent. In the South, local departments tend to be organized on a county basis. And there are in-between arrangements, as in Pennsylvania, in which there is provision for county health departments (but very few in existence), local government (subcounty, town, borough, etc.) units with largely environmental responsibilities, as well as regional state health department offices. In some parts of the country, we find metropolitan and other kinds of multijurisdictional departments, that is, multicounty or combined city-county departments. How much autonomy the local (county, town, city, or multijurisdictional) department has from the state authority will vary from state to state and even within the state, depending on the extent of state support, the dynamism of the local health officer, the relative political strengths of the different local governments, as well as the administrative style of the state health agency leaders.

The state health department sets the minimum standards for local department operations. Typically, the local units submit their budgets and plans to the state authority for review and approval. With state approval, the local department is then approved to receive state funds. In many states, the local unit can, if it wishes, exceed the standards set by the state and use its own resources to accomplish that end. The level of state support will vary from state to state but often is usually based on a minimum program expected of the local unit and funds distributed on some kind of formula basis.

To illustrate the kinds of activities engaged in by a strong local health department, I am reprinting in the next section major portions of the informational brochure *Community Health Services*, which is issued by the Anne Arundel County Health Department of Annapolis, Maryland. It is reprinted with permission of its health officer, Dr. J. Howard Beard.

In fiscal 1978, the Anne Arundel County Health Department served a population of approximately 374,000 people.

LOCAL HEALTH DEPARTMENT SERVICES: ANNE ARUNDEL COUNTY, MARYLAND

Demography*

Between the years 1960 to 1978, Anne Arundel's population increased from 206,634 to 373,560; a total of 166,926 persons or 81%. The current population is composed of 88% white and 12% non-white; persons of American Indian, Filipino, and Oriental ancestry are also included in the latter classification.

The City of Annapolis, one of two incorporated towns, has a population of 42,453, including the U.S. Naval Academy; the other town, Highland Beach, has a population of 6. Large unincorporated areas of the county include: Brooklyn Park, Glen Burnie, Linthicum, Odenton, Severna Park, and Arnold.

Population by Race—July 1, 1978 (projected)

Total	White	Non-White
373,560	328,813	44,747

The density of population for the county as of July 1, 1978 is 698 persons per square mile or 1.26 per acre.

*Source: Anne Arundel County Office of Planning & Zoning.

Population Trends: 1960-1980

Year	Total	White	Non-White
1960	206,634	178,076	28,558
1970	297,539	262,268	34,271
1980	405,145	369,114	30,031

Vital Statistics**
(provisional)

Annual Number and Rate of Births: 1976
(Live)

Number			Rate/1000 Population		
Total	White	Non-White	Total	White	Non-White
4,667	3,991	676	13.6	13.2	16.4

Annual Number and Rate of Deaths: 1975

Number			Rate/1000 Population		
Total	White	Non-White	Total	White	Non-White
1,954	1,708	246	5.7	5.7	6.0

Death Rates for Leading Causes—1975
Rate/100,000 Population
All Causes 570.2

Diseases of the Heart	- 216.5	All Accidents	- 34.1
Malignant Neoplasms	- 131.0	Diabetes Mellitus	- 13.1
Cerebro-Vascular Disease	- 36.5	Influenza and Pneumonia	- 12.8

Cirrhosis of Liver - 11.4

Hospitals Located in County, Type and Bed Capacity: 1978

Anne Arundel General	General	272 beds
North Arundel General	General	228 beds
Crownsville Hospital Center	Mental	725 beds

**Most recent figures available from Maryland Center for Health Statistics—June, 1978.

470

Physicians Practicing in County by Specialty: 1978
(Total: 291)

General Practice	- 54	Family Practice	- 12
Pediatrics	- 22	Radiology	- 10
Obstetrics	- 36	Ophthalmology	- 12
Surgery	- 18	Dermatology	- 9
Psychiatry	- 34	Urology	- 6
Internal Medicine	- 33	Pathology	- 4
Anesthesiology	- 4	Otolaryngology	- 9
Orthopedics	- 12	Plastic Surgery	- 4
Neurology	- 6	Other	- 6

Dentists Practicing in County by Specialty:
1978
(Total: 140)

General Practice	- 98	Pedodontics	- 10
Oral Surgery	- 8	Periodontics	- 5
Orthodontics	- 15	Prosthodontics	- 3
	Endodontics - 2		

Nursing Homes, Types and Bed Capacity: 1978

(S) Skilled (A) Intermediate A

Plaza Manor	- 115 (A)	Bay Manor	- 74 (A)
Annapolis Nursing Center -	76 (S)	Cooper Domiciliary Care	- 26
Knollwood Manor	- 86 (S)	North Arundel Conv. Center - 102 (S)	
	11 (A)	Hammonds Lane	- 80 (S)
Fairfield	- 36 (S)		20 (A)
	34 (A)	Maryland Manor	- 24 (S)
			75 (A)

County Chapters of Voluntary Health Agencies: 1978

American Lung Association	American Cancer Society
Mental Health Association	Planned Parenthood
National Paraplegia Foundation	United Way of Central Maryland
American Red Cross	

Civic Groups Active in Health Programs—1978

Public Health Lay Council
National Council of Jewish
   Women, Annapolis Section
County Counsel of Community
   Services
Rotary Club

Lions Club
Kiwanis Club
Jaycees
Community Health Associations

Woman's Club of Annapolis and Anne Arundel County

Organization of County Health Department

The Anne Arundel County Health Department was organized on a formal basis, in 1930, with the appointment of a physician to serve as full time Health Officer. Currently, the Health Officer serves in a triple capacity: as the County Health Officer (with the County Council as the Board of Health) by provision of the Anne Arundel County Charter; as the Health Officer of the City of Annapolis (with the City Council as the Board of Health) by provision of the Ordinances of the City; and as Deputy State Health Officer by provision of the Maryland State Legislature. The primary responsibility of the Health Officer is the implementation of adequate services to insure the health of the citizens and the enforcement of the health regulations promulgated by these three political subdivisions.

To fulfill these responsibilities, the Department is organized into ten basic operational divisions:

Administration
Preventive Health
Environmental Health
Mental Health
Special Health

Community Health Nursing
Communicable Disease Control
Dental Health
Health Education
Laboratory Services

The director of each division is directly responsible to the Health Officer, while staff members are responsible first to their respective division director, but ultimately to the Health Officer.

The basic philosophy of the Department, since its inception, has been to provide services directly in the communities where the recipients reside. Therefore, many of the services function on a decentralized basis.

> To accomplish this goal, a system of health centers, built and maintained by the communities, but equipped and staffed by the County, has been developed. Currently, the county has thirteen
> (continued on page 476)

Table 10-1. Anne Arundel County Health Department
Summary of Budget by Funding Source
Fiscal Year 1979

Description	Funding Formula	State	County	Federal	Total*
Administration	Case Formula (53.33% state; 46.67% local)	$332,091	$290,619		$622,710
Nutrition		3,984	3,486		7,470
Public Health Nursing	"	192,191	168,189		360,380
Medical Social Work	"	62,023	54,277		116,300
Physical Therapy	"	68,588	60,022		128,610
Occupational Therapy	"	12,202	10,678		22,880
Speech Pathology & Audiology	"	9,063	7,932		16,995
Personal Health—General	"	8,847	7,743		16,590
Child Health Programs	"	213,981	187,259		401,240
School Health Services	"	92,933	81,327		174,260
Maternity & Family Planning	"	92,730	81,150		173,880
Family Planning	"	122,568	107,262		229,830
Crippled Childrens Program	"	63,996	56,004		120,000
Dental Health Program	"	42,312	37,028		79,340
Communicable Disease Program	"	61,314	53,656		114,970
Tuberculosis Control	"	70,353	61,567		131,920
Venereal Disease Control	"	7,213	6,313		13,526
Adult Health Program	"	38,355	33,565		71,920
Chronic Illness Program	"	47,549	41,611		89,160

Table 10-1. (Continued)

Description	Funding Formula	State	County	Federal	Total*
Home Health Services	"	36,046	31,544		67,590
Geriatric Services		336	294		630
Coordinated Home Care	"	(2,933)	(2,567)		(5,500)
Federal Clinic Recovery	"	(15,466)	(13,534)		(29,000)
Environmental Health—					
General	"	82,310	72,030		154,340
Food Protection	"	100,532	87,978		188,510
Housing, Community Conservation and Vector Control	"	74,587	65,273		139,860
Rodent Eradication	"	16,086	14,078		30,164
Animal Control & Protection	"	213	187		400
Health Care Facilities	"	15,682	13,724		29,406
Water Quality & Waste Disposal Control	"	65,025	56,905		121,930
Master Plan for Water & Sewerage	"	39,998	35,002		75,000
Air Quality	(53.33% state; 46.67% local)	97,263	85,117		182,380
Public Health Education		19,984	17,489		37,473
TOTAL CASE FORMULA		$2,071,956	$1,813,208		$3,885,164

Program	Funding Source	State	County/Local	Federal	Total
Infant Stimulation	(53.33% state; 46.67% local)				
Program	100% County		59,000		59,000
Addictions Program	"		25,930		25,930
Front Footage Assessment (Health Centers)	"		6,410		6,410
Cervical Cancer Screening	100% State	6,175			6,175
Blood Pressure Screening	"	14,298			14,298
WIC Program FF	100% Federal			691,218	691,218
Geriatrics Services FF	"			27,754	27,754
Day Care Centers for Mentally Retarded Operations	75% state; 25% County	395,425	131,808		527,233
Transportation	100% State	155,637			155,637
Summer Program	100% State	32,188			32,188
Community Mental Health	90% State; 10% County	571,264	63,474		634,738
Alcoholism Program	100% State	79,992			79,992
Drug Abuse Program	"	96,500			96,500
Air Quality Grant	100% Federal			60,000	60,000
GRAND TOTAL		$3,423,435	$2,099,830	$778,972	$6,302,237

*Amounts are net of revenue—see Table 10.2.

Prepared by Mrs. Kathleen Leibe, Accountant/Auditor for the Anne Arundel County Health Department

Author's Note: The Case Formula is the formula employed by the State of Maryland to determine the amount of State money to be given to county governments for support of public health services. The State portion includes some Federal monies which are given to the states with the Federal requirement that most will be passed on to local health services. The Case Formula provides that the State will pay for half of the total approved budgets for local health services, but the exact percentage paid in each county will vary depending on the economic ability of the county to pay its share as determined by population and assessed value of property in the county. County government may appropriate more than the formula calls for, but when it does, the State will not provide the same matching share.

Table 10-2. Anne Arundel County Health Department
Summary of Budgeted Revenue by Source
FY 79

Item	Amount
Patient Fees—Clinic	$69,980
Medical Assistance Reimbursement—Clinic	67,000
Home Health Fees (92% Medicare)	89,000
Environmental Health Fees	149,000
TOTAL	$374,980

Prepared by Mrs. Kathleen Leibe, Accountant/Auditor for the Anne Arundel
County Health Department

districts, each with a health center from which Clinical, Nursing,
Home, and School Health Services are available. Several of the
centers conduct additional "outreach clinics" in isolated areas of
their respective districts.

Two Community Addiction Centers, for Alcoholism and Drug Abuse,
function in "store front" facilities, the Open Door in Annapolis and

Table 10-3. Full Time Professional Staff

Anne Arundel County Health Department 1/4/79	
Physicians	7
Dentist	1
Community Health Educator	2
Community Health Nurse	74
Psychologist	2
Social Workers & Assistants	14
Physical Therapists	6
Occupational Therapists	3
Speech Pathologist	1
Audiologist	1
Administrative Specialist	1
Accountant Auditor	1
Nutritionist	1
Public Health Engineers	3
Sanitarians	32
Public Health Trainees	2

the Open Door North in Glen Burnie; many of these patients are seen, too, in the health centers in their respective communities.

Recent construction of housing units for the low income and elderly have necessitated the development of nursing stations in the units. Presently, there are two stations in operation to provide health services and education to these residents.

Mental Health Services have been greatly augmented since 1973 by the establishment of Comprehensive Mental Health Units; in Glen Burnie, to serve the northern section of the county, and in the Health Services Building to serve the southern section of the county.

The Department has earned international recognition for the development of this system of providing services to the residents of this county. To date, seven hundred and eighty-nine health officials from ninety-one countries have visited Anne Arundel County to observe the Health Department. The United States Department of State has presented a commendation plaque to the County Health Department for its participation in the training of foreign health officials.

Facilities Utilized by the Health Department (1978)

The concept of community owned health centers, unique to Anne Arundel County, began almost simultaneously with the establishment of the Department as full time unit. Originally, interested citizens formed Community Health Associations to seek adequate facilities from which the Department could function in their respective communities. These facilities have gradually evolved from midwives homes, church halls, school buildings, and store fronts, into Health Centers, built and financed by these Health Associations. Presently, there are eleven centers owned by Associations and utilized full time as the bases from which Community Health services are made available in the districts these centers serve. The eleven centers and the clinic sessions per month, individually, are:

BROOKLYN PARK	- 26	MAGOTHY	- 10
CHURCHTON	- 8	ODENTON	- 21
DAVIDSONVILLE-MAYO	- 11	PAROLE	- 13
GLEN BURNIE	- 33	ST. MARGARETS	- 5
FRIENDSHIP	- 14	SEVERNA PARK	- 13
SOUTH SHORE	- 11		

Two health centers, owned by the County and utilized full time, complete the system of thirteen health districts and the centers serving each:

ANNAPOLIS - Headquarters of the County Health Department. Sixty-eight clinic sessions per month, including eleven evening clinics.

NORTHEAST - Facility provided by Department of Education. Nine clinic sessions per month.

To provide service in the isolated areas of these districts, extension or "outreach clinics" have been initiated and function in quarters provided by the community. These areas include:

Bacontown   Stanton

Services of the Department are available too, in quarters provided in several housing projects of the City and County. To date, these Nursing stations are functioning in:

Meade Village   Robinwood

Two facilities, serving as the centers for the Alcohol and Drug Abuse Programs, have reverted to the use of "store fronts"; the Open Door, 62 Cathedral Street in Annapolis, and the Open Door North, 12 U Crain Highway in Glen Burnie.

FEE FOR SERVICES

The Maryland State Legislature, in 1975, enacted Senate Bill 972 requiring that all County Health Departments establish and collect fees for certain services. Each patient's fee is determined, individually, on the basis of ability to pay. However, no one is denied service if the fee is unaffordable.

Adolescent Clinic	Gynecology
Adult Health	Maternity
Alcoholic Rehabilitation Clinic	Mental Health
Child Health Assessment	Methadone Clinic
Child Health Conference	Occupational Therapy
Dental Clinic	Open Door Addictions Center
Family Planning	Pediatric Consultation
General Diagnostic	Physical Therapy
Geriatric Clinic	Speech Pathology

STAFF

All positions allotted to the Department are classified by the Secretary of Personnel under the Merit System of the State of Maryland. All staff members must possess the required qualifications for their specific position, pass a written examination, and serve a six month probationary period before attaining a permanent appointment.

With the advent of the Comprehensive Education and Training Act, (CETA), federal funds, made available to the County, are utilized to obtain additional personnel for this Department. These employees function on a temporary basis, and must be eligible for Merit System classification prior to attaining a permanent appointment.

> The service and facilities of the Anne Arundel County Department of Health are operated on a non-discriminatory basis. This prohibits discrimination on the basis of race, color, religion, political affiliation or opinion, national origin, age, sex or handicap in the provision of services, use of facilities, opportunity to participate, employment practices and granting of advantages, privileges and accommodations.

Preventive Health Services

Historically, the motto of this Department has been "Tomorrow's Health Depends Upon Today's Prevention." In keeping with this philosophy, a series of services, categorized as Preventive Health Services, is provided consisting of: Maternal Health; Pregnancy Screening; Family Planning; Infant, Child, and Adolescent Health; WIC; School Health; Day Care Supervision; and Crippled Children's Services. Each of these services function in close association with the private practice of medicine, dentistry, and the allied agencies. Preventive Health encompasses too, not only the maintenance of good health, but the necessary follow up procedures to assure that those who are ill or disabled are accorded the opportunity to obtain correction or amelioration of their abnormalities.

MATERNAL HEALTH

The availability and utilization of maternity supervision for every expectant mother is the objective of both the private practice of medicine and the Health Department. To achieve this objective, the Department provides Maternity Clinics on a regularly scheduled basis in each of the thirteen community health centers and for outreach clinics located in the County. Physician service in these clinics is primarily provided by Residents (Obstetrical) from Johns Hopkins and University of Maryland Hospitals.

The frequency of clinic visits is in accordance with the prevailing practice: first to seventh month of pregnancy, visit every month; eighth month of pregnancy, visit every two weeks; and the ninth month of pregnancy, visit every week.

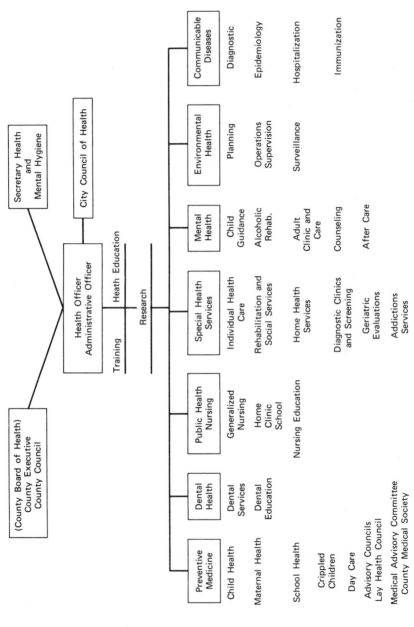

Since laboratory services are a state health department function but only housed in the offices of the county health department, the laboratory unit does not appear on the local organization chart.

480

In sequence, the clinic visit includes a review, with the Community Health Nurse, of the patients' progress to date; a summary of the procedures for the present clinic; the examination and interview by Clinician; consultation with the Nutritionist concerning special diet during pregnancy, the interpretation of the clinic team's recommendation by the Community Health Nurse, and a discussion of plans for delivery in a hospital. Subsequent home visits by the Community Health Nurse implement the planned program of maternity supervision.

The provision of two monthly Obstetrical Consultation clinics (Johns Hopkins Referral Clinic) enables family physicians or the Maternity Clinics to refer expectant mothers with complications of pregnancy for specialized care. Patients with such complications are delivered at the Johns Hopkins Hospital through a special arrangement between this Department and the Hospital.

In the post partum period, each patient returns for a complete examination. The clinicans refer those with complications to the Gynecological Consultation clinics and therapy, where indicated, is performed by the family physician, a specialist, or a hospital service on referral.

Family Planning is emphasized in the post partum period too, and arranged according to the method selected by the patient, to allow those families who desire, to space pregnancies in accordance with socio-economic, physical, and emotional consideration.

Two pregnancy screening clinics, in Annapolis and in Glen Burnie, are held weekly, by appointment only, either on order of a private physician or on a self referral basis. All patients, pregnant or not, are counseled by social workers concerning their individual follow up and all patients receive initial counseling in Family Planning by a Planned Parenthood Volunteer. If Health Department Maternity Services are requested, these services are provided to the patient thru the health center located in the patient's respective community.

Recent innovation to Maternity Health Services is providing "Early Periodic Screening for Diagnosis and Treatment" to all maternity patients under 21 years of age.

Under the W.I.C. Program, dietary supplements are available to the prenatal and lactating mother at all centers.

The recent construction of housing units for the low income and elderly has necessitated the establishment of Nursing Stations in these units. Two stations are currently functioning; both providing Family Planning, Maternity, Child Health, and Nursing Conference clinics on a regularly scheduled basis.

TERMINATION OF PREGNANCY

In accordance with the provision of Maryland State Law, pregnancy can be terminated. Patients may elect therapeutic abortion after a positive pregnancy screening test and consultation with a medical social worker.

Patients without medical complications can visit an approved facility where the workup is performed by the facility staff; patients with complications are referred to the Fertility Control Clinic at The Johns Hopkins Hospital for advice.

FAMILY PLANNING SERVICES

Family Planning Services, available in the thirteen health centers and augmented by outreach clinics in three other communities, are supplemented by the federally funded Family Planning Project, through the State Department of Health and Mental Hygiene. The federal assistance enables this Department to provide thirty clinic sessions each month, five of which are held after 5:00 p.m., for the conveniece of the patients.

A group of volunteers trained by the Planned Parenthood and Health Department personnel, give additional assistance to the nurse by conducting group sessions on methods of Family Planning.

Patients participating in the program receive a complete physical evaluation which entails (1) Health and Medical History; (2) Physical examination; (3) Blood tests (S.T.S., Hgb., Hematocrit); (4) Pap smear and G. C. culture; (5) Urinalysis; (6) Blood pressure; (7) Weight. This evaluation is performed at the time of admittance and annually, thereafter, by the clinic physician.

The monthly Gynecological Consultation clinic is available for patients with problems and if further services are necessary, referral can be made to either the Johns Hopkins Hospital or the University of Maryland Hospital.

INFANT AND CHILD HEALTH

The infant, child, and immunization programs follow the established public health practices of preventive pediatrics. The Child Health Conference (clinic) consists of history; health appraisal; measurements of height, weight and head circumference; developmental testing; speech-language, vision, hearing, and dental screening; tuberculin testing; hematocrit; blood lead level; phenylketonuria; thyroxine; urinalysis for protein and sugar; sickle cell anemia; blood pressure; physical examination; and immunizations against communicable disease. While the majority of these procedures are performed routinely, others are done where applicable. In most instances, parent education and/or consultation is provided.

The Infant and Child Health Services, historically available to all children, became mandatory in 1972, for all individuals age 0 - 6 who were eligible for Medical Assistance (Title XIX, Social Security Act, 1967). Currently, the age limitation has been extended to 21 years; family planning and maternity patients, under 21, are provided these services, too.

The Immunization program, available in these clinics, includes vaccines for diptheria, tetanus, pertussis, poliomyelitis, measles, rubella and mumps. All of these immunizations, with the exception of mumps, are mandatory for any child entering a Maryland school unless a medical contraindication, signed by a physician, or a bonafide religious exemption is presented by the parent.

Patients may be referred to these services by private physician, allied community agencies, self-referral, or as a result of a principal-nurse conference under the School Health Services. Patients requiring follow up are referred to private physicians, dentists, hospitals, or the various specialized clinics offered by this Department, e.g. orthopedic, seizure, cardiac, etc.

The Child Health Conferences are supplemented by Child Health Assessment sessions, wherein the community health nurse administers the vaccines, provides counseling periods, and continues the health appraisal with additional screening procedures when indicated.

ADOLESCENT CLINIC

An innovation in the Preventive Health Services was the establishment of an Adolescent clinic, in 1974, to provide preventive health care to all youth of the County aged 13 to 21 years. The clinic is designed specifically for individuals in that age group with concerns or questions concerning physical, mental, or social health; variations in growth and development; personality problems; or general appearance.

The clinic is staffed by a physician, dentist, nurse, social worker, and vision-hearing technicians, however, other specialized personnel are available for testing, assistance, or referral. The procedure for the clinic includes some or all of the following: history, physical examination, dental evaluation, health appraisal, developmental evaluation, vision-hearing screening, immunizations, tuberculin test, hematocrit, and urinalysis. G. C. cultures, pap smears, and sickle cell screening are provided where applicable. All patients are interviewed by the social worker.

The evening clinics, functioning twice a month in Annapolis, and once a month in Brooklyn Park, are not designed to accept or care for cases of acute illness; they provide counseling, screening, health education, and therapy only.

SPECIAL SUPPLEMENTAL FOOD PROGRAM FOR WOMEN, INFANTS, AND CHILDREN
WIC

The WIC program, funded by the United States Department of Agriculture, enables this Department to provide free supplemental food and nutrition education to eligible participants. Potential participants must: reside in Anne Arundel County; be enrolled in the Health Department clinics; meet specific economic standards; and be confirmed to be at nutritional risk through physical examination at the clinic.

Trained interviewers are present in all Health Department Maternal and

Child Health clinics, located throughout the County, to assist individuals with application procedures. Eligibility is then determined by the WIC Coordinator-Nutritionist on the basis of the application information and clinical data. The food supplements are available to pregnant, lactating, or post partum women; infants; and children up to age five, who have met the eligibility requirements.

SCHOOL HEALTH PROGRAM

School Health Services, the joint responsibility of the Departments of Health and Education, are formulated each year by the Health-Education Council. The council includes representatives from these two Departments, the County Council of P.T.A.'s, the Western Shore Dental Society, and the County Medical Society. In this Department, the specific responsibility for conducting the services is that of the Chief of School Health Services, (a full time pediatrician) and the staff of community health nurses. In the schools, the responsibility rests with the Health Team consisting of the teacher, the counselor, the principal, pupil personnel worker, the community health nurse and/or other appropriate professionals. In every instance, however, the final responsibility must be that of the parent and the family physician.

The segments of the program which this Department provides include health and dental examination, hearing and vision screening, and assessment by the nurses. Many of these evaluations are obtained in the regular Child Health Conferences provided by this Department.

The Health Examination* is encouraged for every pupil prior to entering school for the first time; for every pupil transferring to the County School System for the first time; for every pupil referred by the Health Team; and annually for every participant on an inter-school athletic team in secondary schools.

The Dental Examination* is encouraged for every pupil prior to entering school for the first time; for every pupil entering the seventh grade; for every pupil transferring to the County School System for the first time; and for every pupil referred by the Health Team.

Hearing Screening* is provided for every pupil in kindergarten; grades 1, 3, and 8; those referred from Special Education or speech-language therapy; those receiving itinerant vision resource services; pupils who failed the screening the previous year; and any pupil referred by parent, school or health personnel, or upon self referral.

Vision Screening* is provided for every pupil entering kindergarten or grade

---

* Pupils transferring to the Anne Arundel County School System may be excused from these procedures if written evidence is presented proving that they have undergone these examinations within the past year.

1; grades 3, 6, and 8; those referred from Special Education; those receiving itinerant hearing resource services; pupils who failed the screening the previous year; and any pupil referred by parent, school or health personnel, or upon self referral.

These Vision and Hearing evaluations are performed by full time and part time audio visual technicians on the staff of this Department, and are provided to private and parochial schools, too. Volunteers, trained and supervised by the nurses and technicians, render an invaluable service by participating in these screening sessions. Screening is available to younger children in the E.N.T. Clinics, Day Care Center, Kindergartens, and classes for retarded and handicapped. Children found with deficiencies are being followed and corrections obtained prior to their entrance into the schools.

Physical and Occupational Therapy evaluation and treatment is provided as prescribed by a physician.

Height and weight measurements are taken on any pupil referred by parent, school, or health personnel.

Since January, 1973, it has been mandatory that all pupils admitted to any public or private nursery, kindergarten, or elementary school in the State, furnish evidence of primary immunizations against diptheria, tetanus, pertussis, polio, measles (rubeola) and rubella (German measles) in a manner approved by the County Health Officer. Two exceptions to this regulation are religious conflict or medical contraindications signed by a physician.

The responsibility for enforcing the provisions of the regulation is delegated jointly to the Superintendent of Schools and the Health Officer of the County.

Assessment by the community health nurse is performed on request of the principal of the school concerned or by Pupil Personnel Staff. The nurse provides counseling in the home, too, if requested by the Health Team.

SCHOOL HEALTH AIDE PROGRAM

With the allocation of twenty five CETA positions, this Department, in conjunction with the Department of Education, recruited, trained, and assigned full time School Health Aides to twenty five secondary schools in November of 1977. These aides must successfully complete an extensive orientation course, with major emphasis on first aid, conducted by this Department prior to their assignments. The aides function in the health suite of the school by providing temporary care and first aid to all students reporting to the suite.

SCHOOL HEALTH SERVICES FOR SPECIAL EDUCATION

In accordance with federal legislation (Public Law 94-142) health services have been designed to meet the unique needs of handicapped children who are to receive their education in the Public School System. These services are provided by full time, qualified personnel, in the Oakwood Elementary, Marley Glen, Ft. Smallwood Center, and the Central complex, public schools.

The personnel, on the staff of the Health Department, includes: community healh nurses, physical therapist, occupational therapists, licensed practical nurses, and therapy assistants; the services they provide to the pupils is on specific order of a physician. They are available, too, to provide guidance, as requested, to the teacher in the classroom.

Additionally, an audiologist provides service and counseling to pupils with hearing loss and is available to the school personnel for consultation.

All staff members provide, too, counseling and education to the parents of these children.

DAY CARE CENTERS

The Division of Preventive Health is responsible, too, for the supervision of private and public day care centers, and nurseries. The Day Care Team, consisting of the Chief of School Health Services (a full time pediatrician), the Coordinator of Day Care Licensing (Environmental Health), the Specialist in Early Childhood Development, a part time Community Health Nurse, and an Environmental Health Aide, function in unison to supervise these centers. Major emphasis is placed upon upgrading the standards of day care centers through conferences, workshops, in service training for credits, and consultation. Based upon the recommendations of the Team, this Department issues licenses to those centers (excluding those centers under auspices of Department of Education) meeting the requirements of the Day Care Regulations adopted by the State Department of Health and Mental Hygiene.

The Division provides screening for all children in these centers for Hearing, Vision, and Speech defects. The full range of Preventive Health Services is offered to all children in the Child Development centers operated by both the Department of Social Services and the Community Action Agency.

CRIPPLED CHILDRENS' SERVICES

The Crippled Childrens' Services, available to any youngster up to age 21, are provided thru specialized clinics; specifically: Cardiac; Ear, Nose and Throat; Hearing, Speech-Language; Pediatric Neurology; Orthopedic; Plastic; Seizure; and Vision. All clinicians conducting these specialized clinics meet the eligibility requirements of their specialties and the State Department of Health and Mental Hygiene. Since early discovery and amelioration of deviant health is extremely important, the clinicians in the Child Health or Pediatric Consultation clinics refer all patients with obvious or suspected anomalies to the appropriate specialty clinic outlined above.

Private physicians in the community very frequently utilize the facilities and services of the Crippled Childrens' Program by referring their patients to specific special clinics. The Department of Education, too, utilize these services and referrals are made as a result of teacher nurse, or nurse principal conferences; direct referral by a principal, or referrals may be initiated by Pupil Personnel staff.

Children with apparent or suspected genetic abnormality, (mental retardation or cerebral palsy) can be referred in the same manner and are either seen in the specialty clinic appropriate to their specific problem or by specialized personnel such as a psychologist, vision and hearing technician, speech pathologist, dentist, or multiproblem clinician.

To preserve the quality of service and prevent over-crowding of those highly specialized clinics, all referrals are reviewed by the Director of the Division of Preventive Health. The Director is available for consultation at all of these clinic sessions and arranges, too, for admissions to Baltimore hospitals or private facilities, when the need arises.

The facilities of this Department are augmented by the Diagnostic and Evaluation clinic at the Johns Hopkins Hospital, and the Central Evaluation clinic at the University of Maryland Hospital. Referrals to these clinics are processed through the offices of the Crippled Childrens' Services at the State Department of Health and Mental Hygiene.

MULTIPROBLEM SERVICE

A specialized program of major import is the multiproblem service conducted by the Deputy Director of the Division of Preventive Health. Children referred to this service are predominately of pre-school age with multiple handicaps. These handicaps may be physical, e.g. an orthopedic with a severe vision problem or a combination of physical and mental, e.g. mental retardation with a severe physical handicap. The objective of this service is to accumulate and correlate information; determine the present physical and mental status of the patient; and plan for both immediate and future management. Children with handicapping conditions and who require additional special services can acquire these services through the Crippled Childrens' Program if they meet the eligibility requirements.

SPECIAL FACILITY PLACEMENT

Select representatives from the Departments of Health and Education constitute the Admission, Review, Dismissal Committee to review each child for placement in a special facility (may be out of state). Candidates for these special placements are children with learning disabilities; those classified as educable mentally retarded; those with hearing impairments; the physically handicapped; the emotionally disturbed; and those with communication disorders.

It must be ascertained, too, that there is no program available in the County Public School System to accommodate these children.

Data available on the candidate from the community health nurse, physical therapists, or other members of the staff, are provided to this committee via the Chief of School Health Services who is this Department's representative. The decisions of the committee are forwarded to the Department of Education for appropriate action.

Environmental Health Services

Among the responsibilities of the Health Department are the implementation of services to insure the environmental health and safety of the residents of the County, and the enforcement of State and County Laws, Rules, and Regulations applicable thereto. One hundred thirty specific environmental health services, constituting thirty major program activities, are provided annually through this Department's Division of Environmental Health, and, in every instance of enforcement, educational and informational measures are the primary methods utilized to achieve compliance.

To facilitate the numerous functions of the Division, it is consolidated into four sections: Community Hygiene, Consumer Protection, Sanitary Engineering, and Air Quality Control; radio communication is utilized from field to office; and all data are collected and stored by use of an Electronic Data Processing System.

COMMUNITY HYGIENE SECTION

The responsibilities of this section include Residential Environment, Mobile Home Parks, Rodent and Vector Control, General Nuisance complaints and General Preventive Disease Control. Due to the nature of these services, the section is involved in the legal aspects of code enforcement and each case is setup as a legal case file in the event court action is necessary to achieve compliance.

Residential Environment, the implementation of the County's Housing Maintenance and Occupancy Code, is generally: the investigation of all complaints concerning violations of the Code; housing quality appraisal and code enforcement survey; and the biannual inspection and licensing of all multiple dwellings in the County. Housing information is compiled too, for assistance in developing housing plans and determining needs for the County Office of Planning and Zoning, the Regional Planning Council, and the State Department of Economic and Community Development. Staff members assigned to Housing, work closely with Federal, State, and County agencies, serve on task forces, technical committees and planning groups for determining regional and local housing conditions and needs, and are an integral part of the planning and implementation of the County Community Block Grant Program.

Mobile Home Parks, although basically housing units, are governed by separate and specific State and County Ordinances. Each of the twenty nine parks in this County are inspected approximately four times annually, and a unit-by-unit inspection is made prior to each annual re-licensing period. Drinking water samples are taken monthly from parks with private water systems and the sewage disposal systems are inspected concurrently; plans and specifications for alterations or additions to the parks are reviewed by staff members of this section. When enforcement action is required, it is accomplished in conjunction with the County Department of Inspections and Permits, the Fire Prevention Bureau, and the Office of Planning and Zoning. There are no housing regulations concerning the interior of these mobile homes.

Rodent and Vector Control services are provided by three staff members, certified by the Maryland State Department of Agriculture in the use of rodenticides and pesticides. The service includes bait setting, burrow gassing, and education and counsel to individuals and community groups on the preventive measures to control rodent infestation. Baiting and gassing operations are performed on a massive scale in areas of heavy infestation, and approximately thirty new rodent control provisions have been added to the Housing Code to achieve prevention of infestation in new structures built for human occupancy. Citizen requests for investigation and advice on insect infestations, too, are handled by staff of this section and appropriate referrals made when necessary.

General Nuisance Complaints, classified under Article 43, Sections 49 and 50 of the Maryland State Health Laws, are investigated, evaluated, and abated by this section's personnel. Abatement of these health hazards is very often achieved by mutual action with other County and State agencies as well as a system of informal conferences and hearings with property owners and agency staff. All efforts to abate these hazards are primarily oriented toward advice and health education relating to the particular circumstances, but when necessary, legal action is instituted, with the advice and counsel of the State's Attorney, as the final persuasion to achieve compliance with State and County health codes.

General Preventive disease activities, conducted by trained staff of the Community Hygiene section, involve: occupational health investigations in conjunction with the Maryland Department of Labor and Industry; radiological health services in cooperation with the Maryland State Department of Health and Mental Hygiene; assistance in operation of rabies vaccination clinics; and doing field investigations related to control of rabies; working closely with County Animal Control Agency; supervising the destruction of dangerous drugs and other substances in cooperation with city and county police departments and State's Attorney's Office; site approvals for fumigations conducted by private exterminators; providing photographic services for this Department; and participation in all mass immunization programs conducted by the Health Department.

CONSUMER PROTECTION SECTION

To facilitate the administration for these services, there are five functional units operating within this section: Food Service Facilities, Markets and Food Processing, Institutional Services, Water Quality, and the City of Annapolis.

Perpetual surveillance of Food and Milk products protects the citizens from food borne diseases, fraud, spoilage, and unsanitary practices in the production and distribution of these products. The techniques employed consist of inspections, sampling, plan review, education and consultation, and enforcement of the "Regulations Governing Food Service Facilities" (COMAR 10.03.15) of the State Department of Health and Mental Hygiene. The responsibility for all Food and Milk Control is shared by the Food Service Facilities unit, and the Market and Food Processing unit; these two units inspect and monitor all aspects of food processing and distribution in the County.

The Food Service Facilities unit routinely inspects all public eating and drinking establishments on a biannual basis with reinspection or enforcement action conducted as required (Fig. 10-1). Currently, there are over fourteen hundred such establishments, and grocery outlets operating in the County; for each new or remodeled facility, plans must be reviewed by this section and inspections made at the completion of construction for issuance of Occupany certificates. The Public schools are inspected at least twice per year for proper food handling techniques, in conjunction with an inspection of the premises to determine the general environmental status to insure the safety and health of the student. These inspection results are transmitted as a combined annual report to the Anne Arundel County Board of Education, but items requiring immediate correction are channeled directly.

In addition to the routine inspections of permanent establishments and mobile food trucks, the Food Service Facilities Unit inspects the sites of all special events (carnivals, fairs, crab feasts, etc.) where food is served by non-professional food handlers using temporary facilities. Special attention and considerable counseling is required, in these instances, to ensure that adequate food sanitation is maintained; the staff function after hours and on weekends to accomplish this supervision.

The Markets and Food Processing Unit is responsible for all facets of the food industry related to processing, commercial transportation, warehousing,

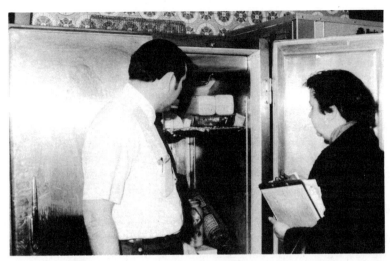

Figure 10—1. Sanitarian inspects restaurant refrigeration equipment. Routine inspection of food-service facilities is an important part of all local health-department work, serving to minimize the danger of disease from food contamination through food handling, processing, and storage. (Courtesy of the Anne Arundel County Health Department.)

and retail facilities in this county; inspections are made in all stores, markets, supermarkets, bakeries, trucks, truck depots, plants or factories in the county. Warehousing and processing plants are inspected in conjunction with the State of Maryland and the Food and Drug Administration to assure compliance with state and federal regulations.

Personnel from this unit monitor, too, the quality of shellfish (oysters, clams, crabs, mussels) and the waters from which they are harvested; all must conform to standards developed by the United States Public Health Service and the State Department of Health and Mental Hygiene prior to this Department granting approval for interstate or intrastate distribution. All shucking and packing plants are inspected and the products sampled on a monthly basis; clam harvesters and shippers are monitored daily throughout the season; all shellfish boats operating in county waters; and all trucks transporting the products are inspected routinely.

This unit functions, also, in Civil disorders or natural disasters by aiding in the determination of safe food sources; the safe destruction of contaminated foods; and public education regarding water purification.

Assistance is routinely provided, by personnel team both the Food Service Facilities Unit and the Markets and Processing Unit, to food service operators for in-service training for their personnel, and/or on site consultation to improve sanitation practices.

The Water Quality Unit endeavors to maintain the quality of the waters of Anne Arundel County, not only for the harvesting of shellfish as required by the National Shellfish Sanitation Program, but for recreational use as well. Under the provisions of the National Shellfish Sanitation Program, the entire shoreline of the County must be minutely surveyed every ten years to detect and correct any source of sewage discharge into the shellfish producing waters. Included in the surveillance of the four hundred thirty one linear miles of shoreline is the weekly sampling of the effluent from all sewage treatment plants discharging into shellfish harvesting waters and the offshore samples collected routinely of the waters over the shellfish harvesting areas. If these samples are below acceptable standards, the areas are closed to harvesting until the source of pollution is located, abated, and the samples again meet acceptable standards.

Recreational water quality is monitored, too, by this unit; during the summer months all public and community beaches are inspected on a monthly basis and weekly water samples are obtained to assure that the quality of water is acceptable for recreational use as well.

In the event of a sewage discharge from a public or private facility, the body of water involved is immediately posted prohibiting water contact activities. All residents of the water front homes concerned, and all Improvement associations are notified by personnel from this unit.

Marinas, too, are monitored by this unit, with emphasis on the cleanliness of their public facilities, adequate sewage disposal, and proper trash collection and removal.

The Institutional Services Unit is responsible for the surveillance of hospitals, nursing homes, penal and mental institutions, halfway houses, day care centers, nursery schools, kindergartens, and placement homes (foster, adoption, family day care). The personnel endeavor to ensure that applicable State regulations and approved public health practices are adhered to by these facilities. In many instances, the unit functions on a consultive basis, providing environmental evaluation of facilities, and/or workshops or in-service training courses in environmental hygiene.

Several staff members from this unit serve, too, as member of this Department's Day Care Team which inspects, supervises, and recommends for licensure, all day care centers and pre-schools operating in the County. Based upon the recommendation of the Team, this Department issues the required license for these facilities to operate in this County.

The City of Annapolis is assigned one senior sanitarian from this section to function exclusively within the City limits. Services provided include the inspection of all food service facilities and schools; the investigation and abatement of nuisance complaints; participation in all Annapolis Urban Development projects; and assistance in the enforcement of the City Housing

Code and Ordinances. The sanitarian is responsible for all Environmental Health programs in the City with the exception of air quality, swimming pools, and institutional services which are referred to the appropriate staff member in the Division of Environmental Health.

SANITARY ENGINEERING

The County Administration's Capital Improvements Program for the construction of public water supply and sewage treatment facilities has progressed; currently, fifty five per cent of the residents are being provided these services. The Sanitary Engineering Section is responsible for monitoring these facilities and for supervising the installation and maintenance of the private facilities upon which forty five per cent of the residents must still depend. Services related to water and sewage are also within the province of this section - namely scavenger operations, swimming pool maintenance, landfill facilities, river water sampling, and complaints incurred by malfunctioning private water supply and sewage disposal systems.

In the effort to assure that all water supplied to residents of the County is both potable and in adequate quantity, specific procedures have been developed. The location of all wells, both private and commercial, is predicated upon the plan review, recommendations and approval of this section prior to the installation, and all new water wells are tested for bacteriological contamination before becoming operational. Public water supplies throughout the County are regularly sampled to guard against bacteriological and chemical contamination, as are all private wells upon the request of the individual using water from this source.

The prevention of sewage contamination in the sources of water supply and the waterways of the County necessitates proper installation and maintenance of all sewage disposal systems and sewage treatment plants. The installation of all individual sewage disposal systems, or the required additions thereto, is approved only after certain criteria are met. The soil in which the system is to function must be permeable as evidenced by the successful percolation test. In areas of the County where a fluctuating high water table is indicated on the Soil Survey maps, percolation tests are performed only between February 1st and April 30th. The building lot must be of sufficient size to accommodate the system planned, considering house size, number of inhabitants, auxiliary disposal equipment (automatic washer, etc), location of adjacent water wells, and adequate area for replacement of the system if ever required. Based upon this data, the system is designed specifically for the individual lot and installed under the general supervision of a staff member from the Compliance Unit of this section to assure that the recommended design, components, size of system, and legal requirements have been adhered to.

Percolation tests are performed, too, on any land scheduled for development, with a minimum of one test per acre required prior to approval of the area for subdivision.

Commercial and/or industrial establishments planned for construction in non-public sewer areas of the County must install either extensive sewage disposal systems or package sewage treatment plants, both of which require the submission of detailed engineering plans for review and approval. The package sewage treatment plants necessarily discharge their effluent into the waterways of the County; it must be ascertained, therefore, that the effluent has been sufficiently treated prior to discharge. This is accomplished by monthly inspections, and sampling of the effluent from each plant; frequent consultations with the operators for improvement of function or the facility; and dye testing or laboratory analysis when indicated.

Closely associated with the maintenance of private sewage disposal systems is the periodic pumping of the septic tanks performed by Septic Tank Cleaning contractors. These contractors, referred to as "scavenger", utilize the content of septic tanks on airtight tank trucks, to remove the content of septic tanks and transport it to approved dumping sites. Services provided to assure the sanitary operation of the scavengers begin with annual inspection of all equipment; the dump sites are initially approved and monthly inspections conducted thereafter to insure efficient functioning. Permits and licenses are issued to all contractors meeting the requirements of State and County laws; additionally, each contractor, under County Regulations, must be bonded to guarantee satisfactory performance. A continual surveillance is maintained to prevent the operation of non-licensed scavengers or the use of illegal dump sites.

Swimming pool construction and maintenance is supervised by personnel of this section in accordance with State and County Ordinances. Both public and private residential pools are included, but with major emphasis necessarily on public pools. Plans and specifications for all pools must be reviewed and approved prior to installation and those functioning with the backwash cleaning of the filters must dispose of the effluent in the same manner as sewage. The County Swimming Pool Ordinance, adopted in 1972 and supplemental to State Ordinances, requires the licensing of all public pools, operators and lifeguards, as well as outlining definite standards for pool operation and penalties for the violation thereof. Of basic importance is the maintenance of the pool waters, therefore, biweekly visits are made to check turbidity, chlorine, and pH with monthly water sampling of both pool and potable water supplies. A complete inspection is performed once per season to assure satisfactory operation; consultations and follow up inspections are utilized if indicated.

Sanitary landfill facilities, the primary method for disposing of solid waste utilized in this County, are issued permits to function after design plans and specifications have been jointly reviewed and approved by representatives from the Sanitary Engineering Section; the Public Works Department; the Office of Planning and Zoning; the State Department of Health and Mental Hygiene; and the State Department of Natural Resources. The operation of the landfill is then supervised by staff from this section in the form of monthly inspections, compilation of reports, and field consultations. Efforts are expended to continually improve landfill operations to meet Health Department standards and while significant progress has been made with most facilities, some have been required to cease operations for continued failure to comply. Landfills function, too, as land reclamation projects, for when the capacity of the area is reached, the land is available for other uses, e.g., golf course, park, etc.

While strict surveillance of all waterways in the County is perpetuated by the Consumer Protection Section, supplementary surveillance of the Patuxent River Watershed and the Severn River Watershed is provided by the Sanitary Engineering Section. Effluent from several major sewage treatment plants is discharged into these watersheds, therefore, State and County Regulations designated definite procedures to insure the quality of these waters. Samples are collected, monthly, of the effluent from the individual treatment plants, and of the water, both upstream and downstream, from each plant's point of discharge. Sample results are compiled and if improvements, additions, or corrections are indicated, they are effected in coordination with the State Department of Health and Mental Hygiene.

Finally, the Sanitary Engineering Section receives all complaints relating to unsanitary conditions involving any of the above areas of responsibility. Each complaint is investigated, and correction achieved through consultation, education, or legal action.

AIR QUALITY CONTROL

The Air Quality Control Section became operational in 1965, when as a result of the Clean Air Act of 1963, the Metropolitan Baltimore Air Quality Survey was initiated. The survey, a joint venture of Anne Arundel County, Baltimore County, Baltimore City, and the State Department of Health, was instrumental in establishing a network of air sampling stations (three in this County) to study the ambient air quality and identify the major pollutant sources in the metropolitan Baltimore area. Data acquired during the survey were utilized in the development of ambient air quality standards and the regulatory methods designed to achieve them.

Currently, this section operates a network of permanent air monitoring stations, with supplementary temporary sites, to determine pollution trends, the effectiveness of control procedures, and the effect of two major metropolitan areas on the quality of the air over the county. These stations, utilizing a variety of methods and equipment, measure both contaminants and meteorology parameters. The contaminants include: particulates (settleable and suspended dusts, dirt, metals, sulfur and hydrocarbon compounds), sulfur dioxide, carbon monoxide, hydrocarbons, nitrogen dioxide, and ozone. The meteorological parameters are: wind speed and direction, and temperatures, measured for correlation with the contaminant levels. Samples are procured for time periods varying from a few minutes to twenty four hour daily; specific instruments operate constantly, thus providing a continuous record of contaminant levels for each day of the year. These stations were recently integrated with a statewide system, AIRMON, which retrieves data from instruments via telephone lines, processes it in a central computer, and sends the information to teletype terminals at local agencies. Information acquired by this network of sampling stations measures long range trends of contaminant levels, detects "hot spots" of pollution, and serves to determine the effectiveness of local, state, and regional abatement efforts.

The Section registers and maintains vigilance, too, on all sizable sources of emissions e.g. existing and proposed industrial, commercial and governmental installations. Presently, over eight hundred fifty installations at three hundred sixty premises are registered. Site inspections are made concurrent with application for registration; thereafter, bi-annual inspections, fuel sampling, observations for visible emission, and stack emission tests are made to insure compliance with applicable regulatory provisions (Fig. 10-2). Establishments found to be in violation are required to correct the deficiencies within an allotted time or suspend operations, many local firms have made significant investments in pollution control equipment resulting in substantial reductions in emission. In exceptional circumstances, however, the regulatory suspension date may be extended if a plan for compliance is negotiated.

A plan for compliance is a time schedule of actions submitted by the installation owner and, upon the recommendation of this Department, approved by the Secretary of Health and Mental Hygiene. To negotiate such a plan, the owner must demonstrate that: a method for expedient abatement is not readily available; design, purchase, and installation of specific equipment over a time period is required; or changes in process and/or materials or fuels are necessary.

To further the reduction of air pollution, effective controls are also maintained on open burning, fugitive dusts, emission from furnaces and automobiles, and the sulfur content of fuels. Open burning for construction land clearing, demolition, or agricultural purposes is allowed only by authorization of the Control Officer (Health Officer). Upon application for a permit to burn, a site inspection is made to determine if minimun distance restrictions and fire prevention requirements can be met; if not, the authorization is denied.

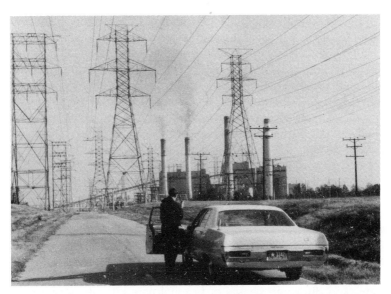

Figure 10–2. Sanitarian monitoring smokestack emissions. Air-pollution control is of growing importance in our industrial society for maintenance of the public's health and the quality of the environment. (Courtesy of the Anne Arundel County Health Department.)

Sulfur content of fuels cannot, by legislation, exceed one per cent by weight limit being burned. Each residual fuel oil and coal user is registered by this section and visited twice during the winter heating season for sampling.

Anne Arundel County is included too, in the federally designated Metropolitan Baltimore Intrastate Air Quality Control Region which encompasses the City of Baltimore and the counties of Baltimore, Carroll, Harford, and Howard. A plan has been instituted to closely monitor and to reverse increasing pollutant levels during period of air stagnation over this region; such periods are termed "air pollution episodes". During these episodes, usually of two to three days duration, periodic bulletins are issued through the news media advising susceptible individuals to take precautionary measures and the general public to curtail their pollution producing activities. Concurrently, section personnel implement prearranged measures with all commercial, industrial and governmental establishments to reduce emissions to the minimum.

Mental Health Services

Mental Health Services, first established by this Department in 1934, are currently designed to foster the prevention and/or early detection and treatment of mental illness in all aspects of personal and community health, and, to provide these services in facilities readily accessible to all citizens.

To facilitate the delivery of services, the Division of Mental Health functions under the direction of a full time psychiatrist; a second psychiatrist serves as full time director of the Glen Burnie Community Mental Health Center, established in 1971. Professional staff assigned to the Division include, in addition, psychologists, psychiatric social consultants, social workers, and community health nurses. Recent additions to the full time staff include two mental health associates and one licensed practical nurse. The part time staff consists of ten psychiatrists, and one pharmacist, who is responsible, in accordance with State law, for the packaging of medications dispensed in the clinics.

The services rendered by this Division are not confined, solely, to treatment, but provide also for diagnostic evaluation and placement of individuals in appropriate therapeutic and rehabilitative regimens, e.g. clinics, day hospital, twenty four hour facility, or education center. Communication is insured, too, between family and patient in community and/or hospital, in pre-admission, admission, and discharge phases of hospital care. To augment the services, provision is made for counseling and educational mental health services to staff members of this Department and personnel from allied agencies, specializing in services for children and families.

MENTAL HEALTH ADVISORY COMMITTEE

The General Assembly, during its 1978 session, repealed and reenacted with amendments, Section 1J of Article 43 of the Annotated Code of Maryland, (1971 Replacement Volume and 1977 Supplement), to be effective July 1, 1978. In compliance with the revised Code, the County Executive appoints a Mental Health Advisory Committee for Anne Arundel County. The Committee is composed of one representative from each: the County Council, the department of education, the department of social services, the practicing phsycians, other mental health professional, the clergy, the legal profession, the Mental Health Association, an individual who has or is receiving mental health care; an individual who is a relative of a mental health care recipient, and at least three members representing the Community. The Health Officer, a representative of Crownsville Hospital Center, and the Regional Mental Health Director, serve as ex-officio members; the Health Officer provides staff service to the Committee.

PREVENTIVE SERVICES

Psychiatric consultation is available to the Department of Social Services for discussion of difficult individual or family situations. The psychiatrist aids the presenting social worker both in understanding the problems and the approaches for satisfactory solution. New social workers and students participate in these sessions as a learning experience. Individual consultation is available, too, for personnel in allied community agencies.

Parents of a child in treatment with a psychiatrist receive simultaneous counseling by a staff social worker. Thus, the knowledge gained concerning the problems of one child, the patient, can be utilized to forestall or alleviate similar problems in the siblings.

The staff is available to meet with community groups, such as P.T.A's, schools, civic, or fraternal organizations, to discuss the problems of mental health, the need for early diagnosis and treatment, and, the services available from this Department to alleviate mental and emotional illness. An innovation to the mental health services has functioned since 1968 when the Health Department, the recipient of a grant, assigned a mental health team (psychiatrist, psychologist, psychiatric social worker) to the Northeast High School. Guidance counselors refer the most difficult cases to the team who evaluate and treat the students on an individual basis initially; later, the students join, under team leadership, group discussions regarding their individual problems. At the completion of several such sessions, the group discusses other topics, e.g., educational matters; student-parent and boy-girl relationships; drug use; smoking, etc. When necessary, parents of the students are invited to join the discussions. A similar program was initiated at the Severna Park High School in 1973.

The personnel of this Division provide consultation and psychiatric evaluations to both the County Detention Center and the Providence Center as requested.

CLINICAL SERVICES

The capability of this Department to increase direct out patient clinic services was enhanced in 1971, when an additional grant was obtained to establish the Glen Burnie Community Mental Health Center (exclusive of inpatient beds).

Concurrent with the establishment of the Glen Burnie Center, the Annapolis Mental Health Center began operations in the Health Services Building in Annapolis; each center is available to approximately one hundred fifty thousand residents or one half the total population of the County.

The two Community Mental Health Centers function in unison with mental health services available from the Brooklyn Park Health Center, the Northeast and Severna Park High Schools; the Annapolis Alcoholic Rehabilitation Clinic, and the Crownsville Hospital Center. The mission of the clinics is to provide direct out patient service to mentally and emotionally disturbed children, adolescents, and adults, including diagnostic evaluation, counseling, therapy, after care services, and referrals to other facilities. Very recently, the capability to provide geriatric evaluations of patients, prior to their entering a mental health facility, has been included in those services.

After care supervision of patients discharged from psychiatric hospitals is a major service provided thru these clinics; because of its availability, periods of required hospitalization and the related expenses are reduced significantly. Patients discharged to after care are seen regularly by the clinic psychiatrists who continue both drug treatment and psychotherapy; the medications are provided at minimal cost to the patient in the effort to preclude re-admission to hospitalization.

ALCOHOLIC REHABILITATION

Since 1953, the Department has sponsored an evening clinic dealing with problems of alcohol abuse. Individual counseling, accompanied by medication when indicated, is combined with group therapy under the guidance of a psychiatrist, psychologist, social worker, and community health nurse. Problem drinkers, recovered alcoholics, spouses and residents of local halfway houses and Crownsville Hospital Center's Alcoholic Rehabiliation Unit are all represented at these weekly sessions.

EMERGENCY SERVICES

Situations constituting an emergency are given priority and dispatched rapidly during daily clinic hours. After clinic hours, any acute case is referred to the emergency room of the general hospital where the physician on duty, after an examination, contacts a psychiatrist practicing in the area to provide the necessary follow up. Priority is given, also, to any patient referred by the court, the police, private physician or allied agency for they too, in many instances, constitute an emergency.

EDUCATIONAL SERVICES

All staff members working with children and adolescents of school age arrange individual conferences with teachers, pupil personnel workers, or school counselors, to discuss these cases in the effort to provide better understanding and maximum assistance for the patient. Conferences are held with school personnel for discussion of more complicated cases and issues pertaining to the services of the Mental Health Division.

Personnel of the Division participate in a preventive program in the community through attendance of monthly meetings of the Council of Services for Families and Children, and the Health-Education Council. Community issues are discussed, improvements are suggested, and brought to the attention of the appropriate individual or agencies.

The Director of the Division participates in community activities too, through membership on the Criminal Justice Coordinating Committee, the Juvenile Rehabilitation Center Board of Directors, the Chesapeake Bay Psychiatric Association, both State and County Mental Health Associations, and the Sub-Area Advisory Council of the Central Maryland Health Systems Agency.

The Community Health Nurse Supervisor (Mental Health) serves on the Maryland State Health Coordinating Committee by appointment by the Governor of Maryland.

Throughout the school year, human service students from Anne Arundel Community College participate in a program of orientation to community mental health services. Field placement, under the guidance of a mental health associate, is then provided for one student per semester at the Glen Burnie Center.

The Mental Health Centers also offer community experience to Crownsville Hospital Center psychiatry residents specializing in child psychiatry as well as to interns from Johns Hopkins Mental Health Counseling Program. Nursing students from Crownsville and the Community College nursing program are regularly oriented to the services by our nursing staff. The nursing staff provides an ongoing training program in Family Systems Theory to other community health nurses and health department personnel.

A community health educator, assigned to the Division, has been most effective in increasing the dissemination of mental health information to both allied community agencies and the general public; thereby enhancing the preventive aspects of mental illness.

CROWNSVILLE HOSPITAL CENTER—HEALTH DEPARTMENT COMMITTEE

Since 1955, the Crownsville Hospital Center—Health Department Committee on Mental Health Services for citizens of Anne Arundel County has had regular monthly meetings. Initially, this committee was concerned with the coordinated plan and services for discharge of hospitalized patients. Subsequently, the development of the day hospital and educational facilities for the emotionally disturbed have been the result of the committee's deliberations. Drugs for patients discharged as well as those prescribed by psychiatrists in the clinics are obtained from the hospital. The exchange of nurses from the Hospital and the Health Department for in-service training and education is a continuing program. Statistical reporting on all services relating to the clinics and Hospital was developed with advice from the State Department of Mental Hygiene.

COMMUNITY HEALTH NURSING SERVICES IN MENTAL HEALTH

All community health nurses participate in the Mental Health program through the referral of patients with psychiatric needs, observed during routine home visits or school health program.

A psychiatrically trained nurse is the liaison between clinicians and the nursing staff and through them, arranges home visits to patients. The nurse assists the clinicians, too, with family interviews, the dispensing of medications, survey of appointments, and telephone information.

Two community health nurses, also trained in psychiatric services, participate with the Crownsville Evaluation Team prior to the release of patients to the community; they visit these patients at home after discharge to continue services or in the event of missed appointments to the after care services.

Special Health Services

The County Health Department makes available a variety of services that function basically for adults; all of which are provided and/or coordinated by the Division of Special Health Services. These services can be classified, generally in the following broad categories: Tuberculosis Control; Indigent and Medically Indigent; Home Health Services; Medical Social Work Services; Addictions and Drug Abuse Services; Rehabilitation Services; Long Term Care; Geriatric Evaluation Services; and the Hypertension Program.

TUBERCULOSIS CONTROL

Anne Arundel County is showing a continuing decline in incidence of newly reported cases of tuberculosis and for 1977 showed an incidence of only 10.0/100,000 population. This compares with the state average (excluding Baltimore which has an incidence of 48.8/100,000) of 12.9 or 19.7 including Baltimore. The national statistics are not available for 1977, but the 1976 national average was 15.0/100,000 with Maryland that year showing an incidence of 22.3.

Services directed toward control of tuberculosis continue to be of major import and are the specific responsibility of the Director, Division of Special Health Services. Currently, these services are devised to detect and manage cases of communicable tuberculosis by means of seven (7) Chest Clinics each month; maintain surveillance over those cases being treated by private physicians; continue efforts at prevention of future cases by means of identifying those who should have a course of INH Preventive Therapy.

Communicable cases of tuberculosis, both new and reinfection, are identified through Health Department Chest Clinic evaluations or diagnosis, and referral by private physicians or other medical facilities. Supervision is assumed by the Chest Clinics with ongoing care and follow up by the Community

Health Nurse, or only surveillance is maintained over continuing management by the private physician, as may be appropriate for each case. It is the responsibility of the Health Department to take measures determine both the source of the infection of the individual cases, if possible, and to conduct as extensive a study of the contacts of the index case as is appropriate, instituting Preventive Therapy when indicated. A Tuberculosis Registry is perpetuated, thereby providing a complete record of all identified communicable cases of tuberculosis during the complete course of therapy which is usually eighteen to twenty-four months.

Tuberculin skin testing is completed on all individuals who have a history of recent exposure to communicable tuberculosis, suggestive findings on chest x-ray film, suggestive symptoms, or as part of an Associate Study. The latter study is conducted under circumstances such as identification of a child with a positive skin test reaction, identification of a recent skin test converter (within previous two years), or on first identification of a positive reactor when the skin test reactions of other household members or close associates are not known. Tuberculin skin tests are routine for all patients admitted to child health, maternity and family planning, and other specialty clinics; and, consideration of Preventive Therapy is made when appropriate.

Four of the local Health Centers have x-ray facilities and chest x-ray clinics are scheduled regularly in each center, with some evening clinics being held in two of the four centers. Two of the centers (Glen Burnie and Annapolis) provide Chest Clinics, with evening clinics available at both, with specialists in chest diseases serving as clinicians.

The Community Health Nurse provides home care instruction to the patient and family after diagnosis or hospitalization, relative to management of tuberculosis, or preventive measures; supervises or gives treatment such as streptomycin injections; and pursues contact studies of the newly identified case. One Community Health Nurse is assigned as coordinator in the Tuberculosis Control program, performing special functions of the program and acting as liaison between the Tuberculosis Control physicians and the various health centers.

A continuing educational program is conducted by the Health Department and the American Lung Association of Maryland to keep the public informed of the importance of prevention as well as early diagnosis and treatment of active disease. Patients and their families are assisted in understanding the nature of the disease and the steps necessary for its management.

INDIGENT AND MEDICALLY INDIGENT

The State of Maryland was a pioneer in the effort to make quality medical care readily available to those unable to pay for it. Historically, both the indigent and medically indigent residents received this care under the provisions of the Maryland Medical Care Program, administered locally by the County Health Department. This Program was supplemented in 1966 by Title XIX of the Social Security Act which authorized the Medical Assistance Program (Medicaid); financed jointly by Federal and State governments.

The County Health Department, under Medicaid, is responsible for the preauthorization of drugs, eye glasses, dentures, and quality medical care; supervision of Title XIX beneficiaries in nursing homes and chronic disease hospitals; the provision of Home Health Services to those beneficiaries who are maintained in the home; and periodic screening, diagnosis, and treatment of beneficiaries, thru age twenty, as described in Infant and Child Health section.

HOME HEALTH SERVICES

Historically, the Community Health Nurses have provided care for the sick in the home, on a limited basis, under the supervision of the attending physician. With the advent of federal health legislation and the extension of the State Medical Assistance Program (Medicaid), it was anticipated that a larger proportion of the community would seek health services within the home. A Home Health Services Program was established to provide services of the community health nurses, physical therapy and speech pathology, with ancillary services of occupational therapy, medical social work, home health aides, or nutritionist available as required.

This Department was certified, in 1966, by the Social Security Administration as a Home Health Agency eligible to participate in the Medicare Program; in 1978, licensure by the State Department of Health and Mental Hygiene became mandatory, too.

In August, 1974, the Department became the first community-based home health agency in Maryland to contract with Maryland Blue Cross, Inc., North Arundel Hospital, and Anne Arundel General Hospital as the provider of home health services to eligible beneficiaries under the Maryland Blue Cross Home Care Program. In January, 1976, these benefits were extended to Federal employees insured by Blue Cross, Inc. In addition, the agency has a contract with the South County Family Health Center for delivery of home health services to their clients for whom that facility is financially responsible for health care services.

An advisory committee with broad community health related agency representation assists in establishing policies and objectives in planning and implementing home health services. The advisory committee, with the Health Officer as Chairman, holds quarterly meetings.

Home Health Services are under the administrative direction of the Director,

Division of Special Health Services; the staff of the Division and the community health nurses provide specific care, prescribed by the attending physician, to the patient in the home on an intermittent basis. Criteria for the acceptance of clients have been developed to include a written plan of treatment prescribed by the attending physician, willingness of client and family to accept the services; adequacy of home facilities for provision of needed services; and feasibility of client's needs being met by provision of such services in the home situation.

A fee schedule has been established on a cost basis. Reimbursement by medicare, medicaid, and other third party providers is dependent upon individual eligibility for benefits. The ability to pay is not a requirement for admission and no one is refused necessary care.

MEDICAL SOCIAL WORK SERVICES

Medical Social Work Services provide both direct casework and group work services to the reahabilitation and prevention programs, in collaboration with other disciplines of the medical and paramedical team of the Health Department. In addition, they are available for consultation to both the Department staff and to allied agencies.

Currently, Medical Social Work staff consists of five (5) Social Workers, each with an M.S.W. Degree, and two (2) Social Work Assistants (C.E.T.A. Program) under the Division of Special Health Services. Of the five social workers, one works exclusively with Geriatric Evaluation Services and one is assigned to Geriatrics. The remaining three social workers and two social work assistants provide generalized services to all of Anne Arundel County. To improve provision of services, the health center districts were divided in 1973 into three (3) geographic areas with a Social Worker responsible for each area.

Casework services are available in medically related situations which involve a need for socio-emotional counseling for personal adjustment problems, family relationship difficulties, and vocational-educational concerns.

Information and referral is provided in cases where there is need for financial resources and medically-related transportation. This coordination of services facilitates maximum utilization of community resources in Anne Arundel County. Coordination is also provided in convalescent and chronic care planning. Consultation on specific socio-social problems is available to Health Department staff and other involved agencies. In keeping the Public Health principle of providing education for prevention of illness, the Social Work Services offers education and information both on individual and a group basis to those who have socio-emotional concerns regarding health issues.

GERIATRIC EVALUATION SERVICES

Further development of evaluation, screening, and placement services for patients age sixty-five and over, was made possible by the establishment of a Geriatric Evaluation Team in January, 1973. The team is composed of a medical social worker, who coordinates the program and functions full time; a registered nurse, who evaluates patients at home as to their capabilities in performing activities of daily living, determines those in need of further diagnostic screening, manages the Geriatric Evaluation Clinic, and functions part time; and a physician, (Assistant Director, Division of Special Health) who conducts medical examinations in the home when required, acts as physician-consultant, and functions on a full time basis in the Department with approximately 20% of her time devoted to the Geriatric Evaluation Services.

The purpose of the evaluation is twofold: to reduce unnecessary admissions to mental hospitals, nursing homes and long term care facilities; and to provide assistance and consultation in finding and utlizing resources in the community to maintain the patient in the home.

Patients evaluated include: mentally impaired, aged sixty-five and over, for whom admission to a state mental hospital is considered; physically or mentally impaired aged persons being considered for long term care; and selected applicants, 60 years of age and over to determine level of care or whether patient could be maintained at home.

Geriatric evaluation is a prerequisite for admission to state mental hospitals, for any patient sixty-five years of age or older, except in a psychiatric emergency situation when the evaluation is necessarily done immediately after admission.

GERIATRIC EVALUATION CLINIC

The Geriatric Evaluation Services were expanded to include comprehensive medical examinations, in a special clinic, to all persons 60 years of age and older, who are not receiving regular medical care by a private physician. The clinic, held the third Friday of each month, includes: physical examination by a physician, dental survey, EKG, vision and hearing screening, physical therapy tests, chest x-ray, blood tests, nutritional evaluation, urine specimen, and medical social consultation. Assistance and consultation is provided, too, in finding and utilizing community resources to aid the individual's specific needs.

ALCOHOL AND DRUG ADDICTIONS

The General Assembly of Maryland, enacted in 1968, the Comprehensive Intoxication and Alcohol Control Law; the first of its kind in the nation. The law removed public intoxication from the criminal code and established a modern public health program for the detoxification of inebriates and the treatment and rehabilitation of alcoholics. To assist in implementing the law and solving the inherent problems of alcoholism, this Department established the Alcoholism Program Committee.

The following year, the General Assembly enacted the Comprehensive Drug Abuse Control and Rehabilitation Act, designed to combat the effects of all forms of drug abuse through a state wide program of education, treatment, rehabilitation, and after care, for drug addicts. The activities of the committee were expanded accordingly and it functioned as the Drug Program Committee.

The Committee members were representatives from the State, County, and City Police; from Anne Arundel and North Arundel General Hospitals; Crownsville Hospital Center; the Department of Education; the State Division of Alcoholism Control; the State Drug Abuse Administration; the Department of Social Services; the State Motor Vehicle Administration; this Department; the District Court; the State's Attorney's Office; two physicians; and two concerned citizens. This committee was instrumental in the formation of the "Open Door"; the Drug Abuse Speaker's Bureau; the Samaritan House; and Raft House.

ALCOHOLISM ADVISORY COUNCIL

The Drug Program committee was superseded in 1977, by an Act of the General Assembly creating the Local Alcoholism Advisory Council, responsible only for activities concerning alcoholism control. Members of the Council, appointed by the County Executive, consist of one representative each from: The County Council; the Departments of Education, and Social Services; practicing physicians; the clergy; the legal profession; two persons currently employed in a local alcoholism treatment program; and at least four additional members from the community as a whole. The Council is empowered to create subcommittees and obtain additional participants as needed. The Health Officer; Director, Open Door; and the Alcoholism Coordinator serve as ex-officio members, with the Health Officer providing staff services to the Council. It is anticipated that the Council may be expanded to function in the Drug Program capacity, too.

COMMUNITY ADDICTIONS CENTER

The first Community Addictions Center, more familiarly known to its patients and the public as the "Open Door", was established in Annapolis in December, 1969. A second facility, the "Open Door North", began functioning in Glen Burnie in October, 1971. These centers are designed to provide counseling, coordination of services, and education, in relation to the use and abuse of alcohol and other addictive or dependency developing drugs. The latter may include the "hard" drugs, e.g. heroin, morphine, or cocaine, the "soft" drugs, e.g. amphetamines, barbiturates, or tranquilizers; and the hallucinogens, e.g. marijuana, LSD, PCP, or glue.

More specifically, the services provided at the centers are: crisis intervention; individual, family, and group counseling; medical and nursing evaluation; diagnostic services; urine surveillance; supportive rehabilitation; coordination of other community services; and preventive educational program. Procedures for Methadone maintenance and/or withdrawal; and transportation are available only at the Annapolis Open Door at the present time.

The staff functioning in the program ranges from the professionally trained social worker, community health nurse, psychiatrist, and physician, to the addictions counselors, who receive specific technical training from the Office of Education and Training for Addictions Services of the Mental Health Administration.

One program, the Driving While Intoxicated/Impaired receives referrals from both the Motor Vehicle Administration and judges hearing cases involving the impaired driver. Persons so referred, attend a 10 week course at the Open Door where they are educated as to the effect of alcohol and other drugs on the driver of an automobile.

The Open Door provides opportunity for volunteer service and for field work for Anne Arundel Community College students.

SAMARITAN HOUSE, INC.

In conjunction with the services of the Addictions Center, "half way houses" are essential in the rehabilitative program for the addicted person. The Health Department was instrumental in organizing a private, non-profit group of concerned citizens, (Samaritan House, Inc.) in February, 1971, to operate such a facility, known as "Samaritan House". With the assistance of an initial grant of $16,500 from this Department, the facility was in operation in slightly more than four months from the date of the organizational meeting of the group. The facility has the capacity of assisting twelve men in their recovery from alcoholism; consideration is being given to the establishment of a second Samaritan House for women.

From 1971 until 1975, funds were provided, to sustain the function of Samaritan House, thru this Department's budget. In fiscal 1976, the corporation became a direct grantee from the State.

RAFT HOUSE, INC.

The total scope of alcoholism necessarily includes a small percentage of chronic alocholics for whom recovery is most unlikely; they too, must be provided supportive services and residential facilities classified as "Shelter Houses". This Department, utilizing a grant from the State, mobilized an interested group of community minded citizens to form a private, non-profit corporation (Raft House, Inc.) to establish and operate a shelter house in Annapolis.

The shelter house offers care and protection to the "skid row alcoholic", for while they are but a very small percentage of the total alcoholic population, until they are under appropriate and contructive social management they have a negative effect on services to treat and rehabilitate the majority. Because they are the most visible and most universally recognized alcoholics, those most frequently in contact with law enforcement, health, and social services agencies, they are taken or referred repeatedly to treatment resources, e.g. emergency rooms, clinics, and especially state mental hospitals.

Raft House, too, was the recipient of sustaining funds from this Department until they also became the direct grantee from the State.

REHABILITATION SERVICES

Services encompassed include Physical, Occupational Therapists, and Speech Pathology treatment, and are provided by a staff of six physical therapists, one physical therapy assistant, one occupational therapist, and one speech pathologist. The therapists function in the local health centers, in the schools, in the home, in skilled nursing facilities, and provide services on an out-patient basis. The Social Security Administration certifies this out-patient program.

Therapy is provided for all Home Health patients and all ages are included upon referral of private physician; emphasis is concentrated on individuals with chronic disabilities rather than acute.

Additionally, the therapists function in several major programs: the Infant Stimulation Program, where the child is assessed in the home environment and provided out-patient care at Oakwood School; the Geriatric Clinic, where patient is evaluated and assessed; the Home Rehabilitation Service, where children awaiting proper school placement receive therapy in the home; and the Adult Day Care program, where patients engage in a generalized exercise class and are provided consultation by physical therapists.

Speech and language treatment services are provided to the patient in both North Arundel and Anne Arundel General Hospitals on referral of the patients' private physician.

LONG TERM CARE

At some point during hospitalization, many patients no longer need the intensive care which a hospital provides, but still need continuous skilled nursing care or therapy for optimum rehabilitation. Such long term care can be provided in a skilled nursing home facility, or a chronic disease hospital.

NURSING HOMES

At the present time, there are six skilled nursing home facilities in the County; all six are certified for participation in both the Medicare and Medicaid programs. The facilities so certified are: the Annapolis Nursing and Convalescent Center, Knollwood Manor, Fairfield, Hammonds Lane, the North Arundel Convalescent Center, and Maryland Manor; Fairfield and Knollwood Manor have contracted with this Department for the provision of medical social services, physical, occupational, and speech therapy. These services are all available under the orders of the patients' attending physician.

There is an additional type of facility available too, classified as "Long Term Intermediate A Level", wherein the nurse available only eight hours per day in lieu of the twenty-four hour per day requirement in the skilled nursing facility. Two facilities in the County function entirely in this category: Bay Manor and Plaza Manor; while Fairfield, Hammonds Lane, Knollwood Manor, and Maryland Manor, each have a specified number of beds in the "Intermediate A" classification in addition to their skilled nursing home rating. One additional facility, Cooper Nursing Home, is certified for domiciliary care only.

Assistance and consultation are given to nursing home personnel by the nursing home coordinator, physical therapist, occupational therapist, and speech pathologist. The Nursing Home Coordinator, an especially trained community health nurse, makes regular visits to all nursing homes and hospitals in the County and is responsible for surveying these facilities to assure that licensure requirements are met.

CHRONIC DISEASE HOSPITALS

There are three chronic disease hospitals operated by the State: Deer's Head, in Salisbury; Western Maryland, in Hagerstown; and Montebello, in Baltimore. Baltimore City Hospital also operates a chronic disease unit; patients from Anne Arundel County can be admitted to any one of the four facilities.

In the interim, the community health nurse makes a home visit to compile a social summary for the hospital; she consults too, with the family and the attending physician in regard to possible utilization of physical therapy or skilled nursing care to prevent further deterioration of the patient while awaiting admission. The nurse further discusses the family's responsibilities concerning transportation to the chronic disease hospital, and the articles needed at the time of admission.

After discharge from the hospital, the community health nurse maintains follow up of the patient. Home visits are made to these patients to teach both patient and family the activities of daily living.

HYPERTENSION SCREENING

Community health nurses have routinely screened all clinic patients for hypertension, as well as "walk ins" on request. Utilizing funds from a federal grant, the Department established a Hypertension Clinic in 1977. The clinic functions twice per month in the Annapolis Center, but the clinic team is available to provide the service at other locations throughout the County. Clinic procedures include: hypertension screening and referral; patient education; follow up to encourage patients with elevated blood pressure to obtain medical care; the recheck of patients with borderline readings; and the regular monitoring of hypertension patients at the request of the patients' physician.

Community Health Nursing Services

Nursing services, although an integral part of all Health Department activities, are administered by the Director of the Division of Community Health Nursing; the Director is directly responsible to the Health Officer.

The Division coordinates a program of nursing services to: emphasize the prevention of disease to achieve optimum health in community; provide professional nursing care to the sick and disabled in the home, under medical supervision; instruct and counsel patients and families to gain maximum potential through rehabilitation; and utilize community resources for continuity of nursing services to individuals and families.

Community health nursing services are generalized and function on a decentralized basis from the thirteen community health centers, the community addiction centers, the comprehensive mental health centers, and the nursing stations in housing units. The leadership, in addition to the Director, includes two assistant directors, nine supervisors, an assistant supervisor in each health center, and two program assistant supervisors, who provide support and guidance to the staff nurses, licensed practical nurses, and aides.

Five supervisors function as coordinators of major programs, e.g. Mental Health; Maternal Health and Family Planning; Child Health, Crippled Children and Mental Retardation; Communicable Diseases (Tuberculosis); School Health and Day Care; Home Health and Hypertension. Professional interest and preparation of individual nurses are considered when assigning special tasks such as Nursing Home licensure and certification, Day Care licensure, Cancer detection in the female, Hypertension screening and Tuberculosis nursing activity, the part time community health nurse is employed to meet needs in this area. The knowledge and skills of all staff nurses are utilized in a continuous and active student program in which nurses preparing for a Master's Degree, from universities, are provided field experience in community health as part of their requirements for that degree. Students from the Anne Arundel Community College, visitors from the States and foreign countries, and all new staff members are also provided orientation in community health by the staff nurses.

The high quality of the community health nursing service is primarily maintained through educational activities. With the active participation of the Health Officer, nurses are encouraged to further their professional education; funds are available to the Department for reimbursement to the individual nurse, at the successful completion of a course. Educational leave for one year is granted to those who wish to complete the requirements of a baccalaureate degree; credit courses are available at several campuses provided by the University of Maryland's "University College" program; and the Anne Arundel Community College is yet another source for further study. In addition, a continuous inservice educational program is planned and implemented with active participation by the staff nurses. In-service education is conducted routinely for the established programs.

The maintenance of high standards is assured, too, by continual evaluation of the utilization of nursing skills and training. Consequently, seven licensed practical nurses and seventeen aides have been appointed to perform those tasks not requiring highly specialized techniques. The community health nursing aides receive their basic training through a very comprehensive course conducted by the staff of this Department; the licensed practical nurses are graduates of accredited schools of practical nursing.

Community health nursing services, as stated previously, are an integral part of all Health Department programs. More specifically, however, the programs and the respective nursing services are summarized briefly in the following paragraphs.

MATERNAL HEALTH

The Community Health Nurse maintains a comprehensive approach in the care of the prenatal patient. Concerns include the total family, plans for delivery, home problems, nurse checks, clinic and home visits during the prenatal period, and post delivery and instruction in care of the infant.

FAMILY PLANNING

Patients are introduced to Family Planning during prenatal clinic visits and are counseled by the nurse and Planned Parenthood Volunteer utilizing pamphlets, charts, and films. The nurse visits the home of patients with complications, dispenses oral contraceptives in the clinic on physician's orders, and assists for sterilization if the patient's condition so indicates.

PREMATURE INFANTS

Premature infants are closely followed by the nurse to evaluate the home situation, to instruct the parents in the care of the infant, and to observe the infant for abnormal symptoms or abnormal growth and development patterns.

INFANT AND CHILD HEALTH

The child, from birth to age 21, requires close nursing follow up to detect abnormalities at the earliest age and to give guidance to the parents. Nursing instructions in growth and development of the young child contributes to parental acceptance of normal behavior in various age groups, and aids in the prevention of emotional problems within the family. Instruction in the need for immunization protects the community from communicable disease, as well as the individual child from chronic illness due to complications from the disease. The adolescent from 13 to 21 years of age is provided nursing assessment and intervention through referral to youth clinic where comprehensive approach to physical, mental and social needs is provided by the Health Team.

NURSING ASSESSMENT

Maternal and Child Health clinics are supplemented by Nursing Assessments, initiated in 1958, when nurses began to administer the immunizations. These sessions now include counseling, continued health evaluations, history, Hearing and Vision screening, and fetal heart checks, all performed by community health nurses in all health centers and satellites.

DAY CARE CENTERS

Community health nurses have, historically, provided services to day care centers on request of the operator of the center. Many of the children in these facilities are already known to the nurse through registration in the Child Health clinics. The Community Health Nurse, in addition to counseling services regarding health, assists in assessing the health component for the licensing procedure of the Day Care Center.

SCHOOL HEALTH

Nursing service to the school is a major function of the generalized community health nursing service; it provides continuity of health supervision for the child and his family. The nurse serves whenever possible the district in which the school is located and is therefore, able to function within the framework of school, home, and community to provide services necessary to obtain maximum health for the child. The extent to which the health program is planned by the Health-Education Council will define the types and amount of nursing services given.

Currently, the community health nurse as a member of the School Health Team, engages in the following activities to provide service.

• Serves as a consultant to principals and teachers in situations concerned with physical or emotional health of students, faculty, parents, or community.
• Arranges conferences in the school with pupils and parents to counsel on matters of health.
• The nurse is a participant in the Team Conference planned by the Board of Education which reviews children referred with suspected health and/or learning disabilities.
• Makes visits to the home to assist parents in planning medical follow up for their children.
• Interprets Health Department Program, provides materials for health education, and acts as a resource person on matters pertaining to health.
• Is available for faculty and P.T.A. meetings.
• Is responsible, with the audio-visual technician, for coordination or re-screening vision and hearing failures and follow up care of children referred by the Health Committee.

Volunteers, often mothers of children in school, are trained and supervised by the nurse in methods of screening in the vision and hearing testing programs, as well as height and weight screening. The use of these volunteers serves a twofold purpose; successful completion of screening procedures and the acquisition of knowledge of the school health program on the part of the workers. A well informed volunteer educates her community.

HOME HEALTH

Community health nursing services are provided in the home to persons with an acute or chronic illness. These services include education of the patient and family, supervision of care, and the performance of nursing procedures for the care of the sick in the home. All nursing procedures are performed under the specific order of the physician.

COMMUNICABLE DISEASE CONTROL

The function of the nurse in the control of communicable diseases entails health education regarding the importance of immunization, case finding, and supervision of patients who have contacted the diseases. Epidemiological investigations are conducted including the administration of tuberculin test and the follow up on the contacts of tuberculosis patients.

MENTAL HEALTH

Patients are referred for nursing care who have mental and/or emotional disorders. Many of these patients are returning to the community after hospitalization and need supportive care to assist them in adjusting to the family and the community. The family too, requires help in understanding the patient's illness; the community health nurse provides this suppportive care.

CHRONIC DISEASE

Patients are followed up after discharge from a chronic disease hospital by the community health nurse. Home visits are made to these patients to teach both patient and family the activities of daily living. The nurse also refers the chronically ill patients to other members of the health team, private physician, and other community agencies.

The Community Health Nurse receives additional instruction in Cancer detection in the female and in Hypertension screening. She participates as the screener in the Cancer Detection clinics and Hypertension clinics which are held throughout the county.

OPEN DOOR

Community health nurses assist in the Methadone Clinic administered through the Open Door. The nurses also serve in a case finding and referral capacity to help meet the health needs of these clients. They act as liaison between Open Door and Health Department clinics.

LOCAL HEALTH ASSOCIATIONS

Eleven of the thirteen health centers in the County are owned by non-profit volunteer Health Associations, adopting the name of the local community in which they are located, e.g. Brooklyn Park Health Association. Effective public relations and community education are established and maintained through the joint efforts of these local volunteer groups and the community health nurses assigned to their centers. The nurses attend the regularly scheduled monthly meetings of the associations to provide current information on the activities of the health center and the Health Department; they participate too, in the fund raising or community education projects conducted by their respective health association and in the recruitment of community leaders as potential association members. Community participation is an essential factor in this unique system of health centers; that it has been successful for over four decades is due largely to the efforts of the community health nurse.

Communicable Disease Control

A major responsibility of the Health Department is the control of communicable diseases; therefore, maximum effort is expended toward the prevention of these diseases. Initially, efforts are concentrated on health education, whereby the public is continually kept informed regarding the signs, symptoms, and current trends in control of communicable disease. Immunizations for protection against diphtheria, whooping cough, tetanus, poliomyelitis, rubella and measles are administered routinely to children attending Child Health Clinics as are periodic health evaluations and guidance as to the prevention of these diseases. Additionally, Environmental Health personnel are constantly alert to prevent the occurrence of these diseases by continued surveillance of waste disposal, water supply, food establishments, and processing plants.

The second phase, or control begins with the reporting of cases of communicable disease as they occur in the County. Absentees, in excess of the normal, are reported to this Department daily from all schools and industries while admissions to hospitals are also considered. The compiliation of these reports provides the Health Officer with such information as the number of cases, location, race, age group affected, and type of disease. From this data, definite control methods can be initiated if the occurrences approach epidemic proportions.

When communicable diseases occur, regardless of the preventive measures, specific procedures are established for control. Investigations or epidemiological studies are conducted on patients to determine the source of infection, the number related to the source, and the method of transmission. The latter, once determined, is interrupted and all contacts of the patient are followed in association with the family physician.

The Health Officer is available too, for consultation with the family physician regarding the confirmation of a diagnosis or in making arrangements for hospitalization. If necessary, specimens may be submitted by the family physician to the Health Department Laboratory to enable a definitive diagnosis to be made.

The community health nurses participate directly in all of the communicable disease control activities and may perform specific services in the home upon the request and direction of the family physician.

MASS IMMUNIZATION PROJECTS

Influenza control measures, instituted annually, consist of the administration of influenza vaccine to essential State, County, and City governmental personnel by the Health Officer. The Department encourages, too, all commercial, industrial, and administrative groups, and individuals with chronic or respiratory disease, to procure effective levels of immunization.

Residents of the County are accorded the opportunity, annually, to obtain Rabies immunizations for their dogs and cats at one of three clinics, functioning on a weekend, usually in the Spring, with follow up in the Fall. The Maryland Veterinary Medicine Association and this Department, cooperate to provide this service; Veterinarians, present in each clinic, administer the vaccine. Certification of vaccination, given to each owner, is required prior to the issuance of a license for a dog. The vaccine immunizes the dog for a three year period, and is so noted on the certificate. Immunization for cats is for a one year period.

VENEREAL DISEASE CONTROL

The control of venereal disease entails case finding, contact investigations, and treatment of the individual patients. These activities are conducted by Health Services Specialist, assigned full time to the County by the State Department of Health and Mental Hygiene; the community health nurses; and one part time physician. A Venereal Disease clinic functions weekly, in conjunction with the General Health clinic in Annapolis, with the part time physician serving as clinician. Patients are referred by the Specialist, the nurses, or are seen on a self referral basis.

Patients with infectious syphilis and gonorrhea are interviewed by the Health Services Specialist for contacts, who, are in turn, referred to the clinic or to their private physician.

Tests for syphilis and gonorrhea are performed routinely on all Maternal and Family Planning clinic patients, as yet another method of case finding.

All patients with reactive tests, reported from the State Laboratory or private laboratories, are investigated to determine their diagnosis and treatment. However, permission is obtained of private physicians to interview their patients.

To facilitate the treatment of patients, one physician in the northern section of the County sees patients in his office on a contract basis.

Military Installations and the Detention Center, located in the County, are visited by the Specialist, and cases of infectious venereal diseases are interviewed for contacts. When the contacts reside outside of this County, the epidemiological reports are forwarded to the appropriate jurisdiction for follow up.

One additional procedure utilized in the control and prevention of venereal diseases is an extensive educational program conducted for the various schools, civic groups, and community associations, to inform the public about the diseases, their consequences, and the control measures available from this Department.

Laboratory Services

The Public Health Laboratory provides essential supportive services to the various programs of this Department; to private laboratories; and to private physicians, practicing in Anne Arundel County. The Laboratory functions as a branch laboratory of the Laboratories and Research Administration, State Department of Health and Mental Hygiene; for twenty-three of the past thirty-five years, the laboratory has been quartered in the Health Department Building, in Annapolis. With the construction of the new Health Services Building, on Harry S. Truman Parkway, larger and more modern facilities were provided for the laboratory, on the first floor of the new structure, thereby, making it more readily accessible to clinic patients, private physicians, environmental health personnel, and the public.

The Laboratory services are provided in three distinct categories: Diagnostic, Clinical, and Environmental; in addition to the routine procedures, each category has the capability to conduct special studies.

DIAGNOSTIC

In this category, a special study is currently in progress concerning asymptomatic gonorrhea cases occurring in females of this County. Routinely, special studies are conducted for the identification of both insects and bacteria. In cases of poisonous insect bites, the insect can be identified; bacteria, isolated in private laboratories, also can be identified through techniques available in the public health laboratory. Additional diagnostic procedures include:

Urine cultures	Gonorrhea cultures
Sputum cultures	Syphilis serology
Abscesses	Intestinal parasites
Blood parasites	Antibiotic sensitivity tests
Fungus infections	Enteric infections—Salmonella,
Eye, Ear, Nose, and Throat cultures	Shigella, and Vibrio

CLINICAL

Under the Clinical category, the Annapolis Laboratory is capable of performing the following procedures:

Blood Glucose	All Blood Indices
Blood Nitrogen	Platelet count
Glucose Tolerance	Differential White Cell count
Hematocrit	Reticulocyte count
Hemoglobin	Sedimentation rate
White Cell count	Pregnancy test
Red Cell count	Urinalysis

In the Environmental category, the laboratory routinely performs bacteriological tests on: Private drinking water wells, Public drinking water supplies, sewage treatment plant outfall, streams, shellfish producing waters, Oysters and Clams in season, crabmeat, swimming pools, and bathing beaches. Bacteriological and chemical analysis (Butterfat content and pasteurization) is performed on Milk and Ice Cream samples collected regularly from the vendors.

Waters from all public bathing beaches and swimming pools are routinely tested weekly during the 10 week period from June 15th through September 1st to insure their safety for recreational use. College students, majoring in Science, are utilized both in the laboratory and for the collection of the water samples, thereby providing them some experience in their chosen profession.

The Laboratory participates, too, in the County's Student Intern Program whereby high school students, with an interest in science are assigned to work in the Laboratory, during a regular semester under the tutelage of the Director and the staff of the Laboratory.

Dental Health Services

The Division of Dental Health is responsible for the development and administration of the Dental Public Health Program; a program designed to combat the nation's most prevalent dental problem—dental caries and periodontal disease.

SCHOOL DENTAL HEALTH PROJECT

Title I Dental Program. Those children designated as Title I pupils are offered complete dental services. These include prophylaxis, radiographs, examination, restorations, oral surgery, endodontics as well as space maintenance. Each pupil is given reinforced oral hygiene instructions (proper brushing, flossing and diet counseling). Transportation is provided from school to the Health Department so that children with working parents will not be deprived of these essential services.

National Children's Dental Health Week Program. There is no better place to provide dental health education than in the classroom. With the help of the Western Shore Dental Society and the cooperation of the Board of Education, we have established a very beneficial National Children's Dental Health Week Program. Elementary school teachers attend oral health workshops staffed by volunteer dentists. Here the teachers are taught preventive dentistry concepts such as proper brushing, flossing and diet counseling. They are also provided with resource material to help them teach these preventive dentistry concepts to their pupils in the classroom. There are also school visitations by volunteer dentists during National Children's Dental Health Week.

Consultant and Resource. The Dental Health Division provides consultation and dental health resource materials to teachers on request.

Dental Health Certificate Program. All pre-schoolers and those entering Junior High School must have these certificates completed by their private dentist.

The Dental Division is working to develop programs and facilities to provide clinical dental services to anyone desiring such services. For those persons who cannot seek private dental care because of a potential financial burden, we have innovated a unique program in conjunction with cooperating dentists from the Western Shore Dental Society, referred to as the "Gray Area Program". Patients are screened for eligibility by the Dental Division and subsequently granted a fee reduction of between 10-35%. They may choose from a list of approximately 73 participating dentists, including such specialists as orthodontists, pedodontists, oral surgeons, etc.

Clinical dental services are offered at the Health Department in Annapolis. Appointments are made on a space available basis with consideration as to age, need, and financial status. Dental services provided include prophylaxis, radiographs, topical fluoride therapy, restorations, endodontics, and limited oral surgery. Each patient undergoes an extensive preventive dentistry program including proper brushing and flossing techniques as well as diet counseling.

The Dental Division is endeavoring to make dental examinations an integral part of other Health Department clinics. At the Youth and Geriatric clinics patients are examined for dental defects and oral hygiene status and appropriate referrals are then made (Fig. 10-3).

Health Education

Health Education is an important aspect of all phases of preventive medicine and public health; it is practiced, to some extent, by every member of the Health Department staff. It is provided by the Community Health Nurses in all clinics, home visits, schools, the care of the chronically ill, etc.; by the Environmental Health personnel in restaurant inspection, communicable disease control, supervision of waste disposal, water supplies, etc. All members of the staff, in addition to providing information concerning their specific fields, endeavor to keep the public informed of the total services available from this Department.

The Health Educators on the staff provide assistance to other personnel with health education problems, health information to the public, prepare news releases and education materials for distribution, and serve as resource persons for slides, films, pamphlets, and other education or audio visual materials.

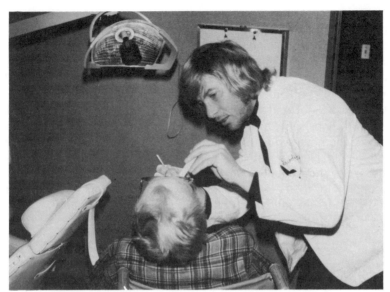

Figure 10-3. Dental care for the elderly is a frequent service of local health departments. This patient is being examined in a dental-geriatric clinic. (Courtesty of the Anne Arundel County Health Department.)

In-service training programs are conducted for all new personnel in order to orient them in every phase of the health department program, and staff meetings are utilized to keep the entire group informed of the latest developments in both public health and the allied programs functioning in the County.

An educational program is carried on, under the direction of the Assistant Director, Division of Community Health Nursing, to provide orientation and field experience for graduate nursing students from the Johns Hopkins University. Orientation to public health is arranged too, for students from Anne Arundel Community College. Formal training programs are developed for community health nursing aides, Family Planning aides, and School Health Aides, who will serve on the staff of this Department. Current information on nursing techniques or medical technology is disseminated to the staff through "cluster courses" held in three locations; subjects have included: hypertension, disaster nursing, and CPR. The CPR course is available to all personnel in the Department.

For visitors from abroad, a program of orientation and observation is conducted, under the supervision of the Health Educator and public health officials from ninety-one countries have participated to date. The Department is approved also as a Residency Training area for physicians, who, under State Department of Health and Mental Hygiene auspices, are endeavoring to achieve certification as public physicians.

Annually, several workshops are held in the County to train the Health Committees of the Parent-Teacher Associations who perform the screening tests in the School under the supervision of the Audio-Vision technicians. These workshops serve to train the new members and also provide a review for those who have served previously.

The Health Department is a participant in the Student Intern Program, sponsored by the County Council, wherein high school students are afforded the opportunity to receive training and work experience, during a regular semester, under the guidance of the Director of the Laboratory.

Vital Records

The County Health Officer is, by law, the ex-officio County registrar of vital records. Copies of the certificates of all births and deaths occurring to Anne Arundel County residents are preserved.

In the event the facts of a birth are made known at a later date and no birth certificate has been filed, the Health Officer investigates the facts and executes the certificate.

The copies of birth certificates preserved by this Department are used for administrative purposes and for the issuance of "Statement of Age" cards. This card verifies the individuals age and is used for employment, application for drivers' licenses, etc.

When it is necessary to disinter a body, this Department issues a Disinterment Permit upon application by the funeral director and a copy of the application is forwarded to the State Department of Health and Mental Hygiene.

Lists of the deaths occurring in this County are furnished to the County Board of Election Supervisors and the Motor Vehicles Administration.

Certified copies of both birth and death certificates must be obtained from the State Department of Health and Mental Hygiene; applications are available from this Department.

Health Mobilization - Civil Defense

The Civil Defense Services in this County include all of the essential components; e.g. medical, fire, communications, etc. In each instance, existing state and local agencies normally engaged in these activities are utilized. As the established practice throughout the country is to assign the medical services organization responsibility to the local health department, the Health Officer of Anne Arundel County is the Director of Medical Services. Operational plans are based upon available personnel, facilities and supplies, both within the County and on a mutual aid basis with Baltimore City and the adjacent counties. All of the community health centers are designed as casualty clearing stations and three high school buildings are equipped for conversion to emergency hospitals. Available personnel inventoried and assigned to these facilities include physicians, clergymen, dentists, pharmacists, veterinarians, morticians, registered nurses, practical nurses, nursing aides, qualified first aid persons, medical administrators, environmental health personnel, cafeteria workers, volunteers for hospital ward duty, and clerk-stenographers.

Facilities such as school buildings, or other public buildings are designed, in relation to location in areas of population concentration and suitability, for ready conversion to a casulty treatment station or an emergency shelter. Supplies available in the local health department, hospital, drug stores and physicians' offices are tabulated and with this information, plans for handling casulties are formulated and kept current.

Currently, this Department is engaged in updating the inventory and assignment of personnel and has recently had radio equipment installed for direct communication with Fire, Police, and Civil Defense headquarters in time of emergency.

FEDERAL-STATE AND STATE-LOCAL RELATIONS

Throughout the world in most all enterprises in which a central authority has local units or branch offices, there is conflict. The branch office typically thinks the head office doesn't know what it is doing, and the head office reciprocates with like attitudes. So, too, in government.

In the federal government, it is not uncommon for federal health officials to speak disparagingly of state health officers and, in state government, officials to speak disparagingly of local health officials and distrustingly of federal officers. What the local health officers think of both the reader can easily guess. These common attitudes stem from the fact that each level of government views the world from a different perspective and with different pressures working on them. Their respective priorities develop accordingly, and it should not be surprising that they often differ. Because the higher level of government tends to have more resources to work with and a stronger bureaucratic structure with the staying power that goes with it, the assessments by the higher government level of the next lower level tend to prevail just as the histories written by victors in wars shape our perspectives on world history. What I hope to suggest by this discussion is that the assessment of local and state health departments by the units of government above them should be treated with caution. They may be valid assessments, but they may also be biased appraisals reflecting age-old styles of bureaucratic in-fighting.

CONCLUSION

Society, as we know it, could not have developed as it did without organized public health programs at the local and state levels. Through a variety of preventive measures, health departments have assured the population of safe drinking water, milk, and other perishable food products and an environment relatively free of harmful substances and elements. They initiated environmental health and personal prevention programs to deal with a variety of communicable and infectious diseases and early on addressed the prevention of problems affecting the poor at points of their greatest vulnerability, that is, in the areas of maternal and child health and school health.

The record of state and local health departments is, on the whole, worthy of praise in most of our states. There are things yet to be done, and old problems sometimes rise again, and other problems sometimes resist even the best of efforts. This is not necessarily a reflection on public health departments, though it may at times be, but more often a result of the inability of public health officials to control all of the variables by the very nature of the variables—the citizens of the areas who are free people and the advance of knowledge and technology that often cause new problems as well as often providing new ways to deal with old problems.

The track record of public health agencies in providing treatment and care services for the mentally ill, mentally retarded, and the poor is not nearly the success record that it is for old-line public health activities. There are, to be sure, state and local governments that have performed well, but all too often the efforts of government in these treatment and care areas have been compromised by the inability and unwillingness to provide the environment within which excellence can emerge in terms of facilities, salary structures, support staff, reimbursement levels for purchased treatment and care services, and bureaucratic rules, regulations, and paper work.

The differences in performance between traditional public health (in the areas of *environmental* and *personal prevention services*) and public health's *treatment and care services* may result from society's perception that in prevention "there but for the grace of God go I," and, therefore, it is for government to do what has to be done, but that in the treatment and care areas the public as a whole will not, or cannot, project itself into the position of those needing publically financed or provided services.

REFERENCES

1. Gossert, D. J. and Miller, C. A.: State boards of health, their members and commitments. *Am. J. Public Health* 83: 1973.
2. Hanlon, J. J.: *Public Health Administration and Practice.* 6th ed. St. Louis, Mosby.
3. Miller, C. A. et al.: A survey of local public health departments and their directors. *Am. J. Public Health* 67: 1977.
4. Miller, C. A. et al.: Statutory authorizations for the work of local health departments. *Am. J. Public Health* 67: 1977.
5. Becker, A. and Schulberg, H. C.: Phasing out state hospitals—a psychiatric dilemma. *New Engl. J. Med.* 294: 1976.

11
Public Health: Federal

Of all monies spent for health in fiscal 1977, the federal government was the source for 28.63% of it*. The federal government paid for 39.18% of the total funds spent for hospital care, 33.32% of the total funds spent for nursing home care, and 18.05% of the total spent for physician services. In terms of research, the federal government accounts for 85.2% of the total expenditures.

It is appropriate to begin this discussion of the federal role in health affairs by citing expenditure statistics, for although the federal government provides some direct services, its chief role has been that of stimulating the development of new and improved services by provision of monies to buy the action it wanted to see developed. Indeed, except in some circumscribed areas, the federal government has no constitutional authority to provide direct health services for people, this being the domain of the states.

THE CONGRESSIONAL ROLE IN HEALTH

For government to do anything requires money that must be raised by some form of taxation. The use of that money, as well as the raising of it, must have a legal base; somewhere in the U.S. Constitution there must be a clause that justifies a law and, in turn, an appropriation, for government to do what it does. This applies to all areas of government activity. And the U.S. Supreme Court is arbiter when otherwise unresolvable disputes arise as to whether or not the activity of the government is in accord with the authorities granted government by the Constitution.

The *Powers of Congress* part of the Constitution (Article 1, Section 8), provides authority to raise and support armies, to provide and maintain a navy, and to make all laws "necessary and proper" for carrying out those powers.

---

* See Table 8-2 in Chapter Eight.

One can quickly see how this justifies the allocation of monies for military and naval and air force hospitals and health services. It requires only a slight extension of logic to justify the VA work in health, whether it is the building of a hospital or clinic for treatment of veterans with service-connected disabilities or the support of medical education to assure an adequate supply of doctors so that there will be enough to meet the manpower needs of the VA system. Similarly, one can justify the developing medical school for the armed forces that is being built on the grounds of the National Naval Medical Center in Bethesda, Maryland.

The Constitution also grants to Congress the power to regulate foreign and interstate commerce. This justifies much of the federal activity regarding regulation of foods, drugs, product and occupational safety, and some environmental health activities because they move in, or affect, interstate or foreign commerce. The power to control federal lands, along with the presidential power to make treaties (with the advice and consent of the Senate) are the sources of federal activity in providing health services for the Indians and Eskimos. Other direct service activities also rely on these clauses for legitimization. But by far the greatest federal influence comes from the distribution of monies to the states, local governments, and nongovernmental agencies. Sometimes these grants of money can be justified as "necessary and proper" for carrying out the specific constitutional powers already cited. An even more significant basis for grant monies derives from the power of Congress "to lay and collect taxes, duties, imports, and excises, to pay the debts and provide for the common defense and general welfare of the United States . . ."

It is the "general welfare" clause that justifies support for medical research, Medicare, Medicaid, health manpower training, health planning, and so on. The power to make monies available for certain general welfare activities also permits the writing of regulations setting out the conditions that must be met in order to get the money. The regulations are applications of the law written by the administering agencies in the executive branch and published in the *Federal Register*, a daily (Monday through Friday) official publication of the U.S. government. Since regulations have force of law, they must follow the intent of Congress. Frequently, litigation revolves around whether or not a regulation has followed the intent of Congress, and this the courts determine, drawing not only on the law itself but also on congressional committee reports that indicate the thinking of the Senate, the House, and sometimes of the conference committee on the bill as each reports it: the House committee report to the House of Representatives, the Senate committee report to the Senate, and the conference committee report to both houses of the Congress. The conference committee is an *ad hoc* group of representatives from the Senate and the House, convened to iron out or resolve different versions of similar bills, one passed by each house.

THE LEGISLATIVE PROCESS

Any proposed law must begin by being introduced in the Senate or the House by one of the respective members. On introduction, it is assigned a number (e.g., HR 1 or S-9, as the case may be). To become a law, a bill must be passed in identical form by both houses of Congress and signed by the president. If the president vetoes the bill, it can become law without his signature if two thirds of both houses vote to override his veto; if the president does not sign the bill or veto it, it can still become law if, after 10 days (Sundays excepted), no such action is taken. If during these 10 days Congress adjourns, then the bill does not become law. The drafting of a bill may be done in the executive branch and given to a member of the Senate and/or House for introduction, or it may be drafted within the legislative branch and introduced by one or more members of the respective houses. Bills may also be drafted by individual citizens or groups and given to a willing member of Congress for introduction.

On introduction, the bill is referred to an appropriate committee for study and for report to the full House. The process in the Senate is very similar to that of the House of Representatives, and each goes through the entire process in considering a bill; each, typically, holds its own hearings on a bill and writes its own report. Neither body defers to the other on such matters.

Many bills die in committee. Some die in conference. More important bills typically have hearings whereby proponents and opponents to the bill may testify to give information to the committee that will help or influence the committee's thinking about the bill. With the benefit of this information and advice from its professional staff, a committee can then decide what action it wishes to take on the bill. It has a report prepared on the bill, a report that accompanies the bill to the full House or Senate. The report will explain what the bill is intended to do. Committee reports can be secured from the respective committees, as can published hearings.

The movement of a bill through the House or Senate is a complicated process, affected by the volume of business before the house as well as political considerations of influential leaders, the administration, interest and pressure groups, and the views of individual members of the house.

There are a number of agencies of Congress that need to be cited because of their key roles in health affairs. These agencies are the key committees of each house and the General Accounting Office (GAO). Some committees not listed below periodically get into health matters, but not in a major way.

Health Committees of the House of Representatives

The *House Ways and Means Committee* is concerned with raising revenue by various tax measures. If a new piece of health legislation is to require new tax monies, then this committee must find the ways and means of securing new monies and so recommend to the full House. The committee might also be concerned with the use of monies previously raised and appropriated and might, therefore, investigate the strengths and weaknesses of what has resulted from its earlier recommendation to the House for authorization of expenditures. A national health insurance bill would undoubtedly have to clear the Ways and Means Committee at some point. To make its work more efficient, the committee has appointed a number of subcommittees that carry out the substantive work. Among its subcommittees is the Subcommittee on Health, which, at the start of the 96th Congress (in 1979), was chaired by Congressman Charles Rangel, Democrat, from New York.

Lines of authority are not always clear, and when fuzzy or overlapping, one sometimes finds committees working together. In 1977, for example, the Subcommittee on Health joined the Subcommittee on Health and Environment of the *Interstate and Foreign Commerce Committee* to investigate Medicare and Medicaid frauds.

The *House Committee on Interstate and Foreign Commerce* also has a health subcommittee to deal with legislative issues, issues that may call for new taxes or simply for new appropriations from existing revenues. This is the Subcommittee on Health and the Environment, chaired at the start of the 96th Congress by Congressman Henry Waxman, Democrat from California. Waxman took over the chairmanship for the first time, succeeding long-time chairman Paul G. Rogers, Democrat of Florida, who retired.

In recent years, this subcommittee has dealt with a large number of health legislative matters. In 1977, for example, it held joint hearings that year with the Subcommittee on Health on the administration's hospital cost containment proposals. It also held hearings, referred to in Chapter 4, on reimbursement of rural clinics under Medicare and Medicaid. Most health legislation comes through this subcommittee.

The Interstate and Foreign Commerce Committee has another subcommittee, the Subcommittee on Oversight and Investigations, which has been chaired for some time by Congressman John E. Moss, Democrat of California. It has been looking at a number of health matters, particularly with regard to unnecessary surgery and medical domination of Blue Shield boards of directors. Congressman Moss retired at the end of the 95th Congress. Whether his successor (Representative Bob Eckhardt, Democrat of Texas) will continue to pursue health issues remains to be seen.

Bills that launch new programs or modify existing programs are substantive legislation that *authorize* the spending of money. The authorization is not, however, an *appropriation*. The appropriation of money is a separate act, and the Constitution provides that money bills must originate in the House of Representatives. The work on appropriations is done by the *House Appropriations Committee* and for health by its Subcommittee on HEW Appropriations, which at the start of the 96th Congress was chaired by Congressman William Natcher, Democrat of Kentucky.

The House Select Committee on Aging has a Subcommittee on Health and Long-Term Care chaired by Congressman Claude Pepper, Democrat of Florida.

Health Committees of the Senate

There are similar committees in Senate. The counterpart of the House Ways and Means Committee is the *Senate Finance Committee.* Its Subcommittee on Health was chaired at the outset of the 96th Congress by Senator Herman E. Talmadge of Georgia. The Senate committee responsible for substantive legislation in health is the *Senate Committee on Labor and Human Resources,* and it works through its Subcommittee on Health and Scientific Research, which Senator Edward M. Kennedy of Massachusetts chairs (Fig. 11-1). The *Senate Appropriations Committee* has a subcommittee on HEW appropriations that is chaired by Senator Warren G. Magnuson of Washington.

Normally, one would expect the Senate Finance Committee to handle national health insurance since NHI will require new taxes. But NHI has been dealt with in the Senate by the Subcommittee on Health and Scientific Research largely because of Senator Kennedy's interest in this subject. Some believe there is the possibility of a jurisdictional dispute erupting and that this may come to pass as Senator Kennedy assumes the chair of the Judiciary Committee.

Not all health matters go to one of these committees. The Senate will

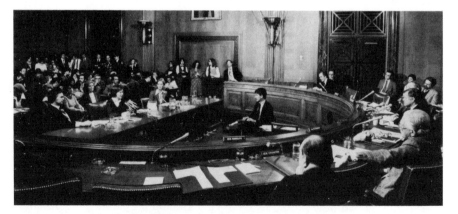

Figure 11–1. Witness testifying in support of mental-health programs before the Senate Subcommittee on Health and Scientific Research. The witness is Mrs. Rosalynn Carter. The subcommittee chairman is Senator Edward M. Kennedy. (Courtesy, the White House.)

occasionally appoint special committees for limited periods of time, such as Senator George McGovern's Committee on Nutrition and Senator Frank Church's Committee on Aging. The latter continues in the 96th Congress under the chairmanship of Senator Lawton Chiles of Florida. In 1974, the Senate Judiciary Committee's Subcommittee on Antitrust and Monopoly conducted an investigation on competition in the health services market. Moreover, one can never be certain when a committee—in the Senate or House—will find an opening in its mandate that permits it to move into a heretofore unexplored channel, unexplored at least for that committee. Sometimes a committee must move into health issues because it is essential to do so to meet its principle obligations. In 1978, for example, the Administrator of the Alcohol, Drug Abuse, and Mental Health Administration testified before the House Subcommittee on Select Education of the Committee on Education and Labor concerning domestic violence. The Deputy Assistant Secretary for Health (Programs) appeared before the House Subcommittee on Domestic Marketing, Consumer Relations, and Nutrition of the Committee on Agriculture. The Assistant Secretary for Health appeared before the House Select Committee on Population and before the Senate Subcommittee on Child and Human Development of the Committee on Human Resources.

The proliferation of committees and subcommittees has always seen a problem for both the Senate and the House. The seeming push and pull in this regard is illustrated by a report in *The New York Times* January 5, 1979 in an account of Senator Edward M. Kennedy's assumption of the chair of the Senate Judiciary Committee. *The New York Times* said:

Senator Kennedy indicated he would take a firmer hand than his predecessors did.

For example, where Mr. Eastland let junior members head subcommittees and run them with a fairly free hand, Mr. Kennedy said he thought there were too many subcommittees now. Heading a subcommittee himself, Mr. Kennedy looked into Watergate, the Vietnam War, and government secrecy with subcommittees.

Adam Clymer of *The New York Times* later goes on to write:

Senator Kennedy said that many complicated pieces of legislation cut across the jurisdictional lines of different subcommittees and could be more productively dealt with in the full committee.

But with somewhat of a bow toward the Democratic senators and their subcommittee staffs, who have been worrying about their roles under his chairmanship, Mr. Kennedy said he planned to have "younger members chairing full committee hearings" on some issues and to create special subcommittees for limited periods of time to consider particular measures.

General Accounting Office (GAO)

The GAO is an agency of Congress. Its job is, in part, to help Congress monitor the performance of federal agencies. It is much more than a bookkeeping operation: It conducts a large number of studies to determine how well the intent of a law is being carried out in terms of program activities, program effectiveness, and program efficiency. As might be expected, its reports are often discomforting to agencies in the executive branch. Recent reports have included:

- *Are Enough Physicians of the Right Types Trained in the United States* (1978)
- *Opportunities to Reduce Administrative Costs of Professional Standards Review Organizations* (1978)
- *Home Health—The Need for a National Policy to Better Provide for the Elderly* (1977)
- *Progress and Problems in Training and Use of Assistants to Primary Care Physicians* (1975)
- *How States Plan for and Use Federal Formula Grant Funds to Provide Health Services* (1975)
- *Comprehensive Health Planning as Carried Out by State and Areawide Agencies in Three States* (1974)

GAO reports are rigorously reviewed for accuracy before release and are the closest the federal government comes to securing independent evaluation of executive branch activities.

HEALTH RESPONSIBILITIES IN THE EXECUTIVE BRANCH

The principal health agency for the federal government is the Department of Health, Education, and Welfare. At the present time (September 1979), it consists of five basic units: Office of Human Development, Public Health Service (PHS), Health Care Financing Administration (HCFA), Educational Division, and Social Security Administration. I say "at the present time (September 1979)" because HEW (sometimes referred to as DHEW) is an agency under almost constant reorganization, units shifting from one area to another, as legislation, priorities, and personalities change. If one accepts this and looks carefully, one finds that HEW's functions are nonetheless evolutionary rather than revolutionary. The evolution continues as this book goes to press: on the President's desk for signature is a bill to remove Education from HEW creating a new Department of Education.

The principal health unit of HEW is the Public Health Service, and the following section describes its history and activities. Issued in September 1976, it is substantially correct as of September 1979 except as noted. Since the section was prepared by PHS, three points should be made. First, note carefully that most of the agency's activities are concerned with helping states and others do the state's and other's work and that most of the help comes from dollars given out in grants. Second, PHS personnel provide considerable consultation to states and communities and, in some cases, personnel are loaned to the states to do work under state direction and supervision. PHS direct services are limited. Third, one should be aware of the language PHS uses, particularly as regards its leadership role. Leadership does not necessarily mean that no one else was doing anything. (Typically, most successful federal activities are the result of successful state and community initiatives more widespread adoption of which the federal government is persuaded to encourage). The federal role of encouragement, and sometimes of facilitation by legislation and/or grants, is what constitutes federal leadership.

The Public Health Service*

Through the years, the Public Health Service has been most vigorous and effective when it was responding to the needs of the society it served and of which it was a part—when it was caring for those not otherwise served, when it was preventing and controlling the spread of disease, when it was stimulating revolution in biomedical research. The history of the Service, then, is essentially the story of society's response to its own most pressing needs. It began, this story, in the year 1798, when President John Adams signed into law an act that provided for the relief of sick and disabled seamen.

---

* The following sections were prepared and published by the U.S. Department of Health, Education and Welfare as *The Public Health Service Today*, September 1976.

At the time there were no doubt other groups of citizens . . . also in need of "relief." But societal pressure for this particular measure, or one similar to it, had been building for nearly a decade.

At the first meeting of the Congress, in 1789, The Marine Society of Boston had proposed the establishment of no fewer than three marine hospitals. Alexander Hamilton had supported this proposal and had carried it a step further, recommending that the hospitals provide services for the "widows and children of those who may have been killed or drowned in the course of their service as seamen."

The case for better health care for seamen and their families was compelling, but not solely for humanitarian reasons. Since the earliest days of the colonies, the merchant fleet had been the young Nation's economic lifeline and a major element of its naval defense. The proponents of the act of 1798—most notably the politically powerful seaboard States and their port cities—also argued that a healthy merchant marine was synonymous with economic prosperity and a strong national defense.

THE MARINE HOSPITALS

The first Marine Hospital was set up within a year of the act of 1798, in an abandoned barracks on Castle Island in Boston Harbor. Soon thereafter, plans were advanced for the construction of a permanent hospital in Boston, and arrangements were made to care for seamen on a temporary basis in boarding houses in Newport, Rhode Island; Norfolk, Virginia; Charleston, South Carolina; Portland, Maine; New London, Connecticut; and Alexandria, Virginia. In Baltimore, a hospital was operated with Federal funds, by the City Board of Health. In New York and Philadelphia, seamen were cared for in the city hospitals.

In 1832, following an outbreak of cholera along the Great Lakes and their drainage rivers, Congress gave the Army the authority to purchase sites for hospitals on Lake Erie and along the Ohio and Mississippi Rivers. Soon, hospitals had been built at ports from New Orleans to Buffalo. A hospital was even erected in Hawaii to care for American seamen plying the whaling trade and other types of commerce in the Pacific.

It was not until 1870, however, that the Marine Hospital Service was formally organized as a national agency with a central headquarters. In April of the following year, the first Medical Officer in Charge, Dr. John Maynard Woodworth, began the tasks of revitalizing the hospitals, many of which had grown obsolete, and of creating a personnel system to staff them.

Dr. Woodworth's efforts, together with new regulations governing the appointment and promotion of physicians in the Marine Hospital Service, paved the way for the statutory establishment, in 1889, of the Commissioned Corps. In 1930, the Corps was first permitted to hire engineers and dentists, and in 1944, this authority was expanded to include research scientists, nurses and a range of other health specialists.

EPIDEMIC CONTROL

In the summer of 1878, the Mississippi River towboat, the John D. Porter, departed New Orleans for Pittsburgh with a string of barges astern and, on board, a passenger with a fever—yellow fever. Within a few days the fever had spread to other passengers and members of the crew, and at each stop along the Mississippi and up the Ohio, the sick and the dead were put ashore. By the time the Porter reached her destination, 23 men had died on board and she had spread infection to nearly 100 towns and cities along the river route. Some accounts say the epidemic of 1878 took 20,000 lives; others claim that as many as 100,000 died.

As early as 1799, Congress had authorized Federal officers to cooperate with State and local authorities in the enforcement of their quarantine laws. And in succeeding years, many short-term laws were enacted, authorizing physicians in the Marine Hospitals to go to the assistance of communities stricken with cholera and yellow fever.

But at the time of the epidemic of 1878, the Nation's quarantine laws and regulations were still the exclusive province of State and local governments and, as such, were far from effective. Cognizant of this situation and its potential for disaster, the Congress, in that same year, moved to give the Marine Hospital Service at least a measure of responsibility for replacing diversity with uniformity. Under the terms of the first Federal Quarantine Act, the Service was authorized to develop quarantine laws for ports that lacked either State or local regulations. Localities that already had laws could cooperate or not, on a voluntary basis. Five years later, however, in 1893, Congress granted the Service full responsibility for foreign and interstate quarantine (Fig. 11-2).

If the great epidemics of the late 1800's helped to prove the need for national quarantine laws, they also pointed up the value of a national health organization, one that could speed assistance to locations that needed it. So it was that when plague was reported in San Francisco in the early 1900's, the Service was prepared to dispatch medical personnel and supplies to the area. The campaign that the Service conducted met with such success that its director, Dr. Rupert Blue, received local and national praise.

A man of considerable ability, both as physician and administrator, Dr. Blue was named Surgeon General in 1911 and immediately undertook campaigns

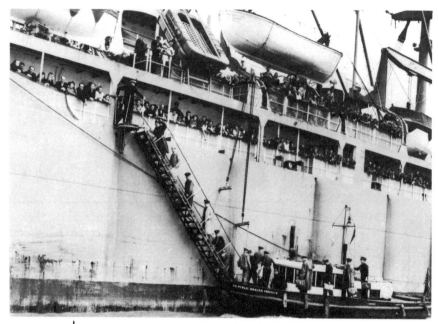

Figure 11–2. Officials of the U.S. Public Health Service, Immigration Service, Customs, and the Department of Agriculture boarding a passenger vessel in midstream in the early part of this century. (Courtesy, Center for Disease Control, Atlanta, Georgia.)

to rid the country of trachoma, typhoid fever and pellagra. His administration is noteworthy, too, for the great emphasis it placed on the organization of county health departments and the employment of full-time health officers.

EARLY RESEARCH AND REGULATION

The last quarter of the 19th Century was a period of steady advance for medical science. In Europe, Joseph Lister had introduced antiseptic surgery. Louis Pasteur had founded the science of microbiology and developed the technic of vaccination by weakened virus. Soon, Robert Koch would discover the tuberculosis and cholera bacilli.

In 1887, one of Koch's students, Dr. Joseph James Kinyoun, set up a one-room laboratory at the Marine Hospital on Staten Island. The purpose of this modest undertaking was to apply the new and still-evolving principles of bacteriology to the study of disease in the United States. The Hygienic Laboratory, as it was called, quickly proved its worth. Four years later, it was moved to Service headquarters in Washington, D.C., where its sections were expanded to include pathology, chemistry, pharmacology and zoology. In 1930, the Hygienic Laboratory would become the National Institute of Health.

By the turn of the century, meanwhile, the production and interstate sale of vaccines, serums and other biologic products had become big business. The Biologics Control Act of 1902 gave the Service responsibility for licensing and regulating the production and sale of biologics in interstate commerce. The Reorganization Act of that same year reflected this broadening of the Service's traditional functions by changing the name Marine Hospital Service to Public Health and Marine Hospital Service. Ten years later, an act of Congress again broadened the responsibilities of the Service, expanding its research program to include conditions other than communicable diseases and specifically authorizing studies of water pollution. This act also required that the Service adopt a new name, one that, as it has turned out, would endure for at least the next 63 years—the United States Public Health Service.

FOODS AND DRUGS

Consumers, today, can hardly imagine the conditions that prevailed in the food and drug industries at the close of the 19th Century. People were moving from the farms to the cities, where they were no longer able to grow their own food, and, as one might expect, the food industry was expanding rapidly, with little or no control. Such chemical preservatives as borax, formaldehyde and salicylates were used extensively in commercial food processing; artificial colors and flavors were indiscriminately employed to enhance the attractiveness of the "embalmed" foods; the country was plagued by insanitary conditions in meatpacking plants.

In that same era, medicines containing opium, morphine and cocaine were sold without restriction at almost any crossroads store. Thousands of so-called patent medicines, such as "Kick-a-poo Indian Sagwa" and "Warner's Safe Cure for Diabetes," were hailed by their makers and promoters as sure cures for every known disease. Only rarely did labels list ingredients, and warnings against abuse were unheard of. What information consumers did receive came, most often, from their own bitter experience.

In 1906, public pressure for change prompted Congress to pass, and President Theodore Roosevelt to sign, the first Federal Food and Drug Act. This law was administered by the Bureau of Chemistry in the Department of Agriculture. The chief of the Bureau was Dr. Harvey W. Wiley, who had worked for more than 20 years for passage of the law.

The Wiley Act defined "adulterated" and "misbranded" foods and drugs and prohibited their shipment across State lines. Following passage of the act, Dr. Wiley and his young staff at the Bureau of Chemistry worked energetically to enforce its provisions, developing scientific methods of investigation, streamlining the legal procedures and the techniques of inspection, applying these procedures and techniques in hundreds of hard-fought court cases, and building strong precedents through administrative decisions and regulations. For their efforts, they won the respect of industry and a high degree of voluntary compliance.

The Wiley Act was a strong law for its times, but the rush of technological change outpaced it. In 1938, following a bitter, five-year debate, a new and stronger Federal Food, Drug and Cosmetic Act was passed. This act covered therapeutic devices and cosmetics and authorized mandatory food standards. A significant provision required that new drugs be approved for safety before going on the market.

Subsequent amendments to the Act of 1938 applied safety controls to a broad spectrum of pesticides, chemicals and colors used in foods, drugs and cosmetics. With this type of industry regulation came new emphasis on scientific research and public education, it being recognized that consumers are best protected by preventing violations of the law, rather than by prosecuting violators afterward.

The Bureau of Chemistry went out of business in 1927, when the Food, Drug, and Insecticide Administration was formed in the Department of Agriculture. Four years later, in 1931, the name was shortened to the Food and Drug Administration.

In 1940, FDA was transferred to the Federal Security Agency, which became the Department of Health, Education, and Welfare in 1953. In 1968, FDA became a part of HEW's Public Health Service.

GROWTH OF THE HEALTH PARTNERSHIP

A major development in the history of the PHS came in 1935 with the passage of the Social Security Act. This legislation, which authorized annual grants to the States for the "investigation of disease and problems of sanitation," greatly facilitated the efforts of the Service to organize and develop the Nation's health resources. In effect, it joined the Federal Government and the States in a partnership to promote and protect the health of the people.

As an immediate result of this act, some 175 new, local health departments were created by the close of the 1936 fiscal year, and, by the end of the following year, the PHS had established consulting services to the States in nutrition, dental hygiene, laboratory methods and accounting.

But the strengthening of local health services was only part of the task at hand, for, by this time, new health problems were pressing heavily upon the Nation. The aging of the population and the spiraling death rates from chronic diseases pointed up the need for a major research effort in the chronic and long-term illnesses.

In 1937, Congress unanimously passed the National Cancer Act. This legislation established the National Cancer Institute and, more significantly, set a national pattern for the Federal support of biomedical research. The act authorized NCI to conduct research in its own laboratories, to award grants to non-government scientists and institutions and to carry out a program of fellowships for the training of scientists and clinicians. It also led to the establishment of a National Advisory Cancer Council, composed of leaders in science, medicine and public affairs, whose job it would be to advise on the grant and training programs.

This comprehensive pattern of support was subsequently applied to all the research programs of the Service. And with the opening, in 1953, of the 500-bed NIH Clinical Center, the Service was able to combine laboratory *and* clinical research into the Nation's major diseases.

The Venereal Disease Control Act of 1938 enabled the Service to launch the first national control program against a specific group of disease—chiefly, in this case, syphilis and gonorrhea. In 1939, as part of the Roosevelt Administration's efforts to consolidate the Federal services, including those in the health, education and welfare sectors, the Public Health Service was made a component of the newly created Federal Security Agency.

During World War II, the Service was given responsibility for a number of emergency health and sanitation functions. These activities contributed substantially to the defense effort but did little to further the development of the kinds of health services programs that the people wanted and that public and medical leaders agreed were badly needed.

At the close of hostilities, therefore, Congress began to enact legislation that, in the years since, has significantly affected the Nation's medical research and training efforts, increased health services in the States and expanded the functions and responsibilities of the Public Health Service.

In 1946, the shortage of hospital and related medical facilities spurred the establishment of the National Hospital Survey and Construction (Hill-Burton) Program, the purpose of which was to provide Federal aid to the States for the construction of hospitals and health centers. Also in 1946, the National Mental Health Act established a National Advisory Council on Mental Health and a broad program of grants for research, training and community mental health services.

The Service's research activities were strengthened in 1948 with the establishment, at the National Institute of Health, of the National Heart Institute, the National Institute of Dental Research and the National Micro-biological Institute. The National Heart Act, which authorized the creation of the Heart Institute, also changed the name of NIH to the National Institutes of Health (plural). Over the next two decades, eight more Institutes were authorized by the Congress and established within NIH.*

A major goal of the Public Health Service during this period of growth in the basic research area was that of putting our new knowledge to work in the Nation's communities. The Community Health Services and Facilities Act of 1961 authorized the Service to support community studies and demonstrations that would lead to new and improved out-of-hospital services, particularly for the chronically ill and aged.

The Mental Retardation Facilities and Community Mental Health Centers Construction Act of 1963 extended this service-development concept to the mentally ill and retarded, authorizing funds for the construction of community-based mental health centers and, generally, emphasizing treatment in the patient's community, rather than custodial care in large institutions. This construction-grant program was expanded in 1965 to include Federal grant support for Community Mental Health Center staffing, as well.

In the field of infectious diseases, the Vaccination Assistance Act of 1962 enabled the Service to help States and communities conduct immunization programs against poliomyelitis, tetanus, diphtheria and whooping cough. The aim of this legislation was to eradicate these preventable diseases in the United States.

Meanwhile, another major campaign was being waged against the health hazards of the environment, from pollution of the air and water to traffic deaths and injuries, and a number of new Public Health Service divisions and laboratories were being created. The Water Pollution Control Act of 1948, for example, launched PHS programs in that field. Environmental health research and training was expanded in 1954 with the opening of the Robert A. Taft Sanitary Engineering Center in Cincinnati.

In 1958, the Division of Radiological Health was created and given the job of coordinating a national program to prevent radiological health hazards. In 1963, the Clean Air Act authorized the development of air quality criteria and limited Federal abatement action in certain problem areas.

Responsibility for the health care of American Indians and Alaska Natives was transferred from the Department of the Interior to the Public Health Service in 1955. Since that time, the PHS has administered a broad program of health services for these groups.

---

*The National Institute of Mental Health, 1949; the National Institute of Arthritis and Metabolic Diseases and the National Institute of Neurological Diseases and Blindness, 1950; the National Institute of Allergy and Infectious Disease, 1955; the National Institute of General Medical Sciences and the National Institute of Child Health and Human Development, 1962; the National Eye Institute, 1968; and the National Institute of Environmental Health Sciences, 1969.

IN RECENT YEARS

Over the last decade, one of the most prominent trends in the healthcare field has been the dramatic increase in both private and public spending for health. Total expenditures for health have grown from almost $39 billion in 1965 to $119 billion in 1975. As part of this total-expenditure figure, the Federal Government in 1965 spent some $5.2 billion for all of its health activities. In 1976, Federal outlays are expected to top $42 billion, which would be an increase over 1975, alone, of approximately $6 billion.

By far the largest share of this dollar growth has occurred in health programs not directly administered by the Public Health Service—Medicare and Medicaid, which were established by the Social Security Amendments of 1965 and which, today, finance a significant share of the health care delivered in this country. In 1976, Medicare outlays of $17 billion will help to meet the medical costs of over 13 million aged and disabled Americans; Medicaid expenditures for some 26 million low-income citizens will top $8 billion.

The role of the Public Health Service in the Medicare and Medicaid Programs has been one of developing, evaluating and recommending standards for health care providers. At the same time, however, the Service has been deeply involved in the health care system in other ways and with other new and innovative programs, many of which, today, are helping to assure that the services financed by Medicare and Medicaid are there for the purchasing, available to all, when they are needed.

THE PROGRAMS

Two important steps were taken in the early 1960's to deal with the shortage of professional health manpower. The Health Professions Educational Assistance Act of 1963 authorized a new program of Federal grants to help build schools of the health professions. It also provided a loan program for medical, dental and osteopathic students. The Nurse Training Act of 1964 authorized Federal aid for the construction and rehabilitation of nursing schools and established a loan fund for student nurses. It also extended the PHS traineeship program for professional nurses, which had begun in 1956, and made aid available to nursing schools for curricula improvement.

The aim of the Heart Disease, Cancer and Stroke Amendments of 1965 was to make the most advanced techniques in the diagnosis and treatment of these "killers" available to physicians and their patients everywhere. These amendments to the Public Health Service Act authorized the Service to create regional programs of cooperation (Regional Medical Programs) in research, training and patient care across the Nation.

Several programs initiated by the Service in recent years have focused on the special health-care needs of communities. The National Health Service Corps, created by the Emergency Health Personnel Act of 1970, recruits and places physicians and other health professionals in areas that have critical shortages of health manpower.

The Health Maintenance Organization Service, established administratively in 1971 (and by the HMO Act of 1973), supports the development of health maintenance organizations, which provide comprehensive health care services on a prepaid basis. HMOs emphasize primary care, preventive services and operational efficiency. The Emergency Medical Services Systems Act, passed by the Congress in 1973, authorizes the Service to provide financial support and technical assistance for the development of better emergency medical services in the Nation's communities.

THE EVOLVING STRUCTURE

The responsibilities that have accrued to the Public Health Service, particularly in the last decade, have been too numerous and complex for detailed discussion in this short history. Much has been omitted. Similarly, the organizational changes that have occurred within the Service in recent years can only be sketched in the narrative that follows.

The Public Health Service Act of July 1, 1944, divided the Service into four bureaus: the Office of the Surgeon General, the National Institute of Health, the Bureau of Medical Services, and the Bureau of State Services. In 1953, PHS, along with other units of the Federal Security Agency, became a component of the newly created Department of Health, Education, and Welfare.

In January of 1967, HEW Secretary John Gardner established a new PHS organization of five bureaus: the National Institutes of Health, the Bureau of Disease Prevention and Environmental Control, the National Institute of Mental Health, the Bureau of Health Services, and the Bureau of Health Manpower. The Surgeon General retained line responsibility for the direction of the Service.

But not for long. In 1968, President Lyndon Johnson again called upon the Secretary, as he had the year before, for a reorganization plan. The objective, the President said, was to "achieve the most efficient and economic operation of the health programs of the Federal Government."

With this mandate in hand, Acting HEW Secretary Wilbur Cohen deemphasized the Office of the Surgeon General and gave line responsibility for the direction of the Service to the Assistant Secretary for Health and Scientific Affairs. He also transferred the Food and Drug Administration (FDA) into the PHS and created a new PHS agency, the Health Services and Mental Health Administration (HSMHA). As part of this restructuring, the Bureau of Health

Manpower and the National Library of Medicine were added to the National Institutes of Health. All other components of what had been the PHS were located in HSMHA, so that by mid-1968 the Federal Government's health functions were consolidated in three agencies, NIH, FDA and HSMHA.

Later that year, under yet another reorganization order, Secretary Cohen created the Consumer Protection and Environmental Health Service (CPEHS), which took from HSMHA its air pollution, urban and industrial health, and radiological health activities, plus certain other functions of its National Communicable Disease Center, and also, for a short while, became the parent organization of the Food and Drug Administration.

In January 1970, however, Secretary Cohen's successor, Robert Finch, abolished CPEHS, dividing it into two agencies—FDA and a new unit, the Environmental Health Service. Now, the much restructured Public Health Service consisted of four operating agencies: HSMHA, NIH, FDA and the new EHS. Late in 1970, EHS was abolished when President Nixon created the independent Environmental Protection Agency. Nearly all PHS environmental health programs were transferred to EPA.

The most recent major reorganization of the Service began in the summer of 1973, when HEW Secretary Caspar Weinberger abolished the Health Services and Mental Health Administration and, in its place, created three separate agencies: the Center for Disease Control (CDC), the Health Resources Administration (HRA), and the Health Services Administration (HSA).

In this restructuring, the National Institute of Mental Health, which had been a component of HSMHA, was temporarily transferred to NIH. FDA remained intact. Then, in early 1974, Secretary Weinberger removed the National Institute of Mental Health from NIH, elevated its alcohol and drug abuse programs to the level of its mental health program, and thereby created the sixth and, as of now, last major PHS agency, the Alcohol, Drug Abuse, and Mental Health Administration.

PHS—Transition

The above history describes the evolutionary development of PHS to early 1974. In 1977, a new administration took over in Washington, and President Carter appointed Joseph A. Califano, Jr., as HEW secretary. Shortly after taking office, another reorganization took place with the creation of the Health Care Financing Administration, moving into this new agency Medicaid (formerly administered by the Social and Rehabilitation Service), Medicare (formerly administered by the Bureau of Health Insurance in the Social Security Administration), and the Office of Long-Term Care and the Bureau of Quality Assurance (formerly with the Public Health Service). Figure 11-3 shows the organization of HEW as of 1978. Figure 11-4 shows the structure of PHS as announced in January 1979, the principal consolidation being in the newly established Office of Research, Statistics, and Technology. Figure 11-5 shows the regional grouping of the states by HEW and the cities in which HEW regional offices are located. Some of HEW's technical assistance and grant review are carried out by staff from the regional offices. The authority of the regional offices fluctuates, with delegation of authority, later withdrawal of that delegated authority, delegation again, and so on. In the summer of 1979, President Carter replaced Secretary Califano by the appointment of Patricia R. Harris. How Secretary Harris chooses to re-structure the department, if at all, is not known, but if history is any standard some reorganization would seem inevitable.

PHS—The National Institutes of Health (NIH)

The National Institutes of Health, one of the largest and most prestigious medical research centers in the world, works to improve human health by acquiring new scientific knowledge. What this means, specifically, is that NIH:

. . . conducts research in its own laboratories;

. . . supports research in universities, hospitals and research institutions in this country and abroad;

. . . helps non-profit institutions build and equip biomedical research facilities;

. . . supports the training of young, promising career researchers; and

. . . promotes effective ways to communicate biomedical information to scientists, health practitioners and the public.

NIH is comprised of eleven research Institutes, four Divisions, a research hospital called the Clinical Center, the National Library of Medicine, and the Fogarty International Center, which fosters international cooperation in biomedical research and provides facilities for foreign scholars in residence. With the exception of the National Institute of Environmental Health Sciences, which is located at Research Triangle Park, North Carolina, NIH is headquartered on a 306-acre campus in Bethesda, Maryland (Figs. 11-6, 11-7). There are also smaller installations at other locations in the United States.

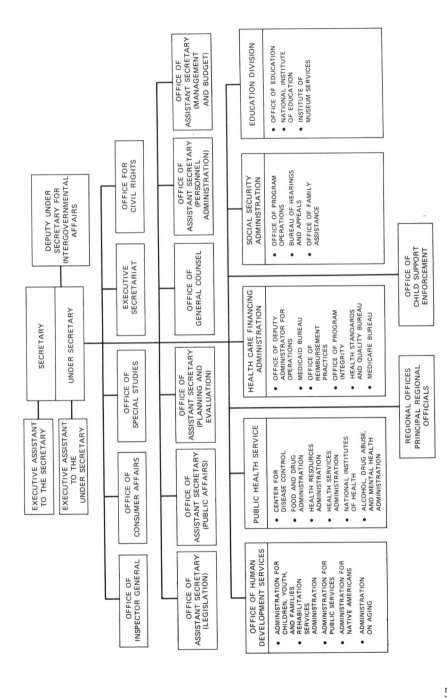

Figure 11–3. Organization chart of the U.S. Department of Health, Education, and Welfare, 1978.

545

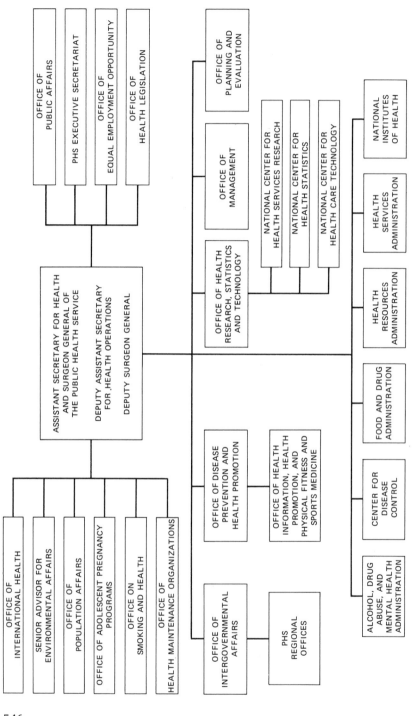

Figure 11-4. Organization chart of the U.S. Department of Health, Education, and Welfare, 1979.

Alaska

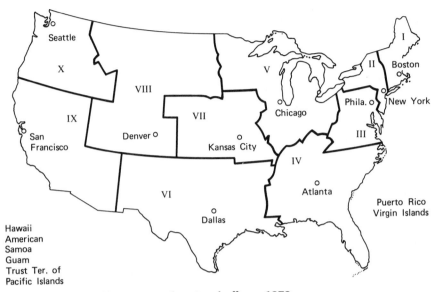

Figure 11-5. HEW regions and regional offices, 1979.

At work in Bethesda and at the other NIH sites are approximately 12,000 persons. Almost half of these people conduct research in the NIH laboratories and clinics. About 2,200 of these workers hold doctoral degrees. More than 1,000 of these are physicians, dentists and veterinarians. Together with nearly 3,000 highly skilled technologists, these scientists work to obtain new knowledge that can be used to combat the major killing and disabling diseases. They study the fundamental life processes that underlie these threats to health; they explore human development and the aging process and investigate the relationship of the environment to human health.

At all times, at least 1,400 research projects are underway in the more than 1,000 laboratories on the NIH campus. Members of the scientific staff annually publish more than 3,500 reports of their scientific findings in leading professional journals.

The remainder of the NIH work force is engaged in administrative and support activities—in processing grants for the support of scientists around the globe, for example; in communicating research information to the scientific and general publics; in carrying out an enormous variety of service and maintenance functions, from constructing new laboratory equipment to raising guinea pigs.

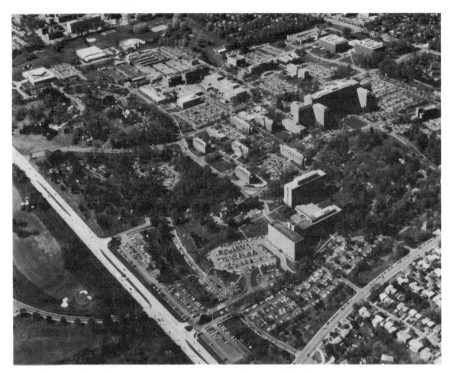

Figure 11—6. The National Institutes of Health in Bethesda, Maryland. Courtesy NIH.

An important resource for the NIH scientific staff is the 14-story, 500-bed Clinical Center, a research hospital with twice as much space devoted to laboratories as to patient care. Unlike most hospitals, the Clinical Center does not offer general diagnostic and treatment services. Patients—about 4,000 annually—are referred by physicians throughout the United States and abroad and are selected for admission solely because they have an illness or disease that is being studied by one or more of the Institutes. The unique design of the Clinical Center, with laboratories and treatment facilities on the same floors, permits bench scientists to work side by side with clinicians who are caring for patients, so that both can work closely together on mutual problems.

NIH also operates the 1,500,000-volume National Library of Medicine, the world's largest, single-subject reference center. The Library publishes the important reference journal *Index Medicus* and numerous other periodicals and materials. It also has pioneered in the automated retrieval of biomedical information [MEDLARS], in computer-assisted publishing and in many other innovative techniques and programs, including the use of communications

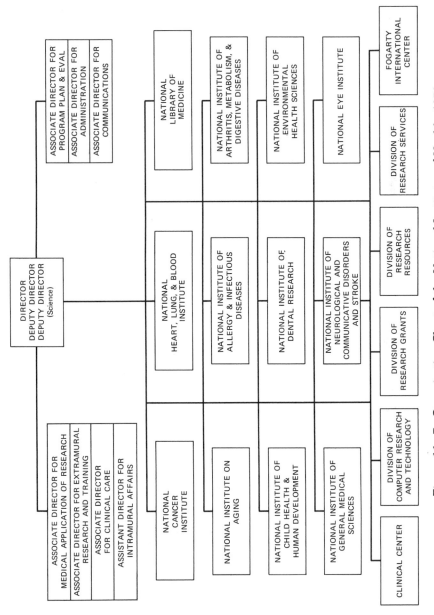

Figure 11–7. Organization Chart of the National Institutes of Health, 1979.

549

satellites, to make its resources available to scientists and practitioners across the country.

The obvious magnitude of its intramural, or in-house, research programs notwithstanding, the fact is that nearly 90 percent of the annual NIH budget of some $2 billion is distributed outside the Institutes, to investigators at universities, in medical centers and hospitals, and in nonprofit research institutions. Today, NIH supports close to 40 percent of all biomedical research and development in this country. More than 2,500 institutions in every State and in several foreign countries receive NIH funds (Table 11-1).

This research investment has produced many outstanding accomplishments, among them the cracking of the genetic code, the discovery of a vaccine against German measles and the development of spare parts for the human body. NIH has supported the work of 58 scientists who have been awarded the Nobel Prize.

Table 11-1. President's 1980 Budget for NIH
Summary of Appropriation
(Amounts in thousands)

	1978	1979*	1980
NCI	$ 871,234	$ 936,677	$ 936,958
NHLBI	447,240	506,384	507,344
NIDR	61,635	65,213	66,118
NIAMDD	260,046	302,767	305,746
NINCDS	178,254	212,365	212,322
NIAID	162,166	191,328	190,202
NIGMS	230,662	277,628	280,378
NICHD	166,255	200,843	204,381
NEI	85,337	105,192	104,528
NIEHS	64,309	78,260	79,012
NIA	37,253	56,911	56,510
DRR	145,046	154,164	154,199
FIC	8,459	8,989	8,989
NLM	37,508	41,431	41,431
OD	19,625	20,427	21,062
Central Services	—	—	—
Buildings and Facilities	65,650	30,950	3,250
Total NIH	$2,840,679	$3,189,529	$3,172,430

*Includes supplemental request for Population; proposed rescission of Child Health Facility; and transfer of OD pay costs.

Source: The NIH Record, National Institutes of Health, February 12, 1979.

PHS—Alcohol, Drug Abuse, and Mental Health Administration (ADAMHA)

The Alcohol, Drug Abuse, and Mental Health Administration (ADAMHA) is the lead Federal agency in the national effort to prevent and treat alcohol abuse and alcoholism, drug abuse, and mental and emotional illness. Much of ADAMHA's work is accomplished through grants and contracts that the agency awards for research, prevention, and training projects, and the delivery of treatment services in community-based programs.

The agency conducts clinical and biochemical research in its own laboratories and provides technical assistance to States and communities to help them establish and operate alcohol, drug abuse, and mental health programs.

All of ADAMHA's varied activities are aimed at reducing—and eliminating where possible—major health problems of alcoholism and alcohol abuse, drug abuse, and mental and emotional illness that bring anguish to millions of individuals and their families. For example, there are more than nine million alcoholic persons and problem drinkers in the United States. Fewer than 10 percent of them are receiving the help and treatment they need. One-quarter to one-half million persons in this country are addicted to narcotics, and a still larger group abuses one or more non-narcotic drugs. Furthermore, approximately one out of every ten Americans suffers from some form of mental or emotional illness, and there are more patients in hospitals receiving treatment for mental disorders than for any other illness.

ADAMHA's responsibilities are shared by its three component Institutes—the National Institute on Alcohol Abuse and Alcoholism, the National Institute on Drug Abuse, and the National Institute of Mental Health.

A short-term goal of the National Institute on Alcohol Abuse and Alcoholism (NIAAA), established in 1971, has been to make the best possible treatment and rehabilitation services available at the community level. In this effort, the Institute has supported nearly 1,000 local programs, helped private industry establish alcoholism services for employees, and financed the training of specialists in the treatment of alcoholism.

The Institute also funds training and education programs aimed at prevention and control of alcohol abuse and operates a major data collection and dissemination facility, the National Clearinghouse for Alcohol Information, and a National Center for Alcohol Education. To determine the causes of alcohol problems and to improve treatment methods, the NIAAA Division of Research supports and conducts scientific investigations of the physiological, environmental, and psychological factors associated with the use and abuse of alcohol.

The long-range goals of the NIAAA are to develop effective methods of preventing alcoholism and to establish, throughout the country, the view that alcohol abuse is a public health problem, not a crime.

Another serious health problem in the United States, particularly among young people, is the abuse of narcotic and dangerous non-narcotic drugs. There is cause for concern, as well, about the growing number of polydrug users—those people who abuse a variety of drugs.

Since its establishment in 1973, the National Institute on Drug Abuse (NIDA) has pursued the goal—now a reality—of making treatment available to all narcotic addicts and drug abusers who want it. In this effort, the Institute has funded more than 300 local programs—programs that, today, can treat nearly 200,000 persons annually. The Institute also has initiated an "outreach" program, which actively seeks out reluctant addicts and encourages them to begin treatment.

The NIDA explores new approaches in the area of prevention through education, and conducts and supports research on the basic chemistry of abused substances and on the many factors that lead to drug abuse and affect its successful treatment. In the NIDA training system, one national and six regional centers train workers in drug abuse prevention and rehabilitation. The Institute's National Clearinghouse for Drug Abuse Information collects data on drug abuse which is available to professionals, students and teachers, and the general public.

The National Institute of Mental Health (NIMH) conducts and supports research into the causes, treatment, and prevention of schizophrenia, severe depression and other mental and emotional disorders. NIMH researchers also explore problems in such special areas as child mental health, the mental health aspects of crime and delinquency, minority group mental health, studies of metropolitan problems, and the mental health of the aging.

Psychopharmacology, or the study and development of drugs that affect behavior, is another important area of NIMH research. In recent years, several major projects, undertaken to improve drug treatment of the severely mentally ill, have found anti-psychotic and anti-depressive medications to be highly effective in preventing relapses among patients previously hospitalized for acute disorders. As a result, drug therapy has become instrumental in helping to stop the "revolving door" phenomenon of mental hospitals.

It is not surprising, then, that recent years have witnessed a steady decline in the inpatient population of the Nation's public psychiatric hospitals. Although this decline can be attributed in part to more effective methods of therapy, it is largely the result of the growth, throughout the country, of community mental health centers. Many mentally ill persons, who once would have been confined to large institutions, today can be treated at one of more than 600 community mental health centers, which have been launched with funds from the National Institute of Mental Health.

In addition to its research and support of treatment programs, NIMH trains all types of mental health workers, distributes mental health information to the professional and general publics, and maintains a national system for the collection, analysis, and dissemination of mental health statistical data. The Institute also administers Saint Elizabeths Hospital, a large, psychiatric hospital in Washington, D.C.

PHS—Food and Drug Administration (FDA)

Day in and day out, the Food and Drug Administration is on the job, carrying out its responsibilities as the oldest and largest consumer protection agency of the Federal Governnent. Is the food that you buy in the supermarket safe? Do the medicines that you purchase in your drug store really work? Is the color TV in your rec room giving off too much radiation? These are among the issues that FDA deals with every day.

FDA enforces a number of laws, four of which authorize most of the agency's activities:

—The Federal Food, Drug and Cosmetic Act, which requires that foods be safe and wholesome, that drugs and medical devices be safe and effective, and that cosmetics be safe. All these products must be truthfully labeled.

—The Fair Packaging and Labeling Act, which requires that labeling enable consumers to compare the values of products they purchase.

—The Radiation Control for Health and Safety Act, which protects consumers from unnecessary exposure to radiation from x-ray machines and such consumer products as microwave ovens and color TVs.

—The Public Health Service Act, one part of which establishes FDA's authority over vaccines, serums and other biological products and is also the basis for FDA programs on milk and shellfish sanitation, restaurant operation and interstate travel facilities.

FDA protects consumers in literally hundreds of ways. Take food products, as one good example of how FDA does its work.

FDA inspectors scrutinize plants in which foods are processed. Their aim is to make sure that good manufacturing and storage practices are observed. FDA scientists test foods and food additives in the laboratory to make certain they're safe and pure and that standards are complied with. Other agency programs check for false or misleading labeling and for deceptive packaging.

FDA also operates nationwide programs to ensure that milk is properly processed, that shellfish is safe, and that foods served on interstate carriers, such as planes and trains, is safe and pure. Together with the food industry, FDA is working on a voluntary program to put nutrient information on food labels, so that you, the consumer, can get the nutritional quality you expect in processed foods.

Medicines are another FDA responsibility. No new drug can be put on the market until its manufacturer provides FDA with evidence of its safety and effectiveness. FDA wants to know that a drug does what it's supposed to do and that its benefits outweigh its risks.

FDA also tests and certifies every batch of insulin and most antibiotic drugs before they are released for sale. Licensing controls that FDA maintains over biological products, such as serums and vaccines, include authority over the Nation's blood banks to insure the safety of transfusions.

And there are other jobs. Eighty percent of the meat-producing animals in the U.S. are raised on medicated feeds. FDA makes sure that such feeds are safe and effective, that farmers understand how to use them and, especially, that meat and other foods that come from animals are free of drug contamination.

FDA also is concerned about drugs used by veterinarians, cosmetics, foreign goods and electronic devices that produce radiation. This concern is evidenced in a variety of ways. For example, FDA sets standards for consumer products—for foods, like peanut butter, that are made according to a set recipe, and for electronic equipment, such as x-ray machines, microwave ovens and color TV's.

The agency issues public warnings when hazardous products have been identified. It can initiate removal of a product from the market when new scientific evidence reveals unacceptable or unexpected risks. FDA can go to court to seize illegal products and to prosecute the manufacturer, packer or shipper of adulterated or mislabeled products. It can take legal action against false and misleading labeling on the products it regulates.

Many of the 6,500 people employed by the Food and Drug Administration are scientists—physicians, chemists, nutritionists, microbiologists, pharmacologists. Their work, which includes laboratory analysis of samples, development of new analytical methods and product standards, review of applications to market new drugs, and research on the effects of substances on animals and humans, forms the foundation for the agency's regulatory activities.

There are also consumer safety officers, who, working out of 19 field stations, inspect manufacturing plants and investigate consumer complaints. And lawyers and compliance officers, who interpret and enforce the laws. In 1973, alone, FDA filed over 1,300 court cases and supervised some 1,500 product recalls. Consumer affairs officers, who are trained to work with you, the consumer, are located in more than 100 offices across the United States. No matter where you live, there's an FDA specialist nearby to serve you.

PHS—Center for Disease Control (CDC)

As its name implies, the Center for Disease Control is responsible for safeguarding the health of the American people by controlling or preventing disease. Since its founding, almost 30 years ago, the Center has led the Nation's attack on communicable and vector-borne diseases—that is, diseases that are transferred from man to man or from animal or insect to man. In recent years, however, the scope of CDC operations has been broadened to include a range of other health problems. As a result, today's Center for Disease Control is concerned not only with infectious diseases but with certain aspects of occupational safety and health, with family-planning program evaluation, birth defects surveillance and leukemia epidemiology, with lead-based paint poisoning, urban rat control and the relationship between smoking and health, and with the health education of the general public.

Originally established as the Communicable Disease Center, on July 1, 1946, CDC is the direct descendant of the World War II agency Malaria Control in War Areas (MCWA). This emergency organization was headquartered in Atlanta, Georgia, primarily because, at the time, malaria was endemic in the southeastern United States. Before its demise, at the end of the war, MCWA had taken on the control of murine typhus fever, a disease transmitted by the bites of infected rodents' fleas, and had established a training program in the laboratory diagnosis of several tropical, parasitic infections to which returning servicemen had been exposed.

The Communicable Disease Center was built around the nuclei of MCWA's disease control specialists. Its first administrators were able t take advantage, as well, of the working relationships that MCWA had established with State and local health departments. As the years went by, CDC added professional and technical personnel, increased its scientific competence, and expanded its training and demonstration programs. At the same time, it applied these resources, with increasing effectiveness, to an ever-widening range of health problems. On June 24, 1970, the name Communicable Disease Center was changed, appropriately, to Center for Disease Control.

Perhaps the best way to discuss CDC's activities is in terms of the health problems that command its attention. Infectious diseases, for instance, account for more than 100,000 deaths in the U.S. each year. Moreover, many chronic conditions begin as infectious diseases. CDC tracks disease incidence and trends and exchanges epidemiological information with health authorities throughout the world, to enable them to take quick action as problems arise and are identified.

In this country, CDC provides State and local health departments with the leadership and specialized services they need to develop and operate immunization and disease control programs. The Center provides laboratory reference diagnostic services for unusual problems; it supplies rare vaccines, immune globulins and therapeutic drugs that are not otherwise available for preventing and treating unusual diseases.

Each year, the Center trains some 11,000 health workers. Annually, too, CDC personnel respond to more than 100 calls from State health departments for epidemic aid and help to control 10 to 20 times that number of local outbreaks of disease (Fig. 11-8).

On the international front, CDC works with foreign governments and with the World Health Organization (WHO) to help eradicate diseases before they can spread from one country to another. In this connection, the Center administers a national quarantine program, which is carried out not only at U.S. ports of entry but at strategic locations overseas, to protect the United

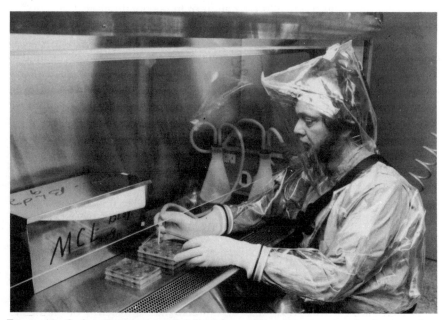

Figure 11–8. A scientist removing fluid from cell cultures under the laminar flow cabinet in Suit Lab, Maximum Containment Lab at CDC (Courtesy, Center for Disease Control, Atlanta, Georgia.).

States against the introduction of diseases from abroad. The Center also provides epidemic assistance and consultation, as requested by foreign health administrations. Seventeen CDC-maintained laboratories have been designated by WHO as national, regional, or international reference centers. There are also, in the CDC disease-fighting arsenal, a center for lipid determination in cardiovascular disease and a center for testing new insecticides.

The safety and health of job-holding Americans is another major concern of the Center for Disease Control. Scientists at the Center's National Institute of Occupational Safety and Health (NIOSH) conduct laboratory research and epidemiological studies to determine hazards in the working environment and the steps that should be taken to eliminate them. The Center recommends to the Secretary of Labor acceptable exposure limits for toxic substances and harmful physical agents that workers may encounter. It also administers a program for examining coal miners for "black lung disease," the objective being to find the disease early and halt its progression.

An inaccurate laboratory diagnosis can be as great a threat to health as an untreated disease or an industrial hazard, which is why CDC licenses clinical laboratories engaged in interstate commerce and administers a comprehensive program to improve the Nation's laboratory services. The Center also administers national programs to eliminate the threat, particularly to children, of lead-based paint poisoning and to reduce the death and disability associated with cigarette smoking.

In the end, of course, individual citizens can do more than anyone else to maintain and improve their own health. But they need to know what to do and how to do it. They need good information, which is the end product of CDC's health education activities. Through its new Bureau of Health Education, the Center coordinates all HEW health education programs, provides technical advice and assistance in the establishment, operation and evaluation of health education activities, and fosters the development of newer and more innovative approaches in this important field.

Because the Center is engaged in such a wide range of activities, it requires the highly specialized services of hundreds of professional men and women in the medical and related fields. Among the 3,600 persons employed by CDC are biologists, entomologists, toxicologists and chemists, physicians, physicists, nurses and writers, education specialists, industrial hygienists, social scientists and statisticians.

Many of these specialists are nationally and internationally recognized experts in their chosen professions. They and their colleagues are backed by a large and versatile staff of skilled technicians and administrative and support personnel.

At any given time, about half of the CDC crew is based at Center headquarters in Atlanta, Georgia, or at one of three CDC installations in the

Atlanta area. The other half, most likely, is scattered far and wide. In addition to those assigned to field stations across the country and in Puerto Rico, many are working on projects of interest to the Center at State and local health departments. Others are stationed abroad, where they are carrying out special surveys and programs.

Still others have been dispatched overseas, on short-term assignments, to help quell an epidemic or to lend a knowledgeable hand at the site of the latest health emergency. And that's the point: year in and year out, across the country and around the world, the Center for Disease Control is on the job, helping people help themselves to better health.

PHS—Health Services Administration (HSA)

HSA has only three basic units: Bureau of Community Health Services (BCHS), Bureau of Medical Services (BMS), and the Indian Health Service (IHS).

Historically, the *Bureau of Community Health Services* has been the source of funds for some of the most creative health service projects in the nation. Its activities over the years have been wide ranging. Presently, its principal foci have been to fund projects directed to improving the access and care of migrant workers, maternal and child health projects in economically depressed areas, and for children afflicted with mental retardation and other crippling conditions, family planning services, and the National Health Service Corps.

The *National Health Service Corps* is a program that seeks to assist medically underserved communities in the development and maintenance of needed primary health services. The corps will recruit and assign physicians, dentists, nurses, and other health professionals to approved community health centers and provide some financial support. The medical and dental assignees were originally assigned for two years in lieu of military service. With the end of the draft, assignees now largely serve for two years in repayment of federal education loans. These primary care centers have met an important need, but they have been troubled by turnover of physicians and dentists, a significant percentage of the centers losing these people every two years, and the centers have been troubled financially in that the communities they serve are often not able to support the level of services that are necessary not only for their health needs but also for retention of professional personnel.

The Bureau of Medical Services has direct medical-care responsibilities that, according to *The Public Health Service Today**:

---

* The following sections were prepared and published by the U.S. Department of Health, Education and Welfare as *The Public Health Service Today*, September 1976.

... can be traced back to the 1798 act of Congress that provided for the "relief of sick and disabled seamen." BMS operates a system of eight Public Health Service hospitals and 26 clinics, located mostly in port cities, that provides medical care for merchant seamen, members of the uniformed services and, increasingly, in recent years, for selected community groups. The Bureau also operates a specialty hospital for Hansen's disease, in Carville, Louisiana, administers the medical programs of the U.S. Coast Guard and the Federal Bureau of Prisons and provides occupational health care and safety services to all Federal employees.

In support of these direct-care operations, BMS conducts clinical and basic research and offers professional training (including residencies in many of the PHS hospitals) to physicians, dentists, pharmacists, nurses, medical record administrators and other allied personnel. The Bureau also trains physician's assistants, medical technologists and many other kinds of technical health aides.

A final responsibility of HSA's Bureau of Medical Services is that of improving the Nation's emergency medical services. Many people, accustomed to seeing well-equipped and highly trained emergency crews in action on television dramatizations, are surprised to learn that emergency medical services are a serious problem. The fact is, however, that in about half of the Nation's communities there isn't even a method—an emergency telephone number or line—for summoning help in a medical emergency. When ambulances do respond to emergencies, only one out of three will be properly equipped, and only one out of four of the personnel operating them will have had the minimum training recommended for emergency technicians. Further, only one out of ten U.S. hospitals has emergency facilities and staff in operation 24 hours a day.

BMS provides financial support and technical assistance for the planning, initial operation and improvement of coordinated emergency medical systems. The Bureau also prepares and disseminates national standards and guidelines for these systems, helps to coordinate the EMS activities of other governmental agencies, consumer groups and professional organizations, and funds the training of emergency technicians, nurses, physicians and other kinds of emergency personnel, including specialists in the planning and management of EMS systems.

The *Indian Health Service* of HSA is another direct health care delivery program with 51 hospitals, 86 health centers, and more than 3,000 field clinics, providing service for some half million American Indians and Alaskan natives (Figs. 11-9 and 11-10).

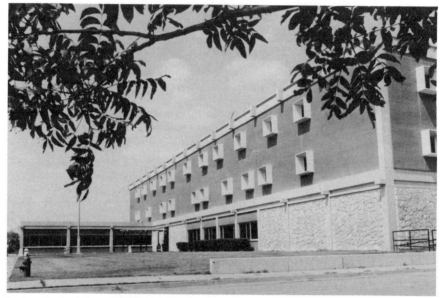

Figure 11–9. The U.S. Public Health Service Indian hospital at Lawton, Oklahoma (Courtesy, Indian Health Service, Health Services Administration, U.S. Public Health Service.).

PHS—Health Resources Administration (HRA)

The HRA housed, until January 1979, four major units: the National Center for Health Statistics (NCHS), National Center for Health Services Research (NCHSR), Bureau of Health Manpower (BHM), and Bureau of Health Planning (BHP). In January 1979, the Secretary of HEW announced another reorganization in which the NCHS and the NCHSR were moved into a new *Office of Health Research, Statistics, and Technology* as part of the assistant secretary's office (See Figure 11-4).

The *Bureau of Health Manpower* (BHM) has been the source of funding for a large number of health education programs in colleges and universities, facilitating the development and/or expansion of programs in medicine, dentistry, nursing, and allied health professions. It has administered loan and scholarship programs as well as institutional grants that enabled the hiring of faculty, construction of buildings, equipment purchases, and the hiring of other support personnel. It has also supported research regarding health manpower education and utilization.

In recent years, questions have been raised within HEW, OMB, and the White House proper regarding future funding levels for many of BHM program

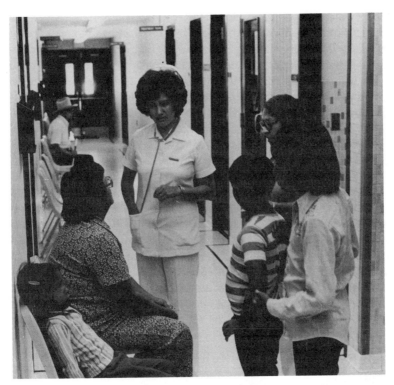

Figure 11-10. A nurse discussing a case with an Indian family at the Indian Health Service clinic at Claremore, Oklahoma (Courtesy, Indian Health Service, Health Services Administration, U.S. Public Health Service.).

funding areas, and cuts have been made. At times, cuts have been proposed by OMB that would virtually abolish BHM. In most cases to date, the cuts have been restored by Congress. There is a spirited controversy in this regard, the administration believing that more trained health professionals add to the heavy cost of health care and that the nation's colleges and universities have trained sufficient people. It is believed that reducing or eliminating federal support will allow for contraction with the residual training efforts more than able to meet the national need. Congress, on the other hand, has felt differently, believing that federal support—and expansion in some academic areas—was essential. Whether the congressional view is based on reasoned analysis or on pressure from the academic institutions that have become dependent on federal dollars is a fair question to ask. Similarly, it is fair to ask whether the administration position is based on reasoned analysis of need or dictated by the felt necessity to curb federal spending and control rising health costs.

BHM is interesting organizationally: Over the years, it has been shunted about between NIH and other units of PHS, its functions remaining largely the same despite its placement administratively within PHS. As indicated earlier in this chapter, the movement of units organizationally within HEW is a continuous process and frequently difficult for outsiders to keep track of. But the reorganizational move can sometimes signal things to come. The movement in January 1979 of the NCHS and the NCHSR to the new secretary's Office of Health Research, Statistics, and Technology had much logic to it, for it consolidated some very important functions that are vital to policy formulation at the secretary's level. The reorganization did, however, seriously weaken HRA, leaving it only with Health Manpower and Health Planning. This will undoubtedly fuel speculation in the months ahead about HRA's long-term survival prospects and, in particular, its Bureau of Health Manpower, which has been under attack, as already noted, by the secretary of HEW, OMB, and the White House proper. Furthering this speculative line are the rumors about Health Planning moving to the Health Care Financing Administration, which also has some logic given the emphasis on cost control by the health planning movement. Should this occur, then the residual Health Manpower activities might well be moved to some other section of HEW. Who knows? Back once again to NIH?

Secretary's Office of Health Research, Statistics, and Technology

Established in January 1979, this office has three basic units: the National Center for Health Statistics (NCHS), the National Center for Health Services Research (NCHSR), and the National Center for Health Care Technology (NCHCT).

NCHS is the focal point for national heatlh statistics. The center works closely with state and local health departments, which are the sources for much of the data, but it also generates significant amounts on its own initiative. As noted in *The Public Health Service Today* *:

The Center designs and operates a number of data collection systems. The Health Interview Survey, for example, is conducted annually in some 40,000 households. It obtains a wide range of data on illness and disability and on the impact of specific health problems and health related practices.

The Health and Nutrition Examination Survey, conducted regularly by

---

* The following sections were prepared and published by the U.S. Department of Health, Education and Welfare as *The Public Health Service Today*, September 1976.

NCHS, compiles important figures on such chronic conditions as heart disease, hypertension, and arthritis among adults, and helps keep tabs on unmet needs for medical care.

Through these means, NCHS gathers a host of statistics that can help in the measurement of the quality of life—the length of life—and the ways in which we become ill. . . .

The Center also conducts research in the development and evaluation of data collection systems and, primarily through the courses presented by its Applied Statistics Training Institute, passes on its expertise to health adminis- trators and statisticians from around the country and abroad.

NCHS also produces data on the availability and use of health manpower. This information is of value to the Bureau of Health Manpower, whose activities affect the flow of personnel into the health-care field, the distribution of the manpower supply, and the quality of its training.

The *National Center for Health Services Research* (NCHSR) provides contract and grant support for*:

. . . analyses and evaluation of the health care system and its financing and underwrites the development and testing of new approaches to improving the distribution, use and cost-effectiveness of services.

The Center is pursuing long-term projects to measure and improve the quality of care; it has supported research and development work in such diverse areas as blood-banking, long-term care of the elderly and health insurance. Its studies of Health Maintenance Organizations have pointed up the strengths and weaknesses of this method of delivering care. Another recent study of emergency medical services resulted in the development of a computerized simulation model that communities can use to analyze and improve their own emergency medical systems.

At its launching in 1968, the center held out the promise of being the source for the most innovative developments within PHS, to stimulate and to support projects that would, in time, rationalize, if not revolutionize, the delivery of health services in the United States. Like so many new agencies, the hoped-for results were not forthcoming. The center supported some very good work, but it never managed to take off. It has, in recent years, been under considerable

---

* The following sections were prepared and published by the U.S. Department of Health, Education and Welfare as *The Public Health Service Today*, September 1976.

bureaucratic and congressional attack, and its growth has been stunted by the criticism and by limited budget.

The *National Center for Health Care Technology* was established to provide guidance to physicians and hospitals on new therapeutic approaches and new technologies. The center does this by convening experts to discuss these developments with the view to reaching some sort of consensus, which judgments can be passed on to physicians and hospitals.

Public Health Service—The Commissioned Corps and the Decline of Professionalism

In most developed countries, health professional and administrative leadership rests with a career civil service. There is political accountability and control through an elected or politically appointed official (e.g., minister of Health, secretary of HEW), but the health service is granted considerable autonomy. It is an area generally thought of as the domain of the health professionals—and mostly physicians—with political interference minimal and political control limited largely to budget and to major policy directions such as the institution of a national health service or a NHI program.

In the United States, the professional elite at the federal level was in the Commissioned Corps, which was almost synonymous with the Public Health Service. The corps was a quasi-military organization headed by a surgeon general (as in the army), with associate surgeon generals and assistant surgeon generals with other ranks below this. The corps had its uniforms, which were worn at many official functions, as well as on duty in some PHS installations. In recent years, the wearing of uniforms has sharply declined. Over the years, the composition of the corps changed with the admission of many health workers who joined the ranks with physicians, dentists, and nurses. But alongside the corps personnel was a large number—and growing number in the years after World War II—of civil servants who did not have the benefits of the corps or its kind of military personnel system. But the corps, until the 1960s, held the key leadership positions. The surgeon general was appointed by the president for a four-year term, but he was normally from the ranks of the corps.

The control of key positions by the corps, as in the army, allowed for the development of a highly professional service with people committed to a lifelong career in the PHS. Presidents would come and go, as would secretaries and assistant secretaries of HEW, but PHS, the corps—like the country—would carry on. This kind of stability tends to build an even-keeled organization. Some would see this as leaning to the conservative side, while others might see it as liberal. But the corps certainly recognized the political constraints under which it operated; while political winds of change might blow, the Constitution and the federal system of government would go on. Corps leaders understood the federal system and the constitutional limits on PHS insofar as what constituted federal authority and what properly belonged to the states. Many in the corps would rotate for limited periods of service to state and local health departments.

Since the end of the Second World War, the expansion of federal programs caused a rapid expansion in the numbers of people needed to run them at the federal level. While corps personnel increased in numbers, the greatest increase came in the Civil Service with physicians, dentists, nurses, health administrators, and others. But the corps occupied the key positions. This caused some resentment, and the resentment played into the hands of elected and appointed officials (some of the latter being health professionals from outside the corps), who held bold new ideas and wanted them put into operation, only to find the corps resisting, not so much as corps but as professionals who will be around long after the political people have gone off to greener, or at least to other, pastures. And this was no small problem, for the U.S. Civil Service system is very open. One can enter at senior levels without previous government experience, let alone federal experience. But because of the ease of entry and because of American high employee mobility, particularly as one rises in positions of responsibility, many entered the Civil Service and worked in PHS and then moved on to other government agencies (federal, state, and local), to medical schools and other university units, to private industry, to professional commissions and associations, and to hospitals. The corps was, however, a stabilizing force, for it was there to keep the service on a steady course after "the best and the brightest" left.

In the late 1960s, the pressures on corps personnel were considerable. There were strong political pressures that proved destabilizing: an enormous number of new programs, aggressive political drives that were altering the very nature of our federal system, whereby the states were becoming increasingly dependent on the federal authority, and agitation by the new people who perceived the corps as stodgy and unprogressive and too conservative. The various pressures, including the upheavals of frequent major reorganizations, prompted many in the corps to leave. Many simply waited until they could take, as in the military, a 20-year retirement. Key offices were increasingly filled by non-corps people, people who appeared more responsive to the political winds of change, and an increasing number who had to pass political screening, that is, political party identification, in order to get their jobs. For several years in the 1970s, there was no surgeon general, only one who was acting and who represented our government in the international arena, but during most of the 1970s the surgeon general had no significant operational responsibility for PHS, this responsibility being assigned to the Assistant Secretary for Health. With the administration of President Carter, the Assistant Secretary of Health also became the surgeon general. He was not only from outside the Commissioned

Corps but also from outside the federal Civil Service. Some see in all this the emergence of new opportunities for aggressive federal initiatives. Others see in this a deprofessionalization of the Public Health Service and the loss of experienced career personnel.

Health Care Financing Administration (HCFA)

HCFA was established in 1977, bringing together the Office of Long-Term Care, the Bureau of Quality Assurance, Medicare, and Medicaid. The Office of Long-Term Care was concerned primarily with the development of standards for nursing homes and ensuring their enforcement. The Quality Assurance Bureau was responsible for administering the End-Stage Renal Disease Program, which paid for the care of nearly all persons with end-stage renal disease, renal dialysis, and renal transplants. The Bureau was also responsible for developing the PSRO program. The functions of the Office of Long-Term Care and of the Bureau of Quality Assurance have been integrated within HCFA.

Medicare was moved to HCFA from the Social Security Administration. Medicaid was transferred from PHS. Both programs were launched in 1966, each funded differently and each designed mostly for different clientele. Both programs are dealt with in Chapter 9. Suffice it to say here that HCFA is the federal focal point for administering these two programs. It is the agency that issues the regulations, oversees the administrations, and deals with the Congress.

Office of International Health (OIH)
Agency for International Development (AID)

OIH is in the office of the secretary of HEW and is the principal health representative of the U.S. government in the international arena. It works directly with foreign governments and with the World Health Organization (WHO). OIH has a particularly close relationship with AID, which is the foreign-aid arm of the State Department. AID is engaged in a wide variety of health projects overseas — financing some projects, sending consulting teams on other projects.

Occupational Safety and Health Administration (OSHA)

The Occupational Safety and Health Act of 1970 was designed "to assure as far as possible every working man and woman in the nation safe and healthful working conditions and to preserve our human resources" (Public Law 91-596). To do this, the law (act) provided that each employer "shall furnish to each of his employees employment and a place of employment which are free from recognized hazards that are causing or are likely to cause death or serious physical harm to his employees." To carry out the mandates of this legislation, OSHA is required to issue legally enforceable standards and regulations that may govern the work environment and the work practices to be employed. OSHA is also responsible for enforcing the standards and regulations; to do this, it carries out periodic inspections of establishments covered by the legislation. OSHA is in the Department of Labor.

It is generally acknowledged that OSHA will play an increasingly important role in health affairs and in the nation's economy, the former because of the growing body of knowledge we have about hazardous substances, practices, and machinery in the work environment and the latter because many of the changes may seriously affect the financial standing of the firm, which, in some cases, may force businesses to close, in other instances, a rise in the cost of the products produced.

Environmental Protection Agency (EPA)

EPA was also established in 1970. Prior to its establishment by presidential order, there were 15 environmental control programs in various federal agencies, including many within HEW. Consolidation of the programs was designed to facilitate an integrated and coordinated attack on the environmental problems of air, water, pollution, solid-waste management, pesticides, radiation, and noise. EPA is a regulatory agency, setting and enforcing standards in the areas mandated. It works through regional offices, and through state and local governments. In some instances, state and/or local governments enforce EPA standards. In other instances, EPA inspects and enforces. As with OSHA, EPA is having a significant impact, both positive and negative. On the positive side, it is orchestrating an effort to improve the quality and safety of the environment in which we live and work. On the negative side, its regulations are forcing businesses and industries to incur costs that either make the enterprises unprofitable (resulting in loss of jobs and taxes) or make the enterprises pass on the costs to the consumer.

Veterans Administration (VA)

The VA reports that there were approximately 29.9 million veterans as of September 30, 1977. Of these, 26.5 million served during war periods. Our government has, over the years, provided a variety of benefits for those who served in the armed forces, and among these is a wide range of health services. Veterans who have some health problems connected with their service in the armed forces are clearly entitled to be cared for by the government for those problems. The emphasis here is *service connected* and *not* war or combat connected. But other veterans and their families are entitled to government health care also—specifically, veterans with non-service-connected disabilities who cannot afford private care, those over 65 regardless of their ability to pay, and also the spouse or child of a veteran "who has a total and permanent disability; *and the widowed spouse or child of a veteran who died as a result of a service-connected disability, or of any condition if totally and permanently disabled*" (italics mine; 1, p.16).

Congress has been sensitive to the government's moral obligation to meet the health care needs of those who served, and it has also been responsive to the veterans' lobby and has, as a result, liberalized, over the years, veteran and veteran family entitlement to VA care. The importance of the VA system is that it is a *total* system as well as a large one which interacts and affects the civilian sector. Moreover, the liberalization by the Congress over the years as to the persons who might have access to VA care, makes the VA system a potentially more pervasive force on the health care scene. This can be seen from the 1977 rise in utilization by aged veterans which the VA surmises as possibly "related to the constantly increasing cost of participating in Medicare, while VA care may be obtained without deductibles or co-insurance charges." In this connection it should be remembered that our population is aging and the bulk of veterans from the Second World War are now approaching retirement age and Medicare eligibility. The Korean War veterans are not far behind. In addition to VA growth resulting from congressional liberalizations, as new facilities are built, access is facilitated and utilization of the VA system might well increase. It will be worth watching in this regard the experience and impact of the new VA hospital at Loma Linda, California.

No matter how one looks at the VA health system, the results are impressive as the following account and accompanying figures and tables indicate (1, pp.9-11,34,39).

The Veterans Administration health care system is the nation's largest. Comprising the system are 171 hospitals (not counting the recently dedicated hospital at Loma Linda, California), 219 outpatient clinics, 89 nursing home care units, and 16 domiciliaries. During the year veterans were also given care under VA auspices in non-VA hospitals and in community nursing homes. In addition the VA authorized on a fee-for-service basis visits to non-VA physicians and dentists for outpatient treatment, and supported veterans under care in 8 hospitals, 33 nursing homes, and 35 domiciliaries operated by 30 States and the District of Columbia [Table 11-2 presents some of the highlights of the VA system].

A record 2,375,000 veterans applied for VA health care. Almost 1,323,000 veterans, also a record, were treated by the VA in hospital or extended care

Table 11-2. VA: Comparative Highlights

Item	Fiscal Year 1977	Fiscal Year 1976	Percent Change
Facilities operating at end of year			
Hospitals	171	171	
Domiciliaries	16	18	
Outpatient clinics	219	215	
Nursing home units	89	88	
Employment (net full-time equivalent)	186,083	181,443	+2.6
Operating costs (in millions)	$4,524.9	$3,974.8	+13.8
Medical care	4,376.3	3,838.8	+14.0
Research in health care	109.6	101.5	+8.0
Other	39.0	34.5	+13.0
Inpatients treated	1,322,773	1,287,125	+2.8
VA facilities	1,239,085	1,208,281	+2.5
Other facilities	83,688	78,844	+6.1
Average daily inpatient census	111.164	113,055	−1.7
VA facilities	91,384	94,347	−3.1
Other facilities	19,780	18,708	
Outpatient medical visits	17,045,079	16,409,740	+3.9
VA staff	14,675,284	14,222,694	+3.2
Fee-basis	2,369,795	2,187,046	+8.4
Outpatient dental care			
VA staff			
Examinations	107,987	93,230	+15.8
Treatment cases completed	100,305	94,097	+6.6
Net authorized on fee-basis	107,265	121,956	−12.1
Prescriptions dispensed	31,935,815	32,043,649	−0.3
Laboratory procedures (unit count)	181,867,305	166,868,618[1]	+9.0
Radiology examinations	5,807,776	5,939,845	−2.2

[1]Revised

Source: Veterans Administration, Annual Report 1977.

facilities, with VA hospitals treating 1,210,000. Visits for outpatient medical care, again a record, amounted to more than 17 million, including 14,675,000 to VA staff and 2,381,000 to private physicians. On any single day, on the average, more than 181,000 individuals received care from the VA.

By the end of the year, more than 205,000 individuals comprising more than 115,000 family groups had established entitlement for medical care at VA expense under the Civilian Health and Medical Program of the Veterans

Administration (CHAMPVA) established by Public Law 93-82. The VA has expended some $74 million on CHAMPVA benefits since the program began in September 1973.

Since the end of FY 1976, a new 500-bed hospital was dedicated at Loma Linda, California, and four new outpatient clinics and one new nursing home were activated. Numerous renovations and expansions were accomplished. At the end of FY 1977, 327 projects were under construction at a total estimated cost of $627 million. Major projects included replacement hospitals at Bronx, New York, Augusta, Georgia, Columbia, South Carolina, Richmond, Virginia, and Martinsburg, West Virginia; a spinal cord injury center at West Roxbury, Massachusetts; and air conditioning of four hospitals. Working drawings for the construction of a new domiciliary at Wood, Wisconsin, the first such facility to be constructed in the VA system since the end of World War II, were completed in June 1977.

The VA reassessed its program of specialized medical services, strenthening programs to assure that every patient receives the highest quality and most modern medical care possible. At the end of the year, there were 1,176 separate programs in operation, including 159 intensive care units, 78 alcohol treatment units, 53 drug dependence treatment centers, 18 spinal cord injury centers, 14 renal transplant centers, and 20 prosthetic treatment centers.

A Rehabilitative Engineering Research and Development Center, the first engineering program in a VA hospital dedicated solely to the problems and needs of the handicapped and disabled veterans, was established at the VA hospital at Hines, Illinois. Its mission will be to conduct research and come up with technological advances designed to replace loss of human function.

The VA conducted an extensive program of education and training for most of the occupations in health care through affiliation with more than 2,300 schools of medicine, dentistry, pharmacy, nursing, social work and other fields. Almost 92,000 individuals were trained in VA hospitals at the graduate or undergraduate levels, close to 5,000 more than in FY 1976. The affiliations include 134 VA hospitals and 38 outpatient clinics with 103 medical schools, and 85 VA hospitals with all of the country's 58 schools of dentistry.

VA spent $109.6 million for health care research and development during FY 1977. Probably no greater recognition of VA's efforts in this area could have been possible than that attained in FY 1977 when two VA career scientists were awarded the coveted 1977 Nobel Prize in the field of medicine. These awards represent one of the few times Nobel awards have ever gone to scientists employed by the U.S. Government, and are the first ever to go to VA medical researchers.

More advances were made by VA's 28 Medical Districts in the regionalization of the management and delivery of health care. Likewise, the program for sharing specialized medical resources between VA and non-VA health care facilities under Public Law 89-785 continued to make progress. Since the end of FY 1976, 93 VA health care facilities entered into 225 sharing agreements with community health care centers . . .

During the year, VA's Department of Medicine and Surgery (DM&S) employed a full-time equivalent of 186,083 persons, including 10,993 physicians, 25,978 nurses, and 972 dentists. In addition, a monthly average of more than 100,000 volunteers gave VA health care facilities almost 10.9 million hours of service. VA's budget for health care programs (excluding construction projects) was $4.5 billion.

PATIENT CARE

During FY 1977, more patients were cared for by the VA than during any other year since the establishment of the Veterans Administration in 1930. As can be seen in the accompanying [figure], an average of 181,186 veterans were under care each day (amounting to more than 66.1 million patient days of care during the entire year)—almost 800 more than the daily average during FY 1976. Of the 181,186, 42.6 percent were patients in VA hospitals or in non-VA hospitals under contract, 8.1 percent were patients in VA or community nursing homes, 5.0 percent were in VA domiciliaries, 6.0 percent were under state home care, and the remaining 38.4 percent were out-patients visiting VA staff or private physicians and dentists on a fee-for-service basis [Fig. 11-11].

During FY 1977, VA received an all-time high of 2,375,000 applications for care—122,000 more than in the previous year. Of the applications processed, 80.3 percent were accepted for care: 41.7 percent for hospital care, 38.2 percent for ambulatory care, 0.1 percent for nursing home care, and 0.3 percent for domiciliary care. The remaining 19.7 percent of the applicants were either found not to be in need of care or their applications were cancelled.

Vietnam era veterans accounted for 19.5 percent of the applications processed and veterans 65 years of age or older for 12.8 percent. The number of applications processed per 1,000 veterans has increased from 41.4 in FY 1970 to 77.2 in FY 1977—from 36.4 to 54.0 for Vietnam era veterans, from 92.7 to 135.4 for veterans 65 years of age or older, and from 37.6 to 80.7 for all other veterans. The smaller rate of applications from Vietnam era veterans is attributed to their younger age.

Hospital Care

On September 25, 1977, a new VA hospital—the Jerry L. Pettis Memorial Veterans Hospital—was dedicated at Loma Linda, California. This 500-bed

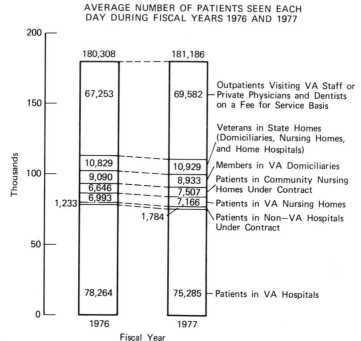

Figure 11–11. Average number of patients seen each day during fiscal years 1976 and 1977 in VA hospitals (*Source*: Veterans Administration, *Annual Report*, 1977.).

general hospital will provide a complete range of acute medical, surgical and psychiatric services either inhouse or by sharing of resources through its affiliation with the Loma Linda University Medical School. An estimated 310,000 veterans living between Los Angeles and the southwestern part of Nevada, will now be able to receive health care services from a major VA facility which will be closer to their homes.

At the end of the fiscal year, VA's 171 hospitals (excluding the new VA hospital at Loma Linda, California, which had not yet begun to receive patients) were operating 91,754 beds—44,495 in medical bed sections, 19,438 in surgical bed sections, and 27,821 in psychiatric bed sections. During the year the average bed occupancy rate was 81.1 percent.

There were more than 1,133,000 patients admitted to VA hospitals and more than 31,000 to non-VA hospitals under VA authorization. Admissions of Vietnam era veterans to VA hospitals amounted to almost 156,000, an increase of 2,000 compared with FY 1976.

The number of patients treated in VA and non-VA hospitals during FY 1977 (i.e., the number of discharges and deaths during the year plus the number on the hospital rolls at the end of the year) totaled more than 1,242,000. Of this number, almost 1,210,000 were treated in VA hospitals— the highest number in VA history and 31,000 more than during the prior year [Fig. 11-12].

The increase in the number of patients treated was accomplished largely by reducing the length of time patients spent in the hospital during an episode of care, thus making beds available for more admissions. The most important factors contributing to this increased pace of care were greater use of ambulatory care and more extensive placement of patients in nursing homes and other extended care facilities.

The VA provided almost 28 million days of care during FY 1977. This represented an average daily census of 76,629 patients, 75,285 of whom were in VA hospitals. . . .

DYNAMICS OF VA HEALTH CARE DELIVERY

Information about the demographic and medical characteristics of patients comes from two sources, the FY 1977 file of patient discharges and the annual census of patients taken on September 29, 1976 and September 28, 1977. All data on patients discharged in FY 1977 exclude approximately 197,000 one-day hemodialysis discharges. All census figures are based on a 20 percent sample of VA hospital and domiciliary patients, and on 100 percent of the VA patients in VA nursing home care units and community nursing homes.

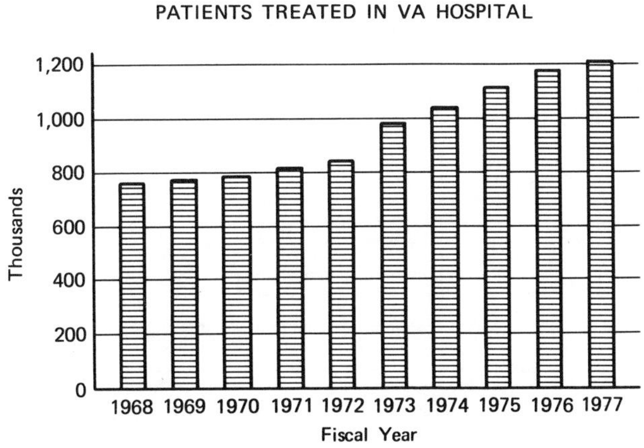

PATIENTS TREATED IN VA HOSPITAL

Figure 11–12. Patients treated in VA hospitals. (*Source:* Veterans Administration *Annual Report*, 1977.)

Age

The utilization of VA hospitals increases as does veterans' age. This is demonstrated in the accompanying chart which shows by age the total number of discharges from VA hospitals during FY 1977 per 1,000 living veterans [Fig.11-13].

This age related phenomenon occurs also among veterans who use VA domiciles and who are VA patients in VA and community nursing homes. It is most marked among the nursing home patients. The accompanying table shows the number of discharges during FY 1977 per 1,000 living veterans [Table 11-3].

During 1966, when Medicare became law, and the following 4 fiscal years the number of discharges from VA hospitals of veterans aged 65 or more decreased both absolutely and per 1,000 living veterans aged 65 or more.

This trend of decreasing use of VA hospitals was related to the declining number of living veterans, the exercise by eligible veterans of their new financing option—Medicare, the emergence of VA nursing home care and expanding ambulatory care programs.

Beginning in FY 1971 this pattern reversed and each year since has seen

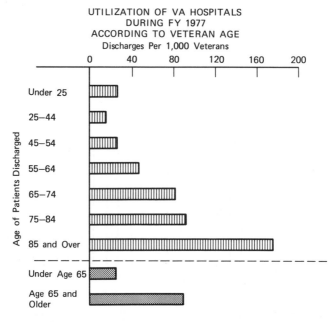

Figure 11−13. Utilization of VA hospitals during FY 1977 according to veteran age (*Source*: Veterans Administration, *Annual Report*, 1977.).

Table 11-3.

Age	Veteran Population on 3/31/77 (Thousands)	Discharges from VA Hospitals FY 1977		Discharges from VA Domiciliaries FY 1977		Discharges from Nursing Homes FY 1977			
		Number	Rate per 1,000 Veterans	Number	Rate per 1,000 Veterans	VA Nursing Homes	Community Nursing Total	Total	Rate per 1,000 Veterans
Total	29,765	942,075	31.7	7,945	0.3	3,300	14,127	17,427	0.6
Under 25	1,340	35,537	26.5	30	†	3	25	28	†
25-44	11,764	194,228	16.5	714	0.1	104	444	548	0.1
45-54	8,481	231,357	27.3	2,333	0.3	412	1,390	1,802	0.2
55-64	6,006	285,052	47.5	2,989	0.5	863	3,343	4,206	0.7
65-74	1,266	103,001	81.4	1,174	0.9	630	2,782	3,412	2.7
75-84	796	72,810	91.5	577	0.7	916	4,541	5,457	6.9
85 and over	112	19,556	174.6	128	1.1	372	1,602	1,974	17.6
Unavailable		534							
65 and over	2,174	195,367	89.9	1,879	0.9	1,918	8,925	10,843	5.0
Under 65	27,591	746,174	27.0	6,066	0.2	1,382	5,202	6,584	0.2

†Less than 0.1

Source: Veterans Administration, Annual Report 1977.

increasing utilization until by FY 1977 the rate of utilization of VA hospitals by aged veterans in terms of discharges per 1,000 living veterans had increased, again, to the level observed prior to the enactment of Medicare. This trend reversal may well be related to the constantly increasing cost of participating in Medicare, while VA care may be obtained without deductibles or coinsurance charges. . . .

Service Connected and VA Pensioners

Less than half (47 percent) of the hospital discharges in FY 1977 involved veterans who had a service connected disability or who were in receipt of a VA pension. The accompanying chart indicates a leveling off in the declining proportion of hospital discharges involving veterans who have a service connected condition or who receive a VA pension [Fig. 11-14].

Of the 75,058 patients in VA hospitals on September 28, 1977, 56 percent were veterans who had a service connected disability or who were receiving a VA pension. The accompanying table indicates the percentage distribution of patients in VA hospitals on the census days of 1971 through 1977, according to their compensation and pension status. The percentage of VA hospital patients receiving care for a non-service connected disability and who are not receiving compensation or pension dropped slightly from 1976 to 1977 [Table 11-4].

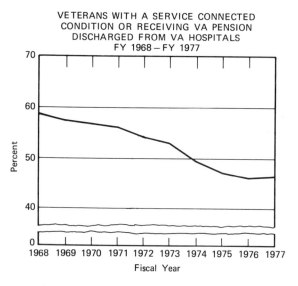

Figure 11–14. Veterans with a service-connected condition or receiving VA pensions discharged from VA hospitals FY 1968–FY 1977 (*Source*: Veterans Administration, *Annual Report*, 1977.).

Table 11-4.

Compensation and Pension Status	Percent Distribution of Patients in VA Hospitals on Census Day					
	1977	1976	1975	1974	1973	1972
Receiving care for a service connected disability	16.9	16.8	19.2	18.8	19.1	19.8
Receiving care for a nonservice connected disability and has a service connected disability which does not require medical care	12.4	10.4	9.9	10.6	11.1	12.1
Total service connected	29.3	27.2	29.1	29.4	30.2	31.9
Receiving care for a nonservice connected disability and on VA pension rolls	26.5	27.0	27.6	27.8	29.9	30.7
Receiving care for a nonservice connected disability and not on VA compensation or pension rolls	43.8	45.3	42.9	42.3	39.4	36.8
Non-veterans	0.4	0.5	0.4	0.5	0.5	0.6

Source: Veterans Administration, Annual Report 1977.

The fact that the percentage of patients with service connected disability or receiving VA pension remaining in hospital is higher than the percentage of such patients discharged during the year is a reflection of the longer term nature of service connected veterans remaining.

Diagnoses

Diagnoses are classified as either principal or associated by the Veterans Administration. The principal diagnosis is the one that the discharging physician considers to be responsible for the major part of the patient's length of stay. The associated diagnoses are all others for which the patient has been treated up to the time of discharge. The VA statistical system permits the reporting of a maximum of eight diagnoses per patient discharge. Hence, a count of total diagnoses includes the principal diagnosis and up to seven associated diagnoses.

Five major diagnostic categories accounted for the majority of principal diagnoses among patients discharged from VA hospitals during the past 5 fiscal years. When both principal and associated diagnoses are considered, and attention is focused on more specific diagnostic categories, the two most common are heart disease and alcoholism, accounting for 25 and 18 percent of total diagnoses, respectively [Table 11-5].

. . . As in previous years, general medical and surgical patients tend to be older—31 percent are over 65 years of age, and patients with psychoses tend to be younger—only 18 percent are over 65 years of age.

Duration of Stay

There has been a steady decline in average length of stay of patients discharged from VA hospitals over the past several years; FY 1977 continues that trend. The average length of stay of patients discharged from VA hospitals in FY 1977 was 32.3 days, down from 33.8 days in FY 1976. Similarly, the median length of stay has decreased from 12.2 days in FY 1976 to 11.7 days in FY 1977. Again the most notable change was among psychotic patients, where the average length of stay dropped from 137.8 days in FY 1976 to 122.9 days in FY 1977. Among general medical and surgical patients, who accounted for 70 percent of all the FY 1977 discharges, the average length of stay, 20.0 days, was only slightly less than the FY 1976 average, 20.4 days. The accompanying table shows the median length of stay of patients discharged, by type of patient during 1970, 1976 and 1977 [Table 11-6].

The complex combination of long and short term and acute and chronically ill patients who receive VA hospital care means that a single measure of duration of stay, such as average or median, may obscure as well as explain the process.

Table 11-5.

Major Categories of Principal Diagnosis (ICDA)[1]	Percent of Patients Discharged from VA Hospitals				
	FY 1977	FY 1976	FY 1975	FY 1974	FY 1973
Mental Disorder	23	24	25	25	24
Circulatory	15	15	15	15	15
Neoplasms	10	9	8	8	8
Digestive	9	9	9	9	10
Respiratory	6	7	7	7	7

[1]International Classification of Diseases

Source: Veterans Administration, *Annual Report 1977.*

Table 11-6.

Type of Patient	Median Length of Stay of Patient Discharged From VA Hospitals (in Days)		
	FY 1977	FY 1976	FY 1970
All patients	11.7	12.2	16.5
General medical & surgical	10.4	11.0	14.3
Psychoses	24.9	26.1	49.6
Other psychiatric	13.8	13.7	20.3
Neurological	14.5	15.2	20.5
Tuberculosis	21.7	23.8	52.3

Source: Veterans Administration, *Annual Report 1977.*

During FY 1977, 81 percent of the 942,075 discharges spent 30 days or less. These patients accounted for only 25 percent of the 30,721,000 days of care received since admission by all the discharges. Lastly these short term patients had an average stay in hospital of only 9.7 days [Table 11-7].

At the other extreme of stay, 0.8 percent of the discharges had been in a hospital more than one year and received 32 percent of all days of care of the discharges. Their average stay was 1,317 days. . . .

The percentage of patients resident in VA hospitals on successive census

Table 11-7.

Type of Patient	Age Distribution of Patients in VA Hospitals on Septermber 28, 1977				
	Total	Under 45	45-54	55-64	65 and Over
All patients[1]	75,058	15,355	19,970	22,765	18,967
General medical & surgical	33,975	4,023	7,525	11,977	10,450
Psychoses	20,027	6,272	5,188	4,971	3,597
Other psychiatric	12,954	3,706	3,363	3,314	2,571
Neurological	7,455	1,260	1,722	2,253	2,220
Tuberculosis	645	95	172	252	126

[1]Figures may not equal sum of component parts due to machine rounding of sample data.

Source: Veterans Administration, *Annual Report 1977.*

days who have been patients for 90 days or less has shown a slight upward trend over the past years. As shown in the accompanying table, 67 percent of all patients in the 1977 census had been hospitalized less than 90 days, compared with about 63 percent in 1973 [Table 11-8].

Disposition Status

Of 934,200 patients discharged from VA hospitals in FY 1977 for whom disposition data are available, 88.6 percent returned to the community. Although this overall percentage has changed little over the past 5 fiscal years, two of its components have changed. The percent of patients discharged for further care as VA outpatients has increased progressively from 50.5 percent in FY 1973 to 64.5 percent in FY 1977. Correspondingly, the percent discharged for no further care has decreased from 32.2 percent to 18.6 percent in the 5 year period [Table 11-9].

As shown in the accompanying table, 6.7 percent of the FY 1977 discharges were for further inpatient care in another VA hospital, a VA domiciliary, a VA nursing home, or a community nursing home. Deaths accounted for 4.7 percent of the discharges. The percentage of patient deaths and patient discharges for further inpatient care in another VA facility have remained roughly constant since 1973.

Over the years, the VA health system has improved considerably. Prior to the Second World War, most VA hospitals were scattered in various congressional districts and often in rural settings. Because of their location and low salary structure, the hospitals had difficulty recruiting top-flight personnel. The remote locations became dysfunctional as medical science developed and was able to do more to help ill persons and also as the population shifted to more urban settings. To address these developments, the VA began to shift its facility

Table 11-8.

| Type of Patient | Percent of Patients in VA Hospitals with Less than 90 Days of Attained Stay on Census Day | | | | |
	1977	1976	1975	1974	1973
All patients	66.9	65.0	64.9	64.3	62.7
Psychoses	36.4	32.6	32.9	32.9	30.5
General medical & surgical	87.5	87.7	87.7	87.9	87.2

Source: Veterans Administration, *Annual Report 1977.*

Table 11-9.

Manner of Disposition	Discharges from VA Hospitals During FY 1977	
	Number	*Percent of Total*
Total	934,200[1]	100.0
To community	827,833	88.6
Further care as VA outpatients	602,973	64.5
No further care	173,909	18.6
Irregular, refuse care, neglect or obstruct treatment, AWOL, regulatory offense, etc.	47,520	5.1
Release of committed or institutional award cases for trial in community	3,431	0.4
To further inpatient care	62,241	6.7
Another VA hosptal	31,293	3.4
VA nursing home or community nursing home	22,287	2.4
VA domiciliary	8,661	0.9
Deaths	44,126	4.7

[1]*The total number of discharges excludes 7,875 cases with missing data on manner of disposition. Data varies slightly from reports based on all discharges.*

Source: Veterans Administration, *Annual Report 1977.*

construction to more urban settings and, wherever possible, to affiliate the hospital with teaching hospitals and medical schools. The VA had the support in this effort not only of the AAMC but also of the AMA.

As with other hospitals—government and voluntary and proprietary—scandals sometimes erupt that point to deficiencies in the quality of care provided by VA hospitals. In any large system, there are bound to develop weaknesses, failings by therapists as well as by administrators and governing bodies, not to be condoned but to be prevented when possible and certainly to be corrected when they come to our attention. The VA system seems to have done well in this regard. Out of 171 hospitals in 1977, 135 were affiliated with medical schools, and all of the 171 were involved with the education and training of other health personnel in affiliation with those educational institutions. Cotton Lindsay, in an evaluation study of VA hospitals, wrote in 1975, when there were only 167 hospitals (2, p.19):

By objective standards, medical care provided by Veterans Administration hospitals appears to be of good quality. Not one of the 167 hospitals in the system has failed to receive accreditation by the Joint Commission on Hospital

Accreditation. Admittedly many of the facilities are old, inconvenient, and difficult to maintain. In comparison to the sparkling new facilities springing up across the country that have been financed through the Medicare-Medicaid programs, the VA system is clearly "taking a back seat" with regard to federal health care dollars. Nevertheless, the Veterans Administration has continued to deliver care that is not demonstrably inferior in a therapeutic sense to that provided through other health care delivery institutions in the United States. Though evidence has been offered that VA hospitals utilize less manpower per patient than other hospitals do, detractors have failed to establish that this impairs the ability of these hospitals to care for patients.

Federal Trade Commission (FTC)

The FTC was established to protect the public against anticompetitive behavior and against unfair and deceptive business practices. Its rulings affect such things as advertising practices (no deceptive advertising) and warranties and consumer rights for refunds.

In recent years, it has moved against what it perceives to be anticompetitive forces in the health field, such as the AMA's role in medical school accreditation through the Liaison Committee on Medical Education, the AMA's Code of Ethics, which the FTC ruled in late 1978 created an unfair practice because it effectively banned advertising and patient solicitation (which the AMA vows to fight), and the restrictive practices of the American Society of Plastic and Reconstructive Surgeons (ASPRS) in allowing, among other things, only board-certified specialists into the society and setting standards for notices and advertisements in its journal. The ASPRS has also actively promoted the notion that only board-certified specialists should be permitted to perform plastic surgery, and this the FTC also does not like. The ASPRS position here is in part a jurisdictional dispute with the otolaryngolists. The president of ASPRS wrote society members, commenting that the FTC preliminary consent order draft (3, p.26):

---

states that board certification by the American Board of Plastic Surgery can no longer be used as an essential condition for membership in ASPRS. This, in essence, would mean that anyone calling himself a plastic surgeon—regardless of training and background—would have to be considered for full active membership. The FTC further complains of the unduly high standards in plastic surgery.

ASPRS members immediately began contributing to a fund to fight the FTC if necessary. In an editorial in *Medical World News,* editor in chief Dorsey W. Woodson argued that "in general, codes of ethics, accreditation, and board certification have helped protect the public, not exploit it" (4, p. 7). Woodson went on to argue:

This isn't to argue that medicine should be immune to the antitrust laws. It is arguing that in applying those laws to medicine, the FTC should use more discrimination, precision, and judgment. The FTC's charter does not include the remaking of medicine to satisfy the perceptions of a handful of anti-elitist government attorneys nor does it call for the undermining of the quality of medical care.

Office of Management and Budget (OMB)

OMB is technically part of the White House. Its job is to pull together the budget requests of the various federal agencies and to propose to the president a consolidated budget that falls within presidential policy guidelines. In recent years, OMB has assumed an increasingly influential role. Its choices on which programs to fund and at what levels have a profound effect on health policy. When OMB proposes a cut, the agency can appeal to the president; increasingly, however, the presidents have been relying on OMB choices as the only viable way to control the growing burden on government of health care expenditures. Particularly irksome to HEW has been the tendency for OMB to make the policy choices rather than to let HEW make the choices when budgets must be cut. HEW's view has been that it, and not OMB, should be the principal adviser to the president on health policy, and if a budget cut is necessary, it (HEW) is in a better position to give the president sound advice as to what programs to cut.

There is, here, a basic conflict between the professionals and the president. The former seek to strengthen the health services as they perceive the need and to persuade the president to adopt their advice. The president, on the other hand, knows well that the agency's advice is frequently self-serving and may not, in fact, represent what is best for the country in terms of health or in terms of the relationship of health to the total economy. Hence, the tendency to rely on a more independent body: OMB. This, in turn, prompts the professionals in HEW to employ a variety of strategies to force the president's hand. Among these strategies are the unleashing of outside interest groups to pressure the president and Congress, as well as the outright appeal to congressional committees and individual congressmen—through the subtleties of testimony while "supporting"the president's decision to the "behind-the-scenes" persuasion of key members of Congress.

HOW FEDERAL MONEY IS DISPERSED

Federal monies to the states, to local governments, and to non-governmental agencies are distributed by *grant* or by *contract.*

Contracts are usually thought of as government buying the effort for someone to do specifically what the government wants done. By contrast, a grant is usually viewed as getting money from government to do what the recipient wants to do but which also is in the government's area of interest. The recipient of grant money generally has greater freedom of action.

There are different kinds of grants, but they fall, essentially, within two basic groups: *formula grant* and *project grant.*

A *formula grant* is money distributed to a class of entitled agencies (e.g., state or local governments, universities.) All members of the class are entitled to receive a portion of the total sum appropriated so long as they meet the conditions governing entitlement to the money. The money is distributed on approval of the application on the basis of some mathematical formula, which, with state government, typically is weighted according to population and per-capita income. Other elements may also be factors. With universities, the formula may weigh different factors such as the number of graduates and length of curriculum. The amount distributed to each entitled agency is thus objectively arrived at. *Capitation grants* to universities are one kind of formula grant. *Block grants* are also a kind of formula grant given to cover a wide range of activities, usually with considerable discretion left to the recipient.

Project grants are not entitlements. These are grants awarded on a competitive basis. The applicant develops a plan or proposal stating what is to be done if money is awarded. The applications are reviewed competitively, though, in fact, the government is sensitive to the need to see to it that the awards are spread around. Some grant programs have delegated the review and approval process, and the money, to HEW regional offices. Others are handled centrally with comments from the regions. Still others, particularly NIH research grants, are reviewed without regional comments.

Some grants, both formula and project, require the applicant to match the requested government grant. In other words, the government expects the applicant to contribute some of the agency's funds to the effort. Some *matching grants* have a fixed ratio governing applicant contribution or match; other grants are flexible.

Project grants, whether for research, training, demonstration, or other purpose, have typically been reviewed by outside (peer-review) committees, which make recommendations to the granting authority, the granting authority usually accepting the advice. These outside committees of experts, who are usually peers of the applicant, have been a vehicle for assuring that grant proposals are of high quality and merit support. These committees have also helped government agencies to withstand political pressures to approve certain grants. The bureaucrat can say to anyone applying pressure: This expert committee said that the proposal did not merit support; you would not want us to spend public money for something that is without merit, would you? This is not to say that political pressures do not exist but that they are less because of the peer-review process.

Typically, what happens is that a grant proposal is reviewed by agency staff first. From there, it goes to a peer-review committee. The recommendation to the agency head from the committee may be to disapprove, approve, or approve with certain conditions. The agency head then decides what to do. As indicated, the agency usually accepts the advice, for if it does not usually accept the advice, it won't be long before the committee does not take care in rendering advice because it is usually ignored. Not all projects that are recommended for approval are, in fact, funded. Many are approved but not funded because there is insufficient money available.

The committees are drawn mainly from universities, research institutions, and health agencies from around the country. Expenses and a modest honorarium are paid each member.

There has been, in recent years (1960s and 1970s), pressure on HEW to reduce its dependence on outside committees, to do in-house reviews only. The argument has been that the committees are costly and that the agency probably has or should have enough expertise to do the job. This is very reasonable, though one can appreciate why some agencies, and particularly NIH, have resisted this, for it would open the door wide to the worst of political influence.

With the inflationary period following the Vietnam War, there has been a sharp reduction in the availability of grant funds in many categories. This has proved a problem for agencies and universities that had grown to depend on federal grant monies for their operations. Grant money, from government or foundations, is considered *soft money,* as distinct from *hard money.* Soft money is short-term money, for fixed-project periods—often up to five years. Soft money is not assured. The project period may cover several years, but the money is usually awarded year by year and thus not assured. By contrast, hard money is money that is fairly secure: Legislative annual appropriations to a university and student tuition are fairly reliable sources of funding; hence, the money is hard, albeit not always assured, for a legislature can cut budgets (but not likely the entire budget), and student enrollment can decline (but not likely to ground zero).

The review process for grants can sometimes be very long—a year, and sometimes longer. If an investigator or an agency has a brilliant idea, and it captures the imagination of the granting agency, the agency can sometimes go the contract route rather than the grant route. Getting a contract through the bureaucratic machinery can be fairly simple—a week or two. To use a contract as a substitute for a grant is, of course, expedient, and some agencies have a mechanism for peer review of contracts. But the contract mechanism is also subject to abuse since the money can flow for weak proposals. The government has sought to curb the worst abuses in contract work by requiring that most be awarded on a competitive basis. When this is done, the agency lists the proposed contract in the Commerce Department's *Commerce Business Daily,* a publication that is scanned by many who seek government business. Usually, there is a short description of the proposed contract and an agency contact for more information. The listing in the *Commerce Business Daily* is a call for an *RFP,* which is a *request for proposal,* being a request by the agency that would issue the contract. Not all RFPs are in good faith. Sometimes the agency knows the group that it wants to get the contract and is only advertising to meet the legal requirement to do so. Sometimes, too, the agency has no intention of issuing a contract, but it advertises in order to get some information about a particular subject..

REFERENCES

1. Veterans Administration, *Annual Report: 1977.*
2. Lindsay, Cotton M: *Veterans Administration Hospitals.* Washington, D.C., American Enterprise Institute, 1975.
3. Quoted in *Medical World News,* August 21, 1978.
4. *Medical World News,* January 8, 1979.

12

Health Planning

Health Systems Plan! Annual Implementation Plan! Health Systems Agency! State Health Coordinating Council!

These phrases are part of today's health language. They were legitimized by P.L. 93-641—the National Health Planning and Resources Development Act of 1974. Before this, the language was different: During the late 1960s and early 1970s, the health field knew instead about *a* agencies and *b* agencies and comprehensive health planning.

The language is federal language, the result of a long history of aggressive and expanding federal initiatives in the health field. But it should not be forgotten that the antecedents—the successful demonstrations long before the start of federal initiatives—were many.

The most pervasive organized planning efforts for health had been carried out in America since at least the eighteenth century by local and state boards of health, representing organized community efforts to deal with sanitation and communicable diseases, applying the knowledge of the day in activities that were carefully planned. The record of those planned efforts by public health officials is one of which all can be proud. We have seen, too, in Chapter 1, how leaders in the medical profession planned successfully over the decades to improve the quality of medical education and medical practice: In each era, the health planners of the day—though they weren't called health planners—successfully applied knowledge and reason with political skill to bring about improvements that contributed to the quality of medical care and—in general—the quality of life. In Chapter 2, we read about the Millis Commission and its report, which was essentially a proposed plan designed to improve the quality of medical training and, in turn, medical practice, and it, too, has been successfully implemented. So long as one doesn't get hung up on the phrase

---

A major portion of this chapter was presented at the annual meeting of the American Public Health Association in 1972.

"health planning," one can find it done throughout history—indeed, from Biblical times and even before that.

While health departments throughout the land planned, and still plan, to deal with the health problems and health opportunities of the day, our conceptualization of health planning began to take on a new look beginning in 1938 with the formation of the Hospital Council of Greater New York. Population growth and new medical advances led the hospitals of the New York metropolitan area to band together voluntarily to coordinate their development through area-wide planning. The idea took hold, and before long hospital planning groups were organized in Baltimore, Birmingham, Buffalo, Chicago, Cleveland, Columbus, Detroit, Kansas City, Los Angeles, Pittsburgh, Rochester, Scranton, and elsewhere. On a voluntary basis, the hospitals got together, collected data and talked about that data, negotiated differences, and agreed on planned, orderly development of facilities. Sometimes their plans were faulty; sometimes participants ignored them. On the whole, however, they demonstrated that organized community efforts could be good for the communities and the hospitals that served them, just as the health departments with their boards of health were doing in connection with the environment and personal preventive services and, in some areas, with medical care for the poor.

The federal government entered the voluntary and state-local arenas with the Hospital Survey and Construction Act of 1946, better known as the Hill-Burton Act. This legislation required that each state develop, and update annually, a plan for health facility construction that would serve as a basis for allocation of federal construction grants. The work of the state Hill-Burton agencies (many of which were in the state health departments) was facilitated by the voluntary area-wide or metropolitan hospital planning councils, and the number of these councils grew.

In 1964, the Hill-Burton Act was amended by the Hill-Harris amendments, which sought to stimulate the further development of voluntary area-wide health facility planning agencies by making federal support money available under section 318 of the Public Health Service Act.

Federal stimuli for health planning by the states also occurred the previous year with passage of the Mental Retardation Facilities and Community Mental Health Centers Act of 1963 (PL 88-164) and, in 1965, with the passage of the Regional Medical Program legislation (PL 89-239). Each of these acts required planning in order to get operational funds. Finally, in 1966, Congress passed the Comprehensive Health Planning Act of 1966 (PL 89-749), which was "designed to bring order into the statewide health planning process which is now spotty and fragmented . . . Comprehensive health planning is a process which depends on, complements, and links up existing and varied health program planning activities"(1).

COMPREHENSIVE HEALTH PLANNING (CHP)

Congress believed that the fulfillment of the national purpose depended on "promoting and assuring the highest level of health attainable for every person . . ." and that "attainment of this goal depends on an effective partnership, involving close intergovernmental collaboration, official and voluntary efforts, and participation of individuals and organizations"(1). To achieve this end, Congress went on to authorize the appropriation of funds to establish state and area-wide comprehensive health planning agencies. The state agencies were authorized under section 314(a) of the legislation and hence became known as the (a) agencies; the area-wide agencies were authorized under section 314(b) of the legislation and became known as the (b) agencies.* To assure the *partnership* component, Congress provided that each planning agency would have an advisory council, a majority of its members to be consumers.

Testifying on behalf of this administration bill in October 1966, the Surgeon General, Dr. William H. Stewart, stated(2, p.33):

The bill would . . . enable states to establish state health planning agencies and representative councils, to determine health needs and to develop plans for health services, utilization of health facilities, and health manpower requirements for meeting these needs . . .

The bill is not designed to supplant with new state health planning agencies the existing planning mechanisms in specialized programs—(for example, hospital and other health facilities construction programs, mental retardation programs, or construction of community mental health centers). Rather, it is designed to help bring order into the statewide health planning process, which is now spotty and fragmented. It would provide, for the first time, resources to measure and understand the special health needs of each of the states, and would make it possible to establish priorities for meeting these needs.

Comprehensive health planning is a process which depends on, complements, and links up existing and varied health program planning activities. It

---

*It might be noted that many of the *b* agencies were originally area-wide facility planning agencies funded under section 318 of the Public Health Service Act. Public Law 89-749 transferred their funding base to Section 314 (b), and the agencies were given a few years to go *comprehensive* or get off the federal dole. The agencies, with facility oriented staffs, introduced an orientational bias to the 314(b) movement, and this, in part, accounts for the emphasis on hospitals and nursing homes and the lesser emphasis—if any at all—on public health services, environmental health services, and mental health services.

is not limited in time, or to a particular set of disease entities, or to a segment of the health services system, or to a collection of health programs. This essential process provides the mechanism through which:

All health planning can be linked and strengthened and clear purpose secured; health status can be measured, goals and objectives defined, priorities set, and actions planned for; service, manpower, and facility needs can be identified and interrelated and program accomplishments assessed.

The intent of the House and of the Senate echoed the Surgeon General's words, their reports, in fact, containing essentially the same language(3).

Elaborating on the aims of this new legislation, the Surgeon General said in March 1967 before the National Health Forum(4):

... planning is neither magic nor menace. It is not magic because there is no guarantee that it will be done well and still less assurance that even the best-laid plans will not go agley, as Burns said, during the difficult translation into action. It is not a menace to liberty because planning itself dictates nothing—it merely proposes reasoned courses of action . . .

Planning begins . . . with the aspirations of society. The first step is to articulate these aspirations into meaningful goals . . .

Once a set of goals has been agreed upon, the second step in the planning process is to break these down into a set of objectives—definable targets toward which we can aim specific efforts . . .

The product of the planning process at any point in time is the presentation of these choices. The decision is made, the course of action selected, by the decision-making processes of a democratic society. Thus planning, far from restricting freedom, provides a rational basis for the exercise of freedom.

Later in the address, the Surgeon General returned to this point:

As I have tried to make abundantly clear, the kind of planning we envision provides coherent information on which to base democratic decision . . .

As for the role of government in the process, it is the servant and not the master. Government in the city, the state or the Nation can be, first, an effective instrument for gathering pertinent information; second, an instrument for assembling and allocating resources; third, an instrument for assessing progress and reflecting changes in social aspirations. But the broad decisions are made by the people themselves, and the operating decisions are made by those who are charged with doing the work. Government can synthesize and catalyze; it cannot dictate.

It was a time of great expectations. Nearly everyone in the health field "knew" that the delivery system was breaking down. There were shortages of trained health workers and of dollars. What existed was sometimes dysfunctional from duplication of effort, lack of coordination, gaps in services, rising costs. At the same time, new opportunities were being proposed. CHP thus loomed as a panacea, as a way to bring order out of the chaos that many felt existed, a bringing about of order through reasoned analysis and negotiation and not by direction.

But the legislation never accomplished what it was designed to do. The seeds of decay were, in part, built into the original legislation—perhaps innocently—when Congress specified that grant monies given out by sections 314 *d* and *e* of the act had to be for health services that were "in accordance with such plans as have been developed" by the *a* agency. This seemed harmless enough at the time, for the monies in those sections were small, and they went heavily to state (and from state to local) health departments. In most states, moreover, the *a* agency was a unit in the state health department and would be hard put to recommend a denial of federal funds to its own agency, funds that largely went to support the same programs that were operational and federally supported before the passage of PL 89-749. Less onerous was the requirement of many federal grant programs that applications for grant support be submitted to the *a* and *b* agencies *not* for approval but for *review and comment* before sending them on to HEW. (This did not apply to NIH research grant proposals.) Some of these requirements stemmed from presidential orders in the form of directives from the White House's Office of Management and Budget (OMB). The idea of forcing a dialogue by submitting grants to the *a* and *b* agencies had considerable logic. The same kind of logic applied a year later when the 1967 amendments to the act specified that each state CHP agency (the *a* agency) had to give planning assistance to health facilities in its state, although this was not to become a vehicle for control of the capital expenditures of any institution. This was all in keeping with the principle of stimulating good planning by hospitals and others and to better link those efforts so that the democratic process could work more effectively without weaknesses from spotty and fragmented efforts. The overall effect, however, put the planning agencies in the position of reviewing specific proposals and formulating ideas about them.

It was clear to the *a* and *b* agencies that their review efforts were only coordinative and advisory and that their efforts could be, and were, easily ignored. Not only could funding agencies fund as they saw fit, but also health facilities could develop in any way they wished, if not with Hill-Burton money, then with bank loans or public subscriptions. This freedom of action from the advice of the *a* and *b* agencies was very frustrating to the agencies, many of which had come to view themselves as appropriate decision-making bodies, perhaps because they had taken time to review the proposals and had formulated perspectives and positions on them. The planning agencies responded to the free-acting health agencies and facilities by arguing that only with approval authority could they be effective as planners. They wanted, as they often expressed it, "clout." But the planning agencies were still neophytes (save a few old-line agencies that grew out of the hospital facility planning group). They had no track record that would encourage established health facilities and agencies to have confidence in *a* and *b* agency advice, competence, and fairness.

The health planning agencies also complained about other things: insufficient staff, fund-raising chores (a *b* agency lament), the need for more and more data, and the time demands on existing staff resources of the *review and comment* function. How burdensome the review and comment activities were was reported to HEW in 1971 from a consultant group. It found that the typical *b* agency devoted:

---

approximately one-third of its time to planning activities, almost thirty percent of its time to conducting review and comment for facilities applications, about twenty percent of its time to activities aimed at fostering better relations with other health-related agencies in the community, and slightly more than ten percent of its time to fund raising.

The burden of review and comment was made heavier in 1972 when Congress amended the Social Security Act and mandated the 1122 review process, which required that the *a* agency review all health facility plans that exceeded $100,000. The aim of this amendment was not to strengthen the health planning movement as a planning movement but to enable the planning agencies to help government contain rising health care costs under Medicare and Medicaid. Under this amendment (section 1122; hence, the 1122 review process), the secretary of HEW would determine, if the proposed expenditures were certified as *not* in accord with the state plan, whether to allow Medicare and Medicaid reimbursement for use of those beds. Congress and the administration thus found in the developing health planning movement a vehicle for altering its mission into a control agency. This played right into the hands of those *a* and *b* agencies that wanted clout. In some states, the agencies got even more clout when the legislatures and state administrations felt moved to contain Medicaid costs and did it by adopting certificate-of-need legislation years before there was federal legislation on this matter. Once the health planning agencies got *review and approval* authority via issuance of the certificate-of-need, the pressures on the agencies increased, for if they erred, the political and legal pressures could be enormous. The danger was that the planning agencies would devote so much time to review of proposals that they would have no time to do planning, and this was borne out in practice as we shall see.

Although the health planning agencies acquired greater influence from the above congressional, federal agency, and state actions and laws, the complaints against the agencies grew. They came from providers and from federal officials. One HEW official in September 1972, for example, spoke to a state CHP group and said that he supports continuation of CHP, although some of his colleagues believed it should be abandoned. He gave as his reason for continued support: It would cost too much to start over. Provider complaints varied but focused heavily around the lack of good planning by the agencies. In one state, for example, although the *a* agency was responsible for administering a certificate-of-need law, it had not published a state plan. Complaints from providers forced the legislature to order the agency to produce the plan so that the providers would know what it was and be able to act accordingly. On receipt of the legislative mandate, the agency found it did not have the capacity to do what it had been set up to do. Its solution was to let a contract to a university to produce the' plan. In other states in which there were certificate-of-need laws, health facilities began to circumvent the planning agencies by a variety of devious means.

The authorizing legislation for CHP was due to expire in 1973. The secretary of HEW requested that Congress extend the CHP authority for three years. His letter of request was quite remarkable on a number of points, as the following excerpt illustrates. For our purposes here, however, we note that it included a rather frank assessment of the CHP movement(5, pp. 11-12):

Although we propose to extend the legislation under which we foster comprehensive State and areawide health planning, we do so with awareness that the comprehensive health planning system is beset with weaknesses that interfere with its effectiveness. One significant problem with comprehensive health planning, for example, is that the legislation and the accompanying rhetoric have articulated very ambitious missions which, by and large, the CHP system has been unable to carry out. Moreover, Federal implementation of program requirements has not been effective to assure an open public planning process or consumer participation in that process. The degree to which some CHP agencies are accountable to the local public has therefore been compromised.

Despite the widespread disenchantment with the CHP system that these problems, among others, have engendered, the evidence is persuasive that unconstrained health resource development, particularly of inpatient facilities, contributes significantly to the problem of excessive and unnecessary increases in health care costs. The lack of effective competition, the dependence of patients on the judgment of their physicians regarding their health care needs (and the consequent capability of supply to generate its own demand), the predominance of cost reimbursement as a means of paying for institutional health care services, and pressures for institutional aggrandizement in a noncompetitive economy, combine to offset normal competitive constraints on building surplus capacity. Thus, unless or until reasonably effective competition is established, there is a need to maintain some effective control over construction or expansion of health care institutions.

The Congress granted a one-year extension.

General Accounting Office Review of CHP Activities

The GAO review was made because congressional authority for the CHP activity expired on June 30, 1974.

The report confirmed many of the problems cited in earlier studies. It is interesting, moreover, to note the extent to which the report reflects the changes in the CHP field from 1966 to 1973. GAO's digest of its findings and conclusions were(5, pp.1-3):

The comprehensive health planning (CHP) agencies reviewed by GAO have had beneficial impact on the health care delivery system, mostly by

— fulfilling responsibilities to review and comment on federally financed projects for delivery of health services.
— performing review and approval functions for health facility construction, and
— reacting to health problems brought to their attention by various sources rather than through a systematic planning process . . . .

The Maryland CHP agency, for example, through its review and approval function, stopped construction from July 1970 through November 1972 of four unneeded health facilities valued at $10.8 million and approved, after such modifications as eliminating unnecessary equipment, facilities, and services, 29 projects valued at $129.3 million.

The organization and planning activities of the agencies reviewed centered around advisory councils and working committees comprising volunteers representing government, provider, and consumer interests. These were assisted by professional staffs which the agency officials considered too small to carry out agency responsibilities effectively.

Attendance at most council meetings was generally less than 50 percent, and only two agencies had consumer majorities in attendance at half the meetings. The councils were not always geographically and socio-economically representative, and two agencies' councils did not have the consumer majorities required by law . . . .

The extent to which the agencies had mature working committees contributing to planning varied. Some had committees still being organized or inactive even though the agencies had been operating for several years.

Although the use of volunteers for CHP functions is consistent with the partnership arrangement envisioned by the Congress in enacting CHP legislation, the result in practice has made the decision-making process inherently cumbersome and slow . . . .

Some of the areawide agencies had significant problems raising required local matching funds. This activity requires much staff and volunteer time and also affects the agencies' abilities to recruit and retain qualified staffs. Most of the agencies said they did not have sufficient Federal and local funds to provide staffs to assist the volunteer councils and committees. Some donors stopped or reduced contributions or threatened to do so because of positions taken by the agencies.

The Maryland agencies, however, did not have fund raising problems because the State contributed most of the local matching funds.

One State agency and three areawide agencies had developed comprehensive health plans, but these plans needed refining and revising before they could be used for implementing actions. Other agencies had made little progress toward developing comprehensive health plans . . . .

Establishing a health planning process and developing related plans have been impeded also by shortcomings in available data, ineffective working relationships between State and areawide agencies, and geographic makeup of planning areas.

Control functions (review and comment or review and approval) of CHP agencies showed mixed results. On the one hand they had a beneficial impact on the health care delivery system. On the other, they sometimes were performed without following systematic procedures and without being based on developed plans.

In addition, review and comment requirements were disjointed, some agencies were not aware of projects they should have been reviewing and have not always been given opportunities to comment on proposed projects . . . .

HEW assistance to State and areawide agencies in planning techniques has been limited, and its review and monitoring responsibilities have not always been effective, because of insufficient staff and the desire to not interfere with functions considered to be State and local matters . . . .

HEW's recently established agency assessment program should give agencies the needed guidance and technical assistance . . . .

Looking at the extent to which comprehensive health plans had been developed and how the CHP agencies handled both *review and comment* and *review and approval*, GAO reported(5, pp.17-22):

Before a CHP agency can develop a comprehensive health plan or effectively perform its review and comment and review and approval responsibilities, it must assess area health needs.

In a previous review* we found that in responses to a questionnaire on health facilities:

— Less than half of 163 health planning agencies (131 of which received some funds under section 314(b) of the Public Health service Act) indicated knowledge of 1972 needs for types of inpatient and extended and ambulatory care facilities and beds.
— The number knowing 1975 bed needs was even lower.
— Most knew the number of existing health facilities . . . .

Our review showed that, nationally, few State and areawide agencies had actually prepared comprehensive health plans. A private health consultant's report stated, however, that most CHP agencies were developing such plans, though little agreement existed as to the nature, purpose, or content of the plan document. On the basis of information provided by private consultants studies and our interviews with HEW officials, it appears that the prepared plans are not comprehensive in scope and are so general they cannot be used in making decisions or recommendations.

Of the CHP agencies we reviewed, only the California State CHP agency and three areawide agencies (two in California and one in Maryland) had prepared health plans, all of which need refining and revising before they can be used for implementing actions. The Salisbury areawide agency was in the organizational phase at the time of our review . . . .

----

*"Study of Health Facilities Construction Costs" (B-164031(3), Nov. 20, 1972).

REVIEW AND COMMENT

Through Federal laws and HEW program regulations and guidelines, CHP agencies have been given review and comment responsibility for various health programs financed by HEW and other Federal agencies. In addition, Office of Management and Budget Circular A-95 requires that CHP agencies review and comment on applications for financial assistance for health-related projects under certain Federal programs before the applications are submitted to the responsible Federal agency. CHP agencies are also requested occasionally to comment on projects not covered by these requirements. The purpose of the review and comment is to insure that proposed projects are consonant with the goals, priorities, and needs of the local community as seen by the CHP agencies and to assist Federal agencies in making this determination.

A private consulting firm under contract with HEW completed a study in November 1972 of areawide agency performance of review and comment functions. The firm collected plans, procedures, and criteria that 109 areawide agencies used as guides in review and comment functions and assessed the completeness and quality of documentation available. The study concluded that, in general, the completeness and quality of documentation reviewed was only fair and recommended that:

— The agencies begin immediately to develop quality baseline areawide comprehensive health plans. The plans should be supported by supplementary documentation articulating and defining review and comment procedures and identifying evaluation criteria for assessing project applications.
— HEW strengthen and refine its review and comment guidelines.
— Regional directives implement these improved guidelines as soon as they are established.

REVIEW AND APPROVAL

CHP agencies' review and approval responsibility for health facility construction projects comes through certificates of need legislation, which is enacted by the States primarily to insure that health facilities are properly distributed and to prevent unneeded facilities and services. There is little uniformity among these laws, but they all include CHP agencies in the certification process through the review and approval function. This allows agencies to prevent unnecessary construction of health facilities and to direct (i.e., by proposing alternate actions) available financial and other resources to areas of greater health needs. For example, an agency could disapprove a hospital's proposed construction of additional bed space by suggesting that the available resources be used to improve outpatient services.

Because the judgments of need must be sound and legally defensible, the review and approval function—as well as the review and comment function—makes it imperative that CHP agencies develop formal health plans and other criteria upon which to base decisions on the need for health facility construction or other changes in the health care delivery system. Unless the CHP agencies develop such plans and criteria, their judgments are subject to challenge.

As of February 1973:

— 21 States had enacted certificate of need legislation giving CHP agencies varying degrees of control over construction of health care facilities.
— 7 States had legislation pending.
— 6 States had drafted legislation.
— 10 States had considered but not passed legislation.
— 5 States had taken no action.
— North Carolina's legislation had been declared in violation of the State constitution.

Of the three States included in our review, Maryland and California have enacted certificate of need laws and in both States the certificate is a requirement for licensure.

Further controls over constructing hospitals and other health facilities were established recently by a provision in Public Law 92-603, which amended title XI of the Social Security Act and which will be administered by the CHP Service.

Under this law, operators of health care facilities will not be reimbursed by Medicare, Medicaid, or the Maternal and Child Health programs for depreciation, interest, or return on equity capital (for proprietary facilities) for capital expenditures not first recommended by a designated State agency. The law applies to capital expenditures which exceed $100,000, change the bed capacity of the facility, or substantially alter the services provided.

The law provides that the State planning agency designated by the Governor shall inform the Secretary of HEW of proposed capital expenditures by or for health facilities or health maintenance organizations which are inconsistent with plans for meeting the communities' facilities needs. The designated agency may be the State CHP agency; however, if it is not, the designated agency must consult with the State CHP agency before it makes a recommendation to the Secretary of HEW. The appropriate areawide agency will also have an opportunity to participate in the review process. An appeals mechanism is provided for at both the State and Federal levels. In California, Maryland, and Ohio, the State CHP agencies have been designated to make the reviews required by Public Law 92-603.

For this legislation to be fully effective, the designated review agency must, in our opinion, develop a sound plan for health facility needs. Without it, the agency may be unable to adequately defend decisions which are appealed.

With regard to Federal leadership at HEW, the General Accounting Office stated (5, p.32):

We found that the CHP Service had done little to provide program leadership, maintain liaison with other Federal agencies and national organizations, provide technical assistance to HEW regional offices, or assess the progress of State and areawide agencies, primarily for the reasons stated above.

THE NATIONAL HEALTH PLANNING AND RESOURCES DEVELOPMENT ACT OF 1974—PUBLIC LAW 93-641

PL 93-641 revamped the CHP movement and tidied up the various federally funded planning efforts in the states. Each state was asked to designate a State Health Planning and Development agency to carry out the various health planning functions and the old Hill-Burton work. These new agencies were generally the old a agencies. Replacing the a agency advisory council was a State Health Coordinating Council (SHCC) with membership and responsibilities spelled out more precisely than under PL 89-749. SHCC was to have at least 16 members, a majority of whom had to be consumers. Appointments to SHCC were to be by the governor from nominees submitted by each of the areawide health systems agencies (HSAs), which were the successors to the b agencies and RMPs. The governor might also appoint government officials to SHCC, but they were not to exceed 40% of the total SHCC membership.

SHCC's responsibilities are specified: review and approval of the state health plan, review and approval of HSA plans, review and approval of grant applications under a number of congressional acts. Despite the specifity as to its functions, there is still potential for conflict with the state agency because of the ambiguity as to its role as against that of the agency.

The extent of the authority granted to the agency can be found in Section 1523 of the act, which states that the state agency shall:

Serve as the designated planning agency of the State for the purposes of section 1122 of the Social Security Act . . . and . . . administer a State certificate of need program which applies to new institutional health services proposed to be offered or developed within the State and which is satisfactory to the Secretary . . . In performing its functions under this paragraph the State Agency shall consider recommendations made by health systems agencies . . . .

In addition to this federal mandate that the states begin to regulate the development of health services (if they have not already done so) with the secretary of HEW monitoring their performances, Section 1523 all provides for

Review on a periodic basis (but not less often than every five years) all institutional health services being offered in the State and, after consideration of recommendations submitted by health systems agencies . . . respecting the appropriateness of such services, make public its findings.

The legislation does not provide specifically for closing facilities or for denial of payments under Section 1122 of the Social Security Act if a negative finding is made, although the threat of possible coercion is there and, as we shall see later, has been clearly stated by a congressional aide. The Senate report accompanying the bill states, however (6, p.53):

Although no sanction is required by the proposed legislation with respect to modifying or eliminating services in institutions found to be unnecessary, it is hoped by the Committee that the act of reviewing services periodically will in itself result in the elimination of unnecessary or duplicative services or facilities.

It will be interesting to observe the administrative burden and resulting costs that this will impose on health facilities, particularly hospitals, as they are forced periodically to justify every service.

Health systems agencies under PL 93-641 (205 in all) are to cover the entire nation and to replace the CHP b agencies and RMPs. In many instances, the b agencies merged with the RMPs, sometimes creating staff dislocation in the process. Each HSA must have a consumer controlled governing board, but consumer representatives may not exceed 60% of the membership. Of the provider members at least one-third of them must be direct service providers, that is, physicians, nurses, and other health practitioners, and the administrators of health facilities or institutions such as hospitals, long-term-care facilities, and so on. Indirect providers include health product suppliers and health insurance company personnel.

Each HSA is called on to develop and seek to implement a Health Systems Plan (HSP) and an Annual Implementation Plan (AIP), as well as to assist the state agency in carrying out its functions. The role of the HSA in review and approval (or disapproval) of certain federal grant programs is explicitly stated.

To a very large extent, the key actors at the state and area-wide levels are the same people who were in leadership roles under the earlier legislation.

The thrust of PL 93-641 is clearly directed toward cost containment and the maldistribution of services. The latter is typically cited to support the argument that we have enough—we just have to alter the distribution of what we have, and, therefore, no or few expansions are necessary. The Senate Committee on Labor and Public Welfare stressed these points as it reported the bill to the full Senate(6, p.39):

The need for strengthened and coordinated planning for personal health services is growing more apparent each day. In the view of the Committee the health care industry does not respond to classic marketplace forces. The highly technical nature of medical services together with the growth of third party reimbursement mechanisms act to attenuate the usual forces influencing the behavior of consumers with respect to personal health services. For the most part, the doctor makes purchasing decisions on behalf of the patient and the services are frequently reimbursed under health insurance programs, thus reducing the patient's immediate incentive to contain expenditures.

Investment in costly health care resources, such as hospital beds, coronary care units or radio-isotope treatment centers is frequently made without regard to the existence of similar facilities or equipment already operating in an area. Investment in costly facilities and equipment not only results in capital accumulation, but establishes an ongoing demand for payment to support those services. There is convincing evidence from many sources that over-building of facilities has occurred in many areas, and that maldistribution of high cost services exists.

A recently published study indicates that by 1975, over 67,000 unneeded hospital beds will be in operation throughout the United States.

Hospital beds, though unused, contribute substantial additional costs to the health care industry. It is estimated that a hospital bed, full or empty, costs ⅓ its initial cost each year to operate. Each $1,000 invested in hospital expansion requires approximately $333 each year in operational financing. This operating cost exists whether or not the bed is occupied at a particular time. The same is true with respect to other medical facilities and services. A coronary care unit with a low rate of utilization, or an open heart surgery team which performs relatively few operations a year requires a substantial proportion of the support required by similar services with a high utilization rate.

Widespread access and distribution problems exist with respect to medical facilities and services. In many urban areas, hospitals, clinics and other medical care institutions and services are crowded into relatively tiny sectors, while large areas go poorly served or completely unserved. Many rural communities are completely without a physician or any other type of health care service, while adjacent urban areas are oversupplied.

But perhaps the bluntest statement was made before the American Health Planning Association by Brian Biles, M.D., a staff member for the Senate committee. As reported in *Hospitals*, the Journal of the American Hospital Association(7, p.18):

"Costs are the number one problem and the number one justification for the planning program," Biles said. "Unless the planning program can control health care costs, the program itself is unjustifiable," he said.

With regard to the need to control health care costs, Biles predicted that "we will see recommendation for decertification"—the closing of unneeded beds—and greater emphasis on prospective rate setting through the states or the federal government when Public Law 93-641, the national health planning law, comes up for renewal next year. He also predicted that "the focus will be on moving hospitals to a regional system" and that "we'll have to see national standards" on the number of beds per thousand persons. "Health Systems Agencies [HSAs] are the mechanism that's been chosen to deal with the cost problem," Biles said. "We can't sit by and watch the Medicaid program bankrupt our states."

Some Responses to PL 93-641

American society is becoming increasingly litigious, more prone than ever before to seek the solution to problems through the judicial process. But, in a very real sense, litigation, like war, represents a failure on the part of parties to resolve their differences through negotiation.

Legal challenges (23 as of May 1978) came from many sources, including the National Association of Regional Councils, the AMA, and a number of state governments, among them being North Carolina, Missouri, and Nebraska. Seven of the suits questioned the constitutionality of the legislation, seven challenged the process by which the health service areas were designated, six challenged the designation of the health systems agencies, seven challenged the validity of the selection of the health system agency governing bodies, and four challenged the validity of HEW regulations. In late 1977, the states of North Carolina and Nebraska, challenging the act's constitutionality, lost their case before the U.S. District Court in Raleigh and were later unsuccessful in an appeal to the U.S. Supreme Court. But which party wins in this case, as in the others, is not as important as is the overriding failure of the federal government to be able to resolve the outstanding issues with state governments and major interest groups without both of the latter being forced to litigate.

Behind the litigation, and the political maneuvers of many groups, is an uneasiness, if not distrust, of the federal authority, a fear that it will abuse power, that it will encroach upon the legitimate prerogatives of those outside the federal government, and that the federal government's primary concern is not on value but on cost. Historical (evolutionary) development in the health sector lend some support to these views: Certainly the evolution of health planning from the CHP days in 1966 to the present is that of a progressive alteration by planners, bureaucrats, and politicians of what was widely viewed as an open, democratic process to an increasingly regulatory process. Most scholars, moreover, would point out that planning should be an advisory process to decision makers and that regulation, like cost containment, is not an appropriate planning function. How much things have changed can be seen in GAO's 1978 assessment of PL 93-641.

PROBLEMS TO BE OVERCOME: GAO ASSESSMENT OF PL 93-641 (8,p.25-41)

The impact of areawide health systems agencies and State health planning and development agencies in restraining increases in health care costs and improving accessibility to health services cannot be determined because these agencies have been in existence for only a short time. The impact of these agencies in accomplishing these two goals probably will not be known for several years.

In order for areawide and State health planning agencies to have an impact on the health care system, meaningful, specific, and thorough areawide and State health plans that are supported by both consumers and providers, as well as local governmental entities, will be needed. Without such plans and support, areawide and State health planning agencies will experience serious problems in achieving these goals.

At the time of our review, areawide and State planning agencies were limited in developing the necessary quality health plans because

— limited useful data was available on the existing health care system and status of health of residents;

— no approved national standards or criteria were available regarding the appropriate supply, distribution, and organization of health resources and services;

— adequate numbers of qualified staff were not available in some areas; and

— timely guidance on health plan development from HEW and regional centers for health planning had not been provided.

The development of adequate health systems plans was impeded indirectly because

— responsibilities of HSAs and SHPDAs had not been clearly defined, especially in States with statewide HSAs;

— HSA board members were not optimistic about achieving the goals of restraining health care costs and improving accessibility to health care, they believed additional legislative authority was needed; and

— controversy existed over the compatibility of the objectives of the act.

In addition, local health professional groups and public officials doubted that the goals of the act could be achieved and questioned the authority and ability of areawide HSAs to accomplish the goals. Many of these problems are similar to those identified in our 1974 report to the Congress on the former Comprehensive Health Planning program . . .

Limited Data Availability

All of the 15 HSAs we visited were experiencing some difficulty in obtaining the data necessary to develop their health systems plans. Data sharing relationships between HSAs and PSROs were uncertain. In some cases, needed data was not available, current, or in the necessary form. As a result, existing information may not have accurately reflected the actual health status of area residents and the health resource needs of the area.

HSA/PSRO Cooperation

HSAs and PSROs share certain common long-range goals, such as to improve quality of care and to contain health care costs. They are also charged with improving the health care system, though in different ways. Consequently, HSAs and PSROs need to cooperate and coordinate their efforts with each other. The most basic and initial need is to share data.

PSROs have data available which can assist HSAs in determining the hospital bed and other facility needs. Such data would include routine information on hospitalizations, including the diseases and surgical operations involved and the lengths of stay in hospitals.

At the time of our review, HSAs were experiencing some difficulty in obtaining data from PSROs primarily because of data confidentiality provisions in the PSRO authorizing legislation. Since that time, the President has signed Public Law 95-142 which provides for the sharing of data by PSROs with HSAs. Implementation of this law should resolve PSRO/HSA data sharing problems.

Other Data Problems

Data problems were particularly apparent at HSAs having no prior health planning experience. For example, one such HSA cited the following problems regarding health data.

— Almost no morbidity data existed on a State or county level.
— Physician manpower data was imcomplete and unreliable.
— Admission and discharge data from hospitals by service or diagnosis was not available.
— Financial data on costs of services was difficult or impossible to obtain.
— Environmental and occupational health information was not collected by any health agency.
— No centralized statewide health data bank existed.
— Data on private services, facilities, and unlicensed health personnel was almost nonexistent.

Other HSAs noted that they rely too often on outdated or unreliable health data from Federal, State, and local agencies. For example, one HSA we visited was using data developed by a regional council of governments which was more than 3 years old. An official at another HSA told us that only between 10 and 20 of 200 health status indicators were going to be used in its health system plan because data for most of the indicators was not available. Another HSA had to limit its health planning activities because of the quantity and quality of health data.

Officials at several HSAs noted that the act itself makes it difficult for an HSA to develop its own data. Section 1513 (b) requires that existing data be used to the maximum extent possible.

Need for Standards and Criteria For Health Resources and Services

The health systems plan is the HSA's statement of desired achievements for improvements in the health status of area residents and in the health systems serving that population. The plan should provide a basis for the HSA to promote a healthful environment, to review proposed health systems changes, to reduce documented deficiencies and inefficiencies within the area, and to foster desired achievements which meet identified health needs of the community. In order for HSAs to efficiently and effectively plan health delivery systems and to judge the proposed changes to the system, standards and criteria for the various types of health resources and services are needed. The act recognizes the need for such standards in section 1501 (b) which directs the Secretary of HEW to include in the National Guidelines for Health Planning "Standards respecting the appropriate supply, distribution, and organization of health resources."

HEW awarded contracts costing about $1.4 million to develop standards and criteria for 17 different types of health services for the use of HSAs. These standards and criteria were distributed informally to HSAs with the stipulation that they were not endorsed by HEW and were to be used at their own discretion. According to an HEW official, HEW was reluctant to endorse these standards and criteria because in some cases they did not reflect HEW policy and in other cases HEW had not yet established policy.

Several HSAs indicated the need for national standards and criteria. One HSA official said that until such standards and criteria are available, he would not review proposed health services because legal actions challenging the basis of the HSA's decision could occur. According to the HSA executive director, these actions could tie up a considerable amount of the HSA's resources.

On March 28, 1978, subsequent to the completion of our review and almost 2 years after most of the HSAs had been designated, HEW issued final national guidelines for health planning in nine types of health services and facilities. HEW is developing further guidelines setting forth national health planning goals and additional standards.

Project Review Experience

We obtained statistics from several of the States on the approval rate of applications for new institutional services under certificate of need programs and section 1122 project review responsibilities . . . As the table . . . following . . . shows, the approval rate was about 92 percent. We believe that one reason for the high approval rate is the lack of standards and criteria on which to evaluate these applications.

Summary of Project Applications Reviewed and Approved by 10 State Health Planning Agencies During Calendar Year 1976

State	Projects Reviewed	Projects Approved	Percent Approved
Colorado	54	48	89
Wyoming	13	13	100
Utah	31	30	97
Florida	176	165	94
Alabama	159	150	94
Arizona	35	35	100
Maine (note a)	18	15	83
New Hampshire	18	16	89
Massachusetts (note b)	71	57	80
Virginia (note a)	61	55	90
Total	636	584	92

a/Review period covered 7/1/76-3/31/77.
b/Review period covered 7/1/76-1/31/77.

Many applications for new or expanded facilities or services are never submitted because of project review procedures. Several HSAs, as well as HEW, brought this fact to our attention.

The need for timely standards and criteria is particularly important when new technology is developed. For example, considerable concern has recently been expressed about the number of computerized tomography[1] scanners being acquired throughout the country. In the absence of standards and criteria, HSAs and SHPDAs have little basis to disapprove a hospital's request for one of these expensive ($400,000-$700,000) machines. As a result, the health care system could be buying unnecessary scanners which could cause increased health care costs.

The schedule below shows the approval rate of applications to purchase scanners.

[1]The computerized tomography scanner is a relatively new radiological (X-ray) device that is based on the same principles as conventional X-ray techniques but collects and processes information using a computer to transmit three dimensional "pictures" of the body. It has been hailed as the greatest advance in radiology since the discovery of X-rays.

State	Applications	Number Approved	Percent Approved
Florida	17	16	94
Alabama	7	7	100
Colorado	16	15	94
Wyoming	1	1	100
Utah	7	7	100
Maine	3	2	66
New Hampshire	1	1	100
Massachusetts	3	2	66
Virginia	21	20	95
Total	76	71	93

Need for More Timely Guidance on Developing Health Systems Plans

HEW did not provide guidelines for developing health systems plans until late in December 1976, almost 2 years after the act's passage.

Several of the HSAs we visited indicated that the lack of formal guidelines from HEW has delayed them from preparing their health systems plans. The delays had not yet affected some of the remaining HSAs because their activities were centered on hiring staff and other organizational and administrative functions, and plan development was in the preliminary stages.

. . . at least one HEW regional office provided HSAs guidance on health systems plan development that was not consistent with the December 1976 HEW guidelines. More timely HEW guidance may have prevented this inconsistency from occurring and eliminated the confusion that exists as a result of not having HEW guidelines.

Staffing Problems

Some of the HSAs we visited were experiencing difficulty in employing health planning staff. Limited numbers of persons having experience in health planning were available in certain areas and, in some cases, HSAs had been unable to offer salaries that would attract potential employees. Also one HSA official indicated that qualified persons were reluctant to work for HSAs because of the uncertainty surrounding the continuance of the program.

To assist HSAs in employing qualified staff, HEW awarded a 2-year $215,000 contract in August 1975 to the American Association for Comprehensive Health Planning. The purpose of this contract was to (1) design and operate a program for recruiting persons with certain professional skills and competencies in the health planning area to be used by HSAs in meeting their staffing requirements and (2) design and operate an employment referral service as a national focal point to provide linkage between qualified candidates for jobs in health planning agencies and those health planning agencies seeking employees. As of April 30, 1978, the Association had placed about 220 persons at HSAs and SHPDAs.

Several HSAs said that their inability to offer competitive salaries had seriously hindered them in employing qualified staff. Salaries for HSA executive directors of the 15 HSAs ranged from about $19,300 to $35,000. Salaries of subordinate staff were generally in the $13,000 to $25,000 range.

Adequacy of HSA Funding

Officials at only 6 of the 15 HSAs said they were satisfied with the funding they received during the first year grant period. One of these officials anticipated returning about $200,000 of the first year grant to HEW.

Officials at six other HSAs said that funding levels were inadequate for the first year, while officials at several HSAs complained that the method used by HEW regional offices to award grant funds on an incremental basis caused problems, particularly in hiring needed staff at an early date.

For example, one HSA applied for $1.1 million for its initial 1-year grant period. The initial grant received from HEW, however, amounted to only about $325,000. Because of this low funding level, this HSA, which was a former comprehensive health planning agency, had to lay off nine staff members and stretch out its work program. Five months after this HSA received its initial grant award, HEW increased the grant by about $311,000 bringing the first year funding to a total of about $636,000.

Several HSAs noted that the incremental grant funding also caused their budgets and workplans to be revised.

Need to Clarify HSA and SHPDA Functions

The act requires that HSAs and SHPDAs perform many similar functions. For example, both develop comprehensive health plans, review projects, and periodically review the appropriateness of existing institutional health services. Relationships between HSAs and SHPDAs in several of the States visited need to be clarified, particularly in States having statewide HSAs. There are 12 States that have such HSAs.

Health Systems Plan Development Activities

Several SHPDAs had agreements with their respective HSAs regarding the format and methodology to be used in developing health systems plans. This is particularly important so that the State health plan can be readily developed from the local health systems plans.

The HSAs and SHPDAs in one State, however, were proceeding initially with health systems plan development efforts in a manner that appeared to be inconsistent with the intent of the act. Sections of the State plan were to be developed for all three HSAs by an individual HSA. For example, one HSA was responsible for developing the burn care section of plans for the other HSAs. According to a SHPDA official, this process was being considered to avert problems associated with combining the health systems plans prepared by the individual HSA into the State health plan.

During our visit to the SHPDA, a new agency director was hired. At the conclusion of our review, the new director was reconsidering the methodology to be used in developing the State health plan.

We believe that the initial methodology which was to be used in developing the State plan was inconsistent with the goals and objectives of the act. The autonomy of the HSAs in the State could be jeopardized because of its limited influence over health systems plan development within its own health service area if this methodology is used.

Single State HSAs

Some statewide HSAs and their respective SHPDAs were having difficulty in communicating. Officials from both agencies were concerned about potential conflicts and duplication of effort because of their similar responsibilities. HEW has provided little assistance to statewide HSAs and their SHPDAs in dealing with this situation.

A SHPDA official in a State having a statewide HSA was concerned about the power which the HSA could execute through its representation on the SHCC. The act requires that the SHCC be representative of at least 60 percent of the HSAs in the State, which in the case of a State having only one HSA, would give the HSA a majority on the SHCC. The SHCC advises the SHPDA and has final approval of the State health plan.

Project Review Cooperation

The executive director at another HSA brought another problem to our attention. He said that the SHPDA in his State was consistently overruling HSA recommendations on new health service applications. He said that the SHPDA often gave little justification of its decision to the HSA. He was also concerned that if this trend continues, the effectiveness of the HSA would be minimal and that applications for new services would place little importance on the HSA review and recommendation.

In one State having a statewide HSA, conflict had developed regarding the certificate of need law. Both the HSA and the SHPDA submitted bills to the

State legislature. The HSA bill provided for joint HSA/SHPDA determination of project review procedures, standards, and criteria. It also allowed the HSA to decide what questions would be asked of applicants and the scope of the review process. The SHPDA bill, however, provided that the State would be responsible for the project review procedures and that only the State should have final authority to set review procedures, standards, and criteria.

Authority Over Federal Health Facilities

The act did not provide HSAs and SHPDAs the authority to control Federal health care facilities. HEW has interpreted this silence as an expression of congressional intent not to provide HSA jurisdiction over Federal health care facilities. HEW's interpretation follows the Supreme Court statement in *Federal Power Commission v. Tuscarora Indian Nation*, 362 U.S. 99, 120 (1960):

> "The law is now well settled that:

> 'A general statute imposing restrictions does not impose them upon the Government itself without a clear expression or implication to that effect.' *United States v. Wittek*, 337 U.S. 346,358-359."

Our legislative review of the act provided no indications as to congressional intent regarding the question of Federal health facilities.

The act, however, does provide that if a health service area includes a Veterans Administration health care facility, the HSA's governing board must include a Veterans Administration representative as an ex-officio member.

Approximately 10 percent of all general medical-surgical hospital beds in the Nation are under the authority of the Veterans Administration, Department of Defense, and Public Health Service. Most of the HSAs we visited had Federal health care facilities within their health service areas.

Generally, HSA officials did not consider the exclusion of Federal health facilities from their authority to be one of the major problems confronting them at the time of our review. Several, however, stated that to have a meaningful health planning system, Federal health care facilities should have the same restrictions as other health care facilities. The expansion of Federal health care facilities or the purchase of new technology could have a significant impact on the non-Federal system, particularly where the non-Federal system has been providing services to Federal beneficiaries. According to an Institute of Medicine study entitled, "Controlling the Supply of Hospital Beds," over 3 million dependents of military personnel are now covered in a program that purchases health care in the private sector—the Department of Defense's Civilian Health and Medical Program of the Uniformed Services, more commonly known as CHAMPUS.

The Veterans Administration announced in 1976 that it planned to replace seven hospitals and construct one new hospital for about $850 million. The Department of Defense's Five Year Military Department Medical Construction Programs dated June 1, 1977, included plans to replace 10 hospitals and construct 3 new hospitals for about $758 million.

Among the national health planning goals identified in the act are

— developing multiinstitutional systems to coordinate or consolidate institutional health services.
— developing multiinstitutional arrangements to share support services necessary to all health institutions, and
— developing health service institutions which can provide various levels of care on a geographically integrated basis.

We believe that including Federal health care facilities in the health planning system authorized by the act could further the achievement of these national goals, as well as assist in restraining increases in health care costs.

Lack of Optimism in Achieving Goals of the Act

In order for HSAs to have a positive effect on improving accessibility to health care and restraining increases in health care costs, persons involved in the process should believe that these goals can be achieved. HSA board members and staff, however, were generally not optimistic about the success of the health planning program authorized by Public Law 93-641.

In a questionnaire, we asked the board members of each of the 15 HSAs to what extent their HSA could accomplish several objectives associated with health planning. The table below summarizes the results of 462 board members' responses (83.1 percent of those queried).

HSA Board Members' Perceptions About Achieving Objectives of Public Law 93-641

Objectives	Very Large Extent	Substantial Extent	Moderate Extent	Some Extent	Little or No Extent
			Percent		
Contain overall health care costs	2.3	13.1	27.2	28.7	28.7
Improve access to health care	6.0	17.6	27.8	27.0	21.6
Restrain construction of unneeded health facilities	18.1	38.7	21.6	11.4	10.2

Objectives	Very Large Extent	Substantial Extent	Moderate Extent	Some Extent	Little or No Extent
Restrain acquisition of unneeded equipment	13.4	31.4	26.4	15.9	12.9
Educate the public in use of health care system	15.0	24.9	22.4	22.2	15.5

While these statistics can be interpreted several ways, we believe that they show that members felt the goals could not be accomplished. This is noteworthy when it is acknowledged that the health planning program is relatively new and that under such a circumstance more optimism could be expected. The responses to containing health care costs and improving accessibility to health care are particularly alarming since these are the primary objectives of the act.

As shown below, provider board members were slightly less optimistic than consumers about HSAs achieving these two goals.

Comparison of Responses of Consumer and Provider HSA Board Members on the Ability of HSAs to Contain Costs and Improve Accessibility to Health Care

Objective		Responses (Percent)				
		Very Large Extent	Substantial Extent	Moderate Extent	Some Extent	Little or No Extent
Contain overall health care costs	Consumers	3.4	14.2	27.5	26.5	28.4
	Providers	1.0	11.9	27.0	31.1	29.0
Improve access to health care	Consumers	8.6	18.6	29.7	26.8	16.3
	Providers	3.1	16.5	25.8	27.3	27.3

There are many possible reasons for this apparent lack of optimism of board members in accomplishing the goals of the act. One is the perceived lack of authority on the part of HSAs. The following schedule summarizes the responses to questions regarding the authority given to HSAs to contain health care costs and improve access to health care.

Board Members Perception of Authority to Contain Costs and Improve Health Care Accessibility

	Responses (Percent)				
Question	Much More Authority Than Necessary	More Authority than Necessary	Just the Right Amount of Authority	Less Authority than Necessary	Much Less Authority than Necessary
In your opinion, have HSAs been given the necessary authority to achieve the goals of:					
containing health care costs	4.6	4.4	24.9	43.7	22.4
improving access to health care	2.7	4.1	30.3	46.7	16.2

As can be seen, HSA board members believed that the act did not provide sufficient authority to accomplish these goals.

Officials at several HSAs were also not very optimistic about the success of HSAs in achieving these two goals of the act. Some HSAs believed project review activities would reduce the unnecessary construction of health facilities and the purchase of unneeded expensive medical equipment. One HSA official, however, described the project review process as "putting a band-aid on the problem of cost escalation" since HSAs have no authority over the activities of private clinics and physicians' offices. Also, several HSA officials said that State agencies have too much authority in the project review process. One HSA official said that the project review functions were often meaningless because the State agency had final approval and that such decisions were often made without regard to the HSA's recommendations. Another HSA official said that the greatest benefit his HSA can presently provide is to educate the public in the availability and use of the health care system and solicit the involvement of the community in health planning through subarea councils.

HSA officials noted that the act does not provide authority over health manpower distribution or the purchase of expensive medical equipment by physicians, both of which can effect the cost and accessibility of health care. One official said that HSAs should have hospital rate review authority in order to have a positive influence on health care costs.

Support of Local Governmental, Community, and Professional Groups to Health Planning

The involvement of local consumers, providers, and government officials in the health planning system is provided through their memberships on HSA governing boards. The support of the health planning activities directed by HSA governing boards, particularly the approval and support of the health systems plan by local consumers and health professional groups and local governmental entities, will be needed if HSAs are to be successful in achieving the act's goals.

We asked consumers, health professionals, and local government representatives in the health service areas their opinions regarding the ultimate success of HSAs in achieving the goals of the act. Generally, they believed that HSAs have not yet established the needed credibility in the community and, thus, have not gained the confidence and support of the above groups.

Some of the concerns brought to our attention were:

— HSA staffs in general have no real knowledge of the operation of the health care system.
— HSAs seem to be dedicated to the destruction of the existing health care system.
— HSAs are not accountable to the people and, thus, should not be making decisions that elected officials are responsible for.
— Health providers will dominate and control HSAs, thus reducing their effectiveness in controlling costs.
— The methodologies needed to measure cost, availability, accessibility, and quality of health care have not been developed.
— HSAs do not have enough power to contain health care costs and improve accessibility.
— The goals of containing health care costs and improving accessibility to the health care system conflict with one another.
— Medical standards and criteria are the responsibility of the medical profession, not HSAs.
— HSAs' reviews and comments on new projects will not be an effective means of containing health care costs.
— The savings attributable to preventing the construction of unnecessary health care facilities or the acquisition of unneeded equipment may be offset by the costs associated with preventing such expenditures.

Several groups had not formulated opinions and were waiting to see what will happen in the next few years. They acknowledged that HSAs will experience difficulties in improving the health care system without the support of consumers, providers, and local governments.

Compatibility of the Act's Objectives

Since the passage of the National Health Planning and Resources Development Act of 1974, considerable concern has been expressed regarding the compatibility of providing access to quality health care and restraining increases in health care costs. Some Federal, State, and local officials have agreed that the objectives are not compatible because costs cannot be restrained while the health care system is being expanded to provide access to all persons.

An HSA official was confused as to where emphasis should be placed—improving access or restraining costs. HEW has provided limited guidance in regard to this question. The HEW guidelines on developing health systems plans do, however, state that HSAs should "place priority on restraining cost increases." The guidelines also state that "efforts should be made to estimate current needs of area residents to reduce the inequity in the provision of care."

While the legislative history of the act is not explicit as to congressional intent regarding the question of health care accessibility and containment of health care costs, section 1502 does list first, as 1 of the 10 national health priorities, "the provision of primary care services for medically underserved populations, especially those which are located in rural or economically depressed areas." Several of the remaining nine priorities also deal with accessibility to health care.

We believe that health systems plans can emphasize accessibility to primary care as a priority (for example, an economically depressed area), while at the same time stress that increased costs from such things as overbedding, the questionable purchasing of expensive equipment, or duplicating certain services such as intensive care or cardiac care units should be minimized. Therefore, in our opinion, the act's objectives of cost containment and health care accessibility need to be addressed by health systems agencies.

Conclusions

The HSAs in our review were concerned, as were their predecessor local Comprehensive Health Planning agencies, with the availability and adequacy of data on which to develop a health systems plan. At the time of our review, agreements between HSAs and PSROs were being formalized but little data was being exchanged. A recent amendment to the PSRO authorizing legislation provided for the exchange of data between PSROs and HSAs and should resolve the problems HSAs were encountering.

HSAs were being hampered in making project reviews because of a lack of standards or criteria on which to make decisions. HEW's slowness in developing guidelines had also delayed the preparation of health systems plans.

Since our review, HEW has issued national standards and criteria for nine types of health services and facilities for use in the development of areawide and State health plans. HEW should continue to expedite the issuance of national guidelines and standards so that they can be used by HSAs and SHPDAs in developing health plans and making judgments on proposed changes to the health care system.

Concern about the adequacy of salaries and whether the health planning program will be continued hampered HSAs in their ability to attract qualified staff. The job faced by HSAs is at best a difficult one; without adequate staff it may well be an impossible one.

In those States having only one HSA, the HSA was confused about its responsibilities as opposed to those of the State health planning agency. This situation exists in 12 States. We see no need for having a State health planning agency and an HSA which covers the entire State. The provisions of section 1536 of the act could be expanded to allow more States to have only a State health planning agency. Another alternative would be to require States to have at least two HSAs.

In passing the National Health Planning and Resources Development Act of 1974, the Congress did not provide HSAs with any specific authority over Federal health facilities. Since these facilities are an important part of our national health resources and serve millions of people, these facilities cannot be disregarded by HSAs. If the health planning program is to become the vital force that the Congress expects it to become and to have a major impact on containing costs and improving accessibility to health care, then we believe the institutions created to achieve those objectives must interact with all parts of the health care system. To specifically exclude Federal facilities from the national health planning program, in our opinion, is to seriously impede the ability of the local and State health planning agencies to carry out the responsibilities given to them by the Congress.

The extent to which HSAs will be successful is largely dependent upon their board members and their attitudes. Recognizing that their task is not an easy one, we were disappointed to see the relatively low level of optimism expressed by HSA board members in achieving the goals in the act. In some respects, board members seemed to feel they were faced with impossible and sometimes conflicting objectives. We believe the goals of containing health care costs and improving accessibility are not necessarily conflicting. In many health service areas, there are areas where duplicative health services are available and other areas where services are not available. In these situations, we believe HSAs could be active in attempting to redistribute or reallocate resources. In our opinion, HEW should provide HSAs with additional guidance in this area.

If HSAs are to achieve their objectives, they must have the support of local governments, community and professional groups, private health care providers, and others working in the health care field. As could be expected, this support has been slow in developing, and many look upon the health planning agencies with distrust and suspicion. We believe that HSAs must establish their credibility in the health care field as soon as possible. The longer this process takes, the less likely success will be achieved. Consequently, we believe HEW should stress the importance of each HSA developing positive relationships with all who are active in the health care field. If fear and mistrust can be successfully overcome, then HSAs will have a much greater chance of succeeding.

HEALTH PLANNING PROSPECTS

Since the GAO report there has been some tidying up of the health planning system. Federal challenges of some of the Health Systems Plans (HSPs) has led many of the HSAs to produce more complete and meaningful documents, but in many instances the plans do not enjoy the support of those institutional providers whose cooperation for implementation is vital. Some HSAs have been de-certified by HEW and lost their funding because of various shortcomings. Other HSAs are threatened with de-certification, and others have had their conditional designation extended. These threats should prompt more positive agency responses to federal guidelines and directives. At least one SHPDA in a large state has also been threatened with de-certification but whether HEW will actually move to de-certify is questionable both politically and constitutionally. Legal actions continue by various parties—legal challenges to the law, and challenges to the way the law is being implemented by the federal and state governments and by HSAs. HSAs continue to agonize over the problem of structuring representative boards and committees. Conflicts continue between HSAs and SHPDAs especially with regard to CON decisions. Agency staff time continues to be heavily committed to the project review process, and is likely to be more so as federal guidelines become more specific especially with regard to intitutional services.

On the most important issue there is also no change. Developing a positive relationship with health providers, eliminating the widespread fear and mistrust, continues to elude the HSAs and SHPDAs. Their dilemma is that establishing a positive relationship with the providers is extremely difficult, if not impossible, so long as the agenda is pre-set with the charge of cost containment and regulation. Both the HSAs and SHPDAs, under federal pressure, continue to urge hospitals, nursing homes, physicians, and others to support and to conform to the federal guidelines, and to meet the specifications of new federal regulations. Challenges are being made by the health planning agencies to continuance of some existing services, and further challenges can be anticipated as the process accelerates for reviewing the appropriateness of all institutional services and facilities. Proposed new services and facilities are, moreover, subject to intense scrutiny by the planning agencies and to frequent challenge. The result of these activities has a dampening effect if only because it takes much longer now to get something approved, and in the delay inflation may make a project too costly for the agency which wishes to initiate it. In a perverse sort of way this all serves the federal objective of slowing down the rate of growth. But the administrative burden on hospitals, nursing homes, and other providers in terms of the delays and costs of special studies and preparing reports to justify proposed as well as existing activities is considerable; the federally threatened HSAs and SHPDAs, however, have the leverage of the 1122 review process and CON laws, so the tendency for the health service agencies is to grin and bear it. Relatively few litigate. Understandably, many health service providers see their agencies under attack and consequently feel compelled to defend and to protect their domains at all costs.

How vastly different is the climate today from that contemplated by PL 89-749: health planning as a democratic process involving a *partnership* between government, providers, and consumers employing reasoned analysis, negotiation, and compromise seems forgotten.

The prospects, moreover, for lasting cost containment via the HSAs and SHPDAs are not bright: First, although politicians and bureaucrats are loathe to concede this, the rising cost of health services are, by and large, outside the control of the health industry. As the minimum wage goes up, as fuel and food costs go up, as the costs of regulation increase, and as the inflationary spiral continues, health services costs must go up. Alternatively, consumer ease of access to care and quality of care are likely to suffer. Second, as new technology is developed which will contribute to improved quality of care, physicians and then the consumers will demand access to that technology, despite what the HSAs, state agencies, and the federal government say. Third, elected officials at the state and federal levels will continue to insist on the development of projects in which they have a special interest (often from political popularity or usefulness) sometimes without even consulting the planning agencies. Finally, people are ingenious and will find ways to beat the system which they believe to be irrational, oppressive or unfair. Paul Ward, president of the California Hospital Association, speaking of the proposed *cap* or *lid* on hospital charges, was quite blunt when he said, "we'll find ways to get things out from under the lid—we always have" (9, p.37). Or as one hospital administrator put it as someone marveled at the new hospital with its huge lobby, "See that wall over there? On the other side is the fastest growing department in this hospital.

When I have to expand it, I only have to move the wall, taking off some of my expendable lobby. Funny thing, when the HSA approved the plans for this hospital, they looked at everything—the number of beds, size of the lab, radiology and other departments, but they didn't pay any attention to the lobby." Or as the administrator in another state put it when asked why the hospital was building an extended care wing, "In this city that's the only thing the HSA will approve these days."

GAO in its report urged HEW to stress the importance of HSAs developing a positive relationship to the health care field, and overcoming the field's fear and mistrust. Though successful health planning is dependent on this occurring, it might fairly be asked: given the constraints of the law(s) and federal regulations and administrative processes, is this goal within the power of the HSAs.

REFERENCES

1. *Comprehensive Health Planning and Public Service Amendments of 1966.* Public Law 89-749.
2. *Hearing before the Committee on Interstate and Foreign Commerce.* House of Representatives, 89th Congress, second session, October 11, 1966, serial # 89-52.
3. *House Report No. 2271 Accompanying HR 18231.* Committee on Interstate and Foreign Commerce, 89th Congress; *Senate Report No. 1665* Commitee on Labor and Public Welfare, 89th Congress.
4. Presented March 21 at the 1967 National Health Forum, *Planning for Health,* Chicago.
5. *Report to the Congress: Comprehensive Health Planning as Carried Out by State and Areawide Agencies in Three States,* Comptroller general of the United States, General Accounting Office, 1974.
6. Senate Report No. 93-1285 accompanying S. 2994. Committee on Labor and Public Welfare, 93rd Congress, second session.
7. *Hospitals,* JAHA, August 16, 1976.
8. *Report to the Congress: Status of the Implementation of the National Health Planning and Resources Development Act of 1974,* Comptroller general of the United States, General Accounting Office, HRD-77-157, November 2, 1978.
9. *Hospitals,* JAHA, November 1, 1977.

13
Conclusions

I

Dr. K. Birkum Petersen met me at the railroad station at Sorø in Denmark. He was the local health officer who had been asked by the government to arrange a program for me. It was mid-October 1978, and it was the start of a delightful, informative day visiting general practitioners and specialists, a general hospital, and a nursing home. We talked during the day about health services in Denmark and the problems that confronted physicians, hospitals, politicians, and the public. I was particularly interested in how Denmark planned health services and how the nation resolved differences between levels of government and between various contesting provider and consumer groups. I was struck by the absence of contention. I said to Dr. Birkum Petersen that I didn't detect rancor: the medical association seemed to have harmonious relations with the central government, and both parties viewed the other as a positive force; similarly, industrial relations were without militancy and there was no evident hostility between central and county governments or between physicians and politicans and hospital administrators. I asked why this was so, and I shall never forget Birkum Petersen's reply: "We are a small country, and everyone knows each other."

There were disagreements in Denmark over health policy. There were differing viewpoints, but the Danes had reached a consensus about the importance of being civil. They seemed to be saying, and Birkum Petersen's words so aptly set the tone, that they are a community in which there were a variety of interests and leadership groups; no useful purpose would be served by tearing the body politic to pieces over issues that, though important, were not so important as to allow them to destroy the social fabric, the Danish community. When he said, "We are a small country, and everyone knows each other," my host was also saying: We are one community, one family, and we must understand each other and get along with each other. He also seemed to be saying that the various actors will discuss and discuss and reach agreement through compromises. And, indeed, at the national level, one of the country's chief health planners noted that there were disagreements between central and county governments over health affairs, but he could recall no instance in which the disagreements had degenerated to the point at which the parties were polarized.

What a contrast, I thought, to the American scene in which the American Academy of Family Physicians is contemplating a lawsuit against the JCAH over the latter's refusal to let the AAFP become a partner in JCAH along with the other groups; the FTC is attacking the codes of professional ethics and the propriety of medical school accreditation by the Liaison Committee on Medical Education; the chiropractors sue to gain admission to hospitals; some radiologists threaten to sue the AMA over its proposed settlement of a chiropractic suit; state governments challenge in court the legality of federal health planning legislation; the Pennsylvania Medical Society sues the state, asking the court to force the state to do its job in monitoring quality of medical practice; President Carter castigates the AMA at a news conference; medical schools refuse capitation grants because of onerous conditions attached to them by the Congress; medical societies challenge in court the PSRO legislation; consumers sue over a variety of health policy issues. Invective and court battles seem to be the rule in America. But the question might fairly be asked, Are we any better off for the adversary system on which we now seem to be hooked? Every group seems determined to insist that the game be played according to its rules—and now! There is impatience and there is an unwillingness to wait, to take a step at a time, to compromise. What is ultimately gained by scoring political points, by winning court skirmishes? Wounds are inflicted. Distrust is created. And health agencies simply devise strategies to beat the system to get what they want.

I thought, too, how different things were in the nineteenth and early half of the twentieth centuries when enormous strides were made toward improving the quality of medical care, hospital practice, and medical education—not perfection but clearly steady progress. And as I thought about this, I couldn't escape the feeling that even today's progress—when progress can be measured—comes about when the actors have reached a consensus as to what needs to be done. If this observation is correct, and it is only from a study of history that this can be determined, then serious question can be raised over the actions of so many groups today, including government agencies. Perhaps each should pause and hearken to the words of Oliver Cromwell: "I beseech you . . . think it possible you may be mistaken."

II

In the final chapter to a book, an author frequently avails himself or herself of the opportunity to scatter pearls of wisdom and to provide solutions to some of society's most vexing problems. The temptation to do this is considerable, and in the preceding section I succumbed to what some, I hope, at least may perceive to be wisdom. The temptation to do likewise in offering solutions also exists, but on this, the author can resist.

This is not to deny the existence of problems, for they are many. Rising health costs seem to be the most pressing issue, for they spawn or touch on an array of other problems relating to such areas as health insurance, length of hospital stay, unnecessary surgery, codes of medical ethics, malpractice insurance rates, new technology, new drugs, and easy access to the highest quality of health service.

We are troubled as a people, for example, about health insurance—its cost, its shortcomings, and the advisability of adopting some sort of national health insurance system. We are concerned about how long patients stay in hospital, for the extra day or two ultimately affects either the taxes we pay or the cost of our own health insurance policies. Added unnecessary days, moreover, may lead to the building of costly new facilities that are not really needed. The question of unnecessary surgery not only concerns us because of the effects on hospital and physician utilization and costs but because of the unnecessary risk to patients and our individual confidence in physicians and particularly surgeons, if we need care. The codes of medical ethics raise questions about their use to maintain a monopoly, which leads to unnecessarily high costs and the exclusion of competitors, whether they are other physicians or other health practitioners. Concern is felt by others that the very processes of accreditation—of hospitals and of medical and other health education programs—have the potential for interfering with the supply, efficiency, and cost of services and care. The cost of malpractice insurance not only affects the cost of care, for the insurance and the settlements are eventually passed on to the patients, but also the cost and litigation raise troublesome questions about how safe and effective our health system is. New technology and new drugs are always being developed; and the cost is high. To what extent do we have built-in obsolescence, and can we really afford the rush to production with early "models", and to what extent should every village have these around the corner? Perhaps such ease of access, while convenient, is not cost effective. We wonder to what extent rural people should be denied access or be required to travel great distances because it would be uneconomical to disperse the new technology or the hospital beds or the medical specialists. And the problems posed by the aged, the mentally ill, and the mentally retarded are enormous in terms of the facilities available for their care—both supply and quality—and of the services in general to meet their needs.

These are only a few of the troublesome questions we face. Each relates to real problems in our health system. What an opportunity an author has with the bold stroke of the pen to solve these all by suggesting any variety of mechanisms that, when stated, seem so obvious a solution: a national health insurance system, a national health service (socialized medicine), or deregulation to allow full competition to reign! But these solutions are simplistic, and I, for one, have no final solution to offer. There are many steps that might be taken to address these problems, but there is, in my judgment, no "quick fix." The problems and issues are complex, and complex matters, by their very nature, do not lend themselves to easy solutions.

Yet group after group yearns for a quick and easy solution. Pronouncements are made. Invectives are hurled. Witnesses before congressional committees are scored. Legal challenges are made. Confrontation politics, which is really what was described in the first section of this chapter, is perhaps a more serious problem than rising costs, access to care, and the problems they spawn. If there are no simple solutions because of the complexity of the issues, including the insufficiency of data, then little hope can come from the tactics currently in use as regards meaningful, long-term solutions. Securing trust through the greater use of reasoned analysis, negotiation, and compromise is perhaps our greatest need and in its absence our greatest health problem. Without trust we will persist in not developing long-term solutions to complex problems because in our desire to score points and win skirmishes, we shall always miss central issues.

Acronyms in Common Use

AAFP	American Academy of Family Physicians
AAFPRS	American Academy of Facial Plastic and Reconstructive Surgery
AAGP	American Academy of General Practice
AAMC	Association of American Medical Colleges
ABMS	American Board of Medical Specialties
ACP	American College of Physicians
ACS	American College of Surgeons
ADA	American Dental Association; American Dietetics Association; American Diabetes Association
ADAMHA	Alcohol, Drug Abuse, and Mental Health Administration
AFDC	Aid to Families with Dependent Children
AHA	American Hospital Association
AHEC	Area Health Education Center
AHME	Association of Hospital Medical Education
AHPA	American Health Planning Association
AID	Agency for International Development
AIP	Annual Implementation Plan
AJPH	American Journal of Public Health
AMA	American Medical Association
ANA	American Nurses Association
AOA	American Osteopathic Association
APHA	American Public Health Association
APhA	American Pharmaceutical Association
ARC	Appalachian Regional Commission
ASPRS	American Society of Plastic and Reconstructive Surgeons
ASTHO	Association of State and Territorial Health Officers
AUPHA	Association of University Programs in Health Administration
BC	Blue Cross
BCHS	Bureau of Community Health Services
BHM	Bureau of Health Manpower
BMS	Bureau of Medical Services

625

BS	Blue Shield
BSN	Bachelor of Science in Nursing
CAHEA	Committee on Allied Health Education and Accreditation
CAT	Computerized Axial Tomography
CCME	Coordinating Council on Medical Education
CDC	Center for Disease Control (formerly, Communicable Disease Center)
CETA	Comprehensive Education and Training Act
CHAMPUS	Civilian Health and Medical Program of the Uniformed Services
CHAMPVA	Civilian Health and Medical Program of the Veterans Administration
CHP	Comprehensive Health Planning
CME	Council on Medical Education; Continuing Medical Education
CMSS	Council of Medical Specialty Societies
CON	Certificate of Need
COPA	Council on Postsecondary Accreditation
COTRANS	Coordinated Transfer Application System
CPHA	Commission on Professional and Hospital Activities
CPR	Cardiac Pulmonary Resuscitation
CT	Computed Tomographic
DC	Doctor of Chiropractic
DDS	Doctor of Dental Surgery
DHEW	Department of Health, Education, and Welfare
DMD	Doctor of Dental Medicine
DO	Doctor of Osteopathy
DPM	Doctor of Podiatric Medicine
DRG	Division of Research Grants
ECFMG	Educational Commission on Foreign Medical Graduates (formerly, Educational Council for Foreign Medical Graduates)
EENT	Eye, Ear, Nose, and Throat
EMS	Emergency Medical Services
ENT	Ear, Nose, and Throat
EPA	Environmental Protection Agency
EPSDT	Early and Periodic Screening Diagnosis and Treatment
ESP	Economic Stabilization Program
FAH	Federation of American Hospitals
FDA	Food and Drug Administration
FHA	Federal Housing Authority
FIC	Fogarty International Center
FLEX	Federation Licensing Examination
FMG	Foreign Medical Graduate
FSMB	Federation of State Medical Boards
FY	Fiscal Year

GAO	General Accounting Office
GHA	Group Health Association
GNP	Gross National Product
GP	General Practioner
GYN	Gynecology
H-B	Hill-Burton Act
HCFA	Health Care Financing Administration
HEW	Health, Education, and Welfare
HIAA	Health Insurance Association of America
HII	Health Insurance Institute
HIP	Health Insurance Plan of New York
HMO	Health Maintenance Organization
HRA	Health Resources Administration
HSA	Health Systems Agency
HSA	Health Services Administration
HSP	Health Systems Plan
HUP	Hospital Utilization Project of Pennsylvania
HURA	Health Underserved Rural Areas
ICF	Intermediate Care Facility
IHS	Indian Health Service
JAMA	The Journal of the American Medical Association
JCAH	Joint Commission on Accreditation of Hospitals
JME	The Journal of Medical Education
LCCME	Liaison Committee on Continuing Medical Education
LCGME	Liaison Committee on Graduate Medical Education
LCME	Liaison Committee on Medical Education
LCSB	Liaison Committee for Specialty Boards
LPN	Licensed Practical Nurse
LVN	Licensed Vocational Nurse
MAP	Medical Audit Program
MCAT	Medical College Admission Test
MCH	Maternal and Child Health
MD	Doctor of Medicine
Med	Medicine
MEDLARS	Medical Literature and Analysis Retrieval System
MH	Mental Hygiene or Mental Health
MR	Mental Retardation
NBME	National Board of Medical Examiners

NCHS	National Center for Health Statistics
NCHSR	National Center for Health Services Research
NCHCT	National Center for Health Care Technology
NCI	National Cancer Institute
NEI	National Eye Institute
NEJM	The New England Journal of Medicine
NHC	Neighborhood Health Center
NHI	National Health Insurance
NHLBI	National Heart, Lung and Blood Institute
NHSC	National Health Service Corps
NIA	National Institute on Aging
NIAAA	National Institute on Alcohol, Abuse and Alcoholics
NIAID	National Institute of Allergy and Infectious Diseases
NIAMDD	National Institute of Arthritis, Metabolism and Digestive Diseases
NICHD	National Institute of Child Health and Human Development
NIDA	National Institute on Drug Abuse
NIDR	National Institute of Dental Research
NIEHS	National Institute of Environmental Health Sciences
NIGMS	National Institute of General Medical Sciences
NIH	National Institutes of Health
NIMH	National Institute of Mental Health
NINCDS	National Institute of Neurological and Communicative Disorders and Stroke
NIOSH	National Institute of Occupational Safety and Health
NIRMP	National Intern and Resident Matching Program
NJPC	National Joint Practice Commission
NLM	National Library of Medicine
NLN	National League of Nursing
NLRB	National Labor Relations Board
NMA	National Medical Association
NRMP	National Residency Matching Program
OB	Obstetrics
OD	Doctor of Optometry
OEO	Office of Economic Opportunity
OIH	Office of International Health
OMB	Office of Management and Budget
OSHA	Occupational Safety and Health Administration
PA	Physician Assistant
PAHO	Pan American Health Organization
PAS	Professional Activity Study
PHR	Public Health Reports
PHS	Public Health Service
PHSA	Pennsylvania Hospital Services Association

PL	Public Law
PMA	Pharmaceutical Manufacturers Association
PNHA	Physicians National Housestaff Association
PSRO	Professional Standards Review Organization
RFP	Request for Proposal
RHI	Rural Health Initiative
RMP	Regional Medical Program
RN	Registered Nurse
SHPDA	State Health Planning and Development Agency
SHCC	State Health Coordinating Council
SHUR	System for Hospital Uniform Reporting
SMI	Supplementary Medical Insurance
SMSA	Standard Metropolitan Statistical Area
SNF	Skilled Nursing Facility
SSA	Social Security Administration
SSI	Supplementary Security Income
TB	Tuberculosis
UCR	Usual, Customary and Reasonable
UR	Utilization Review
USMG	United States Medical Graduate
VA	Veterans Administration
VD	Venereal Disease
VE	Voluntary Effort
VQE	Visa Qualifying Examination
VNA	Visiting Nurse Association
WHO	World Health Organization
WIC	Women, Infants and Children

Index

631

About the Author

Marshall W. Raffel is Professor of Health Planning and Administration at The Pennsylvania State University. He has had extensive experience in the health field, first as a corpsman in naval hospitals during the Second World War, later with Blue Cross and Blue Shield in New York City, then in industrial health and safety programming for the Baltimore and Ohio Railroad, followed by four years as the principal health planner for the Maryland State Planning Commission. After a stint teaching political science in New Zealand and doing research on the health services of that country, he returned to the United States to serve as Chief for Program Research and Development in the United States Surgeon General's Office of Comprehensive Health Planning. At Penn State he pioneered in developing the baccalaureate program in Health Planning and Administration, and continued his research interests in New Zealand health services (to which he returned briefly in 1975 for field research) and in health manpower education. In 1973, he served as a consultant to the World Health Organization in India and Nepal, and in 1978 he was a World Health Organization travel fellow, studying the health services of England, Denmark, Sweden, and Czechoslovakia. Under sponsorship of the United States and Yugloslav governments, he also spent time studying the health services of Yugoslavia. Returning to Penn State, he put the finishing touches on his book, *The U.S. Health System: Origins and Functions,* and is currently directing a Robert Wood Johnson Foundation grant concerned with the development and maintenance of primary care services in rural areas.

A graduate in philosophy from the University of Illinois, Dr. Raffel holds a Ph.D. in political science from the Victoria University of Wellington, New Zealand.